Medicinal Chemistry: Research and Innovation

Medicinal Chemistry: Research and Innovation

Editor: Thomas Haldane

NY RESEARCH PRESS

New York

Published by NY Research Press
118-35 Queens Blvd., Suite 400,
Forest Hills, NY 11375, USA
www.nyresearchpress.com

Medicinal Chemistry: Research and Innovation
Edited by Thomas Haldane

International Standard Book Number: 978-1-63238-549-9 (Hardback)

Cataloging-in-Publication Data

Medicinal chemistry : research and innovation / edited by Thomas Haldane.
    p. cm.
Includes bibliographical references and index.
ISBN 978-1-63238-549-9
1. Pharmaceutical chemistry. 2. Pharmaceutical chemistry--Research. 3. Pharmaceutical chemistry--Technique.
4. Toxicity testing--In vivo. 5. Pharmacology. I. Haldane, Thomas.
RS403 .M43 2017
615.19--dc23

Printed in the United States of America.

Contents

Preface

This book has been a concerted effort by a group of academicians, researchers and scientists, who have contributed their research works for the realization of the book. This book has materialized in the wake of emerging advancements and innovations in this field. Therefore, the need of the hour was to compile all the required researches and disseminate the knowledge to a broad spectrum of people comprising of students, researchers and specialists of the field.

Medicinal chemistry is the research and study of drug design and development. It is a synthesis of organic chemistry and pharmacology. Research in medicinal chemistry focuses on the discovery of new drugs as well as improvements on older therapeutic drugs. Topics included in this text discuss the synthesis of new chemical elements to transform them into medicinal products. This book is a valuable compilation of topics ranging from the basic to the most complex advancements in this field. It aims to present researches that have transformed this discipline and aided its advancement. As this field is emerging at a fast pace, this book will help the readers to better understand the concepts of medicinal chemistry. With state-of-the-art inputs by acclaimed experts of this field, this book targets students and professionals.

At the end of the preface, I would like to thank the authors for their brilliant chapters and the publisher for guiding us all-through the making of the book till its final stage. Also, I would like to thank my family for providing the support and encouragement throughout my academic career and research projects.

Editor

Mechanism of 150-cavity formation in influenza neuraminidase

Rommie E. Amaro[1], Robert V. Swift[1], Lane Votapka[1], Wilfred W. Li[2], Ross C. Walker[3] & Robin M. Bush[4]

The recently discovered 150-cavity in the active site of group-1 influenza A neuraminidase (NA) proteins provides a target for rational structure-based drug development to counter the increasing frequency of antiviral resistance in influenza. Surprisingly, the 2009 H1N1 pandemic virus (09N1) neuramidase was crystalized without the 150-cavity characteristic of group-1 NAs. Here we demonstrate, through a total sum of 1.6 µs of biophysical simulations, that 09N1 NA exists in solution preferentially with an open 150-cavity. Comparison with simulations using avian N1, human N2 and 09N1 with a I149V mutation and an extensive bioinformatics analysis suggests that the conservation of a key salt bridge is crucial in the stabilization of the 150-cavity across both subtypes. This result provides an atomic-level structural understanding of the recent finding that antiviral compounds designed to take advantage of contacts in the 150-cavity can inactivate both 2009 H1N1 pandemic and avian H5N1 viruses.

[1] Department of Pharmaceutical Sciences, Computer Science and Chemistry, University of California, Irvine, California 92697, USA. [2] National Biomedical Computation Resource, University of California, San Diego, La Jolla, California 92093, USA. [3] Department of Chemistry and Biochemistry, San Diego Supercomputer Center, University of California, San Diego, La Jolla , California 92093, USA. [4] Department of Ecology and Evolutionary Biology, University of California, Irvine, California 92697, USA. Correspondence and requests for materials should be addressed to R.E.A. (email: ramaro@uci.edu).

Understanding the structural dynamics of the influenza glycoproteins has been a long-standing goal because of their direct impact on public health. The two major influenza glycoproteins, hemagglutinin (HA) and neuraminidase (NA), control entry and exit of the viral particles from the host cell, respectively. HA binds to sialic acid surface receptors on the host cell, whereas NA cleaves the terminal sialic acid receptor linkage, facilitating viral shedding. The nine NA alleles have been divided into two groups based on phylogenetic analysis (group-1: N1, N4, N5, N8; group-2: N2, N3, N6, N7, N9)[1]. During the last century, influenza viruses carrying N1 (H1N1) or N2 (H2N2, H3N2) alleles have circulated in humans, first as pandemic strains and then, after subsequent adaptation to humans, as seasonal epidemic strains. Thus, a better understanding of the structural dynamics of N1 and N2 is particularly relevant for antiviral design.

Oseltamivir (Tamiflu) and zanamivir (Relenza), which target the NA, are currently the only antivirals approved by the FDA for the prophylaxis and treatment of influenza. These drugs, developed against available group-2 NA structures, represent some of the first successful rational structure-based drug development efforts[2]. The crystal structures of group-1 NAs revealed a never-before-seen 150-cavity adjacent to the sialic-acid-binding site[1]. It has been hypothesized, and very recently shown[3], that targeting the 150-cavity may allow the development of new antivirals with increased specificity and potency against group-1 enzymes. The increasing frequency of oseltamivir resistance in pre-2009 seasonal H1N1 viruses[4] and the occasional observation of oseltamivir resistance among 2009 H1N1 pandemic viruses motivates new antiviral development. Having additional antivirals in our treatment arsenal would be advantageous, and potentially critical, if a highly virulent strain, for example, H5N1, evolved the ability to undergo rapid transmission among humans or if the already highly transmissible 2009 H1N1 pandemic virus was to evolve resistance to existing antiviral drugs.

Recently, it was revealed that the structure of the 2009 pandemic H1N1 NA lacked a 150-cavity, despite being a group-1 NA[5]. This surprising finding suggested that the 2009 pandemic N1 protein was structurally more similar to the group-2 NAs than to the group-1 NAs. Based on alignments of sequences representing all available NA crystal structures, highly conserved residues in the 150-loop and the 430-loop (residues 147–152 and 429–433, respectively, in N2 numbering) were hypothesized to functionally determine the structure of the 150-cavity[5]. In particular, I149 was found to be common between the 2009 pandemic N1 and group-2 NAs, whereas V149 was conserved among the other group-1 NAs. In the two solved N2 structures, which have somewhat atypical sequences, a salt bridge between D147 and H150 appeared to prevent the opening of the 150-loop, despite the presence of V149.

Here we test the hypothesis that position 149 is critical for determining the open or closed status of the 150-cavity. Our alternative hypothesis is that cavity status is plastic in the absence of a D147-H150 salt bridge, being dependent on loop conformations that are themselves flexible. Earlier computational studies of N1 from avian H5N1 showed that this isolate exhibited remarkable flexibility in the 150-loop[6]. The same avian N1 was also reported to contain a closed 150-loop under certain crystallization conditions[1] and additionally shown to be able to switch to a closed loop position during a molecular dynamics (MD) simulation initiated from the co-crystallized oseltamivir-bound open-150-loop configuration[6]. The understanding that emerged was that the avian N1 was able to adopt a wide range of configurations in the 150-loop region, favouring an open conformation of the 150-cavity overall. We examined the flexibility of the 150-cavity area in the 09N1 crystal structure through molecular dynamics simulations using 09N1 and other available structures of N1 and N2 alleles derived from human clinical isolates. In combination with the simulations, an extensive bioinformatics analysis for these alleles in the 150- and 430-loop regions offers new clues as to the controlling features of 150-cavity formation in these critical enzymes. Ultimately, we found that a key salt bridge appears to control the 150-cavity formation in both group-1 and group-2 enzymes, both of which are able to adopt flexible loop conformations in this critical region. We propose that this new structural understanding can be related to antiviral design for any of the influenza NA enzymes.

Results

Molecular dynamics simulations. To probe the effect of sequence on the atomic-level structure and dynamics of these critical enzymes, we performed four separate 100-ns molecular dynamics simulations for four tetrameric NA enzymes: (1) A/California/04/2009, an H1N1 virus isolated early in the 2009 pandemic (09N1, Protein Data Bank (PDB) accession code: 3NSS)[5]. We note that the N1 allele in the pandemic strain had recently evolved from an Eurasian-lineage H1N1 swine virus[7]. (2) A mutant N1 that we engineered *in silico* from A/California/04/2009 by substituting Val for Ile at position 149 (09N1_I149V). (3) A/Vietnam/1203/04, an avian-derived H5N1 virus isolated from a human (VN04N1, PDB accession code: 2HTY)[1]. (4) A/Tokyo/3/67, a seasonal human H2N2 virus (N2, PDB accession code: 1NN2)[8]. We note that the I149V mutation in A/Tokyo/3/67 is atypical for a human N2 allele (Table 1; Supplementary Table S1).

The homotetramer configuration of NA allows us to take advantage of multicopy simulation sampling[9], amounting to the equivalent of nearly half a microsecond (400 ns) of sampling for each NA monomer, while accounting for realistic neighbouring subunit effects within the structural dynamics. Alpha-carbon root mean square deviation (RMSD) plots for the tetramer systems and individual monomer chains exhibit stability over 100 ns, and there is good agreement between experimental and simulation-derived B-factors (Supplementary Figs S1–S3).

Pandemic 2009 H1N1 exhibits open 150-cavity. Our simulations reveal that the pandemic 09N1 NA is able to adopt open 150-cavity conformations in normal solution dynamics, and, in contrast to the crystal structure, it appears to favour an open 150-cavity conformation overall (Fig. 1; Table 1). In the simulations of 09N1, the 150-loop transitions to an open configuration by 50 ns in all chains of the tetramer (Supplementary Fig. S4). As a reference for open- and closed-loop structures, the PDB accession codes 2HTY and 2HU4 were utilized, respectively. The open 150-cavity crystal structure (2HTY with hydrogen atoms added) exhibits a 150-cavity volume of 36 Å[3] as computed by POVME[10] (Supplementary Table S3). Closed 150-cavity crystal structures (1NN2, 2HU4, 3NSS with hydrogen atoms added) were used as references and uniformly exhibit a volume of 0 Å[3]. To quantify the extent to which structures within the dynamical ensemble adopt either a closed or open 150-cavity conformation, a time series of the pocket volume was computed over the course of the trajectory (Fig. 2a; Supplementary Fig. S5). Structures were subsequently classified as open or closed based on 150-cavity volume, that is, cavities with volumes greater than or equal to 18 Å[3], or at least half of the crystal structure open-cavity volume, are considered 'open.' Through this method, we determined that the 09N1 system adopts an open 150-cavity during the majority of the simulation (60.8%, Table 2). We note that longer simulation times may further increase the percentage of 09N1 in the open conformation, overcoming the structural bias due to the simulation being initiated with a closed 150-cavity.

RMSD-based clustering of the 150-loop residues enables an atomic-level population-based structural analysis. Although the most populated cluster, that is, the cluster that comprises at least 33% of the sampled ensemble, has a closed 150-loop configuration, structures within the next two most populated clusters adopt open 150-cavity configurations (Fig. 1; Supplementary Table S2). Figure 2 clearly shows that the second most dominant cluster from the 09N1

Table 1 | Variation in the 150- and 430-loops of N1 and N2 NA alleles of avian, swine and human influenza viruses.

Host	N1 and N2 alleles	N	150-loop			430-loop		
			147	149	150	430	431	432
Swine N1	N1 swine H1N1 classic lineage consensus	158	G	V	K	Q	P	K
	N1 swine H1N1 Eurasian lineage consensus	165	G	I/V	K	R	P	K
Human N1	**N1 human H1N1 2009 pandemic consensus and A/California/04/2009**	**1,806**	**G**	**I**	**K**	**R**	**P**	**K**
	N1 human H1N1 seasonal 2007–2009 consensus	1,809	G	V	K	L	P	R
	N1 human H1N1 seasonal 1950–2007 consensus		G	V	K	R	P	R
	N1 human H1N1 seasonal 1930–40s consensus		G	V	K	R	P	K
	N1 human H1N1 1918 pandemic		G	V	K	Q	P	K
Avian N1	**N1 avian consensus and A/Vietnam/1203/2004**	**2,141**	**G**	**V**	**K**	**R**	**P**	**K**
Human N2	N2 human H3N2 seasonal mid-2000s-present consensus	1,727	N/D	V	R	R	K	E
	N2 human H3N2 seasonal 1990-mid 2000s consensus		D	V	H	R	K	Q/E
	N2 human H3N2 seasonal 1970–80s consensus		D	I	H	R	E	Q
	N2 human H3N2 1968 pandemic (NA of human H2N2 origin)		D	I	H	R	K	Q
	N2 human H2N2 seasonal A/Tokyo/3/1967 (atypical 149V)		**D**	**V**	**H**	**R**	**K**	**Q**
	N2 human H2N2 seasonal 1960s consensus	88	D	I	H	R	Q/K	Q
	N2 human H2N2 1957 pandemic (NA of avian origin)		G	I	H	R	P	Q
Avian N2	N2 avian polymorphisms seen since the mid-1990s	1,743	G	T/A/S	H	R	P	K/Q
	N2 avian consensus		G	I	H	R	P	Q

Consensus sequences contain amino acids at a frequency of at least 80%. Sequences in bold font correspond to structures simulated in this paper. Table entries are single-letter amino acid codes .

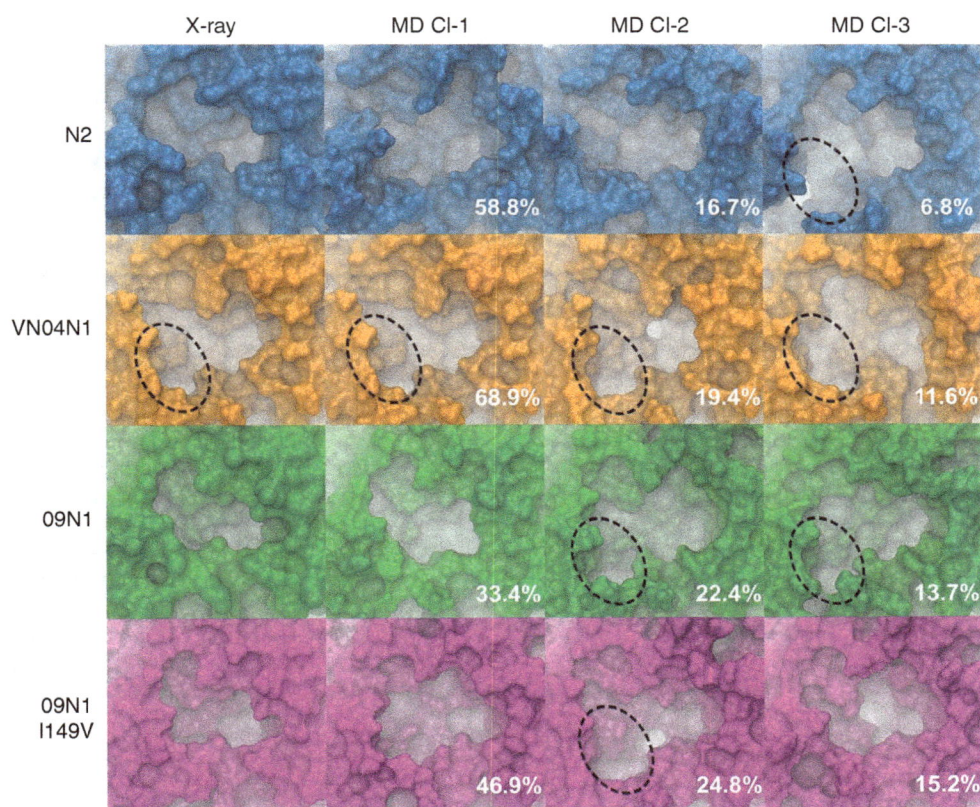

Figure 1 | Solvent accessible surface area of NA-binding site. The solvent accessible surface area of the NA-binding site is shown, as computed by the MSMS[30] program, for the X-ray structure, and top three most dominant central member cluster structures (population percentages indicated in white text for each cluster), shown for A/Tokyo/3/67 (N2), A/Vietnam/1203/04 (VN04N1), A/California/04/2009 (09N1) and the 09N1_I149V mutant strain. The open 150-cavity, where present, is outlined with a dotted circle.

simulations has an open 150-loop, highly similar to the open 150-loop of VN04N1. By comparison, the VN04N1 150-cavity is consistently open throughout the simulations, being present for 93.4%

of the trajectory (Figs 1 and 2b; Table 1; Supplementary Fig. S6). The formation of a stable and open 150-cavity in 09N1 indicates that the structural dynamics of the recent pandemic strain appear to be more similar to the classic group-1 isolates than to the group-2 isolates, in contrast to what the static crystal structure suggests. This finding provides an atomic-level structural understanding of how antiviral compounds designed to take advantage of contacts in the 150-cavity can be active against both the 2009 H1N1 and 2004 Vietnam H5N1 isolates, as very recently shown in ref. 3.

150-Cavity formation controlled by a conserved salt bridge. The dynamics of the N2 strain reveal that a key salt bridge between conserved residues D147 and H150 controls the formation of the 150-cavity in N2. This ionic contact locks I149 in the space of the 150-cavity (Fig. 3), as suggested in ref. 5. However, in each chain of the N2 tetramer simulation, this salt bridge intermittently breaks and then reforms; in chain C, at 60 ns the contact is lost again, after which the open 150-cavity forms, and contact to the 430-loop is lost (Fig. 2c; Supplementary Fig. S7). The loss of the D147-H150 salt bridge allows the 150-loop to move to the open position, even wider than the VN04N1 open 150-loop structure (Fig. 2). RMSD-based clustering of the 150-loop indicates that while both the first and second most dominant configurations remain closed, the third most dominant configuration, representing 6.8% of the trajectory, exhib-

its an open 150-cavity (Fig. 1). Volumetric calculations of the 150-cavity confirm that the open-cavity conformation is present in 10% of the simulation and has a volume of 284 Å³. For the remainder of the simulation, the salt bridge does not reform, and the wide-open 150-cavity therefore persists in one chain of the N2 tetramer.

The spontaneous loss of this key contact under 'physiologically relevant' simulation conditions provides a clear atomic-level model for 150-cavity formation in the N2 clinical isolate. The loss of the salt bridge reduces the rigidity of the 150-loop, enabling the loop to sample more open conformations. Contacts with the neighbouring 430-loop are simultaneously lost, and significant expansions of both the 150- and 430-cavities occur (Figs 1, 2C and 3; Supplementary Table S3 and Supplementary Fig. S8). Although the open 150-loop is energetically accessible in the N2 structures, its low population during the simulation makes it unlikely that this open 150-cavity would appear in X-ray crystallography experiments. Such a cavity would be able to accommodate compounds targeting the 150-cavity, albeit with a lower affinity, as very recently shown in ref. 3. In all the N1 proteins, D147 is replaced with an uncharged G147, and therefore no salt bridge is present to lock I/V149 in the 150-cavity space. This may explain why an open 150-cavity is characteristically observed in crystals, even in 09N1, which is able to adopt a stable open 150-cavity conformation. It also underscores the importance of considering solution-phase dynamics for these enzymes and not only crystallographic information, which is generally only able to provide one low-energy snapshot of the dynamic protein complex under crystalline conditions.

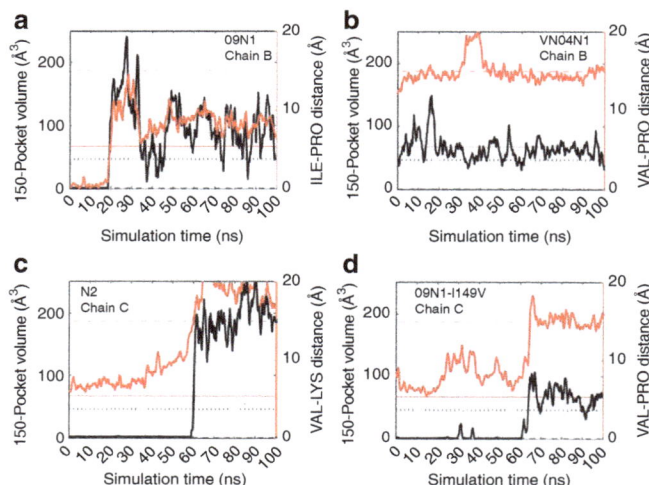

Figure 2 | Time series analysis of 150-cavity volume and width for a particular monomer in each of the simulated systems. On the left-side y axis, the volume of the 150-cavity is computed over the course of simulation. The distance between alpha-carbon of residue 431 (PRO in **a**, **b**, **d**; LYS in **c**) and the closest side-chain carbon of residue 149 (Val149 panels **b**, **c**, **d**; ILE in **a**) is computed and shown in red and the right-side y axis. The black and red dotted lines correspond to the open crystal structure (2HTY) volume and distance, respectively; whereas the black dashed and red solid lines correspond to the closed crystal structure (2HU4) volume and distance, respectively. The systems shown are A/Tokyo/3/67 (N2), A/Vietnam/1203/04 (VN04N1), A/California/04/2009 (09N1) and the 09N1_I149V mutant strain.

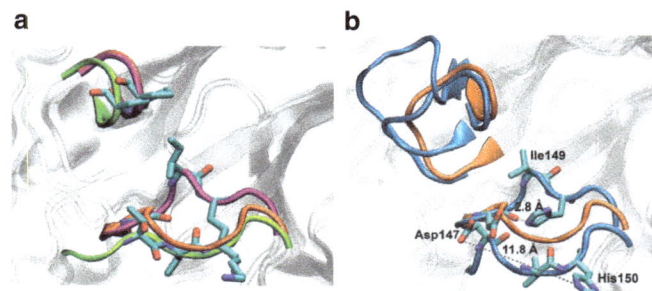

Figure 3 | Structural variation in N1 and N2 clinical isolates. (a) The 150- and 430-loop structures are shown for 09N1 crystal structure (purple), 09N1 second most dominant molecular dynamics (MD) cluster representative structure (green backbone) and VN04N1 crystal structure (orange), indicating that the pandemic N1 adopts an open 150-loop conformation. Gly147, Ile149, Lys150 and Pro431 are shown in stick representation. (**b**) N2 150- and 430-loops from crystal and most dominant cluster representative structures are shown in blue, and open VN04N1 crystal structure are shown in orange. The D147-H150 salt bridge spontaneously ruptures in chain C of N2, extending its initial contact from 2.8 Å in crystal structure to 11.8 Å in the most dominant MD-generated cluster structure, revealing a wide-open 150-cavity.

Table 2 | Population analysis based on open or closed 150-cavity.

System (crystal structure)	Crystal structure state of 150-cavity	147.149,150...431	Total open (%)	Total closed (%)
N2 (1nn2)	Closed	D.VH...K	202 (10.1%)	1,798 (89.9%)
VN04N1 (2hty)	Open	G.VK...P	1,867 (93.4 %)	133 (6.6%)
09N1 (3nss)	Closed	G.IK...P	1,215 (60.8 %)	785 (39.2%)
09N1_I149V (3nss*)	Closed	G.VK...P	742 (37.1 %)	1,258 (62.9%)

*3nss accession code with the I149V mutation introduced in silico.

Among N1 alleles for which structures exist, the 2009 H1N1 pandemic isolate uniquely contains an I149. Thus, Li *et al.*[5] hypothesized that the additional extension of the I149 side chain, compared with V149, may be a compensating factor in controlling the closed-loop structure, despite strict conservation of all other residues in this area. Structurally, the longer side chain of I149 may facilitate van der Waals contacts to the neighbouring 430-loop, and shift the population to a more closed 150-loop state; a V149 mutation would facilitate loss of contact between the 150- and 430-loop, shifting the population to a more open 150-cavity state. To test this hypothesis, we created the 09N1_I149V mutant strain *in silico* and performed an identical 100 ns simulation. Our results indicate that the effect of this mutation on 150-cavity status varies due to 150-loop flexibility. The time series data indicate that the I149V mutation caused chain D to open almost immediately, chain C to open after 60 ns, chain A to open intermittently and had almost no effect on chain B (Supplementary Fig. S9). Overall, the 09N1_I149V mutant is actually more closed, exhibiting the open 150-cavity less frequently, in only 37.1% of the simulation, compared with the normal 09N1 strain with the I149 present (Table 2, Fig. 2d; Supplementary Fig. S9). Moreover, only one of the three most dominant structures, cluster 2, presents the open 150-cavity, and thus, the V149 by itself cannot explain the behaviour of the 09N1_I149V.

Analysis of sequence conservation in the 150-loop region. To date, the evolutionary distribution of the 150-cavity among NA alleles has been inferred primarily from crystallographically resolved structures, which represent a limited subset of the genetic variation of NAs in nature. Based on those analyses, it seemed logical to attribute the occurrence of an open 150-cavity to having a V or I at position 149, and by extension, to membership, in the group-1 or group-2 NAs, respectively, as shown in figure 3 of Li *et al.* Our dynamical analyses suggest that I/V149 is not as critical to 150-cavity status as the D147-H150 salt bridge, which warrants re-examination of the association of cavity status with NA group membership. We determined the distribution of genetic variation in the 150 and 450 loops among all avian, human and swine N1 and N2 sequences that had been deposited in GenBank and Global Initiative on Sharing Avian Influenza Data (GISAID) as of 12 August 2010 using phylogenetic analysis to construct consensus sequences for each major clade (Supplementary Methods for methodological details).

Our phylogenetic analyses (Table 1) show that no single amino acid position in the 150- or 430-loops clearly differentiates the N1 and N2 alleles, which are in group-1 and group-2, respectively. The D147-H150 salt bridge is not a defining characteristic of N2 alleles, as it is not present in avian viruses, which were the source of the N2 allele in the 1957 H2N2 human pandemic strain. Nor is the salt bridge found in human H3N2 viruses that have been circulating since 2008, due to fixation of a D147N mutation. Thus, neither the amino acid at position 149 nor the salt bridge is fixed characters that differentiate group 1 and group 2 NAs. Nor do they, at least by themselves, characterize viruses capable of infection of humans. Additional tests of our hypothesis require the acquisition of crystal structures of additional NA alleles, most critically, an N2 allele that contains both the D147-H150 salt bridge and I149.

Discussion

Our results highlight the importance of interpreting influenza NA sequence and structural data in light of the dynamical ensemble of conformations that are accessible to each NA protein. This work shows for the first time that both N1 and N2 clinical isolates exhibit flexibility in the 150-cavity neighbouring the conserved sialic-acid-binding site. Although it remains possible that the open and closed conformation observed in crystal structures may be due to differences in crystallization conditions or procedures, our results indicate that the presence of the 150-cavity is not a strictly defining

characteristic for group-1 or group-2 NA enzymes. Instead, it appears that both N1 and N2 enzymes are able to adopt an open 150-cavity within their solution phase structural ensemble, in various relative populations, which appear to be predominantly controlled by the presence of the D147-H/R150 salt bridge. This suggests a new paradigm for the understanding of the presence of the 150-cavity in both group-1 and group-2 NAs. The inherent flexibility of the 150- and 430-loops may have a role in full glycan receptor recognition, and in particular, with facilitating recognition events with the distal sugar residues of different glycan receptors. It is likely that the opening and closing of the 150-cavity is required for natural sialoglycan substrates to fit into the active site, given the bulky nature of these glycans.

This study additionally underscores the need to consider dynamics in rationalizing the structure–function relationships of various antiviral–NA pairs. Ensemble-based drug discovery approaches[11] that account for full-receptor flexibility towards NAs that do not contain the D147-H150 salt bridge will likely present additional advances in the design of compounds that selectively target the 150-cavity, opening the possibility for receptor-specific inhibitors. In closing, we note that whether the flexibility of the NA-binding site has an impact on receptor specificity, virus transmissibility or pathogenicity remains to be seen and will likely require a better understanding of HA receptor-binding domain dynamics for each of the NA/HA pairs found in humans[12].

Methods

Simulation protocol. System setup was performed as follows for all simulated systems. Atomic coordinates were taken from 2HTY for A/Vietnam/1203/04 (VN04N1)[1], 3NSS for A/California/04/2009 (09N1)[5] and 1NN2 for A/Aichi/3/67 (N2)[8]. Protonation states for histidines and other titratable groups were determined at pH 6.5 by the PDB2PQR[13] web server using PROPKA[14] and manually verified. All crystallographically resolved water molecules and calcium ions were retained where possible and taken by homology from 2HTY if not present. The system was setup using the AMBER11[15] program xLeap using the AMBER99SB force field[16]. Disulphide bonds were properly enforced using the CYX notation in AMBER. A 10–12 Å pad of TIP3P waters was added to solvate each system. Neutralizing counter ions were added to each system. In order to mimic experimental assay conditions, a 20 mM NaCl salt bath was introduced. System details and additional methodological information can be found in the Supplementary information.

N1 and N2 tetramer simulations were performed with a version of the PMEMD module from AMBER 11 that was custom tuned for these specific simulations and the NICS Cray XT4 and SDSC Trestles supercomputers by SDSC under the NSF's TeraGrid Advanced User Support Program. The N1 and N2 apo tetramer complexes were minimized and equilibrated as follows: in order to alleciate any steric clashes before performing molecular dynamics, the structures were minimized in a number of stages in which harmonic restraints of initially 5 kcal mol^{-1}Å^{-2} on all non-hydrogen protein atoms were slowly reduced over ~40,000 combined steepest descent and conjugate gradient minimization steps.

Following minimization, the system was linearly heated to 310 K in the canonical NVT ensemble (constant number of particles, N; constant volume, V; constant temperature, T) using a Langevin thermostat, with a collision frequency of 5.0 ps^{-1}, and harmonic restraints of 4 kcal mol^{-1}Å^{-2} on the backbone atoms. Then, a further three 250 ps long runs at 310 K were conducted in the NPT ensemble with the restraint force constant being reduced by 1 kcal mol^{-1}Å^{-2} each time and pressure controlled using a Berendsen barostat[17] with a coupling constant of 1 ps and a target pressure of 1 atm. A final 250 ps of NPT dynamics was run at 310 K without restraints and a Langevin collision frequency of 2 ps^{-1}. Production runs were then made for 100 ns duration in the NVT ensemble at 310 K. As with the heating, the temperature was controlled with a Langevin thermostat (but with a 1.0 ps^{-1} collision frequency). The time step used for all stages was 2 fs and all hydrogen atoms were constrained using the SHAKE algorithm[18]. Long-range electrostatics were included on every step using the Particle Mesh Ewald algorithm[19] with a 4th order B-spline interpolation, a grid spacing of < 1.0 Å, and a direct space cutoff of 8 Å. For all trajectories, the random number stream was seeded using the wall clock time in microseconds. The production trajectories for each monomer of the tetramer were extracted and concatenated to approximate 400 ns of monomer sampling.

RMSD clustering. RMSD clustering was performed as implemented in the rmsdmat2 and cluster2 programs of the GROMOS++ analysis software[20]. A total of 500 tetramer structures were collected by sampling at 200 ps intervals. Monomer structures were then concatenated together, yielding a total of 2,000 structures. Before clustering, external translational and rotational motions were removed by minimizing the RMSD distance of the alpha-carbon atoms of the sampled structure to the equivalent atoms of the first frame of chain A. Using a 2.6 Å cutoff, clustering was then performed using the GROMOS + + clustering algorithm[21] in Gromacs[22] on the alpha-carbon atoms of the 6-residue subset, 146–152, which comprise the 150 loops. Each cluster contains a central structure, or 'cluster representative member,' called the 'centroid,' whose RMSD is equidistant to all other cluster members. The cluster representative's structural properties are considered characteristic of all cluster members. Cluster results are summarized in Table 2.

RMSD and B-factor calculations. B-factor calculations, as well as tetramer and monomer RMSD time series, were performed using the ptraj analysis tool in the AMBER 10 program suite[23]. Structures were sampled at 20 ps intervals. Before performing each calculation, external translational and rotational motions were removed by minimizing the RMSD distance of the alpha-carbon atoms to the equivalent atoms of the first frame of the trajectory. RMSD and B-factor values were calculated for alpha-carbon atoms.

09N1 RMSD 150-loop measurements. RMSD values were measured using a custom, hand-written script in the VMD TCL-TK console[24]. Structures were sampled at 20 ps intervals. Sampled structures of each monomer were RMSD-aligned by alpha-carbon to the equivalent alpha-carbon atoms of the 'reference' structure: chain A of PDB ID 2HTY, open reference; or chain A of PDB ID 2HU4, closed reference. Following alignment, the RMSD of the 150 loop of each monomer was measured with respect to the 150 loop of each reference structure. The 150 loops were defined as residues 146–152 for the 09N1 monomers, as well as for the open and closed reference structures.

Interatomic distance measurements. The distance separating the salt bridge pair ASP147 and HIS150 was measured using a custom, hand-written script in the VMD TCL-TK console. Structures were sampled at 20 ps intervals. The distance between the two residues was defined as the distance separating centres of mass of the heavy atoms of the ASP147 carboxylate and the HIS 150 imidazole. The distance between residues 149 and 431 were measured for each step using a custom VMD script.

Neuraminidase volume population analysis. The numbers of open or closed 150-cavity conformations out of a total of 2,000 snapshots were computed. Any instantaneous volume equal to or greater than half the volume of the crystal structure of canonical group-1 serovar (2HTY exhibits a total 150-cavity volume of 36 Å[3]) is considered to be 'open'. Otherwise the 150-cavity is considered 'closed' (that is, when it exhibits < 18 Å[3]). The volume of the 150-cavity was measured for each step by using POVME[10]; a pocket volume measuring algorithm. To measure the volume, we used a single inclusion sphere that encompassed the 150-cavity. The POVME algorithm neglected the volume occupied by NA atoms and not spatially contiguous with a point specified within the 150-cavity. By rotating 90° around the NA tetramer central axis, each of the other three 150-cavity sites were specified. The volume was thus measured for every snapshot of the simulation on all four chains of each NA.

Figures and plots. Matlab was used to generate all plots and molecular images were created using VMD[24].

Consensus sequences. We downloaded all influenza A N1 and N2 gene sequences from humans, avians and swine that were > 600 bp in length from GenBank and GISAID on 12 August 2010. We aligned sequences using ClustalX 2.0 (ref. 25) and constructed phylogenetic trees using MrBayes version 3.1.2 (ref. 26) using the GTR + I + gamma model, as suggested by jmodeltest version 0.1.1 (ref. 27) under the Akaike Information Criterion. All other MrBayes parameters were set to the default. We allowed MrBayes to run, sampling every 1,000 trees, until the Monte Carlo Markov chains converged as determined by Tracer software version 1.5 (ref. 28). We discarded the burn-in as determined by Tracer. Similar results were obtained using the neighbour-joining routine of PAUP* 4.0b10 (ref. 29; results not shown). Consensus sequences containing amino acids found at a frequency of at least 80% were constructed for each major evolutionary clade. Results are shown, along with samples sizes, in Table 1.

References

1. Russell, R. J. et al. The structure of H5N1 avian influenza neuraminidase suggests new opportunities for drug design. *Nature* **443**, 45–49 (2006).
2. von Itzstein, M. The war against influenza: discovery and development of sialidase inhibitors. *Nat. Rev. Drug Discov.* **6**, 967–974 (2007).
3. Rudrawar, S. et al. Novel sialic acid derivatives lock open the 150-loop of an influenza A virus group-1 sialidase. *Nat. Commun.* **1**, 113 (2011).
4. Dharan, N. J. et al. Infections with oseltamivir-resistant influenza A(H1N1) virus in the United States. *JAMA* **301**, 1034–1041 (2009).
5. Li, Q. et al. The 2009 pandemic H1N1 neuraminidase N1 lacks the 150-cavity in its active site. *Nat. Struct. Mol. Biol.* **17**, 1266–1268 (2010).
6. Amaro, R. E. et al. Remarkable loop flexibility in avian influenza N1 and its implications for antiviral drug design. *J. Am. Chem. Soc.* **129**, 7764–7765 (2007).
7. Garten, R. J. et al. Antigenic and genetic characteristics of swine-origin 2009 A(H1N1) influenza viruses circulating in humans. *Science* **325**, 197–201 (2009).
8. Varghese, J. N. & Colman, P. M. Three-dimensional structure of the neuraminidase of influenza virus A/Tokyo/3/67 at 2.2 A resolution. *J. Mol. Biol.* **221**, 473–486 (1991).
9. Caves, L. S., Evanseck, J. D. & Karplus, M. Locally accessible conformations of proteins: multiple molecular dynamics simulations of crambin. *Protein Sci.* **7**, 649–666 (1998).
10. Durrant, J. D., de Oliveira, C. A. & McCammon, J. A. POVME: an algorithm for measuring binding-pocket volumes. *J. Mol. Graph. Model.* **29**, 773–776 (2011).
11. Amaro, R. & Li, W. W. Emerging ensemble-based methods in virtual screening. *Curr. Topics Med. Chem.* **10**, 3–13 (2010).
12. Wagner, R., Matrosovich, M. & Klenk, H. D. Functional balance between haemagglutinin and neuraminidase in influenza virus infections. *Rev. Med. Virol.* **12**, 159–166 (2002).
13. Dolinsky, T., Nielsen, J., McCammon, J. & Baker, N. PDB2PQR: an automated pipeline for the setup, execution, and analysis of Poisson–Boltzmann electrostatics calculations. *Nucleic Acids Res.* **32**, W665–W667 (2004).
14. Li, H., Robertson, A. D. & Jensen, J. H. Very fast empirical prediction and rationalization of protein pKa values. *Proteins* **61**, 704–721 (2005).
15. Newhouse, E. I. et al. Mechanism of glycan receptor recognition and specificity switch for avian, swine, and human adapted influenza virus hemagglutinins: a molecular dynamics perspective. *J. Am. Chem. Soc.* **131**, 17430–17442 (2009).
16. Hornak, V. et al. Comparison of multiple Amber force fields and development of improved protein backbone parameters. *Proteins* **65**, 712–725 (2006).
17. Berendsen, H. J. C., Postma, J. P. M., Gunsteren, W. F. V., DiNola, A. & Haak, J. R. Molecular dynamics with coupling to an external bath. *J. Chem. Phys.* **81**, 3684 (1984).
18. Andersen, H. C. Rattle: a 'velocity' version of the Shake algorithm for molecular dynamics calculations. *J. Comput. Phy.* **52**, 24–34 (1983).
19. Darden, T., York, D. & Pedersen, L. Particle mesh Ewald: an N [center-dot] log(N) method for Ewald sums in large systems. *J. Chem. Phys.* **98**, 10089–10092 (1993).
20. Christen, M. et al. The GROMOS software for biomolecular simulation: GROMOS05. *J. Comput. Chem.* **26**, 1719–1751 (2005).
21. Daura, X., Jaun, B., Seebach, D., van Gunsteren, W. F. & Mark, A. E. Reversible peptide folding in solution by molecular dynamics simulation. *J. Mol. Biol.* **280**, 925–932 (1998).
22. Lindahl, E., Hess, B. & van der Spoel, D. GROMACS 3.0: a package for molecular simulation and trajectory analysis. *J. Mol. Mod.* **7**, 306–317 (2001).
23. Xu, D. et al. Distinct glycan topology for avian and human sialopentasaccharide receptor analogues upon binding different hemagglutinins: a molecular dynamics perspective. *J. Mol. Biol.* **387**, 465–491 (2009).
24. Humphrey, W., Dalke, A. & Schulten, K. VMD: visual molecular dynamics. *J. Mol. Graph.* **14**, 33–38, 27–38 (1996).
25. Thompson, J. D., Gibson, T. J., Plewniak, F., Jeanmougin, F. & Higgins, D. G. The CLUSTAL_X windows interface: flexible strategies for multiple sequence alignment aided by quality analysis tools. *Nucleic Acids Res.* **25**, 4876–4882 (1997).
26. Ronquist, F. & Huelsenbeck, J. P. MrBayes 3: Bayesian phylogenetic inference under mixed models. *Bioinformatics* **19**, 1572–1574 (2003).
27. Posada, D. jModelTest: phylogenetic model averaging. *Mol. Biol. Evol.* **25**, 1253–1256 (2008).
28. Rambaut, A. & Drummond, A. J. Tracer v. 1.4 (http://beast.bio.ed.ac.uk/Tracer 2007).
29. Swofford, D. L. Sinauer Associates. *PAUP*: Phylogentic Analysis Using Parsimony* (Sinauer Associates, 1998).
30. Sanner, M. F., Olson, A. J. & Spehner, J. C. Reduced surface: an efficient way to compute molecular surfaces. *Biopolymers* **38**, 305–320 (1996).

Acknowledgements

This work was funded in part by the National Institutes of Health through the NIH Director's New Innovator Award Program, 1-DP2-OD007237 and a NIH Career Transition Award 1-K22-AI081901 to R.E.A. This research was also supported in part by the NSF through TeraGrid Supercomputer resources provided by a directors discretionary grant from the National Institute for Computational Science (TG-CHE100128) and the San Diego Supercomputer Center (TG-MCB090110) and by NSF SI2-SSE (NSF1047875) and University of California (UC Lab 09-LR-06-117792) grants to R.C.W. W.W.L. is funded in part by NIH P41 RR08605. R.M.B. is supported by National Institute of General Medical Sciences MIDAS grant U01-GM076499. The authors thank Baotran Le for help with the analysis.

Author contributions

R.E.A., W.W.L. and R.B. designed the experiments. R.E.A., L.V., R.C.W. and R.M.B. performed the experiments. R.E.A., R.V.S., L.V., W.W.L. and R.M.B. performed the analysis. R.E.A., W.W.L. and R.M.B. wrote the paper. All authors contributed to the editing of the paper and to scientific discussions.

Additional information

Competing financial interests: The authors declare no competing financial interests.

2

Direct synthesis of imino-C-nucleoside analogues and other biologically active iminosugars

Milan Bergeron-Brlek[1], Michael Meanwell[1] & Robert Britton[1]

Iminosugars have attracted increasing attention as chemical probes, chaperones and leads for drug discovery. Despite several clinical successes, their *de novo* synthesis remains a significant challenge that also limits their integration with modern high-throughput screening technologies. Herein, we describe a unique synthetic strategy that converts a wide range of acetaldehyde derivatives into iminosugars and imino-C-nucleoside analogues in two or three straightforward transformations. We also show that this strategy can be readily applied to the rapid production of indolizidine and pyrrolizidine iminosugars. The high levels of enantio- and diastereoselectivity, excellent overall yields, convenience and broad substrate scope make this an appealing process for diversity-oriented synthesis, and should enable drug discovery efforts.

[1] Department of Chemistry, Simon Fraser University, Burnaby, British Columbia, Canada V7G 1S2. Correspondence and requests for materials should be addressed to R.B. (email: rbritton@sfu.ca).

Iminosugars are naturally occurring carbohydrate mimics that inhibit many enzymes of medicinal interest[1]. Their biological activity is often attributed to a structural resemblance to the oxacarbenium ion-like transition states that occur during the enzymatic hydrolysis of carbohydrates[2]. As such, many iminosugars are potent inhibitors of glycosidases and glycosyltransferases[1], and have been highlighted as lead candidates for the treatment of a variety of diseases, including cancer, diabetes, viral infections and lysosomal storage disorders (for example, Gaucher and Fabry disease)[1,3]. The most common naturally occurring iminosugars possess a polyhydroxylated pyrrolidine core and may be additionally annulated as in the pyrrolizidines (for example, 2, Fig. 1), indolizidines (for example, 3), or nortropanes[4]. A growing number of unnatural analogues of these compounds have also been reported as leads for drug discovery, including the imino-C-nucleosides developed by Schramm (for example, 1)[5,6] and β-hexosaminidase inhibitors developed by Wong[7,8]. Unfortunately, the incorporation of pyrrolidine iminosugars into chemical screening libraries or diversity-oriented synthesis (DOS) campaigns is problematic, as their syntheses are often lengthy, low-yielding, cost-intensive and limited by reliance on carbohydrate building blocks[9]. Thus, while several such pyrrolidine iminosugars have emerged as clinical candidates or drugs[1], fundamental tools for their high-throughput synthesis are lacking. In fact, much of the success in imino-C-nucleoside synthesis[10–14] (for example, 1 (ref. 6) and 4 (ref. 5)) has relied on the common building block 5 (refs 14–16). As evidenced by step counts provided in Fig. 1, the synthesis of pyrrolizidine- and indolizidine-based iminosugars (for example, 2; (ref. 17) and 3; (ref 18)) also remains a significant synthetic challenge.

We have reported preliminarily that when mixtures of the dioxanone 8, an aliphatic aldehyde 6 and N-chlorosuccinimide (NCS) are treated with (S)-proline, a series of well-orchestrated reactions occur[19]. First, the aldehyde undergoes α-chlorination[20], producing a racemic mixture of α-chloroaldehydes 7. Second, an enantioselective proline-catalysed aldol reaction occurs between the dioxanone 8 and the α-chloroaldehyde (R)-7. Importantly, proline also catalyses racemization of the α-chloroaldehydes 7 and, consequently, this second step effects a dynamic kinetic resolution (DKR)[19]. Thus, this one-pot reaction transforms commodity chemicals 6 and 8 into carbohydrate

building blocks 9 in excellent yield, diastereoselectivity and enanantioselectivity. Considering the spatial relationship between the chloromethine and carbonyl functions in 9, these aldol adducts may also serve as building blocks[21–24] for the synthesis of polyhydroxypyrrolidines via a reductive amination–annulation sequence (see grey box, Fig. 2). Such a strategy would allow for the conversion of virtually any acetaldehyde derivative 6 into an iminosugar 10 in two straightforward transformations from commodity chemicals, thus enabling their integration with modern high-throughput screening technologies.

Here we demonstrate that the reductive amination of a wide range of ketochlorohydrins 9 provides a rapid route to pyrrolidine iminosugars[8,11,25–32], such as those depicted in Fig. 1. Importantly, this unique two- or three-step process requires no cryogenic, anhydrous or otherwise complicated experimental conditions. The demonstration of this strategy in several short syntheses of biologically active imino-C-nucleoside analogues, and indolizidine and pyrrolizidine iminosugars highlights its adaptability for DOS and the rapid preparation of iminosugar-based screening libraries[26].

Results

Reductive amination of α-chlorination-DKR aldol products.
The utility of the synthetic strategy outlined in Fig. 2 relies intimately on a diastereoselective reductive amination of aldol adducts 9. Enders has reported[27] that the reductive amination of related aldol adducts that lack a chloromethine function were non selective (dr < 2:1) using $NaB(OAc)_3H$. Likewise, Madsen found similar selectivities in the reductive amination of the corresponding syn-aldol adduct[33]. Bearing this in mind, we began by screening solvents and reducing agents, as well as the addition of acetic acid to the reductive amination of ketochlorohydrin 11 (Table 1) (ref. 19). In all cases, an excess of amine was required for complete imine formation and avoidance of competing ketone reduction (entry 1). As indicated in entry 2, the conditions reported by Enders[27] delivered the amino alcohols 12a and 12b in good yield (82%), albeit low diastereoselectivity. The relative stereochemistry of 12a was assigned based on analysis of $^3J_{H,H}$ coupling constants and NOESY spectra recorded on the cyclic carbamate derived from the reaction of 12a with carbonyldiimidazole. Use of $NaB(CN)H_3$ resulted in an improved diastereomeric ratio of these products (dr ~ 6:1) in both CH_2Cl_2 and MeCN (entries 3 and 4) and in tetrahydrofuran (THF) the 1,3-syn amino alcohol 12a was produced as the only detectable diastereomer in near quantitative yield (entry 5). As

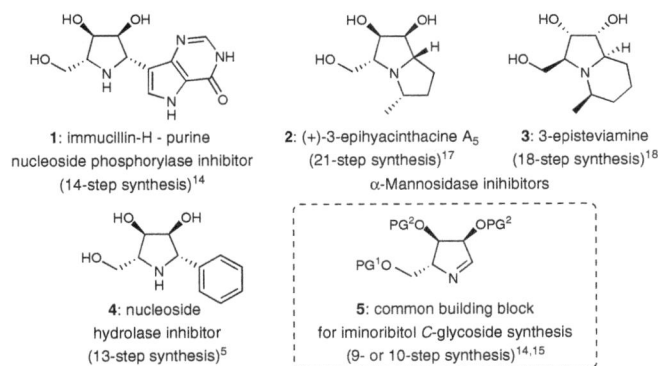

Figure 1 | Biologically active iminosugars and the common building block 5 for imino-C-nucleoside synthesis. Immucillin-H (1) is a potent transition-state analogue inhibitor of purine nucleoside phosphorylase and a lead for the treatment of human T-cell leukaemia and lymphoma. The structurally related imino-C-nucleoside analogue 4 inhibits nucleoside hydrolase. In addition, the pyrrolizidine and indolizidine iminosugars 2 and 3 inhibit α-mannosidase, an enzyme target for anticancer therapies. The number of steps required to synthesize each of 1–4 and the synthetic building block 5 highlight the challenges faced when incorporating pyrrolidine iminosugars into chemical screening libraries and medicinal chemistry campaigns.

Figure 1 labels:
1: immucillin-H - purine nucleoside phosphorylase inhibitor (14-step synthesis)[14]
2: (+)-3-epihyacinthacine A₅ (21-step synthesis)[17]
3: 3-episteviamine (18-step synthesis)[18]
α-Mannosidase inhibitors
4: nucleoside hydrolase inhibitor (13-step synthesis)[5]
5: common building block for iminoribitol C-glycoside synthesis (9- or 10-step synthesis)[14,15]

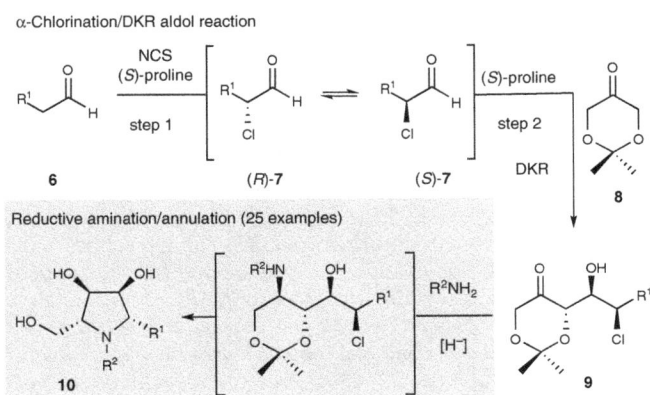

Figure 2 | A convenient synthesis of polyhydroxypyrrolidine iminosugars. Organocatalytic tandem α-chlorination-DKR aldol reaction coupled with a reductive amination/annulation sequence to access iminosugars 10.

Table 1 | Reductive amination of ketochlorohydrin 11.

11
1 step from pentanal
(62%, 94% ee)

12a: R = Bn
13a: R = allyl
14a: R = propargyl

12b: R = Bn
13b: R = allyl
14b: R = propargyl

Entry	Reducing agent	Solvent	R	Products (% yield)*
1	NaBH$_4$[†]	CH$_2$Cl$_2$	Bn	**12a** (17), **12b** (28)[‡]
2	NaB(OAc)$_3$H[†,§]	CH$_2$Cl$_2$	Bn	**12a** (36), **12b** (46)
3	NaB(CN)H$_3$[§]	CH$_2$Cl$_2$	Bn	**12a** (85), **12b** (13)
4	NaB(CN)H$_3$[§]	MeCN	Bn	**12a** (83), **12b** (15)
5	NaB(CN)H$_3$[§]	THF	Bn	**12a** (98), **12b** (<2)[‖]
6	NaB(CN)H$_3$[§]	THF	allyl	**13a** (85), **13b** (<2)[‖]
7	NaB(CN)H$_3$[§]	THF	propargyl	**14a** (83), **14b** (<2)[‖]

a) 2.5 Equivalents of amine is added to stirred solution of **11** at room temperature, after 1 h reducing agent is added and mixture is stirred for an additonal 1 h.
*Isolated yield.
[†]Reaction stirred for 12 h.
[‡]Accompanied by significant amounts of carbonyl reduction products.
[§]1 equiv. of HOAc added.
[‖]Not detected in ^{1}H-NMR spectra recorded on crude reaction product.

3-step total synthesis of nucleoside hydrolase inhibitor **4** (96% ee)

Figure 3 | Synthesis of pyrrolidine iminosugars and imino-C-nucleoside analogues. A highly diastereoselective reductive amination of chlorohydrin aldol adducts followed by brief heating in methanol or toluene with NaHCO$_3$ provides rapid access to native or differentially protected iminosugars. Reductive amination of the benzyl chloride-containing aldol adduct **17** leads directly to the protected iminosugar **18**, a precursor to the potent nucleoside hydrolase inhibitor **4**.

summarized in entries 6 and 7, this optimized protocol proved general and also provided access to the corresponding N-allyl and N-propargyl amines **13a** and **14a**, in excellent yield and diastereoselectivity.

Synthesis of pyrrolidine iminosugars. While the amino-chlorohydrin **12a** did not cyclize directly, its high-yielding conversion into the pyrrolidine iminosugar **15** simply required heating in methanol, which also promoted acetonide removal (Fig. 3). Alternatively, this cyclization could be effected by heating **12a** in toluene with excess NaHCO$_3$, which provided the orthogonally protected iminosugar **16**. Anticipating that the increased reactivity of a benzylchlorohydrin would favour a one-pot reductive amination–annulation process, the readily available aldol adduct **17** (ref. 19) was also treated with NaB(CN)H$_3$ in a mixture of THF/HOAc. Following this optimized procedure, the orthogonally protected iminosugar **18** was produced directly and in excellent yield. Removal of both the acetonide and benzyl-protecting groups by hydrogenolysis in acidic methanol gave the imino-C-nucleoside analogue **4**. Considering the aldol adduct **17** is available in one step from phenyl acetaldehyde[19], this three-step synthesis of **4**, a potent ($K_i = 170$ nM) transition-state analogue inhibitor of nucleoside hydrolase[5], represents a significant advance.

Scope of direct iminosugar synthesis. To further evaluate the scope of this direct iminosugar synthesis, we repeated the reactions described in Fig. 3 with several additional alkyl- and aryl-substituted ketochlorohydrins prepared in one step using our (S)-proline-catalysed α-chlorination-DKR aldol reaction[19]. It is noteworthy that the enantiomeric ketochlorohydrins are also readily prepared using the corresponding (R)-proline-catalysed reaction[19]. As indicated in Fig. 4, the reductive amination-annulation process is general and delivers a wide range of polyhydroxypyrrolidines **22–43** in good to excellent overall yield. A number of the orthogonally protected iminosugars depicted in Fig. 4 are crystalline and their structures were confirmed by X-ray crystallographic analysis (Supplementary Information). As expected (*vide supra*), the synthesis of alkyl-substituted iminosugars required an additional cyclization step, whereby

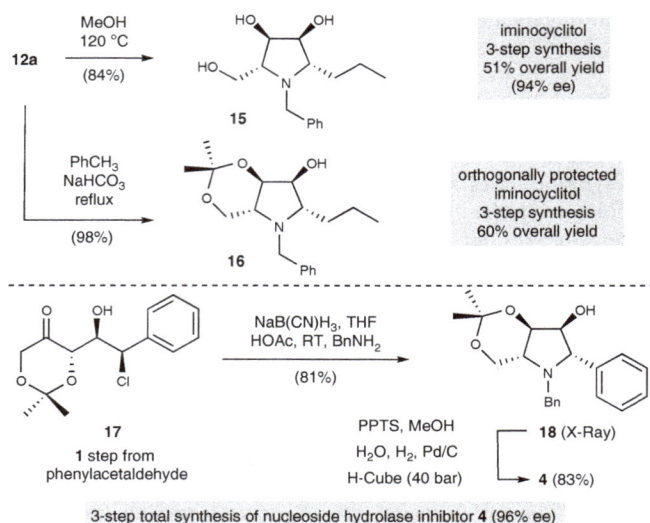

the product of reductive amination was heated in MeOH or toluene with NaHCO$_3$. Thus, this convenient process can be tailored for the production of orthogonally protected (**22, 24, 26, 28** and **30**) or native iminosugars (**23, 25, 27, 29** and **31**). Conversely, reductive amination of aryl-substituted chlorohydrins provided the corresponding iminosugars **18** and **36–39** directly and in excellent yield. It is notable that both the one- and two-step iminosugar syntheses proved tolerant of various functional groups. For example, electron deficient aryl (**36** and **37**), electron rich aryl (**38**) and heteroaryl substituents (**39**) were readily incorporated. Likewise, alkyl (**22–35**), branched alkyl (**24**), silyloxy alkyl (**32**), allyl (**26**), propargyl (**28**), primary alkyl chloride (**33**) and benzyl (**30**) groups were all compatible with the reaction sequence. The use of benzyl amine (**22–39**), allyl amine (**40–41**) or propargyl amine (**42–43**) also highlights the utility of this process for DOS and the potential for further elaboration of these iminosugars through metathesis, click, or cross coupling reactions. Finally, the mild reaction conditions and the protecting-group compatibility deserves note, as the 1,3-dioxane function in **34** and **35**, silyl protecting group in **32** and **43**, and acetonide function (conditions a)) in all substrates remained intact throughout the reaction sequence. Importantly, these readily available iminosugars share many features considered optimal for lead identification[34–37], including MW <350 DA, CLogP <2, multiple chiral centres, heterocyclic rings and H-bond donors/acceptors. In addition, the ease with which the amine function and ring substituent (R^1 and R^2 in **20**) can be differentiated provides unique opportunities for further diversification.

Short syntheses of polyhydroxy pyrrolizidines and indolizidines. Figure 5 highlights the further application of this convenient strategy to the rapid preparation of several structurally complex polyhydroxy indolizidine and pyrrolizidine alkaloids, including analogues of the glycosidase inhibitors hyacinthacine and steviamine. While several strategies could be exploited for

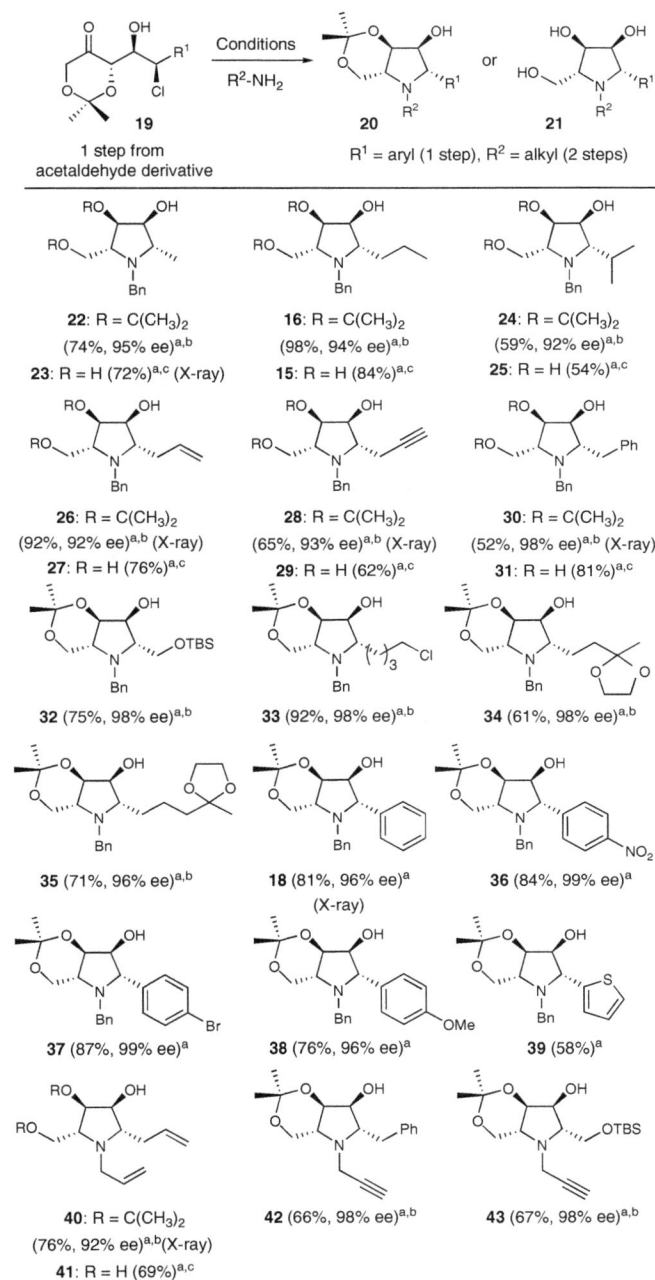

Figure 4 | Scope of iminocyclitol synthesis. (**a**) amine (2.5 equivalents), AcOH, 4-Å mol sieves, THF; then NaB(CN)H₃, room temperature; (**b**) NaHCO₃, PhMe, 105 °C; (**c**) MeOH, 120 °C, (microwave reactor).

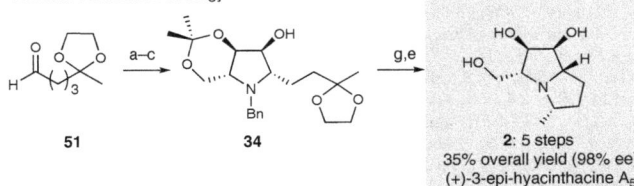

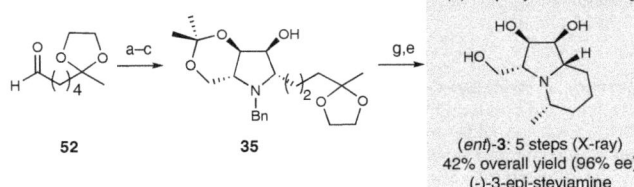

Figure 5 | Total syntheses of indolizidine and pyrrolizidine iminocyclitols. (**a**) NCS, dioxanone **8**, (S)-proline (80 mol%), CH₂Cl₂, room temperature (RT); (**b**) benzyl amine or allyl amine (2.5 equivalents), AcOH, 4-Å mol sieves, THF; then NaB(CN)H₃, RT; (**c**) NaHCO₃, PhMe, 105 °C; (**d**) Hoveyda–Grubbs cat (2nd generation, 5 mol%), PhMe, 60 °C, 2 h; (**e**) H₂ (90 bar), MeOH, 60 °C (H-Cube); (**f**) NaHCO₃, MeOH, 80 °C, 16 h; then PPTS; (**g**) PPTS (cat), H₂O, MeOH, 100 °C, 0.5 h (microwave reactor). NCS, N-chlorosuccinimide, PPTS, pyridinium p-toluenesulfonate.

the second annulation event, ready access to the N-allyl pyrrolidine **40**, alkyl chloride **33** and protected ketones **34** and **35** suggested annulation events involving ring closing metathesis[38,39], alkylation[24,40,41] or reductive amination[17,42]. For example, heating the dienylpyrrolidine **40** with the Hoveyda–Grubbs 2nd generation catalyst[43] in toluene provided the unsaturated indolizidine **45** in excellent overall yield from 4-pentenal (**44**). Alternatively, starting with 6-chloropentanal (**46**) or 5-chloropentanal (**48**), α-chlorination-DKR aldol reactions[19] followed by reductive amination and cyclization provided the chloroalkylpyrrolidine **33** and pyrrolizidine **49**, respectively. Conversion of **33** into the corresponding indolizidine **47** (ref. 44) required hydrogenolytic removal of the benzyl-

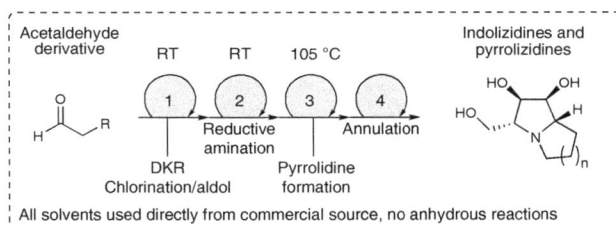

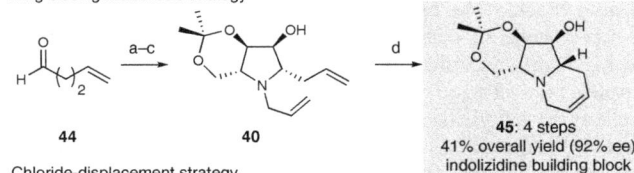

protecting group and brief treatment with base. Completion of the total synthesis of 7a-epi-hyacinthacine A₁ (**50**)[45,46] simply involved hydrogenolysis of **49** in acidic media.

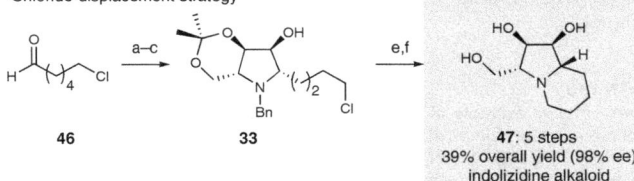

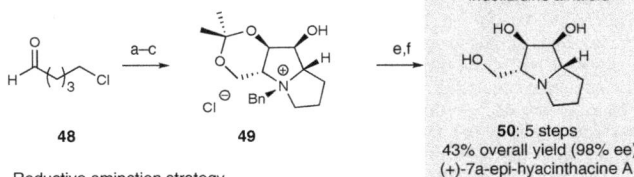

The reductive amination strategy was explored in short syntheses of the hyacinthacine and steviamine analogues **2** (ref. 17) and ent-**3** (ref. 18). In both cases, the ketone function in the readily available pyrrolidines **34** and **35** was unveiled in concert with hydrogenolytic cleavage of the N-benzyl group, and the resulting iminium species (not shown) was reduced in situ to afford the products depicted as single diastereomers. Importantly, each of the total syntheses depicted in Fig. 5 requires 5 steps or less, originates with inexpensive and readily available chemicals, and is completed in a matter of days, which compares well with the reported syntheses of these and related compounds (see for example, Fig. 1).

Discussion

In summary, a highly convergent synthesis of iminosugars has been developed that converts a wide range of acetaldehyde derivatives into polyhydroxypyrrolidines in two or three straightforward reactions and does not rely on carbohydrate building blocks. The application of this cost-effective process to the rapid synthesis of indolizidine and pyrrolizidine iminosugars also highlights its utility for the preparation of more structurally complex natural products and their analogues. Importantly, the excellent overall yields, diastereoselectivity and enantioselectivity, coupled with tunability of pharmacophoric features make this process well suited for chemical screening library and DOS campaigns.

Methods

Representative example of reductive amination/annulation sequence.
Synthesis of aminochlorohydrin 18 and iminocyclitol 4. To a stirred solution of 17 (ref. 19; 130 mg, 0.457 mmol) in THF (4.55 ml) was added $BnNH_2$ (125 µl, 1.15 mmol) and glacial acetic acid (27.0 µl, 0.457 mmol), and the resulting mixture was stirred at 20 °C for 1 h. $NaB(CN)H_3$ (72 mg, 1.15 mmol) was then added and the mixture was stirred for one additional hour. The reaction mixture was then diluted with CH_2Cl_2 to a concentration of 0.05 M and treated with water. The layers were separated and the organic layer was washed with brine, dried ($MgSO_4$) and concentrated under reduced pressure. Purification of the crude product by flash chromatography (pentane-EtOAc 8:2) afforded pyrrolidine 18 (126 mg, 81% yield) as a crystalline solid. mp = 108–111 °C (EtOH); R_f (pentane-EtOAc 6:4) 0.81; $[\alpha]_D^{20} = +11$ (c 0.70 in CHCl₃); infrared (neat): $v = 3444, 2988, 2874, 1454, 1381, 1210, 1048, 853, 753$ and $700\ cm^{-1}$; ¹H-nuclear magnetic resonance (¹H-NMR; 600 MHz, CDCl₃): $\delta = 7.53$ (d, J = 7.4 Hz, 2H), 7.38 (t, J = 7.5 Hz, 2H), 7.31–7.20 (m, 6H), 4.03 (d, J = 4.4 Hz, 1H), 3.90 (d, J = 12.9 Hz, 1H), 3.74 (s, 1H), 3.74 (dd, J = 4.5 Hz, J = 9.6 Hz, 1H), 3.47 (d, J = 12.8 Hz, 1H), 3.46 (dd, J = 10.5 Hz, 1H), 3.25 (dd, J = 4.1 Hz, J = 10.5 Hz, 1H), 2.89 (ddd, J = 4.1 Hz, J = 10.5 Hz, 1H), 2.31 (s, 1H), 1.42 (s, 3H) and 1.40 p.p.m. (s, 3H); ¹³C-NMR (151 MHz, CDCl₃): $\delta = 141.3, 139.2, 128.9, 128.5, 128.2, 127.4, 127.4, 127.3, 100.3, 76.9, 76.8, 74.1, 67.2, 59.6, 58.7, 29.2$ and 19.8 p.p.m.; HRMS ESI (high-resolution mass spectrometry electrospray ionization) m/z calcd (calculated) for $C_{21}H_{26}NO_3$ $[M+H]^+$ 340.1907, found 340.1886.

Preparation of the imino-C-nucleoside analogue 4. A solution of 18 (20 mg, 0.059 mmol) and pyridinium p-toluenesulfonate (15 mg, 0.059 mmol) in 1:1 H_2O/MeOH (4.0 ml) was added to a microwave vial. The vial was sealed in a CEM Discover LabMate microwave reactor and the resulting mixture was heated at 100 °C (as monitored by a vertically focused infrared temperature sensor) for 30 min. The resulting solution was concentrated under reduced pressure and the crude product was used in the next reaction without further purification. A solution of the crude iminocyclitol p-toluenesulfonate salt in MeOH (20 ml) was passed twice through an H-Cube continuous-flow reactor using a 30 mm 10% Pd/C cartridge. Conditions: temperature = 35 °C; flow rate = 0.8 ml min⁻¹; H_2 pressure = 40 bar. The resulting mixture was stirred with DOWEX 1X8-100 (HO⁻ form) for a further 30 min and the resin was removed by filtration. Concentration and purification of the crude product by flash chromatography on C_{18} silica gel (H_2O) afforded iminoribitol 4 (10 mg, 83% yield over 2 steps) as a colourless oil. $[\alpha]_D^{20} = -31$ (c 0.48 in MeOH); infrared (neat): $v = 3306, 2918, 1560, 1494, 1454, 1406, 1347, 1081, 951, 757$ and $699\ cm^{-1}$; ¹H-NMR (400 MHz, CD₃OD): $\delta = 7.45$-7.42 (m, 2H), 7.37–7.32 (m, 2H), 7.27 (ddt, J = 1.4 Hz, J = 6.4 Hz, J = 8.5 Hz, 1H), 4.01 (d, J = 7.2 Hz, 1H), 3.97 (dd, J = 4.7 Hz, J = 6.0 Hz, 1H), 3.86 (dd, J = 6.1 Hz, J = 7.2 Hz, 1H), 3.74 (d, J = 4.5 Hz, 2H) and 3.15 p.p.m. (q, J = 4.5 Hz, 1H); ¹³C-NMR (151 MHz, CD₃OD): $\delta = 142.6, 129.5, 128.5, 128.1, 79.2, 73.6, 68.1, 66.8$ and 63.2 p.p.m.; HRMS (ESI) m/z calcd for $C_{11}H_{15}NO_3$ $[M+H]^+$ 210.1125, found 210.1111.

References

1. Compain, P. & Martin, O. *Iminosugars from Synthesis to Therapeutic Applications* (Wiley, 2007).
2. Lillelund, V. H., Jensen, H. H., Liang, X. & Bols, M. Recent developments of transition-state analogue glycosidase inhibitors of non-natural product origin. *Chem. Rev.* **102**, 515–553 (2002).
3. Asano, N. Naturally occurring iminosugars and related compounds: structure, distribution, and Biological activity. *Curr. Top. Med. Chem.* **3**, 471–484 (2003).
4. Asano, N. in *Glycoscience*. (eds Fraser-Reid, B., Tatsuta, K. & Thiem, J.) 1887–1911 (Springer-Verlag, 2008).
5. Horenstein, B. A., Zabinski, R. F. & Schramm, V. L. A new class of C-nucleosides. 1-(S)-aryl-1,4-dideoxy-1,4-imino-D-ribitols, transition state analogue inhibitors of nucleoside hydrolase. *Tetrahedron Lett.* **34**, 7213–7216 (1993).
6. Kicska, G. A. *et al.* Immucillin H, a powerful transition-state analog inhibitor of purine nucleoside phosphorylase, selectively inhibits human T lymphocytes. *Proc. Natl Acad. Sci. USA* **98**, 4593–4598 (2001).
7. Liu, J. S., Shikhman, A. R., Lotz, M. K. & Wong, C.-H. Hexosaminidase inhibitors as new drug candidates for the therapy of osteoarthritis. *Chem. Biol.* **8**, 701–711 (2001).
8. Liang, P.-H. *et al.* Novel five-membered iminocyclitol derivatives as selective and potent glycosidase inhibitors: new structures for antivirals and osteoarthritis. *ChemBioChem* **7**, 165–173 (2006).
9. Hong, Z., Liu, L., Sugiyama, M., Fu, Y. & Wong, C.-H. Concise synthesis of iminocyclitols via petasis-type aminocyclization. *J. Am. Chem. Soc.* **131**, 8352–8353 (2009).
10. Compain, P., Chagnault, V. & Martin, O. R. Tactics and strategies for the synthesis of iminosugar C-glycosides: a review. *Tetrahedron: Asymm.* **20**, 672–711 (2009).
11. Stocker, B. L., Dangerfield, E. M., Win-Mason, A. L., Haslett, G. W. & Timmer, M. S. M. Recent developments in the synthesis of pyrrolidine-containing iminosugars. *Eur. J. Org. Chem.* **9**, 1615–1637 (2010).
12. Yokoyama, M. & Momotake, A. Synthesis and biological activity of azanucleosides. *Synthesis* **9**, 1541–1554 (1999).
13. Merino, P., Tejero, T. & Delso, I. Current developments in the synthesis and biological activity of aza-C-nucleosides: immucillins and related compounds. *Curr. Med. Chem.* **15**, 954–967 (2008).
14. Evans, G. B., Furneaux, R. H., Hausler, H., Larsen, J. S. & Tyler, P. C. Imino-C-nucleoside synthesis: heteroaryl lithium carbanion additions to a carbohydrate cyclic imine and nitrone. *J. Org. Chem.* **69**, 2217–2220 (2004).
15. Evans, G. B., Furneaux, R. H., Gainsford, G. J., Schramm, V. L. & Tyler, P. C. Synthesis of transition state analogue inhibitors for purine nucleoside phosphorylase and N-riboside hydrolases. *Tetrahedron* **56**, 3053–3062 (2000).
16. Evans, G. B. *et al.* Addition of lithiated 9-deazapurine derivatives to a carbohydrate cyclic imine: convergent synthesis of the aza-C-nucleoside immucillins. *J. Org. Chem.* **66**, 5723–5730 (2001).
17. Izquierdo, I., Plaza, M. T., Tamayo, J. A., Rodríguez, M. & Martos, A. Polyhydroxylated pyrrolizidines. Part 8: enantiospecific synthesis of looking-glass analogues of hyacinthacine A₅ from DADP. *Tetrahedron* **62**, 6006–6011 (2006).
18. Ansari, A. A. & Vankar, Y. D. Synthesis of dihydroxymethyl dihydroxypyrrolidines and steviamine analogues from C-2 formyl glycals. *J. Org. Chem.* **78**, 9383–9395 (2013).
19. Bergeron-Brlek, M., Teoh, T. & Britton, R. A tandem organocatalytic α-chlorination-aldol reaction that proceeds with dynamic kinetic resolution: a powerful tool for carbohydrate synthesis. *Org. Lett.* **15**, 3554–3557 (2013).
20. Halland, N., Braunton, A., Bachmann, S., Marigo, M. & Jørgensen, K. A. Direct organocatalytic asymmetric α-chlorination of aldehydes. *J. Am. Chem. Soc.* **126**, 4790–4791 (2004).
21. Britton, R. & Kang, B. α-Haloaldehydes: versatile building blocks for natural product synthesis. *Nat. Prod. Rep.* **30**, 227–236 (2013).
22. Draper, J. & Britton, R. A concise and stereoselective synthesis of hydroxypyrrolidines: rapid synthesis of (+)-preussin. *Org. Lett.* **12**, 4034–4037 (2010).
23. Dhand, V., Draper, J. A., Moore, J. & Britton, R. A short, organocatalytic formal synthesis of (-)-swainsonine and related alkaloids. *Org. Lett.* **15**, 1914–1917 (2013).
24. Dhand, V., Chang, S. & Britton, R. Total synthesis of the cytotoxic anhydrophytosphingosine pachastrissamine (jaspine B). *J. Org. Chem.* **78**, 8208–8213 (2013).
25. Crabtree, E. V. *et al.* Synthesis of the enantiomers of XYLNAc and LYXNAc: comparison of β-N-atecylhexosaminidase inhibition by the 8 stereoisomers of 2-N-acetylamino-1,2,4-trideoxy-1,4-iminopentinols. *Org. Biomol. Chem.* **12**, 3932–3943 (2014).
26. Saotome, C., Wong, C.-H. & Kanie, O. Combinatorial library of five-membered iminocyclitol and the inhibitory activities against glycol-enzymes. *Chem. Biol.* **8**, 1061–1070 (2001).
27. Enders, D., Paleček, J. & Grondal, C. A direct organocatalytic entry to sphingoids: asymmetric synthesis of D-arabino- and L-ribo-phyto sphingosine. *Chem. Commun.* **6**, 655–657 (2006).
28. Brandi, A., Cardona, F., Cicchi, S., Cordero, F. M. & Goti, A. Stereocontrolled cyclic nitrone cycloaddition strategy for the synthesis of pyrrolizidine and indolizidine alkaloids. *Chem. Eur. J.* **15**, 7808–7821 (2009).
29. Medjahdi, M., González-Gómez, J., Foubelo, F. & Yus, M. Stereoselective synthesis of azetidines and pyrrolidines from N-tert-butylsulfonyl(2-aminoalkyl)oxiranes. *J. Org. Chem.* **74**, 7859–7865 (2009).
30. Davis, F. A., Yang, B. & Deng, J. Asymmetric synthesis of cis-5-tert-butylproline with metal carbenoid NH insertion. *J. Org. Chem.* **68**, 5147–5152 (2003).

31. Dangerfield, E. M., Timmer, M. S. M. & Stocker, B. L. Total synthesis without protecting groups: pyrrolidines and cyclic carbamates. *Org. Lett.* **11**, 535–538 (2009).

32. Dekeukeleire, S., D'hooghe, M., Törnroos, K. W. & De Kimpe, N. Stereoselective synthesis of chiral 4-(1-chloroalkyl)-β-lactams starting from amino acids and their transformation into functionalized chiral azetidines and pyrrolidines. *J. Org. Chem.* **75**, 5934–5940 (2010).

33. Lauritsen, A. & Madsen, R. Synthesis of naturally occurring iminosugars from d-fructose by the use of a zinc-mediated fragmentation reaction. *Org. Biomol. Chem.* **4**, 2898–2905 (2005).

34. Lovering, F., Bikker, J. & Humblet, C. Escapade from flatland: increasing saturation as an approach to improving clinical success. *J. Med. Chem.* **52**, 6752–6756 (2009).

35. Walters, W. P. Going further than Lipinski's rule in drug design. *Exper. Opin. Drug. Discov.* **7**, 99–107 (2012).

36. Feher, M. & Schmidt, J. M. Property distributions: differences between drugs, natural products, and molecules from combinatorial chemistry. *J. Chem. Inf. Comput. Sci.* **43**, 218–227 (2003).

37. Pascolutti, M. & Quinn, R. J. Natural products as lead structures: chemical transformations to create lead-like libraries. *Drug Discov. Today* **19**, 215–221 (2014).

38. Verhelst, S. H. L. *et al.* A Short route toward chiral, polyhydroxylated indolizidines and quinolizidines. *J. Org. Chem.* **68**, 9598–9603 (2003).

39. Jiangseubchatveera, N. *et al.* Concise synthesis of (–)-steviamine and analogues and their glycosidase inhibitory activities. *Org. Biomol. Chem.* **11**, 3826–3833 (2013).

40. Parmeggiani, C., Cardona, F., Giusti, L., Reissig, H.-U. & Goti, A. Stereocomplementary routes to hydroxylated nitrogen heterocycles: total syntheses of casuarine, australine, and 7-*epi*-australine. *Chem. Eur. J.* **19**, 10595–10604 (2013).

41. Wardrop, D. J. & Bowen, E. G. Nitrenium ion-mediated alkene bis-cyclofunctionalization: total synthesis of (–)-swainsonine. *Org. Lett.* **13**, 2376–2379 (2011).

42. Randl, S. & Blechert, S. Concise enantioselective synthesis of 3,5-dialkyl-substituted indolizidine alkaloids via sequential cross-metathesis-double-reductive cyclization. *J. Org. Chem.* **68**, 8879–8882 (2003).

43. Garber, S. B., Kingsbury, J. S., Gray, B. L. & Hoveyda, A. H. Efficient and recyclable monomeric and dendritic Ru-based metathesis catalysts. *J. Am. Chem. Soc.* **122**, 8168–8179 (2000).

44. Gómez, L. *et al.* Chemoenzymatic synthesis, structural study and biological activity of novel indolizidine and quinolizidine iminocyclitols. *Org. Biomol. Chem.* **10**, 6309–6321 (2012).

45. Izquierdo, I., Plaza, M. T., Tamayo, J. A., Franco, F. & Sánchez-Cantalejo, F. Total synthesis of natural (+)-hyacinthacine A$_6$ and non-natural (+)-7a-*epi*-hyacinthecine A$_1$ and (+)-5,7a-di*epi*-hyacinthacine A$_6$. *Tetrahedron* **66**, 3788–3794 (2010).

46. Brock, E. A., Davies, S. G., Lee, J. A., Roberts, P. M. & Thomson, J. E. Asymmetric synthesis of polyhydroxylated pyrrolizidines via transannular iodoamination with concomitant N-debenzylation. *Org. Lett.* **13**, 1594–1597 (2011).

Acknowledgements

This work was supported by an NSERC Discovery Grant to R.B., a Michael Smith Foundation for Health Research Career Investigator Award to R.B., a Multi-Investigator Research Initiative grant (funded by Brain Canada, Genome BC, Michael Smith Foundation for Health Research; and the Pacific Alzheimer Research Foundation), an NSERC PGSD for M.B.-B.; and a NSERC USRA for M.M.

Author contributions

R.B. and M.B.-B. conceived the experiments and R.B. prepared the manuscript. M.M. assisted with the experiments.

Additional information

Accession codes: The X-ray crystallographic coordinates for structures reported in this study have been deposited at the Cambridge Crystallographic Data Centre (CCDC), under deposition numbers 1038918-1038924. These data can be obtained free of charge from CCDC via www.ccdc.cam.ac.uk/data_request/cif.

Competing financial interests: The authors declare no competing financial interests.

3

Tetrasaccharide iteration synthesis of a heparin-like dodecasaccharide and radiolabelling for *in vivo* tissue distribution studies

Steen U. Hansen[1],*, Gavin J. Miller[1],*, Claire Cole[2], Graham Rushton[2], Egle Avizienyte[2], Gordon C. Jayson[2] & John M. Gardiner[1]

Heparin-like oligosaccharides mediate numerous important biological interactions, of which many are implicated in various diseases. Synthetic improvements are central to the development of such oligosaccharides as therapeutics and, in addition, there are no methods to elucidate the pharmacokinetics of structurally defined heparin-like oligosaccharides. Here we report an efficient two-cycle [4 + 4 + 4] tetrasaccharide-iteration-based approach for rapid chemical synthesis of a structurally defined heparin-related dodecasaccharide, combined with the incorporation of a latent aldehyde tag, unmasked in the final step of chemical synthesis, providing a generic end group for labelling/conjugation. We exploit this latent aldehyde tag for ^{3}H radiolabelling to provide the first example of this kind of agent for monitoring *in vivo* tissue distribution and *in vivo* stability of a biologically active, structurally defined heparin related dodecasaccharide. Such studies are critical for the development of related saccharide therapeutics, and the data here establish that a biologically active, synthetic, heparin-like dodecasaccharide provides good organ distribution, and serum lifetimes relevant to developing future oligosaccharide therapeutics.

[1] Faculty of EPS, School of Chemistry, Manchester Institute of Biotechnology, The University of Manchester, 131 Princess Street, Manchester M1 7DN, UK. [2] School of Cancer and Enabling Sciences, The University of Manchester, Wilmslow Road, Manchester M20 4BX, UK. * These authors contributed equally to this work. Correspondence and requests for materials should be addressed to J.M.G. (email: gardiner@manchester.ac.uk).

Heparin and heparan sulphate (H/HS) are ubiquitous linear polysulphated oligosaccharides of the glycosaminoglycan (GAG) family, comprising a repeating disaccharide unit. Because of its structural heterogeneity, H/HS is crucially involved in regulating a myriad of cell signalling pathways through modulation of interactions between cytokines and their receptors. This is typified through its involvement in the mediation of fibroblast growth factor (FGF)-regulated cell phenotypes, such as proliferation, adhesion, motility and angiogenesis[1–7].

Although methods for the isolation of natural H/HS samples from biochemical degradation processes are well-established[8,9], synthetic access to structurally defined H/HS mimetics has also received very significant attention[10–36]. Synthetic access is essential to provide structurally defined H/HS oligosaccharide sequences to interrogate the chemical biology of H/HS-mediated processes, a better understanding of which also offers the potential to aid development of new disease treatments[37–41]. The potential development of such oligosaccharides as therapeutics is also dependent on developing tools to determine the pharmacokinetics, distribution and organ availability of these synthetic species. To date, the limitations of synthetic access to suitable tools has precluded such developments for bioactive lead oligosaccharide structures. This presents the need to develop an efficient procedure for the synthesis of longer bioactive heparin-like oligosaccharides, which also provide efficient access to derivatization/conjugation of structurally defined, biologically significant synthetic H/HS sequences[42–45].

Our previous in vitro and in vivo anti-angiogenic assessments of size-fractionated digests[46–51] and subsequent evaluation of a matrix of structurally defined synthetic oligosaccharides[52] indicated that longer [GlcNS-IdoA2S]-containing species were more effective inhibitors of FGF2, and identified the methyl glycoside analogue of dodecasaccharide 1 ([GlcNS-IdoA2S]$_6$-OMe) as the optimum lead FGF2 and vascular endothelial growth factor antagonist[52] (ex vivo evaluation of the synthetic dodecasaccharide [GlcNS-IdoA2S]$_6$-OMe confirmed that at biologically active concentrations inhibiting FGF signalling, there was no statistically significant impact on anticoagulation, an important feature required for potential development of therapeutic synthetic saccharides of this type).

Here we report a powerful addition to the field of synthetic heparanoid chemistry, which demonstrates an efficient chemical synthesis of this structurally defined [GlcNS-IdoA2S]$_6$ heparin-like lead dodecasaccharide 1, bearing a terminal latent aldehyde tag (LAT), in just two iterative cycles and four steps from a precursor tetrasaccharide. Concomitant LAT release in a final-step modification of the oligosaccharide is applied to ^{3}H radiolabelling of dodecasaccharide 1 with minimal structural impact. This demonstrates the viability of the approach for rapid, iterative synthetic access to large oligosaccharides on useful scales, which are suitable for biological conjugations and labelling. The tritium radiolabelled analogue 1, which provides a new tool to determine the pharmacokinetics of the synthetic oligosaccharide and establish the organ distribution and in vivo lifetime of the lead dodecasaccharide 1, critical factors for the potential development of HS oligosaccharide therapeutics.

Results

Strategy and end labelling. The end modification of oligosaccharides (via ring opening of the terminal acetal unit, for example, for attaching fluorophores) is an established method for labelling native heparin and related GAGs to facilitate their separation or analysis[53,54]. A number of examples have also employed amide derivatization of the uronic carboxylates to introduce fluorescent or spin labels, or to attach conjugates[55,56].

There are also a range of uses of modified O-glycosides recently employed for conjugation, surface and nanoparticle/dendrimer attachments[42–45], including applications of click chemistry, in particular the Huisgen reaction.

However, an alternative approach was needed to ensure compatibility with the deprotection/labelling conditions during synthesis and introducing minimal change to the polarity/functional groups of the oligosaccharide. Thus, a 1,2-diol moiety at the reducing end was incorporated as an LAT. Having an additional O4-sulphate at the non-reducing end of the deprotected dodecasaccharide would allow complete selectivity in a final-stage periodate-mediated cleavage of the LAT to liberate a reactive aldehyde tag (RAT) directly on the final oligosaccharide, thus allowing facile reductive labelling or facilitating other conjugations. Our approach was to develop this LAT incorporation concurrently with the aforementioned tetrasaccharide iteration strategy (Fig. 1).

Synthesis of tetrasaccharide building blocks. The synthetic strategy envisaged using one precursor disaccharide building block, 2, to provide a single tetrasaccharide unit, 7, which would function both as an iterative donor (as its O4-trichloroacetyl derivative 8) and as an immediate precursor to an LAT-bearing tetrasaccharide, serving as the initial acceptor tetrasaccharide.

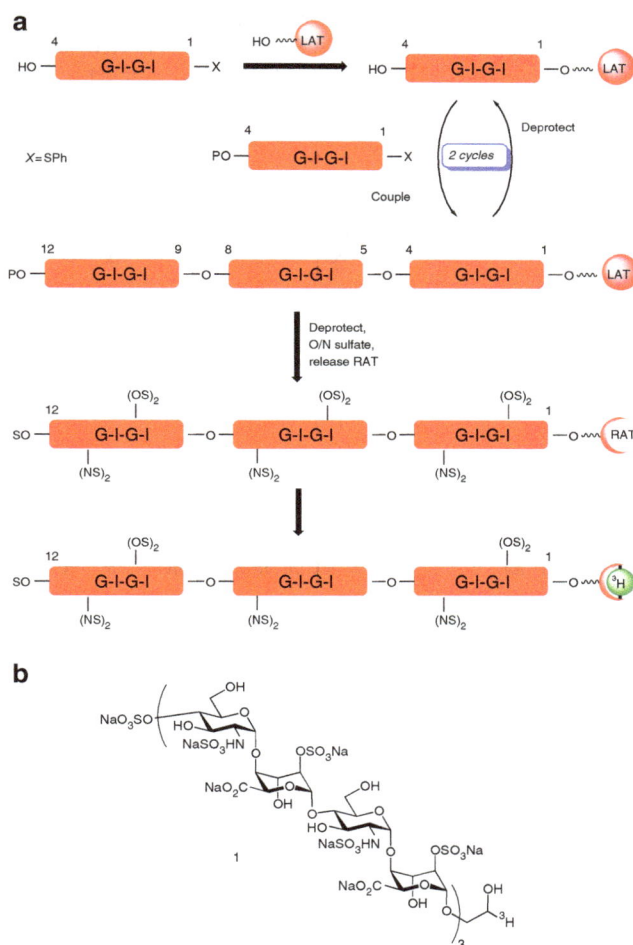

Figure 1 | Strategy for synthesis of end-labelled dodecassacharide.
(**a**) Iterative [4 + 4 + 4] oligosaccharide synthesis strategy with final step RAT release and labelling. G, Glucosamine unit; I, iduronate unit; P, trichloroacetyl; S, SO$_3$Na; LAT, latent aldehyde tag; RAT, reactive aldehyde tag. (**b**) Structure of radiolabelled dodecasaccharide.

Disaccharide **2** was prepared as reported previously, exploiting our scalable iduronate thioglycoside acceptor capabilities for constructing such reagents[57,58], and is a reverse of the common IdoA-GlcN disaccharide repeat unit seen in several previous heparin-related syntheses[10-36]. Disaccharide **2** was divergently elaborated into trichloroacetimidate donor **4** (see Supplementary Figs S5–S12) via free sugar disaccharide **3** (see Supplementary Figs S1–S4) and acceptor **5**, with these two building blocks then efficiently coupled to afford tetrasaccharide **6** (Fig. 2; see Supplementary Figs S13–S17). Deprotection at the non-reducing end terminus of **6** then provided the required tetrasaccharide **7** (see Supplementary Figs S18–S22), which was also protected as its O4-TCA derivative **8** (see Supplementary Figs S23–S31), thereby providing two potential tetrasaccharide donor modules (**6** and **8**), differing only in their non-reducing terminal O4-protecting group.

Synthesis of tetrasaccharide **6** was similarly efficient whether thioglycoside acceptor α-**5** or β-**5** was employed, providing access to either tetrasaccharide α-**7** or β-**7**, respectively, both of which can function in the subsequent iterative homologations to effect the same α-selective glycosylations of the desired oligosaccharide acceptor. These tetrasaccharides can readily be accessed on hundreds of milligram to multigram scale.

Notably, and further enhancing the overall synthetic efficiency, although **7** has both acceptor (4-OH) and donor (1-SPh) functionality, this material could be directly glycosylated at the reducing terminus without the need for protection at O4. The installation of the required LAT was thus effected using a dibenzylated glycerol unit, designed for its ultimate deprotection to the required diol concomitant with the penultimate debenzylation of the protected heparin oligosaccharide. Hence, **7** was glycosylated with (S)-2,3-dibenzyloxy propanol affording the reducing end-modified tetrasaccharide acceptor **9** (see Supplementary Figs S32–S36) directly, with the non-reducing terminus already in place as an acceptor for the first tetrasaccharide homologation (Fig. 3).

Coupling of acceptor **9** and tetrasaccharide donors **6** or **8**, hence, generated the octasaccharides **10** (see Supplementary Figs S37–S39) and **11** (see Supplementary Figs S40–S44), respectively, with complete α-anomeric selectivity. This now further establishes that the iduronate donor-terminated tetrasaccharides can function as efficient oligosaccharide homologation building blocks using longer acceptors (a previous GlcN-GlcA-GlcN-IdoA tetrasaccharide had been shown to be effective as a donor for monosaccharide acceptors)[24] and compliments such a capability exploited using GlcN donor systems[24,44]. This also thereby underpins a capability to now access other long [GlcN-IdoA]n-based sequences using such an accelerated iterative strategy.

Synthesis of oligosaccharide via [4 + 4 + 4] two-cycle iteration. During the deprotection of O4 of octasaccharide **10**, it was found that the ceric ammonium nitrate mediated p-methoxybenzyl removal gave a mixture of products, although the TCA group of analogue **11** could be removed in excellent yield using novel mild conditions. Combined with the higher glycosylation yields obtained, this led to selection of the O4-TCA tetrasaccharide **8** for further iterations. Deprotection of octasaccharide **11** provided

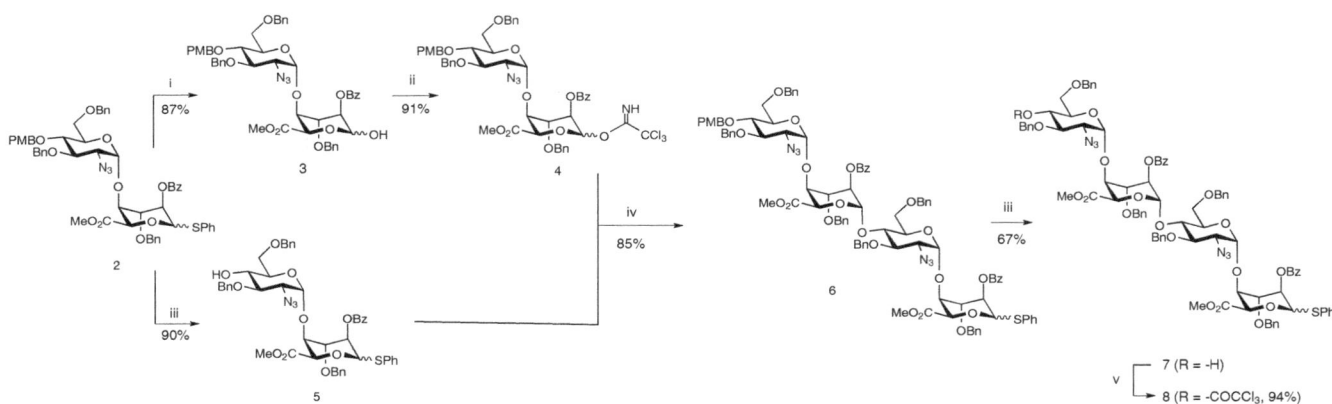

Figure 2 | Synthesis of core tetrasaccharide donor/acceptor modules. (i) NBS, acetone. (ii) CCl3CN, DBU, DCM. (iii) CAN, CH3CN/H2O. (iv) TMSOTf, DCM. (v) CCl3COCl, pyridine, DCM.

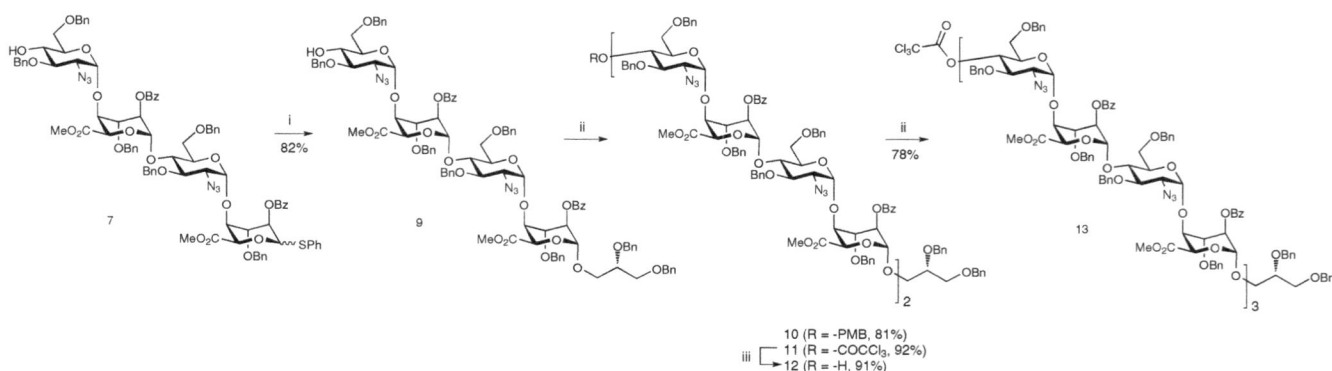

Figure 3 | Iterative [4 + 4 + 4] dodecasaccharide synthesis. (i) (S)-2,3-bis(benzyloxy)propanol, NIS, AgOTf (cat.), DCM. (ii) **6** or **8**, NIS, AgOTf (cat.), DCM. (iii) MeOH/pyridine (5:2).

acceptor octasaccharide **12** (see Supplementary Figs S45–S49) as a substrate, enabling a second cycle of iterative coupling with donor module **8**, providing thereby protected dodecasaccharide **13** (see Supplementary Figs S50–S54) and completing the efficient and rapid two-cycle iteration. The overall four-step yield from tetrasaccharide **7** to protected dodecasaccharide **13** was 54%, yielding around 300 mg of this oligosaccharide, a significant scale for such rapid dodecasaccharide assembly.

From protected dodecasaccharide **13**, concurrent saponification, *O*-sulphation, debenzylation/azide reduction and finally *N*-sulphation provided the fully deprotected and regiospecifically sulphated dodecasaccharide **14** (see Supplementary Figs S59–S64) bearing the free 1,2-diol LAT unit at the reducing terminus (Fig. 4).

Nuclear magnetic resonance provides unambiguous definition of the complete *N*-sulphation, evidenced by the clear difference in shift of the H-2 protons on converting the 2-amino to 2-NS functionality (Fig. 5). Differentiation of the NS of the non-reducing terminal glucosamine 2-NS is evident (the only ring with O4-S) and confirmed by clear correlation spectroscopy correlations (see Supplementary Fig. S60). The clear resolution of signals for the reducing terminal iduronate is clear, and on oxidative cleavage the spectrum for the RAT-terminated dodecasaccharide shows a clear set of two doublets (1.3:1) for the RAT methylene. These are not mutually coupled and the non-equivalent integration would also be consistent with these arising from acetal formation, transiently retaining the LAT aldehyde in a seven-membered ring hemiacetal. This is also consistent with changes in the shifts of H5 and H2 of the reducing terminal iduronate. In addition, the H-5 of ring A is well separated and the small coupling constant for those protons, also evident for the other overlapping H5 protons, shows that these long sulphated oligosaccharides do sit largely in the ido $^1C_4$ conformation.

Oxidative cleavage was effected in near-quantitative yield with sodium periodate, unveiling the target-reducing end aldehyde in the form of reactive conjugate, **15** (see Supplementary Figs S65–S67).

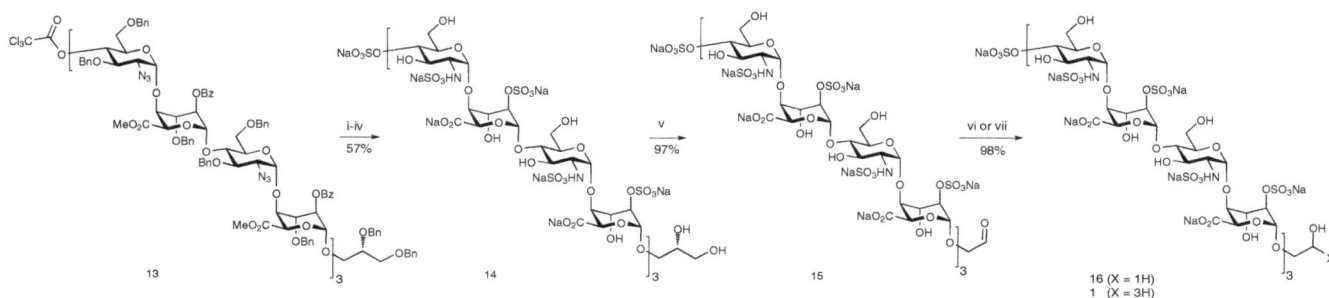

Figure 4 | Dodecasaccharide deprotections and end labelling. (i) LiOH, tetrahydrofuran (THF)/MeOH/H$_2$O, 74%. (ii) Py.SO$_3$ complex, pyridine, 80%. (iii) H$_2$, Pd(OH)$_2$/C, MeOH/THF/H$_2$O 2:1:1, 96%. (iv) Py.SO$_3$ complex, NaHCO$_3$, H$_2$O, 100%. (v) NaIO$_4$, H$_2$O. (vi) NaBH$_4$, H$_2$O. (vii) NaB^{3}H$_4$, H$_2$O.

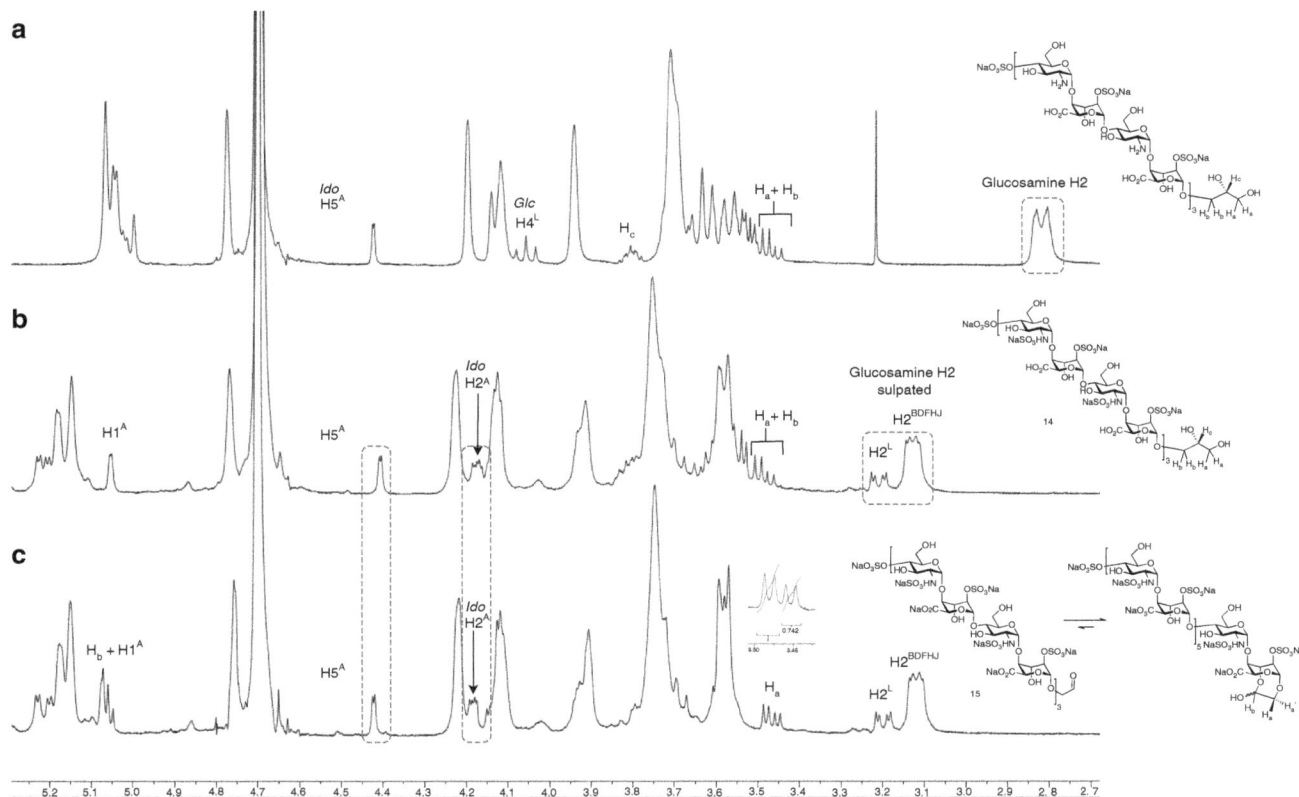

Figure 5 | Nuclear magnetic resonance confirmation of dodecasaccharide *N*-sulphation and comparisons of diol LAT and oxidatively cleave RAT.
(**a**) Intermediate amino containing dodecasaccharide. (**b**) *N*-sulphated dodecasaccharide. (**c**) Oxidatively cleaved RAT-terminated oligosaccharide.

To introduce the tritium label, **15** was then treated with NaB^{3}H$_4$ under basic conditions at 45 °C (following cold-label method evaluations on a disaccharide model and the unlabelled reduction of **15** to **16** (see Supplementary Figs S68–S70)).

After ensuring the reaction was complete by addition of excess NaBH$_4$ and quenching, the sample was desalted on Sephadex G-25 to remove excess reducing agent. Radiolabelled **1** was then further purified by size-exclusion chromatography (Fig. 6) and

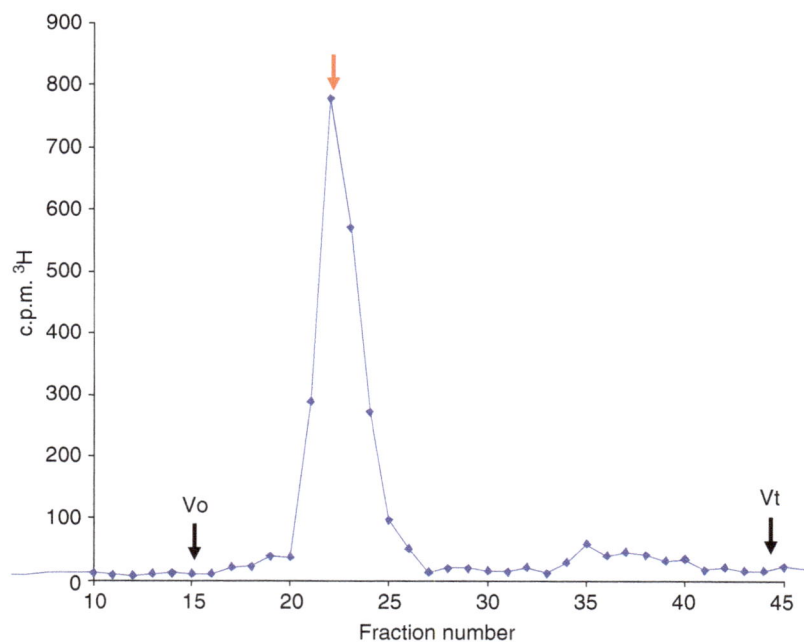

Figure 6 | HPLC size-exclusion chromatogram of 1 on Superdex. To confirm the oligomer size of ^{3}H-**1** HPLC size-exclusion chromatography on Superdex 75 indicated the ^{3}H-**1** elutes (red arrow) at position identical to de-6-O-sulphated dodecasaccharide heparin standard. Vo, excluded volume; Vt, total column volume.

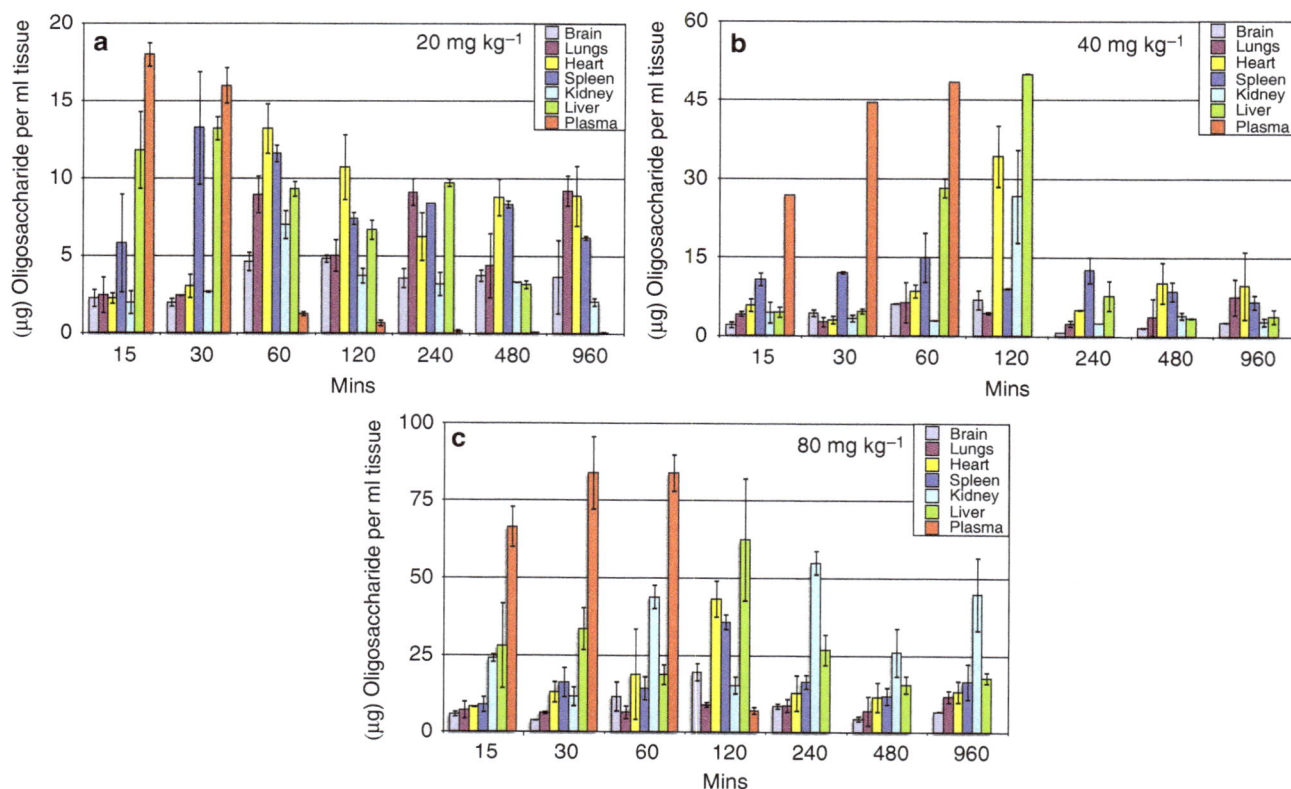

Figure 7 | Tissue localisation of 1. Mice (two) were injected with 20 (**a**), 40 (**b**) or 80 mg kg^{-1} (**c**) of **1**. Tissue quantities are presolublization. Error bars represent the s.e.m. of c.p.m. converted to oligo weight using specific activity.

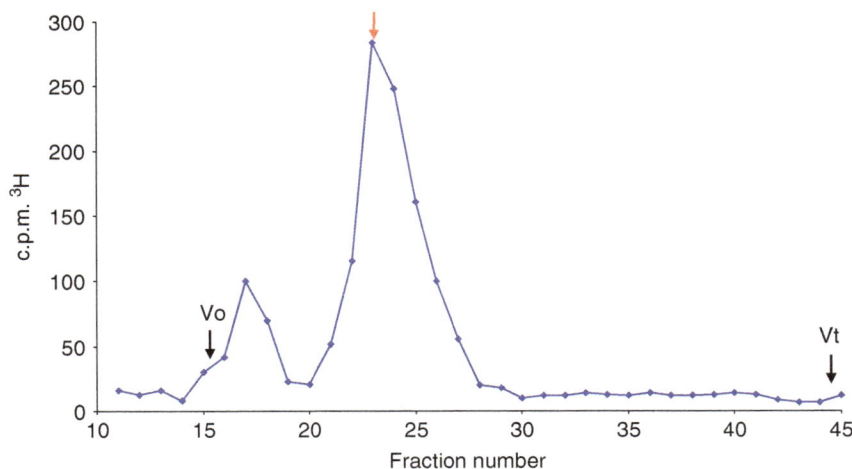

Figure 8 | HPLC SEC of 1 injected s.c. into mice and then extracted and purified from kidneys 4 h after injection. Radiolabelled oligosaccharide **1** was injected s.c. into mice and then extracted and purified from kidneys 4 h after injection (see Methods). Radiolabelled oligosaccharide **1** was subjected to HPLC chromatography on a Superdex 75 size-exclusion column. Red arrow shows elution of ^{3}H-**1** (see Fig. 5). Vo, excluded volume; Vt, total column volume.

was eluted from the column in good accordance with an established de-6-*O*-sulphated dodecasaccharide heparin standard. The specific activity of **1** was determined to be 5.5×10^6 c.p.m. mg^{-1} of oligosaccharide, suitable for the required *in vivo* evaluations.

Applications of radiolabelled heparin dodecasaccharide *1*. Radiolabelled heparin-mimetic **1** was thus employed to determine its *in vivo* clearance and tissue distribution in mice (the biological efficacy of the OMe analogue of which we had previously established *in vitro*)[52].

The mice were dosed subcutaneously (s.c.) with 20, 40 and 80 mg kg^{-1} of oligosaccharide spiked with 140,000 c.p.m. of ^{3}H-12-mer **1** as a radiotracer. Tissue concentrations were determined from the level of radiolabelled oligosaccharide in tissue samples of known mass during a 16-h period (Fig. 7). A maximum plasma concentration of 18 µg ml^{-1} was observed 15 min after dosing mice with 20 mg kg^{-1} of oligosaccharide (Fig. 6a). When dosed with 40 or 80 mg kg^{-1}, maximum plasma concentrations of 44.8 and 84.0 µg ml^{-1}, respectively, were observed after 60 min (Fig. 6b,c). Critically, these data demonstrate that the plasma concentration of oligosaccharide *in vivo* was sufficient to inhibit the biological activity of FGF2 based on *in vitro* data[52].

All tissues, except lungs, showed a time-dependent accumulation of **1** at all doses, and the maximum concentrations increased with a higher initial dose (Fig. 6). The highest concentration of **1** was detected in tissues when mice were treated with 80 mg kg^{-1}. In addition, all tissues, except the liver, attained maximal levels of **1** by 120 min. The tissue distribution data described here show that at 40 and 80 mg kg^{-1}, biologically active concentrations[52] were achieved in the liver, lungs and spleen within a 2-h period. The half-life of oligosaccharides in mice was estimated to be ~2 h. As murine clearance is so rapid, this result is particularly encouraging for the development of oligosaccharide therapeutics.

From the results shown in Fig. 6, there is good evidence for sustained plasma concentrations of **1** up to around 1 h at the two higher dose levels and that the oligosaccharide is well retained in the plasma at these concentrations. At lower doses, there is a more even distribution among the examined tissues, suggesting that higher doses would be needed to sustain sufficient oligosaccharide concentration in plasma.

To assess the metabolic stability of **1** *in vivo*, we extracted and purified ^{3}H-12-mer **1** from mouse kidney after a 4-h treatment, to determine the extent of any degradation or metabolism. The majority of the material eluted in a single peak of 3,500 Da, which corresponds to a mass of dodecasaccharide **1** (Fig. 8).

Discussion
This [4 + 4 + 4] iterative oligosaccharide approach thus provides an efficient two-cycle synthesis of a structurally defined HS dodecasaccharide, illustrating that iduronate donor tetrasaccharides function as effective and selective glycosyl donors with extended saccharide acceptors. The reduction here in the number of synthetic steps taken to assemble these longer heparanoids significantly enhances their accessibility, and the inclusion of the end label via glycosylation (avoiding O4 protection) to directly afford an end-tagged tetrasaccharide acceptor also adds to the abbreviation of the synthetic route. Notably, homologation here using 4-mer and 8-mer acceptors with this longer donor is shown to perform with an efficiency that remains high, even for a [4 + 8] coupling. The efficiency of this tetrasaccharide-iteration-based synthetic route also facilities the viability of new opportunities for sequence versatility and applications to other diverse conjugation targets.

The synthesis and inclusion of the LAT described here offers a unique strategy for discrete end labelling of this heparin-like structure, such that the label will not interfere with the ligand-binding potential of the molecule, and the small structural change would be anticipated to minimize effects on pharmacokinetics. The end-terminal latent tag offers generality for incorporation into other heparanoids.

Utility of this end group for radiolabelling provides the first example of using a structurally defined heparin-like dodecasaccharide to quantify *in vivo* tissue distribution and metabolic stability. Conventional pharmacological development of heparin has relied on its anticoagulant properties that can be measured in patients using universally available tests of the clotting cascade. However, the lack of anticoagulant activity of structurally defined synthetic HS oligosaccharides, although important for non-anticoagulant drugs, also presents the problem of how to measure the pharmacokinetics and metabolism of such novel synthetic heparin-like oligosaccharides *in vivo*. Here we report for the first time a novel solution to this problem that should greatly assist the preclinical and clinical development of potential oligosaccharide therapeutics. In this dodecasaccharide case, this study has shown that the dodecasaccharide has good *in vivo* stability, and strongly indicates that oligosaccharide drugs of this type have a high prospect of effective dose distribution and stability on therapeutically valid timescales.

Methods

Synthesis of dodecasaccharide 12. Octasaccharide **11** (346 mg, 0.10 mmol) was dissolved in a mixture of MeOH/pyridine (5 ml per 2 ml) and heated to 50 °C for 4 h. The solvents were evaporated and coevaporated with toluene (2×20 ml). The crude product was purified using flash column chromatography (EtOAc/hexane 1:2 and 3:5). This yielded **12** (300 mg, 91%) as a white foam, along with recovered starting material (20 mg, 5%). R_f 0.10 (EtOAc/hexane 1:2). $[\alpha]_D^{20} = +9.8$ ($c = 0.32$, CH$_2$Cl$_2$). Mass spectrometry (MS) matrix-assisted laser desorption/ionization–time of flight: *m/z*: calcd for C$_{181}$H$_{184}$N$_{12}$NaO$_{47}$ $[M + \text{Na}]^+$: 3300.2; found: 3300.2. Elemental analysis calcd (%) for C$_{181}$H$_{184}$N$_{12}$O$_{47}$: C 66.29, H 5.66, N 5.13; found C 66.57, H 5.98, N 4.96 (see Supplementary Methods for further characterization data).

Synthesis of dodecasaccharide 13. Acceptor **12** (252 mg, 0.077 mmol) and donor **8** (175 mg, 0.100 mmol) were dissolved in dry dichloromethane (DCM) (4 ml) under N$_2$. Freshly activated 4 Å powdered molecular sieves (222 mg) were added and the solution cooled to 0 °C in an ice bath. After 10 min NIS (47 mg, 0.21 mmol) was added, and after another 10 min AgOTf (catalytic amount) was added. The suspension changed colour from pale yellow to deep red and was stirred for a further 35 min. The reaction was quenched into a separating funnel containing a mixture of DCM (50 ml), saturated aqueous NaHCO$_3$ (50 ml) and Na$_2$S$_2$O$_3$ (5 ml, 10% aqueous). After shaking until the iodine colour was removed, the suspension was filtered through a short pad of Celite washing with water and DCM. The layers were separated and the aqueous layer extracted with DCM (10 ml). The organic layers were combined, dried (MgSO$_4$) and the solvent removed *in vacuo*. The crude product was purified by silica gel flash column chromatography (EtOAc/hexane 7:13) to yield **13** (295 mg, 78%) as a white foam (recovered acceptor (37 mg, 15%)). $[\alpha]_D^{20} = +18.1$ ($c = 0.68$, CH$_2$Cl$_2$). MS matrix-assisted laser desorption/ionization–time of flight: *m/z*: calcd for C$_{265}$H$_{265}$Cl$_3$N$_{18}$NaO$_{70}$ $[M + \text{Na}]^+$: 4946.7; found: 4946.6. Elemental analysis calcd (%) for C$_{265}$H$_{265}$Cl$_3$N$_{18}$O$_{70}$: C 64.58, H 5.42, N 5.12; found C 63.91, H 5.41, N 5.06 (see Supplementary Methods for further characterization data).

Synthesis of dodecasaccharide sodium salt 14. *Saponifications.* Dodecasaccharide **13** (257 mg, 0.052 mmol) was dissolved in tetrahydrofuran (5 ml) and MeOH (1.5 ml), and then cooled to 0 °C in an ice bath. Then, LiOH.H$_2$O (55 mg, 1.30 mmol) dissolved in 1 ml water was added dropwise over 10 min. The solution was stirred for 5 h at 0 °C, and then at room temperature for another 19 h. The solution was then extracted with EtOAc (2×50 ml) and HCl (0.2 M, 40 ml), dried (MgSO$_4$), filtered and evaporated. The crude product was purified using flash column chromatography (DCM/MeOH 30:1). This yielded the carboxylic acid dodecasaccharide intermediate product **A** (174 mg, 74%) as a white solid. R_f 0.18 (DCM/MeOH 20:1), then used directly in the next step.

Sulphation of hydroxyls. The dodecasaccharide intermediate **A** (170 mg, 0.042 mmol) was dissolved in dry pyridine (5 ml), pyridine sulphur trioxide complex (140 mg, 0.88 mmol) added and then heated to 50 °C in an oil bath for 8 h. The solution was stirred at room temperature for another 12 h. The reaction was quenched with MeOH and then evaporated. The crude product was redissolved in MeOH/DCM (10 ml/5 ml), stirred with Amberlite IR-120 Na$^+$ resin (1.3 g) for 8 h, filtered, resin washed with MeOH (2×5 ml) and the filtrate evaporated. This residue was then purified using flash column chromatography (DCM/MeOH 20:1). This yielded 2-*O*-sulphated dodecasaccharide intermediate **B** (160 mg, 80%) as a white solid.

Hydrogenolysis of benzyls and azides. The IdoA2S benzylated 2-azido-containing dodecasaccharide intermediate **B** (132 mg, 0.027 mmol) was dissolved in a mixture of MeOH/tetrahydrofuran (4 ml/2 ml), and NaHCO$_3$ (14 mg, 0.165 mmol) dissolved in 2 ml of water was added, atmosphere exchanged for nitrogen and Pd(OH)$_2$/C (120 mg, 10–20%) added, and again flushed with nitrogen. The nitrogen balloon was replaced with a hydrogen balloon and atmosphere replaced with hydrogen. The reaction was heated to 40 °C in an oil bath for 48 h with vigorous stirring. The product mixture was filtered through Celite, washed with MeOH/water (3×3 ml) and water (3×3 ml). The combined filtrate was then evaporated to give dodecasaccharide amine intermediate **C** (78 mg, 96%) as a glassy solid (see Supplementary Methods).

Sulphation of amines. The dodecasaccharide amine (65 mg, 0.022 mmol) was dissolved in water (4 ml), NaHCO$_3$ (108 mg, 1.29 mmol) and pyridine sulphur trioxide complex (97 mg, 0.61 mmol) was added with vigorous stirring.

This procedure was repeated after 1.30, 3.30, 5.30, 17.30 and 19.30 h (NaHCO$_3$: 109, 121, 113, 110 and 110 mg; Py.SO$_3$: 92, 88, 111, 100 and 70 mg). After 24 h, the mixture was evaporated. The crude containing Na$_2$SO$_4$ salts was redissolved in minimum amount of water and purified by passage through a Sephadex G-25 column (40 ml) by eluting with water. The fractions containing oligosaccharide were pooled and evaporated to yield **14** (78 mg, 100%) as a glassy solid. High-resolution MS (Fourier transform MS): *m/z*: calcd for C$_{75}$H$_{111}$N$_6$Na$_4$O$_{102}$S$_{13}$ $[M-15\text{Na} + 8\text{H}]^{-7}$: 462.4234; found: 462.4244 (see Supplementary Methods for structures of intermediates **A**, **B** and **C**, and further characterization data for **B**, **C** and **14**, and Supplementary Figs 56–59 for spectra of **A**–**C**).

Synthesis of dodecasaccharide aldehyde 15. The dodecasaccharide **14** (61 mg, 0.017 mmol) was dissolved in water (1 ml) and sodium periodate (3.9 mg, 0.018 mmol) was added and stirred for 6 h. The crude was purified by passage through a Sephadex G-25 column by eluting with water. The fractions containing oligosaccharide were pooled and evaporated to yield 58 mg (97%) of **15** as a glassy solid (see Supplementary Methods for characterization data).

Synthesis of ^{3}H-labelled dodecasaccharide 1. Three micrograms of ^{3}H-labelled sodium borohydride (1 mCi) was reacted with 1.2 mg of aldehyde-bearing dodecasaccharide **15** in 20 µl of 50 mM NaOH in a sealed reinforced glass Reacti-Vial at 45 °C for 2 h. To ensure that all aldehyde was reduced, an excess of unlabelled 1 M sodium borohydride was then added and sample incubated for a further 2 h at 45 °C. Reaction was halted by the addition of 5 µl of 1 M sulphuric acid. Tritium-labelled oligosaccharide was then desalted on PD-10 (G-25) column that was pre-equilibrated with water and 0.5 ml fractions were collected. Labelled oligosaccharide **1**, which eluted in fractions 10–14, was collected and freeze-dried. To confirm the size of radiolabelled material, the ^{3}H-dodecasaccharide **1** was subjected to HPLC size-exclusion chromatography on an Agilent 1200 HPLC system. The sample was run on a Superdex 75 column (10 mm × 300 mm; GE Healthcare) in PBS at 0.5 ml min^{-1}. Aliquots from 0.5 ml fractions were taken, mixed with 2 ml of Hisafe scintillation fluid (Perkin-Elmer) and ^{3}H level was counted on a Wallac 1400 scintillation counter. An unlabelled de-6-*O*-sulphated heparin dodecasaccharide (Iduron), which is approximately the same size as synthetic dodecasaccharide **1**, was used to calibrate the column and was monitored at 232 nm by an in-line ultraviolet detector. Fractions containing ^{3}H-dodecasaccharide **1** were collected, desalted, freeze-dried and weighed. Specific activity was determined as 5.5×10^6 c.p.m. mg^{-1} of oligosaccharide.

Pharmacokinetic study of ^{3}H-labelled dodecasaccharide 1 in mice. ^{3}H-Labelled dodecasaccharide **1** was administered to SCID-*bg* female mice s.c. as a single dose at 20, 40 and 80 mg kg^{-1} and animals were culled at 0.25, 0.5, 1, 2, 4, 8 and 16 h after dosing. Two animals per each treatment group were used. At the time of culling, blood was collected by cardiac puncture. The brain, kidney, liver, spleen, heart and lungs were removed and their weight was measured. Samples were incubated overnight at 60 °C in 4 ml of Soluene 350 (Perkin-Elmer). Aliquots of 500 µl of the resultant tissue solution were taken for scintillation counting. Plasma was obtained by centrifuging mouse blood at 1,500 r.p.m. in a bench top Eppendorf microcentrifuge and collecting the supernatant. Plasma (100 µl) was added to 2 ml of scintillation fluid and ^{3}H levels were determined by scintillation counting. Concentration of oligosaccharide in plasma and tissues was derived from the specific activity of the radiolabel (see above).

Extraction and purification of ^{3}H-12-mer dodecasaccharide 1 from mouse kidney. To assess the stability of ^{3}H-dodecasaccharide **1** *in vivo*, one animal was dosed with **1** at 20 mg kg^{-1} for 4 h, and HS was extracted from mouse kidney *post mortem* using a routine method for HS extraction[59]. The kidneys were dissolved for 16 h at 60 °C in 4 M guanidine HCl/8 M urea/1% Triton in 50 mM Tris, pH 8.0. The extract was diluted 1:100 with water and applied to a 1 ml DEAE-Sephacel (Sigma) ion exchange column pre-equilibrated with PBS. The resin was then washed with 5 ml of 100 mM phosphate buffer with 0.25 M NaCl to remove hyaluronan and non-GAG material. The oligosaccharide was eluted with 1 M NaCl in phosphate buffer, concentrated to 1 ml and subjected to size-exclusion HPLC chromatography on a Superdex 75 column in PBS. Fractions (0.5 ml) were collected and counted.

References

1. Casu, B., Naggi, A. & Torri, G. Heparin-derived heparan sulfate mimics to modulate heparan sulfate-protein. *Matrix Biol.* **29**, 442–452 (2010).
2. Bishop, J., Schuksz, M. & Esko, J. D. Heparan sulphate proteoglycans fine-tune mammalian physiology. *Nature* **446**, 1030–1037 (2007).
3. Sasisekharan, R., Shriver, Z., Venkataraman, G. & Narayanasami, U. Roles of heparan sulphate glycosaminoglycans in cancer. *Nat. Rev. Cancer* **2**, 521–528 (2002).

4. Hung, K. W. *et al.* Solution structure of the ligand binding domain of the fibroblast growth factor receptor: role of heparin in the activation of the receptor. *Biochemistry* **44**, 15787–15798 (2005).

5. Olsen, S. K. *et al.* Insights into the molecular basis for fibroblast growth factor receptor autoinhibition and ligand-binding promiscuity. *PNAS* **101**, 935–941 (2004).

6. Seeberger, P. H. & Werz, B. Synthesis and medical applications of oligosaccharides. *Nature* **446**, 1046–1051 (2007).

7. Cole, C. & Jayson, G. C. Oligosaccharides as anti-angiogenic agents. *Expert Opin. Biol. Ther.* **8**, 351–362 (2008).

8. Ikeda, Y. *et al.* Synthesis and biological activities of a library of glycosaminoglycan mimetic oligosaccharides. *Biomaterials* **32**, 769–776 (2011).

9. Zhao, H. *et al.* Oligomannurarate sulfate, a novel heparanase inhibitor simultaneously targeting basic fibroblast growth factor, combats tumor angiogenesis and metastasis. *Cancer Res.* **66**, 8779–8787 (2006).

10. Lubineau, A., Lortat, J.-H., Gavard, O., Sarrazin, S. & Bonnaffé, D. Synthesis of tailor-made glycoconjugate mimetics of heparan sulfate that bind IFN-γ in the nanomolar range. *Chem. Eur. J.* **10**, 4265–4282 (2004).

11. Orgueira, H. A. *et al.* Modular synthesis of heparin oligosaccharides. *Chem. Eur. J.* **9**, 140–169 (2003).

12. de Paz, J. L., Noti, C. & Seeberger, P. H. Microarrays of synthetic heparin oligosaccharides. *J. Am. Chem. Soc.* **128**, 2766–2767 (2006).

13. de Paz, J. L. *et al.* The activation of fibroblast growth factors by heparin: synthesis, structure, and biological activity of heparin like oligosaccharides. *Chem. Bio. Chem.* **2**, 673–685 (2001).

14. Hamza, D. *et al.* First synthesis of heparan sulfate tetrasaccharides containing both *N*-acetylated and *N*-unsubstituted glucosamine—search for putative 10E4 epitopes. *Chem. Bio. Chem.* **7**, 1856–1858 (2006).

15. de Paz, J. L., Noti, C., Böhm, F., Werner, S. & Seeberger, P. H. Potentiation of fibroblast growth factor activity by synthetic heparin oligosaccharide glycodendrimers. *Chem. Biol.* **14**, 879–887 (2007).

16. Tatai, J. & Fügedi, P. Synthesis of the putative minimal FGF binding motif heparan sulfate trisaccharides by an orthogonal protecting group strategy. *Tetrahedron* **64**, 9865–9873 (2008).

17. Poletti, L. *et al.* A rational approach to heparin-related fragments; synthesis of differently sulfated tetrasaccharides as potential ligands for fibroblast growth factors. *Eur. J. Org. Chem.* **14**, 2727–2734 (2001).

18. de Paz, J. L., Ojeda, R., Reichardt, N. & Martín-Lomas, M. Some key experimental features of a modular synthesis of heparin-like oligosaccharides. *Eur. J. Org. Chem.* **17**, 3308–3324 (2003).

19. de Paz, J. L. & Martín-Lomas, M. Synthesis and biological evaluation of a heparin-like hexasaccharide with the structural motifs for binding to FGF and FGFR. *Eur. J. Org. Chem.* 1849–1858 (2005).

20. Terenti, O., de Paz, J. L. & Martín-Lomas, M. Synthesis of heparin-like oligosaccharides on polymer supports. *Glycoconj. J.* **21**, 179–195 (2004).

21. Hung, S.-C. *et al.* Synthesis of heparin oligosaccharides and their interaction with eosinophil-derived neurotoxin. *Org. Biomol. Chem.* **10**, 760–772 (2012).

22. Lee, J.-C., Lu, X.-A., Kulkarni, S. S., Wen, Y.-S. & Hung, S.-C. Synthesis of heparin oligosaccharides. *J. Am. Chem. Soc.* **126**, 476–477 (2004).

23. Lu, L.-D. *et al.* Synthesis of 48 disaccharide building blocks for the assembly of a heparin and heparan sulfate oligosaccharide library. *Org. Lett.* **8**, 5995–5998 (2006).

24. Codée, J. D. C. *et al.* A modular strategy toward the synthesis of heparin-like oligosaccharides using monomeric building blocks in a sequential glycosylation strategy. *J. Am. Chem. Soc.* **127**, 3767–3773 (2005).

25. Hu, Y.-P. *et al.* Synthesis of 3-O-sulfonated heparan sulfate octasaccharides that inhibit the herpes simplex virus type 1 host–cell interaction. *Nat. Chem.* **3**, 557–563 (2011).

26. Tiruchinapally, G., Yin, Z., El-Dakdouki, M., Wang, X. & Huang, X. Divergent heparin oligosaccharide synthesis with preinstalled sulfate esters. *Chem. Eur. J.* **17**, 10106–10112 (2011).

27. Wang, Z. *et al.* Preactivation-based, one-pot combinatorial synthesis of heparin-like hexasaccharides for the analysis of heparin–protein interactions. *Chem. Eur. J.* **16**, 8365–8375 (2010).

28. Czechura, P. *et al.* A new linker for solid-phase synthesis of heparan sulfate precursors by sequential assembly of monosaccharide building blocks. *Chem. Commun.* **47**, 2390–2392 (2011).

29. van Boeckel, C. A. A. *et al.* Synthesis of a pentasaccharide corresponding to the antithrombin III binding fragment of heparin. *Carbohydr. Chem.* **4**, 293–321 (1985).

30. Tabeur, C. *et al.* Oligosaccharides corresponding to the regular sequence of heparin: chemical synthesis and interaction with FGF-2. *Bioorg. Med. Chem.* **7**, 2003–2012 (1999).

31. Karst, N. A. & Lindhardt, R. J. Recent chemical and enzymatic approaches to the synthesis of glycosaminoglycan oligosaccharides. *Curr. Med. Chem.* **10**, 1993–2031 (2003).

32. Arndt, S. & Hsieh-Wilson, L. C. Use of cerny epoxides for the accelerated synthesis of glycosaminoglycans. *Org. Lett.* **5**, 4179–4182 (2003).

33. Yu, H. N., Furukawa, J., Ikeda, T. & Wong, C.-H. Novel efficient routes to heparin monosaccharides and disaccharides achieved via regio- and stereoselective glycosidation. *Org. Lett.* **6**, 723–726 (2004).

34. Zhou, Y., Lin, F., Chen, J. & Yu, B. Toward synthesis of the regular sequence of heparin: synthesis of two tetrasaccharide precursors. *Carbohydr. Res.* **341**, 1619–1629 (2006).

35. Arungundram, S. *et al.* Modular synthesis of heparan sulfate oligosaccharides for structure-activity relationship studies. *J. Am. Chem. Soc.* **131**, 17394–17405 (2009).

36. Xu, Y. *et al.* Chemoenzymatic synthesis of homogeneous ultralow molecular weight heparins. *Science* **334**, 498–501 (2011).

37. Laremore, T. N., Zhang, F., Dordick, J. S., Liu, J. & Lindhardt, R. J. Recent progress and applications in glycosaminoglycan and heparin research. *Curr. Opin. Chem. Biol.* **13**, 633–640 (2009).

38. Dredge, K. *et al.* PG545, a dual heparanase and angiogenesis inhibitor, induces potent anti-tumour and anti-metastatic efficacy in preclinical models. *Brit. J. Cancer* **104**, 635–642 (2011).

39. Johnstone, K. D. *et al.* Synthesis and biological evaluation of polysulfated oligosaccharide glycosides as inhibitors of angiogenesis and tumor growth. *J. Med. Chem.* **53**, 1686–1699 (2010).

40. Zhou, H. *et al.* M402, a novel heparan sulfate mimetic, targets multiple pathways implicated in tumor progression and metastasis. *PLoS ONE* **6**, e21106 (2011).

41. Ferro, V. *et al.* Discovery of PG545: a highly potent and simultaneous inhibitor of angiogenesis, tumor growth, and metastasis. *J. Med. Chem.* **55**, 3804–3813 (2012).

42. Wakao, M. *et al.* Sugar chips immobilized with synthetic sulfated disaccharides of heparin/heparan sulfate partial structure. *Bioorg. Med. Chem. Lett.* **18**, 2499–2504 (2008).

43. Schwörer, R., Zubkova, O. V., Turnbull, J. E. & Tyler, P. C. Synthesis of a targeted library of heparan sulfate hexa- to dodecasaccharides as inhibitors of β-secretase: potential therapeutics for Alzheimer's disease. *Chem. Eur. J.* **19**, 6817–6823 (2013).

44. Baleux, F. *et al.* A synthetic CD4-heparan sulfate glycoconjugate inhibits CCR5 and CXCR4 HIV-1 attachment and entry. *Nat. Chem. Biol.* **10**, 743–748 (2009).

45. Hudak, J. E., Yu, H. H. & Bertozzi, C. R. Protein glycoengineering enabled by the versatile synthesis of aminooxy glycans and the genetically encoded aldehyde tag. *J. Am. Chem. Soc.* **133**, 161119–16126 (2011).

46. Jayson, G. C. *et al.* T. Heparan sulfate undergoes specific structural changes during the progression from human colon adenoma to carcinoma in vitro. *J. Biol. Chem.* **273**, 51–57 (1998).

47. Jayson, G. C. *et al.* Coordinated modulation of the fibroblast growth factor dual receptor mechanism during transformation from human colon adenoma to carcinoma. *Int. J. Cancer* **82**, 298–304 (1999).

48. Whitworth, M. K. *et al.* Regulation of fibroblast growth factor-2 activity by human ovarian cancer tumor endothelium. *Clin. Cancer Res.* **11**, 4282–4288 (2005).

49. Backen, A. C. *et al.* Heparan sulphate synthetic and editing enzymes in ovarian cancer. *Br. J. Cancer* **96**, 1544–1548 (2007).

50. Jayson, G. C. & Gallagher, J. T. Heparin oligosaccharides: inhibitors of the biological activity of bFGF on Caco-2 cells. *Br. J. Cancer* **75**, 9–16 (1997).

51. Hasan, J. *et al.* Heparin octasaccharides inhibit angiogenesis in vivo. *Clin. Cancer. Res.* **11**, 8172–8179 (2005).

52. Cole, C. L. *et al.* Synthetic heparan sulfate oligosaccharides inhibit endothelial cell functions essential for angiogenesis. *PLoS ONE* **5**, e11644 (2010).

53. Babu, P. & Kuberan, B. Fluorescent-tagged heparan sulfate precursor oligosaccharides to probe the enzymatic action of heparitinase I. *Anal. Biochem.* **396**, 124–132 (2010).

54. Xia, B., Feasley, C. L., Sachdev, G. P., Smith, D. F. & Cummings, R. D. Glycan reductive isotope labeling for quantitative glycomics. *Anal. Biochem.* **387**, 162–170 (2009).

55. Fernandez, C., Hattan, C. M. & Kerns, R. J. Semi-synthetic heparin derivatives: chemical modifications of heparin beyond chain length, sulfate substitution pattern and N-sulfo/N-acetyl groups. *Carbohydr. Res.* **341**, 1253–1265 (2006).

56. Park, S., Sung, J.-W. & Shin, I. Fluorescent glycan derivatives: their use for natural glycan microarrays. *ACS Chem. Biol.* **4**, 699–701 (2009).

57. Hansen, S. U. *et al.* Synthesis and scalable conversion of L-idouronamides to heparin-related di- and tetrasaccharides. *J. Org. Chem.* **77**, 7823–7843 (2012).

58. Hansen, S. U., Miller, G. J., Jayson, G. C. & Gardiner, J. M. First Gram-scale synthesis of a heparin-related dodecasaccharide. *Org. Lett.* **15**, 88–91 (2013).

59. Lyon, M. & Gallagher, J. T. Purification and partial characterization of the major cell-associated heparan sulphate proteoglycan of rat liver. *Biochem. J.* **273**, 415–422 (1991).

Acknowledgements

We thank the CRUK (C2075/A9106), MRC (G0601746 and G902173) and Holt Foundation for project grant funding; EPSRC for NMR instrumentation (GR/L52246); and we also thank the EPSRC National Mass Spectrometry Service, Swansea, for MS analyses.

Author contributions

S.U.H. and G.J.M. jointly contributed to the development of iteration and LAT strategies, wrote and finalized manuscript with J.M.G. G.R. conducted the preparation, analysis and purification of tritiated saccharides. C.C. helped in conducting biological experiments. G.C.J. gave overall contribution to project aims. J.M.G. and G.C.J. contributed equally to supervision and planning of this work. E.A., G.R. and G.J. contributed to manuscript biology. J.M.G. supervised synthesis and project planning, and helped in writing and finalizing the manuscript.

Additional Information

Competing financial interests: The authors declare no competing financial interests.

4

In vivo imaging of specific drug–target binding at subcellular resolution

J.M. Dubach[1,*], C. Vinegoni[1,*], R. Mazitschek[1], P. Fumene Feruglio[1], L.A. Cameron[2] & R. Weissleder[1]

The possibility of measuring binding of small-molecule drugs to desired targets in live cells could provide a better understanding of drug action. However, current approaches mostly yield static data, require lysis or rely on indirect assays and thus often provide an incomplete understanding of drug action. Here, we present a multiphoton fluorescence anisotropy microscopy live cell imaging technique to measure and map drug–target interaction in real time at subcellular resolution. This approach is generally applicable using any fluorescently labelled drug and enables high-resolution spatial and temporal mapping of bound and unbound drug distribution. To illustrate our approach we measure intracellular target engagement of the chemotherapeutic Olaparib, a poly(ADP-ribose) polymerase inhibitor, in live cells and within a tumour *in vivo*. These results are the first generalizable approach to directly measure drug–target binding *in vivo* and present a promising tool to enhance understanding of drug activity.

[1] Center for System Biology, Massachusetts General Hospital and Harvard Medical School, Richard B. Simches Research Center, 185 Cambridge Street, Boston, Massachusetts 02114, USA. [2] Dana-Farber Cancer Institute, Department of Pediatric Oncology, 450 Brookline Ave., Boston, Massachusetts 02215, USA. * These authors contributed equally to this work. Correspondence and requests for materials should be addressed to C.V. (email: cvinegoni@mgh.harvard.edu).

Small-molecule therapeutic drugs typically exert their effects through binding to one or a few protein targets. This critical interaction—a prerequisite of therapeutic drug efficacy—is often poorly understood and can generally not be visualized in live cells or entire organisms due to the lack of methods to directly measure drug–target engagement in a biological setting. As a result, most of our knowledge is incomplete, as it relies on target extraction assay systems[1,2] or indirect measurements where critical spatiotemporal information is lost, which further complicates drug development[3].

Recent advances in chemical techniques have allowed the creation of fluorescent drugs, prodrugs and activity-based probes to interrogate target engagement[4–6]. To date, most of these compounds have been used in vitro while a select few have been used in vivo for imaging drug distribution (pharmacokinetics)[7] or tumour detection[8]. However, to realize the full potential of intravital imaging with fluorescently labelled compounds determination of target engagement with subcellular resolution is needed[2,9]. We hypothesized that fluorescence polarization (FP) could be used to accurately measure drug binding in vitro and in vivo through multiphoton microscopy.

FP[10] quantifies the degree of fluorescence depolarization with respect to the polarization excitation plane, providing insight into the state or environment of the excited fluorescent molecule. FP has been extensively used in non-imaging, plate reader and kinetic in vitro assays to measure numerous fluorescent molecule and molecular drug interactions including target engagement[11,12]. Extending FP to optical microscopy imaging modalities could provide spatially and temporally resolved mapping, enabling live cell imaging of target engagement of small-molecule drugs. However, microscopy imaging methods based on FP[13] have been more commonly used to study homo-FRET in membrane dynamics[14–16], structure in ordered biological systems[17,18] and endogenous small molecules[19] or labelled protein interactions[20].

Herein we present multiphoton fluorescence anisotropy microscopy (MFAM) to image intracellular drug–target binding distribution in vivo. Specifically we demonstrate, with a Phase III drug candidate, that our approach is not only applicable to live cultured cells but also enables real-time imaging of drug–target engagement in vivo with submicron resolution.

Results

Fluorescence anisotropy and imaging set-up characterization.
Following photoselection under polarized excitation, all excited fluorophores are aligned with the same emission dipole orientation. However, due to the presence of rotational Brownian motion, fluorophores rotate with a correlation time (τ_θ) dependent on viscosity, molecule size and temperature[21]. If the excited fluorophore is free to rapidly rotate on a timescale that is shorter than its fluorescence lifetime ($\tau_\theta \ll \tau$), emission will be isotropic (depolarized). However, when rotating slowly, the rotational correlation time will increase ($\tau_\theta \gg \tau$) and emission will be preferentially aligned along one axis (Fig. 1a). Furthermore, a change in the fluorescence lifetime will also affect the emission polarization as molecules will have less or more time to rotate before emission. To characterize the extent of linearly polarized emission, fluorescence anisotropy (FA), a dimensionless parameter similar to FP and independent of excitation intensity (Supplementary Fig. 1, Supplementary Methods), can be calculated. Thus, measurements of anisotropy provide insight into the rotational diffusion rate of molecules, which can be used in term to directly determine drug engagement with the target.

Using multiphoton microscopy for anisotropy[22] offers several advantages over other imaging modalities. Extended light penetration depth enables relatively deep imaging in tissues in a physiologically relevant context, while a diminished scattering component in the near infrared reduces tissue scattering[23]. Therefore, multiphoton microscopy, with its low phototoxicity and high axial resolution, is ideally suited for high-resolution drug–target interaction imaging within single cells.

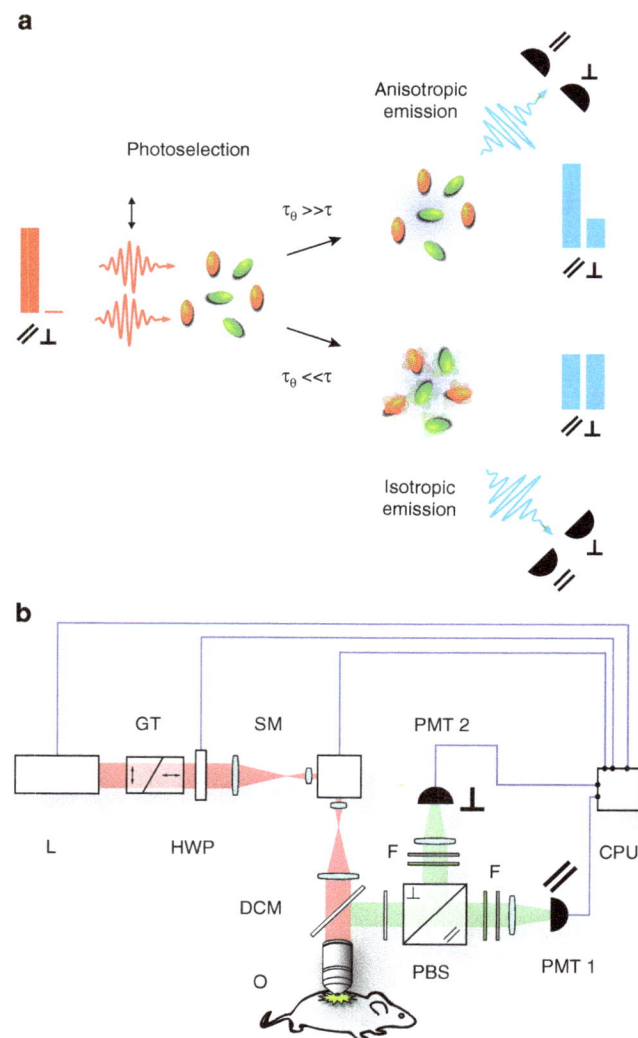

Figure 1 | Imaging set-up. (a) Schematic representation of the two-photon photoselection process in a randomly oriented distribution of fluorophores and the resulting fluorescence emission for low (isotropic) and high (anisotropic) rotational correlation times (τ_θ). Blue bars indicate schematically the distribution of emission along the two orthogonal linear polarization components (||, ⊥) as measured at the two detectors, for the two cases. Orange particles represent excited molecules. **(b)** The optical set-up of the MFAM is based on a custom-modified Olympus FV1000-MPE (Olympus, USA) laser scanning microscopy system equipped with an upright BX61-WI microscope (Olympus, USA). Excitation light (red beam) from a Ti:sapphire laser (L) is filtered to select a linear state of polarization and then focused onto the imaged sample. Emitted fluorescent light (green beam) is epi-collected, separated into two linearly polarized orthogonal components and spectrally filtered before non-descanned detection. GT, Glan–Thompson polarizer; HWP, half-wave plate; SM, scanning mirrors; DCM, dichroic mirror; O, objective; PBS, polarization beam splitter; F, band-pass filters; PMT, photomultiplier tube; CPU, computer.

MFAM imaging was developed using a custom-adapted commercial unit (Fig. 1b). We first tested the imaging system by measuring the viscosity dependence of anisotropy for pentamethyl–BODIPY (Me$_5$–BODIPY), an ideal fluorophore for FA (Supplementary Methods), in increasing concentration of aqueous glycerol (Fig. 2 and Supplementary Fig. 2). As expected, the measured anisotropy increased with increasing viscosity. The superior photoselectivity by two-photon excitation compared with single-photon absorption[24] significantly increased anisotropy values through enhanced photoselection, resulting in increased sensitivity (Supplementary Fig. 3). Although high numerical aperture objectives are well known to produce distorted anisotropy values at the periphery of an image[25] (with small impact on-axis), restricting the field of view eliminates these aberrations (Supplementary Figs 4 and 5, Supplementary Methods).

The resolution of the imaging system was determined using fluorescent microspheres. Both planar and axial measurements of a microsphere point spread function (Fig. 3a) demonstrate the high optical resolution of FA, making MFAM ideal for 3D intracellular imaging. The calculated anisotropy error in each pixel increases at the edges of the microspheres, a consequence of low count rates[26], resulting in some noise artefacts and loss of anisotropy (Supplementary Figs 6 and 7). However, anisotropy remained constant above a threshold that is determined by acquisition parameters and intrinsic noise (Supplementary Fig. 6). Next we exploited the excellent optical sectioning properties for tomographic MFAM imaging of an optical phantom simulating a bound/unbound 3D environment. Two highly homogeneous populations of green-fluorescent microspheres with distinct anisotropy values (Supplementary Figs 8 and 9) were suspended in a 2% agarose solution (Fig. 3b). In both the 3D FA colour-coded reconstructions and the optically sectioned planes, the two populations of microspheres are distinguishable throughout the entire phantom depth (ca. 90 μm) and assigned the correct anisotropy-based colour (Fig. 3b and Supplementary Fig. 8b).

Imaging drug–target engagement in live cells. FA has traditionally been used to measure binding of small fluorescent molecules to a larger target biomolecule[27]. When bound, the increased molecular mass of the probe–target complex will result in a higher rotation correlation time τ_θ limiting molecule rotation and increasing FA (Fig. 4a), while a shift in fluorescence lifetime could also change FA. Depending on its state (bound/unbound) a single fluorescent molecule can produce two values of anisotropy,

and, because anisotropy is an additive property, the measured pixel value in an FA image is the fraction-weighted sum of the two possible anisotropy values within a voxel. MFAM measurements of Me$_5$–BODIPY labelled Biotin (Biotin–BODIPY) indeed show an increase in anisotropy as a function of binding to NeutrAvidin (Fig. 4a) with a similar trend to single-photon measurements (Supplementary Fig. 3), due to a change in τ_θ (Supplementary Methods).

While dyes presenting longer lifetimes could be considered as alternative candidates, BODIPY was chosen due to unique characteristics that allow intracellular imaging. Specifically, (i) BODIPY is relatively non-polar with the chromophore presenting electrical neutrality, therefore minimizing perturbation to the modified drug; (ii) the relatively long lifetime (the BODIPY we use here has a measured lifetime ∼4.0 ns) makes it particularly suitable for fluorescence polarization-based assay; (iii) BODIPY is highly permeant to live cells, easily passing through the plasma membrane, where it accumulates over time; (iv) it has a high extinction coefficient (EC > 80,000 cm^{-1} M^{-1}) and a high fluorescence quantum yield (often approaching 1.0, even in water); (v) it presents a lack of ionic charge and spectra that are relatively insensitive to solvent polarity and pH; and, (vi) finally, it has a large two-photon cross section. Although most BODIPY dyes enjoy a relatively long lifetime, dyes such as Cy3

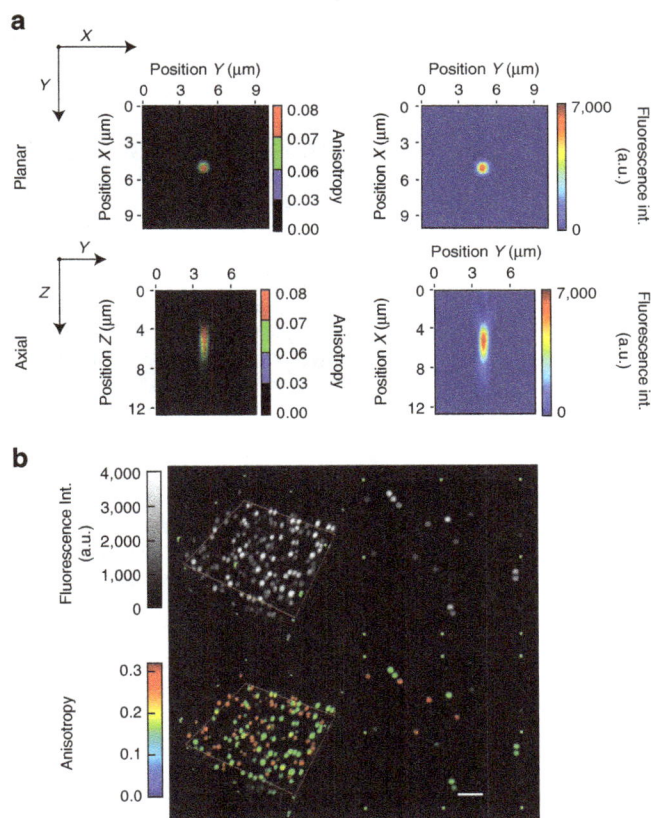

Figure 3 | Optical characterization of MFAM. (**a**) MFAM point spread function characterization. Planar and axial microscope FA and plain fluorescence images of a fluorescent microsphere. (**b**) 3D reconstructions of a mixture of two fluorescent microspheres populations with high and low anisotropy suspended in agarose, with the respective planar images obtained across the transversal plane indicated by the orange line. Anisotropy images colour-coded based on anisotropy values. Right: planar images across the transversal plane indicated (orange line). Top, fluorescence. Bottom, anisotropy. Scale bar, 20 μm.

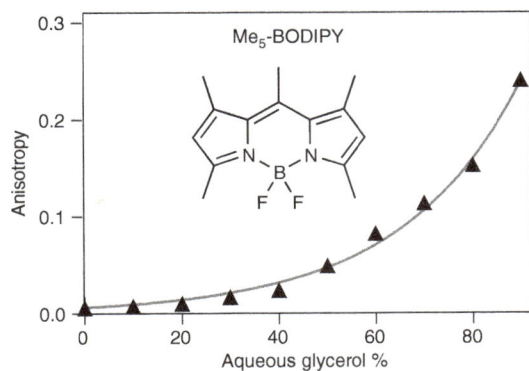

Figure 2 | Anisotropy measurement. Me$_5$–BODIPY anisotropy dependence on viscosity, as measured in glycerol with MFAM. Measurements are obtained from two-photon images of sample drops of Me$_5$–BODIPY and calculating the anisotropy of each pixel. Average ± s.d. ($n = 6$), fitted curve added for trend visualization.

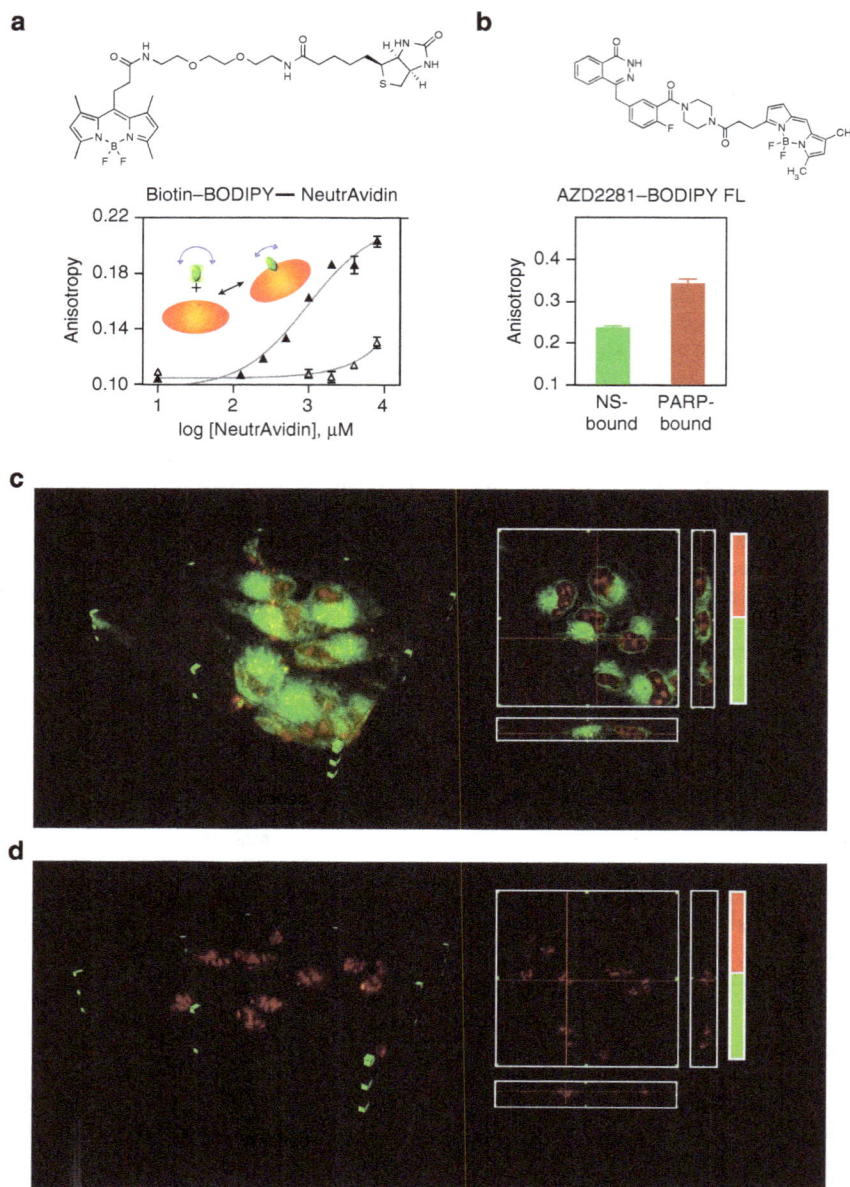

Figure 4 | Live cell imaging of target engagement. (a) The anisotropy value of Biotin–BODIPY (MW 676.62) increases as a function of binding to NeutrAvidin (MW 60 kDa) (filled triangles), which is suppressed in the presence of 10 × unlabelled biotin as competitor (open triangles). Shown are average ± s.d. (n = 3); curve fits added for trend visualization. Inset illustration: comparison between the rotation of a free fluorophore in solution and a fluorophore bound to a protein. Owing to the large difference in size of the ligand and the receptor, the increase in FA following binding is large. **(b)** Average ± s.d. anisotropy of non-specifically interacting (green) and PARP bound (red) AZD2281–BODIPY FL (n = 3). **(c)** 3D anisotropy image and corresponding planar and axial cross sections of live HT1080 cells loaded with AZD2281–BODIPY FL. Green corresponds to fluorescent drug molecules that are non-specifically bound. Red corresponds to fluorescent drug molecules with high anisotropy suggesting target (PARP) binding. Normal fluorescence images are shown in Supplementary Fig. 18. Scale bar, 16 μm. **(d)** 3D anisotropy image and corresponding planar and axial cross sections of live HT1080 cells loaded with AZD2281–BODIPY FL and washed for 30 min. Scale bars, 20 μm.

and the Alexa dyes will be inefficient for FA imaging, with their lifetimes so short that the anisotropy of the unbound probe will be near the fundamental anisotropy, and hence indistinguishable from the bound probe. Conversely, fluorophores with extremely long lifetimes, or phosphorescence emission, are also unsuitable as the increase in rotation correlation time will not be large enough to increase the anisotropy. It is therefore important to characterize the lifetime, by fluorescence lifetime imaging microscopy (FLIM), of the possible candidate dyes for drug labelling that could be potentially used for two-photon fluorescence polarization imaging. Also, dyes presenting changes in

their quantum yield upon binding will bias the readout value of total anisotropy affecting the measured binding isotherm.

To test the MFAM imaging approach in a relevant drug–target system, we chose to target poly(ADP-ribose) polymerase (PARP) with the small-molecule inhibitor Olaparib (AZD2281) that had been modified to bear a BODIPY-FL handle[7]. This model system and its cellular location had previously been well validated[7,28]. PARP comprises a family of enzymes that are required for DNA repair[29–31], and therefore present a potential chemotherapeutic target through inhibition. Owing to the high molecular weight of PARP1 (~120 kDa) a significant increase in anisotropy is observed for 'target-bound' over 'free' or 'intracellular drug' AZD2281–BODIPY FL, respectively (Fig. 4b and Supplementary Fig. 10a). An anisotropy threshold can then be assigned to distinguish between the bound states and MFAM intracellular imaging of drug–target engagement can be obtained in 3D (Fig. 4c,d: red, PARP bound; green, 'intracellular drug'). When incubated with AZD2281–BODIPY FL we observed rapid accumulation throughout the entirety of each HT1080 cell. Intracellular drug was present in the cytoplasmic region, while bound drug was present in the nucleus (Fig. 4c and Supplementary Fig. 11), which colocalized with PARP immunostaining[28] (Supplementary Fig. 10b). Following extended washing cycles, the cytoplasmic AZD2281–BODIPY FL is cleared, while the nuclear, bound drug remains (Fig. 4d). Similar nuclear binding of AZD2281–BODIPY FL was observed in other cell lines reported to express PARP as well (Supplementary Fig. 12), as validated previously[28].

Real-time *in vitro* measurements (Fig. 5) show AZD2281–BODIPY FL accumulated in the cytoplasm significantly more than in the nucleus, which is likely the result of interactions with intracellular membranes. Yet, only the nucleus presents high values of anisotropy, suggesting PARP binding (Fig. 5a). The high nuclear anisotropy (Fig. 5a) is not observed in the presence of unlabelled AZD2281 as competitor (5 ×) (Fig. 5b), which further

suggests the high anisotropy measured in the nuclei was due to drug–target binding and not induced by potential artefacts, such as viscosity. In addition, there was no target binding of AZD2281–BODIPY FL in the cytoplasm, as demonstrated by the significant difference between nuclear and cytoplasmic anisotropy throughout the course of loading and washing as well as the insignificant difference between cytoplasmic anisotropy in the non-competitive and competitive experiments (Fig. 6). Constant anisotropy with decreasing intensity in the cytoplasm in both non-competition and competition experiments indicates that homo-FRET was not the cause of the lower anisotropy (Fig. 6). Additionally, high nuclear anisotropy is not caused by the BODIPY FL itself (Supplementary Fig. 13). Finally, there was no significant difference in fluorescence lifetime between nuclear and cytoplasmic regions in loaded HT1080 cells (Supplementary Fig. 14). Through washing and competition experiments, bound and unbound values of anisotropy in the nucleus can be determined, and the percentage of target-bound AZD2281-BODIPY FL can be calculated at any point in time (Supplementary Fig. 15).

In vivo imaging of drug–target engagement. Finally, we used MFAM for *in vivo* imaging applications. In biological diffusive

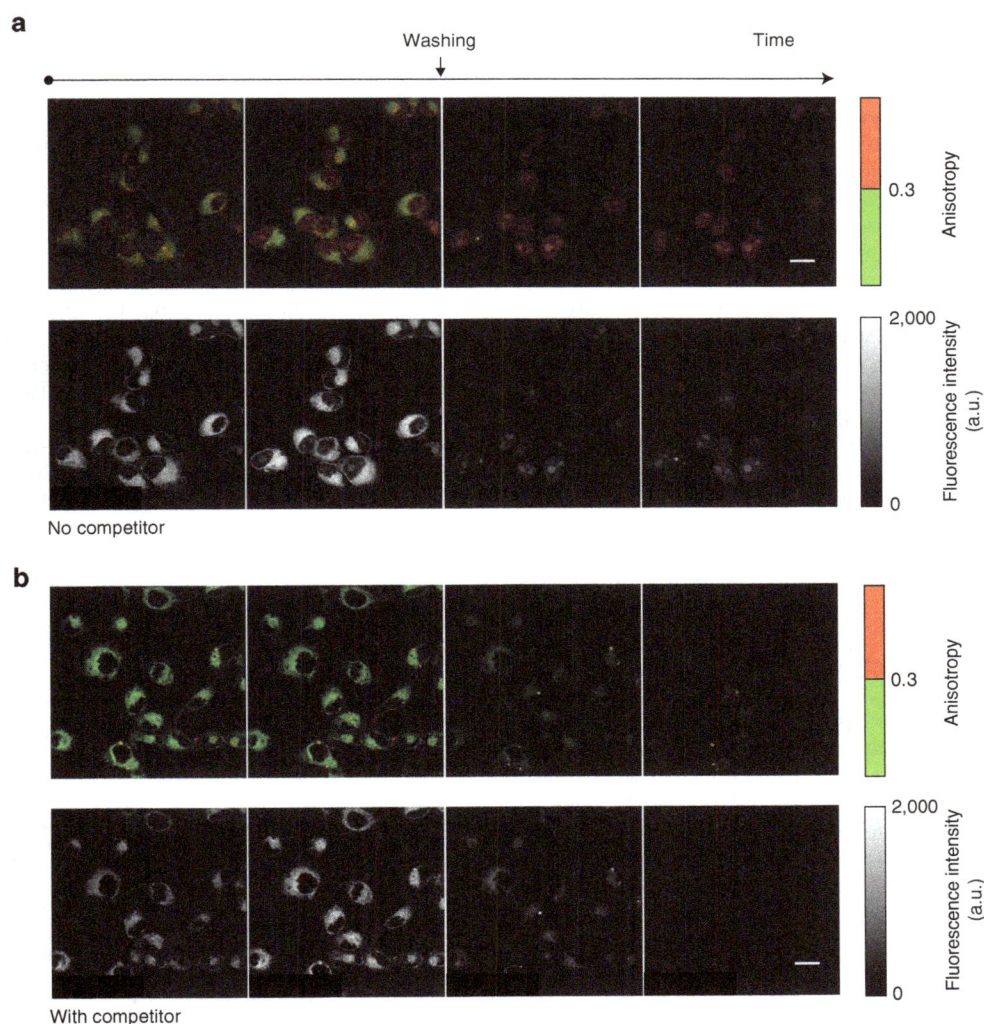

Figure 5 | Imaging target engagement over time. (**a**) Anisotropy and corresponding fluorescence images of AZD2281–BODIPY FL at four representative time points during drug loading and after washing. (**b**) Similar experiment as in (**a**) but in the presence of fivefold higher concentration of unlabelled AZD2281 (competition). Scale bars, 20 μm.

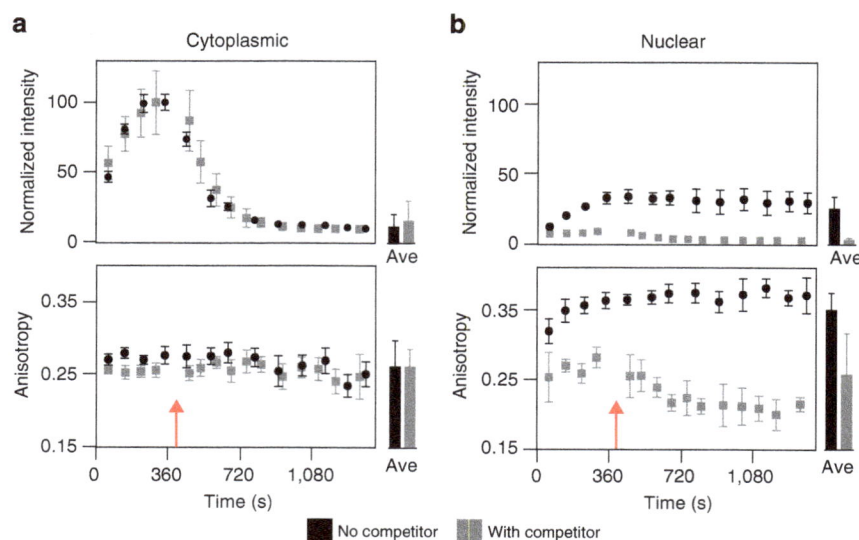

Figure 6 | Real-time imaging of drug–target engagement in live cells. Normalized intensity and anisotropy as a function of time for HT1080 cells loaded with AZD2281–BODIPY FL and washed. Values are measured in both the cytoplasmic (**a**) and nuclear (**b**) regions of the cells in the absence (black circles) and presence (grey squares) of fivefold higher concentration of unlabelled AZD2281 (competition). Points in the graphs refer to a single experiment, average ± s.d. ($n = 6$ cells). Also shown at the right of each figure, average ± s.d. at the end of the wash in the absence (black bars, $n = 42$ cells, seven separate experiments) and presence (grey bars, $n = 36$ cells, six separate experiments) of unlabelled AZD2281 ($5 \times$). Bars are representative of seven and six different experiments, respectively. Red arrows indicate switch from loading to washing. Fluorescence intensity refers to the sum of both perpendicular and parallel channels.

samples multiple scattering events limit the imaging depth by reducing the number of excitation photons in the focal area while decreasing the number of collected photons[32]. A decrease of the degree of polarization with resulting lower values of anisotropy is therefore present as evidenced on tissue phantom measurements (Supplementary Fig. 16, Supplementary Methods). To better characterize how diffusion and absorption limit the effective anisotropy imaging depth we first injected fluorescent microspheres into superficial tissue within a nude mouse dorsal window chamber (Fig. 7a). *In vivo* MFAM measurements indicated a slight depth-dependent loss of anisotropy (Fig. 7b), with a 10% loss at 100 μm, which, based on the anisotropy difference in binding measurements, does not affect target engagement measurements.

After determining that our technique is viable in an *in vivo* setting we measured drug–target engagement in a mouse. Intravenous delivery to an implanted HT1080 cell tumour showed AZD2281–BODIPY FL diffusion into the cancer cells (Fig. 7c). Cells expressing nuclear mApple-labelled H2B, which did not affect AZD2281 anisotropy measurements (Supplementary Figs 11 and 17), were used to locate the tumour[33]. Binding of AZD2281–BODIPY FL to PARP in the nucleus occurred immediately upon drug infusion (Fig. 7d). The bound fraction of the drug was retained in the nucleus while the unbound extracellular and cytoplasmic drug was cleared away over time (Fig. 7d). Both the nuclear and overall fluorescence intensity decreased over time; however, the nuclear anisotropy increased as unbound AZD2281–BODIPY FL was cleared (Fig. 7e).

Discussion

The ability to measure the pharmacology of drugs on a molecular level in live cells represents one of the greatest challenges in chemical biology and drug discovery[9]. Currently, there are no demonstrated methods for direct measurements. Subsequently, all information is based on indirect or artificial approaches that do

not provide the spatiotemporal resolution and accuracy required to establish reliable models and/or do not occur in biologically relevant settings.

Here we have developed a promising novel approach utilizing MFAM, which, for the first time, allows direct visualization of target-bound versus unbound small-molecule drugs in real time. Using a chemotherapeutic compound in Phase III clinical trials, we demonstrate that our approach is not only applicable to live cultured cells but also enables real-time imaging of drug–target engagement *in vivo* and with submicron resolution. Our technique does not require separation between bound and free compound, is not limited to equilibrium analysis and does not affect the biological settings. As such, MFAM offers a new and fundamental imaging platform for accelerating translational drug development through insight into *in vivo* drug activity and inefficacy.

Methods

Cell culture. HT1080 cells (ATCC) stably expressing H2B mApple fluorescent protein[28,33,34] were cultured in DMEM with 10% FBS, 1% pen-strep and 100 μg ml^{-1} geneticin (Invitrogen). HT1080 cells were cultured in DMEM with 10% FBS and 1% pen-strep. MDA-MB-436, HCC1937 and MHH-ES1 cells were cultured in RPMI with 10% FBS and 1% pen-strep. Cells were plated onto 25 mm no. 1 cover glass for *in vitro* imaging.

Tumour model. All animal experiments were performed in accordance with the Institutional Animal Care and Use Committee at Massachusetts General Hospital. Female 20-week-old nude mice (Cox-7, Massachusetts General Hospital, Boston, MA, USA) were used. All surgical procedures were conducted under sterile conditions and facilitated through the use of a zoom stereomicroscope (Olympus SZ61). During all surgical procedures and imaging experiments mice were anaesthetized by isofluorane vaporization (Harvard Apparatus) at a flow rate of 2 l per min of isofluorane: 2 l per mine of oxygen. The body temperature of the mice was kept constant at 37 °C during all imaging experiments and surgical procedures. Dorsal skinfold window chambers (DSC) were implanted 1 day before imaging following a well-established protocol. Briefly, the two layers of skin on the back of the mouse were stretched and kept in place by the DSC. One skin layer was surgically removed and replaced by a 12-mm diameter glass cover slip positioned on one side of the DSC, allowing for convenient access and imaging of the tumour

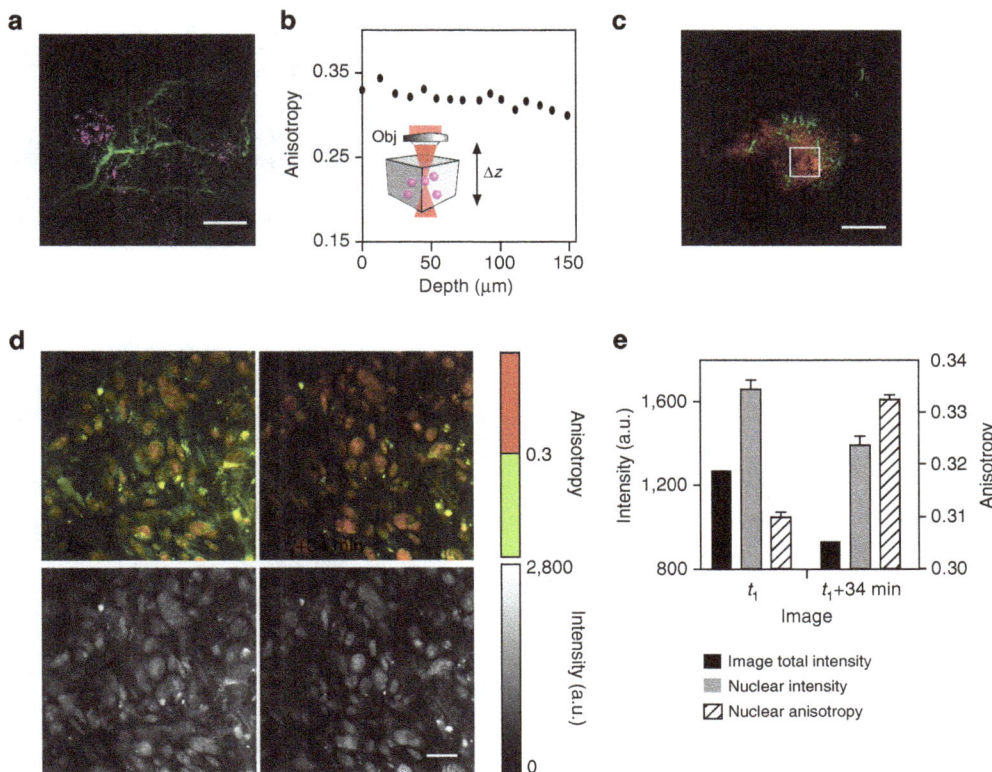

Figure 7 | Imaging of AZD2281–BODIPY FL target engagement in a live mouse. (**a**) *In vivo* fluorescence image of injected fluorescent microspheres (pink) in the vascularized (green) tissue fascia of a mouse DSC. Scale bar, 50 µm. (**b**) Anisotropy of the injected fluorescent microspheres as a function of depth within the tissue fascia. Each point corresponds to a single bead measurement. (**c**) Confocal fluorescence image of HT1080 H2B mApple cells (red) in a mouse DSC. After 1–2 weeks, the tumour area is highly vascularized and, upon intravenous injection, perfused with AZD2281–BODIPY FL (green). The white square indicates the imaged area in (**d**). Scale bar, 100 µm. (**d**) *In vivo* anisotropy (top) and fluorescence (bottom) images of AZD2281–BODIPY FL following intravenous infusion (left) and 34 min later (right). Scale bar, 20 µm (**e**) Overall image intensity (black), nuclear intensity (grey) and nuclear anisotropy (unfilled, striped) as measured from the images in (**d**). Nuclear intensity and anisotropy values are average $\pm$ s.e. ($n = 90$ for image t_1, $n = 102$ for image $t_1 + 34$ min). Fluorescence intensity refers to the sum of both perpendicular and parallel channels.

area. A spacer located on the DSC prevented excessive compression of both tissue and vessel, guaranteeing good vascular perfusion within the tumour region.

HT1080 H2B mApple cells were harvested by trypsinization (0.25% trypsin:EDTA) and resuspended in PBS. Mice were anaesthetized and $\sim 10^6$ cells (100 µl 1 $\times$ PBS) were injected subcutaneously into the back of female *Nu/Nu* mice (Cox-7, Massachusetts General Hospital) aged 20–25 weeks in a 1:1 mixture of Matrigel (BD Biosciences). Cells were injected using a 0.5-ml insulin syringe with the needle bent at 90 degrees to better control the position of the injection site. In order to allow for the tumour to be established and neovascularization to occur, the tumours were allowed to grow for 1–2 weeks before DSC implantation.

Microscope configuration. The optical set-up is based on a custom-modified Olympus FV1000-MPE (Olympus, USA) laser scanning microscopy system equipped with an upright BX61-WI microscope (Olympus, USA) and is illustrated in details in Fig. 1b. Excitation light (red beam) from a Ti:sapphire laser (L) is filtered to select a linear state of polarization and then focused onto the imaged sample. Emitted fluorescent light (green beam) is epi-collected, separated into two linearly polarized orthogonal components and spectrally filtered before non-descanned detection. The MaiTai DeepSee Ti:sapphire pulsed laser (Spectra Physics) had a pulse-width of 110 fs and a repetition rate of 80 MHz. Laser was tuned at 910 nm for two-photon excitation of Me5–BODIPY and BODIPY FL. A Glan–Thompson polarizer (Newport) and a half-wave plate (Thor Labs) were inserted in the laser path toward the objective in order to create a linear state of polarization aligned along a fixed predetermined axis. Light was then focused onto the sample with a $\times 25$ 1.05 NA water-immersion objective (XLPlan N, 2 mm working distance, Olympus). Fluorescence emission was detected in epi-collection mode through the same focusing objective. A dichroic filter (690 nm) diverted the fluorescent light towards a non-descanned detection path, followed by a low-pass filter (685 nm). Along the detection path a polarizing beam splitter (Edmund optics) was inserted to separate the light in two orthogonal states of polarization, each one followed by a band-pass filter (490–540 nm, Chroma). Orthogonal and

parallel linear polarized light was then focused and detected by two separate photomultiplier tubes ($I_{\|}$, $I_{\perp}$). The excitation light was linearly polarized to be parallel and perpendicular aligned to the two PMTs. Dual detector acquisition is recommended to avoid severe anisotropy artefacts induced by intensity fluctuations.

The imaging system was also operated in confocal modality. Me5–BODIPY (Exc: 493 nm; Em: 503 nm), BODIPY-FL (Exc: 503 nm, Em: 512 nm), Fluorescein (Exc: 494 nm, Em: 521 nm) and H2B mApple (Exc: 568 nm, Em: 592 nm) were scanned and excited sequentially using a 473 and a 559-nm diode laser, respectively, in combination with a DM488/559-nm dichroic beam splitter. Emitted light was then separated and collected using an SDM560 beam splitter and BA490-540 and BA575-675 band-pass filters (Olympus, USA). Confocal large field-of-view images were acquired using a $\times 2$ air objective (XL Fluor 2x/340 NA 0.14) and a water-immersion objective with a high numerical aperture (NA) and large working distance (XLPlan N $\times 25$, NA 1.05, w.d. 2 mm, Olympus) were utilized.

3D multichannel serial imaging was obtained through the use of a built-in Z axis motor with a 0.01 µm step size. Different areas along the entire size of the dorsal window chamber were sequentially imaged over time using a microscope-controlled long-range XY axis translation stage.

Optical characterization of the system. All polarizer, optical filters, polarization beam splitter, half-wave plate and Glan–Thompson polarizer were tested and characterized. Light from the laser was first linearly polarized using a Glan–Thompson polarizer and then aligned along a defined arbitrary axis with the use of a half wave plate. Light at the entry of the objective was measured using a polarizer and a photodetector to confirm the state of polarization remained linear along its path to the objective. Photodetectors were tested for any polarization dependence. The path from the objective to the photodetectors was also tested to assure that equal distribution of power is present between the two detectors. Voltage of the two photodiodes was slightly adjusted in order to fine-tune equal signal detection. The noise contribution of the two detectors was equal for all *in vitro* and *in vivo* measurement conditions. The two detectors responded with the same linear curve along the measurement range. Calibration of the MFAM systems was performed using a set of angle-adjustable linear polarizer placed in front of the detectors, and at the entry of the objective. Fluorescein in water at room temperature was used to fine-tune the voltage gains on the two individual PMT sensors. The solution (5 μl) was placed between a microscope slide and a cover glass and imaged. Settings were regulated such that 2 μM fluorescein solution produced an anisotropy of 0.004 after correction of the G factor. The gains settings were then maintained throughout the entirety of all measurements.

To check reproducibility over days, fluorescence slides containing uniformly distributed fluorophores were measured before each imaging session. Images of three different slides (each one with a different fluorophore) were taken during each imaging session to confirm that the measured anisotropy during the session matched the previous measurements. Images of the slides were taken over various time periods and at varying excitation intensity for system characterization.

Thermal variation can cause slight difference on a day-to-day basis. To compensate for them the microscope is located within a thermally stable isolating cage, mounted on an aluminium frame. Measurements over time within the same day and over several days indicate strong reproducibility in FA measurements (Supplementary Fig. 19).

Polarization distortions due to dichroic beam splitter reflections and the objective's high numerical aperture[35], such is the requirement for multiphoton microscopy, can lead to anisotropy artefacts in particular when imaging over the entire objective field of view[36]. While compensation could be used through different calibration methods, images collected over a restricted field of view eliminate any edge artefact (Supplementary Figs 4 and 5, Supplementary Methods).

Me$_5$–BODIPY was brought up in DMSO (Sigma) to a 1 mM stock solution. Solutions of a final concentration of 20 μM Me$_5$–BODIPY in DMSO were mixed with glycerol (Sigma) to create varying concentrations of glycerol. Images of 5 μl drops of solution inserted between the cover glass were taken at each glycerol concentration in triplicate.

3D anisotropy phantom. Six-micrometre green-fluorescent microspheres (InSpeck Microscope Image Intensity Calibration Kits, Invitrogen) were used for demonstrating optical sectioning capabilities. Each kit consists of seven different types of microspheres with fluorescence intensities ranging from very low to very bright (100%, 30%, 10%, 3%, 1%, 0.3% and non-fluorescent). The fluorescence intensity of the microspheres within each vial is defined with respect to that of the microspheres with the highest fluorescence (that is, 100%). We selected one vial containing the brightest microspheres (that is, 100%) and another vial containing the next brightest (30%) microspheres. The fluorescence intensity of the microspheres in each vial is highly homogeneous, as shown in Supplementary Fig. 8. Importantly, their value of anisotropy is not dictated by the lifetime (Supplementary Fig. 9) or mobility of dye within the microspheres, but instead by a concentration-dependent effect (homo-FRET) (see ref. 26 for a detailed explanation of the effect). Owing to homo-FRET, the two populations of microspheres present different values of anisotropy with a highly homogenous distribution (0.274 ± 0.008 and 0.193 ± 0.005; Supplementary Fig. 8). The microspheres are therefore useful for testing anisotropy distributions in phantoms[26]. The two populations of microspheres were mixed in equal proportion, suspended in 2% agarose and allowed to solidify between two pieces of cover glass before imaging.

Point spread function measurements. One-micrometre green fluorescence microspheres (Bangs Labs) on cover glass were also imaged and used for point spread function characterization.

Tissue phantoms. The tissue optical phantoms used for characterization (Supplementary Methods) contained fluorescein (20 μM) (Sigma), which was diluted in 1% Intralipid (10% Solution, Baxter Healthcare) in PBS with varying concentrations of India ink following a well-established protocol[37]. The corresponding scattering coefficient μ'_s was equal to 11 cm^{-1}, a value typically considered for mouse tissue phantoms[37]. Optical densities of ink concentrations in PBS were determined by measuring the absorbance spectrum at 910 nm. Fluorescent images of the solution were taken at 10-μm intervals through the depth of the phantoms.

FLIM measurements. Fluorescence lifetime imaging was performed using a Zeiss 710 confocal NLO laser scanning system on an upright Zeiss Examiner stand with a × 40 NA 1.1 water-immersion LD C-Apochromat objective and a Becker & Hickl TCSPC system. Two-photon excitation was achieved using a Coherent Chameleon Vision II tunable laser (680–1,040 nm) that provided 140-fs pulses at a 80-Mhz repetition rate with an output power of 3 W at the peak of the tuning curve (800 nm). Laser scanning was controlled by Zeiss Zen software and set to a pixel dwell time of 1.58 μs and 0.9-s frame rate at 910 nm wavelength excitation. Enhanced detection of the scattered component of the emitted (fluorescence) photons was afforded by the use of a Becker & Hickl HPM-100-40 hybrid detector, which incorporates the Hamamatsu R10467 hybrid PMT tube. Imaging was performed in the dark with blackout enclosure around the microscope to exclude external sources of light during the sensitive period of FLIM measurement. Emitted

fluorescence was deflected to the non-descanned light path via a 760 + mirror and emission range was limited to 500–550 nm by a Chroma filter in front of the HPM-100-40 detector. Acquisition time was typically 60 s with a count rate of 2–5 × 10^4 photons per second. Photon counting and electronic timing synchronization was controlled and measured with a Becker & Hickl TCSPC electronics (SPC-830) and SPCM software (Becker & Hickl GmbH). Lifetime decay of the fluorescence was analysed with SPCImage software (Becker & Hickl GmbH).

Plate reader anisotropy measurements. Single-photon data were collected in a plate reader set up for fluorescence polarization measurements (Tecan Sapphire 2). A G-factor for the instrument was calculated from 2 μM fluorescein in water. Measurements were performed in 96- or 384-well plates.

Biotin–BODIPY FL and NeutrAvidin binding. Biotin was conjugated to Me$_5$–BODIPY (Biotin–BODIPY) and brought to 1 mM stock solution in DMSO. Biotin–BODIPY (10 μM) was mixed with varying concentrations of NeutrAvidin (Thermo Scientific) in PBS with 1% Triton X (Sigma). Each sample was imaged in triplicate as a drop between a microscope slide and cover glass. Measurements of each sample were also performed using single-photon excitation in a plate reader. Measurements were also made in the presence of 100 μM free Biotin to competitively compete with the Biotin–BODIPY.

Free-molecule anisotropy. AZD2281 labelled with BODIPY FL (AZD2281–BODIPY FL) was prepared as previously described[7,38]. PARP1 (BioVision) was brought up in the manufacturer's recommended solution and added at 1.6 × the concentration of AZD2281–BODIPY FL (5 μM) in imaging media containing 2.5% FBS. Free AZD2281–BODIPY FL (5 μM) (no PARP) in the same imaging media with 2.5% FBS and in DMSO solutions were also prepared. Images were taken of drops of solution between cover glass.

***In vitro* cellular imaging.** Cells on 25 mm cover glass were mounted into a closed bath perfusion chamber (Warner Instruments) and perfused with a custom perfusion system that enabled solution switching in the imaging chamber. Cells were imaged in phenol red-free DMEM with 10% FBS and 1% pen-strep. AZD2281–BODIPY FL (1 μM) was perfused into the imaging chamber followed by a washout with drug-free media. Images were obtained during the entire time interval at regular time points. For competition experiments, free AZD2281 (5 μM) (Selleck Chemicals) was added to the incubating solution before, during and after AZD2281–BODIPY FL addition. Me$_5$–BODIPY was used for fluorophore control experiments.

***In vivo* imaging.** Mice were anaesthetixed as indicated above. When imaged for prolonged period of time, the isoflurane flow rate was reduced to ~1l per min. The DSC was inserted onto a custom stabilization plate to prevent image motion artefacts and axial drifts over the time of the imaging session. Plane tracking to ensure that the same area is imaged repeatedly over the course of the drug uptake measurements was achieved through the use of a built-in Z axis motor. Animals were warmed with a heating plate in order to keep their temperature constant.

Green-fluorescent microspheres (2.5 μm; (InSpeck, Invitrogen) were dried out using an EZ-2 evaporator (Genevac) and resuspended in sterile PBS. After sonication, the microspheres were then injected into the skin tissue of a dorsal window chamber on a nude mouse. Injections were performed with a CellTram vario (Molecular Devices) through pulled glass pipettes. After the skin tissue absorbed the PBS, images of the microspheres were taken at increasing depths. The vasculature in the window chamber was imaged under bright-field with a CCD camera using a × 2 objective and overlaid with a fluorescence image using the same objective.

AZD2281–BODIPY FL (7.5 μl in DMSO) was mixed with 30 μl of 1:1 solutol:dimethylacetamide (Sigma) and slowly added to 112.5 μl of PBS. The drug was injected through a tail vein intravenously and imaged with MFAM using a × 25 objective. Confocal images of drug infusion into the tumour were taken using a × 2 objective.

Image processing. During image acquisition in two-photon microscopy only a small number of photons are typically measured by the photodetectors with numbers ranging from tens to a few thousands with a statistical variation in the recorded number following a Poisson model of the noise. At lower counts per pixel, the error on the calculated anisotropy value will be then increasingly higher, giving rise to images presenting severe noise artefacts (a rigorous treatment on the role of photon statistics on fluorescence polarization can be found in ref. 26). To account for noise-induced variation we decided therefore to statistically weight every pixel anisotropy value within each image by its corresponding total intensity. Intensity-weighted images were created by assigning colours based on anisotropy values, indicated by the scale bar, to each pixel in the fluorescence image. The intensity of the image is therefore dependent on the fluorescence intensity, while the colour is dependent on the calculated anisotropy.

In addition a BM3D collaborative filter was applied on each image[39].

Data analysis. Images were analysed in Matlab (Mathworks) and ImageJ. All anisotropy measurements were calculated from the equation $r = (I_\parallel - I_\perp)/(I_\parallel + 2I_\perp)$. The detector noise of the two photodetectors was subtracted from the whole images before the data were processed. Fluorescence intensity refers to the sum of both perpendicular and parallel channels. Anisotropy values were obtained by defining a region of interest and measuring the average anisotropy within that region. Regions were extended to fluorescent images to calculate the corresponding intensity.

References

1. Adibekian, A. et al. Confirming target engagement for reversible inhibitors in vivo by kinetically tuned activity-based probes. J. Am. Chem. Soc. **134**, 10345–10348 (2012).
2. Martinez Molina, D. et al. Monitoring drug target engagement in cells and tissues using the cellular thermal shift assay. Science **341**, 84–87 (2013).
3. Paul, S. M. et al. How to improve R&D productivity: the pharmaceutical industry's grand challenge. Nat. Rev. Drug Discov. **9**, 203–214 (2010).
4. Edgington, L. E. et al. Functional imaging of legumain in cancer using a new quenched activity-based probe. J. Am. Chem. Soc. **135**, 174–182 (2013).
5. Yang, K. S., Budin, G., Reiner, T., Vinegoni, C. & Weissleder, R. Bioorthogonal imaging of aurora kinase A in live cells. Angew Chem. Int. Ed. **51**, 6598–6603 (2012).
6. Yang, Z. et al. Folate-based near-infrared fluorescent theranostic gemcitabine delivery. J. Am. Chem. Soc. **135**, 11657–11662 (2013).
7. Thurber, G. M. et al. Single-cell and subcellular pharmacokinetic imaging allows insight into drug action in vivo. Nat. Commun. **4**, 1504 (2013).
8. van Dam, G. M. et al. Intraoperative tumour-specific fluorescence imaging in ovarian cancer by folate receptor-alpha targeting: first in-human results. Nat. Med. **17**, 1315–1319 (2011).
9. Simon, G. M., Niphakis, M. J. & Cravatt, B. F. Determining target engagement in living systems. Nat. Chem. Biol. **9**, 200–205 (2013).
10. Perrin, F. The polarisation of fluorescence light. Average life of molecules in their excited state. J. Phys. Radium **7**, 390–401 (1926).
11. Jameson, D. M. & Ross, J. A. Fluorescence polarization/anisotropy in diagnostics and imaging. Chem. Rev. **110**, 2685–2708 (2010).
12. Weber, G. Polarization of the fluorescence of macromolecules. I. Theory and experimental method. Biochem. J. **51**, 145–155 (1952).
13. Bigelow, C. E., Conover, D. L. & Foster, T. H. Confocal fluorescence spectroscopy and anisotropy imaging system. Opt. Lett. **28**, 695–697 (2003).
14. Varma, R. & Mayor, S. GPI-anchored proteins are organized in submicron domains at the cell surface. Nature **394**, 798–801 (1998).
15. Sharma, P. et al. Nanoscale organization of multiple GPI-anchored proteins in living cell membranes. Cell **116**, 577–589 (2004).
16. Weber, P., Wagner, M. & Schneckenburger, H. Fluorescence imaging of membrane dynamics in living cells. J. Biomed. Opt. **15**, 046017 (2010).
17. Vrabioiu, A. M. & Mitchison, T. J. Structural insights into yeast septin organization from polarized fluorescence microscopy. Nature **443**, 466–469 (2006).
18. Kampmann, M., Atkinson, C. E., Mattheyses, A. L. & Simon, S. M. Mapping the orientation of nuclear pore proteins in living cells with polarized fluorescence microscopy. Nat. Struct. Mol. Biol. **18**, 643–649 (2011).
19. Yu, Q. & Heikal, A. A. Two-photon autofluorescence dynamics imaging reveals sensitivity of intracellular NADH concentration and conformation to cell physiology at the single-cell level. J. Photochem. Photobiol. B **95**, 46–57 (2009).
20. Gough, A. H. & Taylor, D. L. Fluorescence anisotropy imaging microscopy maps calmodulin binding during cellular contraction and locomotion. J. Cell Biol. **121**, 1095–1107 (1993).
21. Lakowicz, J. R. Principles of Fluorescence Spectroscopy 3rd edn. (Springer, 2006).
22. Vishwasrao, H. D., Trifilieff, P. & Kandel, E. R. In vivo imaging of the actin polymerization state with two-photon fluorescence anisotropy. Biophys. J. **102**, 1204–1214 (2012).
23. Ghosh, N., Majumder, S. K. & Gupta, P. K. Fluorescence depolarization in a scattering medium: effect of size parameter of a scatterer. Phys. Rev. E Stat. Nonlin. Soft Matter. Phys. **65**, 026608 (2002).
24. Lakowicz, J. R., Gryczynski, I., Gryczynski, Z. & Danielsen, E. Time-resolved fluorescence intensity and anisotropy decays of 2,5-Diphenyloxazole by two-photon excitation and frequency-domain fluorometry. J. Phys. Chem. **96**, 3000–3006 (1992).
25. Axelrod, D. Fluorescence polarization microscopy. Methods Cell Biol. **30**, 333–352 (1989).
26. Lidke, K. A., Rieger, B., Lidke, D. S. & Jovin, T. M. The role of photon statistics in fluorescence anisotropy imaging. IEEE. Trans. Image Process **14**, 1237–1245 (2005).
27. Rossi, A. M. & Taylor, C. W. Analysis of protein-ligand interactions by fluorescence polarization. Nat. Protoc. **6**, 365–387 (2011).
28. Reiner, T. et al. Imaging therapeutic PARP inhibition in vivo through bioorthogonally developed companion imaging agents. Neoplasia **14**, 169–177 (2012).
29. Wahlberg, E. et al. Family-wide chemical profiling and structural analysis of PARP and tankyrase inhibitors. Nat. Biotechnol. **30**, 283–288 (2012).
30. Evers, B. et al. Selective inhibition of BRCA2-deficient mammary tumor cell growth by AZD2281 and cisplatin. Clin. Cancer Res. **14**, 3916–3925 (2008).
31. Gibson, B. A. & Kraus, W. L. New insights into the molecular and cellular functions of poly(ADP-ribose) and PARPs. Nat. Rev. Mol. Cell Biol. **13**, 411–424 (2012).
32. Dunn, A. K., Wallace, V. P., Coleno, M., Berns, M. W. & Tromberg, B. J. Influence of optical properties on two-photon fluorescence imaging in turbid samples. Appl. Opt. **39**, 1194–1201 (2000).
33. Hoffman, R. M. & Yang, M. Subcellular imaging in the live mouse. Nat. Protoc. **1**, 775–782 (2006).
34. Yamamoto, N. et al. Cellular dynamics visualized in live cells in vitro and in vivo by differential dual-colour nuclear-cytoplasmic fluorescent-protein expression. Cancer Res. **64**, 4251–4256 (2004).
35. Bahlmann, K. & Hell, S. W. Electric field depolarization in high aperture focusing with emphasis on annular apertures. J. Microsc. **200**, 59–67 (2000).
36. Schon, P., Munhoz, F., Gasecka, A., Brustlein, S. & Brasselet, S. Polarization distortion effects in polarimetric two-photon microscopy. Opt. Express **16**, 20891–20901 (2008).
37. Baeten, J., Niedre, M., Dunham, J. & Ntziachristos, V. Development of fluorescent materials for Diffuse Fluorescence Tomography standards and phantoms. Opt. Express **15**, 8681–8694 (2007).
38. Reiner, T., Earley, S., Turetsky, A. & Weissleder, R. Bioorthogonal small-molecule ligands for PARP1 imaging in living cells. Chembiochem. **11**, 2374–2377 (2010).
39. Dabov, K., Foi, A., Katkovnik, V. & Egiazarian, K. Image denoising by sparse 3-D transform-domain collaborative filtering. IEEE Trans. Image Process **16**, 2080–2095 (2007).

Acknowledgements

This project was funded in part by Federal funds from the National Heart, Lung and Blood Institute, National Institutes of Health, Department of Health and Human Services (under Contract No. HHSN268201000044C), National Cancer Institute (T32CA079443 and P50CA086355), and from the Institute of Biomedical Engineering (under R01EB006432), and in part by 1R01CA164448-01.

Author contributions

C.V. conceived and designed the study and built the set-up. C.V. and J.M.D. performed the experiments, acquired and elaborated the data, and wrote the manuscript. P.F.F. contributed to the writing of the manuscript and together with C.V. developed the noise-processing algorithm. L.A.C., C.V. and J.M.D. performed the FLIM measurements and L.A.C. contributed also to the writing of the manuscript. R.M. contributed to the experimental planning and the writing of the manuscript. R.W. contributed to the experimental planning, data analysis, funding and writing of the manuscript. All authors reviewed manuscript drafts, provided input on the content and approved the final version.

Additional information

5

Semi-permeable coatings fabricated from comb-polymers efficiently protect proteins *in vivo*

Mi Liu[1], Pål Johansen[2], Franziska Zabel[2], Jean-Christophe Leroux[1] & Marc A. Gauthier[1,3]

In comparison to neutral linear polymers, functional and architecturally complex (that is, non-linear) polymers offer distinct opportunities for enhancing the properties and performance of therapeutic proteins. However, understanding how to harness these parameters is challenging, and studies that capitalize on them *in vivo* are scarce. Here we present an *in vivo* demonstration that modification of a protein with a polymer of appropriate architecture can impart low immunogenicity, with a commensurably low loss of therapeutic activity. These combined properties are inaccessible by conventional strategies using linear polymers. For the model protein ʟ-asparaginase, a comb-polymer bio-conjugate significantly outperformed the linear polymer control in terms of lower immune response and more sustained bioactivity. The semi-permeability characteristics of the coatings are consistent with the phase diagram of the polymer, which will facilitate the application of this strategy to other proteins and with other therapeutic models.

[1] Institute of Pharmaceutical Sciences, Department of Chemistry and Applied Biosciences, Swiss Federal Institute of Technology Zurich (ETH Zurich), Zurich 8093, Switzerland. [2] Department of Dermatology, University Hospital Zurich, Zurich 8091, Switzerland. [3] Institut National de la Recherche Scientifique (INRS), EMT Research Center, Varennes, Quebec J3X 1S2, Canada. Correspondence and requests for materials should be addressed to M.A.G. (email: gauthier@emt.inrs.ca).

Many advances in biotechnology can be linked to the development of robust methods for producing well-defined functional polymers. For instance, anionic polymerization has yielded one of the first well-defined linear polymers, α-methoxy-poly(ethylene glycol) (mPEG), variants of which have profoundly marked the pharmaceutical sector as protective coatings for protein drugs[1–3]. Controlled radical polymerization has also permitted the design of numerous macromolecular drugs, polymer–drug and polymer–protein conjugates[4]. The state-of-the-art of tailored polymer synthesis is currently evolving, the controlled polymerization of functional monomers has become commonplace[5] and new tools for preparing polymers with defined sequences and topologies continue to emerge[6,7]. In comparison to neutral linear polymers, functional and architecturally complex, that is, nonlinear, polymers offer numerous additional opportunities for enhancing the potential of therapeutic proteins, but have only recently drawn attention in therapeutics. Maynard and co-workers have shown that basic fibroblast growth factor could be stabilized by covalent conjugation with a heparin-mimicking polymer containing styrene sulfonate and oligo(ethylene glycol) monomethyl ether methacrylate (OEGMA) units[8]. The conjugate was stable to a variety of environmentally and therapeutically relevant stressors such as heat, acid, storage and proteases. Keefe and Jiang showed how a poly(zwitterionic) polymer grafted to α-chymotrypsin strongly stabilized the latter, even towards strong denaturants, via non-covalent interactions between the polymer and the protein[9]. Unfortunately, in vivo studies are scarce. Leroux and co-workers recently demonstrated that the functionality of different polymers grafted to proline-specific endopeptidases could be manipulated to stabilize and alter the dwell time of orally administered enzymes at different locations in the gastrointestinal tract[10]. Such studies are crucial because trends and observations made in vitro often do not correlate with in vivo observations[11]. This is in part due to the complex and potentially unpredictable nature of the interactions between the conjugate and components of the body.

Our group has recently discovered that comb-shaped poly-OEGMA (pOEGMA) chains with well-defined aspect ratios could generate a molecular sieving effect in vitro when grafted to the surface of a protein[12]. Within a certain regime of polymer characteristics, small molecules could easily diffuse through the coating towards the catalytic site of an enzyme (that is, maintaining high activity), whereas macromolecules were simultaneously blocked. This selective permeability phenomenon, which cannot be emulated with linear mPEG, could be of exceptional value for reducing the immunogenicity of recombinant, non-human-derived therapeutic enzymes without hindering catalytic processing of small molecules. One protein that falls into this category is L-asparaginase (ASNase), an enzyme that is used for treating acute lymphoblastic leukaemia. This protein was one of the first to be modified with mPEG because of its propensity to cause severe hypersensitivity reactions (up to 20–30% of patients)[13] or suffer from 'silent inactivation' by the neutralizing or opsonizing antibodies[14,15]. Modification of ASNase with mPEG in part overcomes these problems[16], however, a key problem is that antibody responses against mPEG–ASNase continue to occur in ∼18% of patients[17–19].

In this study, a molecular sieving pOEGMA coating is optimized for ASNase. In a head-to-head comparison with mPEG–ASNase, pOEGMA–ASNase is ∼100-fold less recognized by anti-ASNase antibodies than mPEG–ASNase and 3,000-fold less than the native protein, with a commensurably low loss of activity. In addition, pOEGMA extends the circulation time of ASNase even in mice previously sensitized to ASNase. The semi-permeability characteristics of the coatings are consistent with the phase diagram of protein-bound pOEGMA, which demonstrates that one can design optimal pOEGMA coatings for proteins with little trial-and-error. Polymer architecture, via the comb-shaped nature of pOEGMA, is a potent parameter for optimizing the bioactivity of therapeutic proteins.

Results

Molecular sieving pOEGMA–ASNase bio-conjugates. ASNase, Fig. 1a, is a tetrameric protein that possesses four identical catalytic sites that transform L-asparagine (Asn) into L-aspartic acid (Asp). As seen in Fig. 1, the solvent-exposed amino groups (lysine and N-termini in red) are uniformly distributed on the surface of the protein and were converted into initiators for atom transfer radical polymerization. Three ASNase macro-initiators bearing on average $x = 24$, 32 and 36 initiators per protein tetramer were obtained. The degree of modification was assessed by matrix-assisted laser desorption/ionization–time of flight mass spectrometry, which showed symmetric distributions near ∼35 kDa (ASNase disassembles into its monomeric form in this experiment; Fig. 1b). The centre of these distributions was taken as the average degree of modification and correlated well with the feed ratios of reactants (Supplementary Fig. 1). Assuming ASNase to be a sphere with a 3.4-nm radius[20], these values of x were targeted based on the expectation that a polymer density of at least one pOEGMA chain per ∼4 nm² of protein surface is required to observe the sieving effect[12]. The polymerization of an OEGMA monomer with eight to ten oxyethylene units was initiated from these sites. Growing polymers directly from proteins is a powerful approach for generating complex bio-conjugates[21–25] and offers the advantage of producing a series of comparable bio-conjugates differing uniquely in the length of the polymer backbone (n). The length of the polymer backbone was varied by allowing the polymerizations to proceed for different times between 30 min and 4 h. The 19 unique bio-conjugates obtained showed monomodal size-exclusion chromatograms (Fig. 1c). The molecular weight characteristics of the pOEGMA chains were determined by three complementary methods and can be found in Supplementary Table 1. One ASNase conjugate bearing ca 42 chains of mPEG (5 kDa), determined by ¹H NMR spectroscopy (Supplementary Fig. 2), was produced for comparison. This grafting ratio is in the range expected of commercially available mPEG–ASNase conjugates (Sigma-Aldrich).

To characterize the molecular sieving characteristics of the conjugates, the conformation of pOEGMA was analysed by ¹H NMR spectroscopy (Fig. 2a,b) and correlated to the catalytic activity of the conjugates (aspartyl transferase assay; Fig. 2c) and their anti-ASNase-binding affinity (sandwich ELISA; Fig. 2d). As a comb-shaped polymer, pOEGMA can adopt either an ellipsoidal or a cylindrical shape as a function of increasing backbone length n (ref. 26). These two states result from the backbone being either in an collapsed or in an extended conformation, a parameter that can be probed by ¹H NMR spectroscopy via peaks 'A' and 'B' (Figs 1a and 2a). As 'A' is in close proximity to the polymer backbone (Fig. 1a), its integrated value, which becomes less than expected in a rigid un-solvated environment, can be used to estimate its mobility. For this, a reference mobile and solvent-exposed group whose integral is expected to be least affected by de-solvation of the main-chain, such as 'B', is required (Fig. 2a). Indeed, Roth et al. have shown that 'B' retained >92% of its integrated value during pOEGMA's soluble-to-insoluble transition in alcohol, whereas peak 'A' was strongly affected[27]. Herein, peak 'B' remained sharp over a wide range of n (12–48; Supplementary Fig. 3). Figure 2b plots the dimensionless flexibility factor F, calculated from A and B

($F = 3A \div 2B$), which varies between 1 when the backbone is fully solvated and flexible to 0 when it is un-solvated and rigid. The abrupt decrease of F followed by an increase as a function of n is characteristic of protein-bound pOEGMA undergoing an ellipsoid-to-cylinder transition. The increase at high n is observed because F reflects the average flexibility of the entire polymer chain, which increases as it extends away from the protein. The transition, identified by arrows in Fig. 2b, is then projected as a dashed line in Fig. 2c,d, which plot catalytic activity and anti-ASNase-binding affinity, respectively, as a function of x and n. Optimal molecular sieving characteristics were previously observed at n just below the transition between these two conformations[12]. Compared with the first values measured at low n, no statistically significant difference in the catalytic activity of the bio-conjugates was observed in the ellipsoidal regime. A decrease was then observed beyond the transition (Fig. 2c; full analysis of variance (ANOVA) table in Supplementary Table 2; fitted parameters in Supplementary Table 3). Shielding of epitopes, assayed via the ability of anti-ASNase antibodies to bind the conjugates, followed a single exponential decay with n (Fig. 2d; fitted parameters in Supplementary Fig. 4). Increasing the complexity of the fit to a double exponential did not improve the quality of the fit. The rate of decay was more pronounced at higher x, although no obvious manifestation of the change of conformation of pOEGMA was evident in these curves. In comparison to native ASNase, mPEG–ASNase was 1.5 times less catalytically active and 25-fold less recognized by anti-ASNase antibodies. A pOEGMA–ASNase conjugate with optimal semi-permeability characteristics ($x = 32$, $n = 17$) was only three times less active than the native protein, but was 3,000-fold less recognized by anti-ASNase. Thus, in relation to the small decrease of activity observed between the mPEG and pOEGMA bio-conjugates, the gain in epitope shielding *in vitro*, and potential for lower immunogenicity *in vivo* (*vide infra*), is enormous. This pOEGMA–ASNase conjugate ($x = 32$, $n = 17$) was selected for *in vivo* analysis because it offered the best compromise between loss of catalytic activity and efficient epitope shielding (Fig. 2c,d).

Circulation time and bioactivity of ASNase *in vivo*. Having demonstrated that grafting of pOEGMA did not eliminate catalytic activity, pharmacokinetic experiments were performed. Here $800\,\mathrm{IU\,kg^{-1}}$ of ASNase, mPEG–ASNase or pOEGMA–ASNase ($x = 32$, $n = 17$) were administered in saline by intra-peritoneal injection to groups of three BALB/c mice. Blood was withdrawn

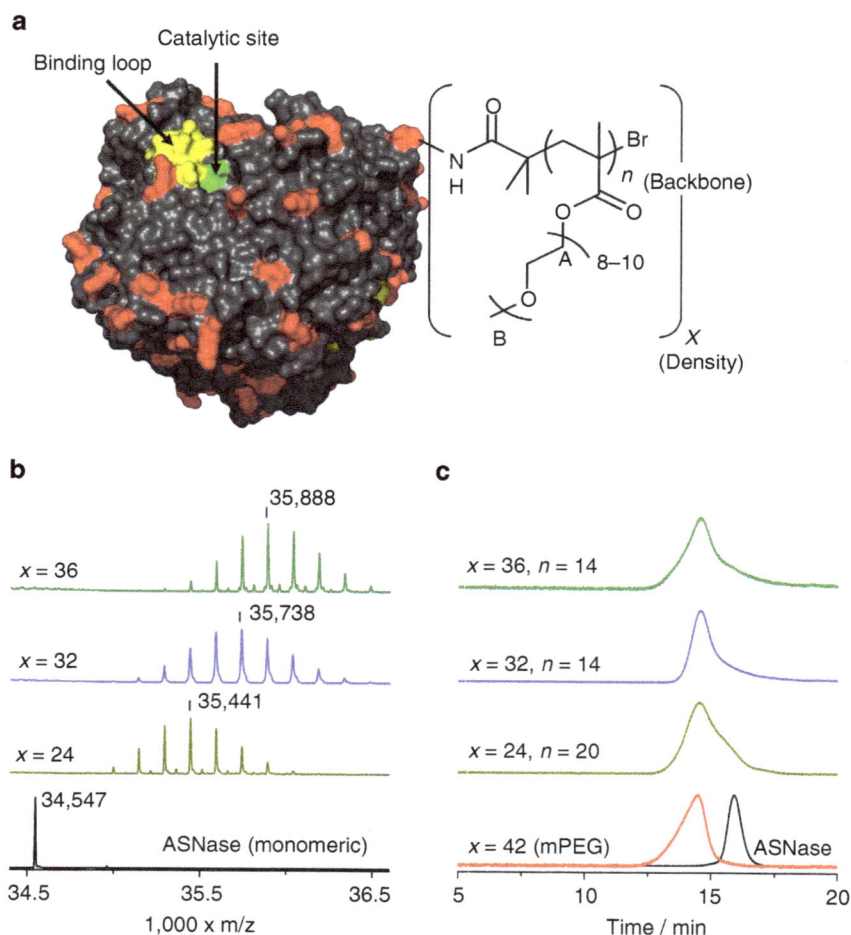

Figure 1 | Preparation of well-defined pOEGMA-ASNase conjugates. (a) Tetrameric ASNase possesses 92 amino groups (lysine residues and N-termini in red) that are evenly distributed on the solvent-exposed surface of the protein. Nineteen unique pOEGMA-ASNase conjugates were prepared by activation of a certain number (x) of these amino groups with 2-bromoisobutyryl bromide, followed *in situ* growth of different length (n) pOEGMA chains by atom transfer radical polymerization. **(b)** Analysis of the molecular weight of ASNase macro-initiators by matrix-assisted laser desorption/ionization–time of flight mass spectrometry to determine the average number of initiating groups per protein. **(c)** Representative size-exclusion chromatograms of pOEGMA-ASNase conjugates, mPEG-ASNase and native ASNase. All conjugates tested displayed monomodal molecular-weight distributions.

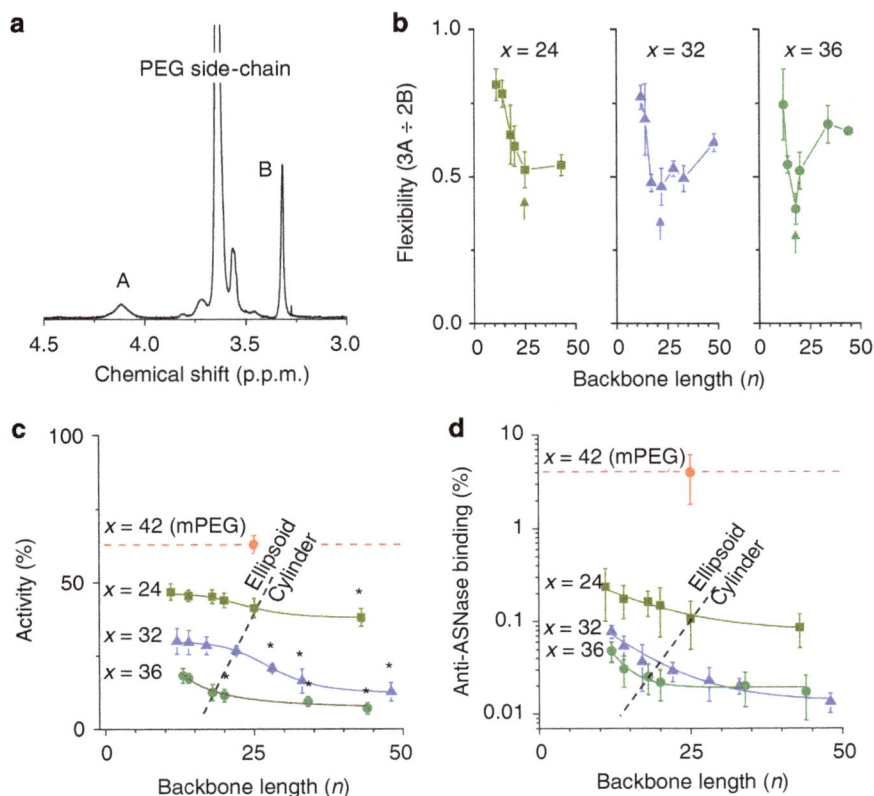

Figure 2 | Molecular sieving characteristics of pOEGMA–ASNase conjugates. (a) Representative ^{1}H NMR spectrum of a pOEGMA–ASNase conjugate with peaks corresponding to 'A' and 'B' from Fig. 1a identified. **(b)** Analysis of the flexibility F of the pOEGMA backbone permits the identification of the transition between ellipsoidal to cylindrical at the local minimum of the curve (arrow). **(c,d)** Enzymatic activity and anti-ASNase-binding affinity of ASNase-polymer conjugates, both relative to native ASNase, plotted as a function of polymer backbone length n. In **c**, star symbols indicate that the measured activity is statistically different from the value at lowest n (ANOVA, Tukey $P = 0.05$; Supplementary Table 2). The sigmoidal curve fit **(c)** and single exponential decay **(d)** used to fit the data are to guide the eye. mPEG-ASNase is shown as a line and a symbol in the centre of the graph for ease of comparison. Mean $\pm$ s.d. ($n = 3$).

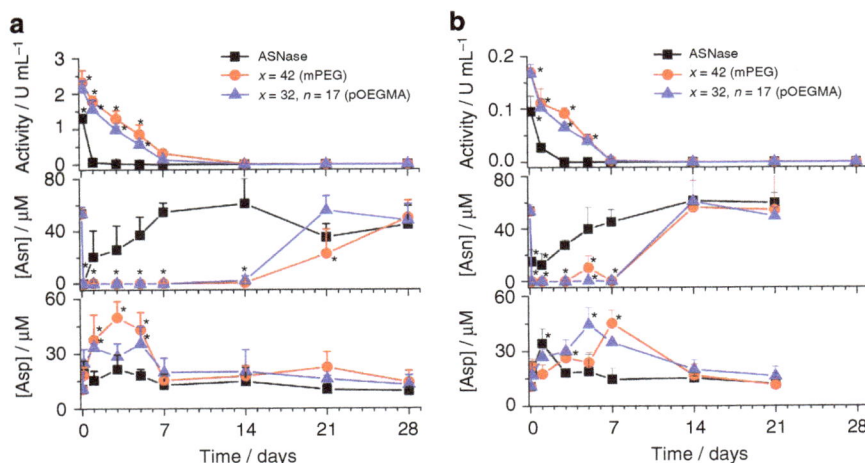

Figure 3 | Pharmacokinetics of ASNase and ASNase bio-conjugates. (a) 800 IU kg^{-1} or **(b)** 80 IU kg^{-1} of ASNase, mPEG-ASNase or pOEGMA-ASNase were administered and the catalytic activity, L-asparagine (Asn) concentration and L-aspartic acid (Asp) concentration monitored in blood samples taken at different intervals. The ASNase bio-conjugates showed similar profiles demonstrating that pOEGMA can convey long circulation to proteins, despite being in a compact conformation. Mean + s.d., $n = 3$. Stars denote statistically significant differences with respect to the natural ASNase activity of blood or to the initial concentration of Asn or Asp (Tukey, $P < 0.05$). When data points are superimposed, only a single star is shown for clarity.

at regular intervals from the tail vein for analysis of residual ASNase catalytic activity and for analysis of the concentration of Asn and Asp. Native ASNase was rapidly cleared from the body, as evidenced by the complete loss of activity within 1–2 days (Fig. 3a). Both mPEG–ASNase and pOEGMA–ASNase displayed

sustained activity and depletion of blood Asn below the limit of detection (250 nM) for ca 14 days. At day 21, mPEG–ASNase was the only sample not to have reached its initial Asn concentration. The longer circulation time of mPEG–ASNase is consistent with its slightly larger hydrodynamic diameter (30 ± 5 and 25 ± 5 nm for mPEG–ASNase and pOEGMA–ASNase, respectively) measured by dynamic light scattering. Thus, despite the expected compact conformation of the pOEGMA backbone in its ellipsoidal state, the hydrodynamic volume of the conjugate is sufficient for extended circulation. A transient increase of blood Asp was observed, consistent with the observations of others[28], indicating that depletion of Asn is occurring according to the expected catalytic mechanism. The observed difference between blood activity and Asn concentration could reflect distribution of the conjugate outside the blood compartment. A lower dose group, receiving 80 IU kg^{-1}, was also investigated and yielded comparable conclusions (Fig. 3b).

Epitope shielding *in vivo*. To assess the efficiency with which the polymers shielded epitopes on ASNase, BALB/c mice were immunized with either ASNase or ASNase bio-conjugates using aluminum hydroxide as adjuvant. Groups of five mice received 20 µg (protein content) of native ASNase, mPEG–ASNase or pOEGMA–ASNase (same conjugates as above) by subcutaneous injections. Analytes were administered on an equal weight (protein) basis to more easily compare their relative ability to generate immune responses. Different results might be expected if the analytes were administered on an equal activity basis, as a lower amount of more active analytes would be administered. For instance, as mPEG–ASNase is twice as active as the selected pOEGMA–ASNase, half as much of it would have been administered. It should also be noted that sensitization was promoted by an adjuvant to test immunogenicity in an accelerated way and that a much lower immune response is to be expected in its absence. Four injections were done with 2-week intervals. Blood was withdrawn on days 28, 42 and 71, and IgG titres towards either ASNase or the bio-conjugate itself were measured. In comparison to the native protein, immunization with mPEG–ASNase and pOEGMA–ASNase conjugates stimulated significantly lower anti-ASNase IgG (Fig. 4a,b; orange bars). The results also revealed that immunization with pOEGMA stimulated ~20-fold lower anti-ASNase IgG titres than immunization with mPEG–ASNase, and ~1,000-fold lower than with the native protein. To compare the relative levels of antibodies raised against the conjugates themselves, ELISA plates were coated with mPEG–ASNase or pOEGMA–ASNase (Fig. 4a,b; blue bars). The amounts of absorbed native ASNase and ASNase conjugates were verified in order to guarantee that the same amount of protein content was coated into each well, which permits comparisons to be made. On day 28, that is, 2 weeks after the second immunization,

low titres of anti-mPEG–ASNase-specific IgG were determined, whereas no pOEGMA–ASNase-specific IgG was detected (Fig. 4a). On day 71, 1 month after four immunizations, low conjugate-specific IgG titres were detected for both formulations, but the titre was approximately 20 times lower in serum from mice immunized with pOEGMA–ASNase. Similar results were observed in serum taken on day 42 (Supplementary Fig. 5). These results demonstrate the effectiveness of the comb-shaped polymer in shielding epitopes of ASNase in the adaptive environment of the body. This result is also interesting in light of reports that antibodies can be raised against the polymer component (for example, mPEG) of bio-conjugates and mPEG–ASNase itself[29,30]. For robustness, the sensitization experiment was repeated by administrating a higher dose of analyte (200 µg protein per injection) into ASNase-naïve mice according to the same schedule as above. The tenfold increase in ASNase dose resulted in a general three- fourfold increase of IgG titres in all samples analysed, but again with pOEGMA–ASNase producing much lower titres than mPEG–ASNase and native ASNase (Supplementary Fig. 6).

Bioactivity of ASNase in ASNase-sensitized mice. Long-term treatment with ASNase can produce unwanted antibody responses against the enzyme. This may compromise the biological activity of the therapeutic enzyme. To assess the biological activity of ASNase in such a sensitization model, mice having received the multiple doses of ASNase, mPEG–ASNase or pOEGMA–ASNase according to the schedule above, then received an intra-peritoneal injection of 800 IU kg^{-1} of the corresponding ASNase formulation 4 weeks after the last of four immunizations. Before injection, Asn concentrations in blood were normal and the sensitizing ASNase preparations had no residual enzymatic activity. As seen in Fig. 4c, neither native ASNase nor mPEG–ASNase were able to maintain full depletion of blood Asn beyond the first 3 h after injection, whereas full depletion was still observed for pOEGMA–ASNase at day 3. Normal Asn levels were observed by day 7 for both native ASNase and mPEG–ASNase and by day 14 for pOEGMA–ASNase. Although the half-lives of both polymer–ASNase conjugates were significantly shorter than those observed in the non-sensitized animals, the longer circulation time of pOEGMA–ASNase vs mPEG–ASNase appears to reflect the lower immune response raised for this conjugate during sensitization and suggests that pOEGMA conveys better stealth-like characteristics to ASNase than does mPEG, even after repeated dosing.

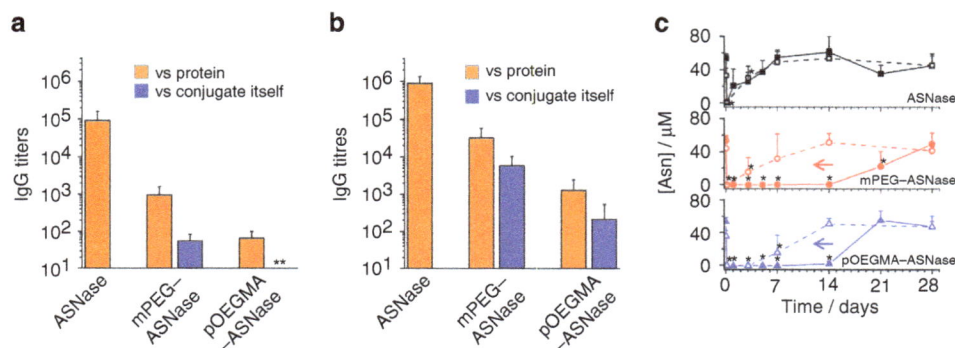

Figure 4 | Development of new antibodies *in vivo*. BALB/c mice were sensitized with either native ASNase, mPEG–ASNase ($x = 42$) or pOEGMA–ASNase ($x = 32$, $n = 17$). (**a,b**) IgG titres at days 28 and 71. Double stars indicates that signal in undiluted serum was undetectable. (**c**) Comparison of pharmacokinetic profiles of unsensitized (filled symbols, from Fig. 3a) and sensitized mice administered ASNase and ASNase bio-conjugates on day 72. Mean + s.d. ($n = 5$). Single star denotes statistically significant differences with respect to the natural concentration of Asn (ANOVA, Tukey, $P < 0.05$). When data points are superimposed, only a single star is shown for clarity. Horizontal arrow indicates shift of the curve because of sensitization.

Discussion

The desire to effectively shield enzymes with polymers, without compromising activity, has driven multiple systematic studies in which the influence of grafting density, polymer molecular weight, polymer type (that is, synthetic, natural), coupling chemistry and so on, have been examined[31,32]. However, studies that directly compare linear polymers to (related) branched ones are rare. In two important studies, Veronese and co-workers compared the activity, pH and temperature stability, and proteolytic digestion of ASNase (from *Erwinia Carotivora*) and three other enzymes modified with either linear mPEG or double-branched mPEG (mPEG$_2$)[33,34]. Although, for the most part, catalytic activity was similar for the mPEG and mPEG$_2$ bio-conjugates, all of the enzymes modified with mPEG$_2$ were more resistant to proteolysis. This is consistent with the more facile diffusion of small vs large molecules through the polymer coating, as observed herein. Furthermore, the antigenicity of the mPEG$_2$–ASNase conjugate was lower than for the mPEG analogue, although the difference was smaller than that observed herein. The present study expands upon these observations and emphasizes how controlling the molecular dimensions of the architecturally complex polymer pOEGMA beneficially reduces the immunogenicity of a subclass of biomolecules with diffusible small molecules as their substrates.

Dense pOEGMA coatings are well-known to efficiently repel the adsorption of proteins to solid surfaces, such as gold[35,36]. However, the application of this strategy to protect proteins themselves has met little attention. The dissuading dogma is the expected strong negative effect multiple polymer conjugation will have on the protein's bioactivity because of obstructed interaction with its binding partners, substrates and so on[31]. To our knowledge, Magnusson *et al.*[37] have presented the only *in vivo* study of the shielding efficacy of multiple pOEGMA chains on a protein, recombinant human growth hormone. The beneficial properties observed, however, were attributed to enhanced stability and prolonged pharmacokinetic profile, which counterbalanced the expected loss of activity, rather than to an intrinsic characteristic of nonlinear polymers or pOEGMA itself. Of course, the mechanism of action of recombinant human growth hormone involves receptor binding rather than enzymatic activity, which is probably why the relevance of the architecture of pOEGMA was not discussed. Other *in vivo* studies have focused on extending the circulation half-life of proteins with single pOEGMA chains[38-40]. Thus, the most significant contribution herein is the demonstration of the particularity of pOEGMA, which can be conveniently and rationally manipulated to address the dogma of loss of activity, even in the complex environment *in vivo*. This is an important finding because many non-human-derived proteins, including ASNase, possess numerous epitopes or enzyme-sensitive segments that can be responsible for treatment failure if they are not adequately shielded[41,42]. In fact, as ASNase is a homo-tetrameric protein, all epitopes are present in four identical copies. Thus, this type of protein absolutely requires multiple polymer conjugation because of the inability of a single (or a few) polymer chains to adequately shield these problematic parts of the protein[43,44]. Finally, it is worth considering that pOEGMA is attached to the protein via an amide bond and is unlikely to be released from the conjugates within the timeframe of the experiments performed. Ultimately, however, one would expect degradation of ASNase, which would release single pOEGMA chains connected to short peptide segments. Considering the molecular weight of the pOEGMA used (that is, $n = 17$ is ~8 kDa), it should ultimately be eliminated by, for example, renal filtration.

In summary, this study is the first *in vivo* demonstration of how polymer architecture, via the comb-shaped nature of

pOEGMA, provides a unique design parameter for optimizing therapeutic proteins. The combined properties of effective epitope shielding with proportionally low loss of activity are inaccessible by conventional 'PEGylation' using linear polymers. Using ASNase as a model therapeutic protein, the designed pOEGMA bio-conjugate outperformed the mPEG–ASNase control (of similar catalytic activity) by being less immunogenic and providing a more sustained activity in sensitized animals. This shows promise for long-term therapies involving pOEGMA-modified proteins. Importantly, observations were consistent with predictions made from the phase diagram of protein-bound pOEGMA[12]. This guided the design of optimal semi-permeable coatings alongside convenient spectroscopic analysis of polymer conformation. This implies that one can easily design optimal pOEGMA coatings for proteins with little trial-and-error. One caveat is the limitation to therapeutic proteins that target soluble substrates small enough to penetrate through the pOEGMA coating. This makes the findings above most applicable to enzymes such as asparaginase, methioninase, arginine deiminase, arginase, uricase and so on[32]. Nevertheless, the presented strategy could also be used to protect and alter the circulation lifetime of emerging classes of therapeutics, such as small-molecule-binding proteins that could be used as drug scavengers[45], and create non-fouling coatings for biosensors that are specific towards small analytes.

Methods

ASNase pOEGMA-ASNase and mPEG-ASNase. *E. coli* ASNase was purchased from Afine Chemicals Ltd and de-salted before use. The synthesis, purification and characterization of ASNase bio-conjugates follow a robust procedure adapted from the original work of Lele *et al.*[22] and is described in detail in the Supplementary Methods.

In vitro **catalytic activity.** ASNase and ASNase bio-conjugate catalytic activities were assayed by the formation of aspartate hydroxamate from Asn and hydroxylamine (aspartyl transferase activity). 20 µl of a 50 µg ml^{-1} (protein) aqueous enzyme solution were added to 1 ml Tris-HCl buffer (100 mM, pH 7.4) containing 20 µM Asn and 400 µM hydroxylamine. The mixture was incubated at 37 °C for 30 min, after which 700 µl of ferric chloride agent (5% ferric chloride, 1 M HCl, 4% trichloroacetic acid) were added. Aspartate hydroxamate forms a coloured complex with ferric chloride that can be quantified at 500 nm (ref. 46).

In vitro **recognition by anti-ASNase antibodies.** Streptavidin-coated 96-well microplates (Pierce) were rinsed with 3 × 200 µl wash buffer (25 mM Tris, 150 mM NaCl, 0.25% bovine serum albumin, 0.05% Tween-20, pH 7.2) after which 100 µl of biotinylated anti-asparaginase antibody (10 µg ml^{-1}) wash buffer were added and incubated for 2 h room temperature. The wells were rinsed with 3 × 200 µl wash buffer after which 100 µl of serial dilutions of native ASNase (1 µg ml^{-1} to 1 pg ml^{-1}) were incubated for 30 min at room temperature to obtain a response curve. Thereafter, 100 µl of either mPEG–ASNase or pOEGMA–ASNase (1 µg ml^{-1}) were analysed in the same manner and the value compared with this response curve. The wells were rinsed with 3 × 200 µl wash buffer, and 100 µl horseradish peroxidase-labelled anti-asparaginase antibody (4 µg ml^{-1} in wash buffer) was added and incubated for 30 min. After a final rinse with 6 × 200 µl wash buffer, 100 µl 1-Step Slow TMB-ELISA Substrate Solution was added. After exactly 10 min, 50 µl 2 N HCl was added and absorbance of each well was measured at 450 nm.

Pharmacokinetics in naïve mice. All animal protocols were approved and conducted according to the guidelines of the Cantonal Veterinary Office Zurich. Groups of three female BALB/c mice (25 g) were administered either 80 or 800 IU kg^{-1} of ASNase, pOEGMA–ASNase ($x = 32$, $n = 17$) or mPEG–ASNase ($x = 42$) in 100 µl sterile saline by intra-peritoneal injection. One international unit (IU) of activity is defined herein as the amount of enzyme that catalyses the formation of 1.0 mmol of Asp per min at 25 °C. Approximately 50 µl blood was sampled from the tail vein repeatedly over 28 days, and was immediately centrifuged for collection of serum that was stored frozen (-80 °C) until analysed.

Sensitization and enzymatic activity in sensitized mice. Groups of five female BALB/c mice were immunized on days 0, 15, 29 and 43 by subcutaneous injections of 100 µl of a sterile saline solution containing either 20 or 200 µg protein content in ASNase, pOEGMA–ASNase ($x = 32$, $n = 17$) or mPEG–ASNase ($x = 42$). All vaccine preparations also contained 0.6 wt% Alhydrogel (Brenntag Biosector). Blood was collected on days 28, 42 and 71 as described above. On day 72, all mice from the low-dose groups were administered $800\,\mathrm{IU\,kg^{-1}}$ of the corresponding ASNase or ASNase bio-conjugate in $100\,\mu l$ sterile saline by intra-peritoneal injection, and blood was sampled for measurement of Asn metabolism as described above.

Blood analysis. Bioactivity of native ASNase and polymer-modified ASNase was measured with an Asparaginase Activity Assay Kit (MAK007, Sigma-Aldrich) according to the manufacturer's recommended protocol. The concentrations of Asn and Asp in mice serum were analysed using pre-column derivatization high-performance liquid chromatography (Supplementary Figs 7 and 8) according to a method modified from Bidlingmeyer and described in the Supplementary Methods[47]. Blood antibody titres were measured by sandwich ELISA as described in the Supplementary Methods.

Statistics. Means from activity tests were compared by one-way ANOVA followed by a Tukey *post-hoc* test. Means from pharmacokinetics data were compared by one-way repeated-measures ANOVA followed by a Tukey *post-hoc* test. Differences were considered significant at $P<0.05$.

References

1. Harris, J. M. & Chess, R. B. Effect of pegylation on pharmaceuticals. *Nat. Rev. Drug Discov.* **2**, 214–221 (2003).
2. Pasut, G. & Veronese, F. M. State of the art in PEGylation: The great versatility achieved after forty years of research. *J. Control. Release* **161**, 461–472 (2012).
3. Alconcel, S. N. S., Baas, A. S. & Maynard, H. D. FDA-approved poly(ethylene glycol)-protein conjugate drugs. *Polym. Chem.* **2**, 1442–1448 (2011).
4. Duncan, R. The dawning era of polymer therapeutics. *Nat. Rev. Drug Discov.* **2**, 347–360 (2003).
5. Matyjaszewski, K. & Tsarevsky, N. V. Nanostructured functional materials prepared by atom transfer radical polymerization. *Nat. Chem.* **1**, 276–288 (2009).
6. Schmidt BVKJ, Fechler N, Falkenhagen, J. & Lutz, J.-F. Controlled folding of synthetic polymer chains through the formation of positionable covalent bridges. *Nat. Chem.* **3**, 234–238 (2011).
7. Kissel, P. *et al.* A two-dimensional polymer prepared by organic synthesis. *Nat. Chem.* **4**, 287–291 (2012).
8. Nguyen, T. H. *et al.* A heparin-mimicking polymer conjugate stabilizes basic fibroblast growth factor. *Nat. Chem.* **5**, 221–227 (2013).
9. Keefe, A. J. & Jiang, S. Poly(zwitterionic)protein conjugates offer increased stability without sacrificing binding affinity or bioactivity. *Nat. Chem.* **4**, 59–63 (2012).
10. Fuhrmann, G. *et al.* Sustained gastrointestinal activity of dendronized polymer–enzyme conjugates. *Nat. Chem.* **5**, 582–589 (2013).
11. Fuhrmann, G. & Leroux, J.-C. *In vivo* fluorescence imaging of exogenous enzyme activity in the gastrointestinal tract. *Proc. Natl Acad. Sci. USA* **108**, 9032–9037 (2011).
12. Liu, M. *et al.* Molecular Sieving on the Surface of a Protein Provides Protection Without Loss of Activity. *Adv. Funct. Mater.* **23**, 2007–2015 (2013).
13. Fu, C. H. & Sakamoto, K. M. PEG-asparaginase. *Expert Opin. Pharmacother.* **8**, 1977–1984 (2007).
14. Müller, H.-J. *et al.* Pharmacokinetics of native *Escherichia coli* asparaginase (Asparaginase medac) and hypersensitivity reactions in ALL-BFM 95 reinduction treatment. *Br. J. Haematol.* **114**, 794–799 (2001).
15. Hak, L. J. *et al.* Asparaginase pharmacodynamics differ by formulation among children with newly diagnosed acute lymphoblastic leukemia. *Leukemia* **18**, 1072–1077 (2004).
16. Avramis, V. I. *et al.* A randomized comparison of native *Escherichia coli* asparaginase and polyethylene glycol conjugated asparaginase for treatment of children with newly diagnosed standard-risk acute lymphoblastic leukemia: a Children's Cancer Group study. *Blood* **99**, 1986–1994 (2002).
17. Asselin, B. L. *et al.* Comparative pharmacokinetic studies of three asparaginase preparations. *J. Clin. Oncol.* **11**, 1780–1786 (1993).
18. Salzer, W. L. *et al.* Intensified PEG-L-asparaginase and antimetabolite-based therapy for treatment of higher risk precursor-B acute lymphoblastic leukemia: a Report From the Children's Oncology Group. *J. Pediatr. Hematol. Oncol.* **29**, 369–375 (2007).
19. Schrey, D. *et al.* Therapeutic drug monitoring of asparaginase in the ALL-BFM 2000 protocol between 2000 and 2007. *Pediatr. Blood Cancer* **54**, 952–958 (2010).
20. Murthy, N. S. & Knox, J. R. Small-angle X-ray scattering studies of *Escherichia coli* l-asparaginase. *J. Mol. Biol.* **105**, 567–575 (1976).
21. Lucon, J. *et al.* Use of the interior cavity of the P22 capsid for site-specific initiation of atom-transfer radical polymerization with high-density cargo loading. *Nat. Chem.* **4**, 781–788 (2012).
22. Lele, B. S., Murata, H., Matyjaszewski, K. & Russell, A. J. Synthesis of Uniform Protein – Polymer Conjugates. *Biomacromolecules* **6**, 3380–3387 (2005).
23. Cummings, C., Murata, H., Koepsel, R. & Russell, A. J. Tailoring enzyme activity and stability using polymer-based protein engineering. *Biomaterials* **34**, 7437–7443 (2013).
24. Murata, H., Cummings, C. S., Koepsel, R. R. & Russell, A. J. Polymer-Based Protein Engineering Can Rationally Tune Enzyme Activity, pH-Dependence, and Stability. *Biomacromolecules* **14**, 1919–1926 (2013).
25. Cummings, C., Murata, H., Koepsel, R. & Russell, A. J. Dramatically increased pH and temperature stability of chymotrypsin using dual block polymer-based protein engineering. *Biomacromolecules* **15**, 763–771 (2014).
26. Cheng, G. *et al.* Small angle neutron scattering study of conformation of oligo(ethylene glycol)-grafted polystyrene in dilute solutions: effect of the backbone length. *Macromolecules* **41**, 9831–9836 (2008).
27. Roth, P. J., Davis, T. P. & Lowe, A. B. Comparison between the LCST and UCST transitions of double thermoresponsive diblock copolymers: insights into the behavior of POEGMA in alcohols. *Macromolecules* **45**, 3221–3230 (2012).
28. Ho, D. H. *et al.* Polyethylene glycol-L-asparaginase and L-asparaginase studies in rabbits. *Drug Metab. Dispos.* **16**, 27–29 (1988).
29. Garay, R. P., El-Gewely, R., Armstrong, J. K., Garratty, G. & Richette, P. Antibodies against polyethylene glycol in healthy subjects and in patients treated with PEG-conjugated agents. *Expert Opin. Drug Deliv.* **9**, 1319–1323 (2012).
30. Armstrong, J. K. *et al.* Antibody against poly(ethylene glycol) adversely affects PEG-asparaginase therapy in acute lymphoblastic leukemia patients. *Cancer* **110**, 103–111 (2007).
31. Gauthier, M. A. & Klok, H.-A. Polymer-protein conjugates: an enzymatic activity perspective. *Polym. Chem.* **1**, 1352–1373 (2010).
32. Pasut, G., Sergi, M. & Veronese, F. M. Anti-cancer PEG-enzymes: 30 years old, but still a current approach. *Adv. Drug Deliv. Rev.* **60**, 69–78 (2008).
33. Veronese, F. M. *et al.* Improvement of pharmacokinetic, immunological and stability properties of asparaginase by conjugation to linear and branched monomethoxy poly(ethylene glycol). *J. Control. Release* **40**, 199–209 (1996).
34. Monfardini, C. *et al.* A branched monomethoxypoly(ethylene glycol) for protein modification. *Bioconjug. Chem.* **6**, 62–69 (1995).
35. Ma, H., Wells, M., Beebe, T. P. & Chilkoti, A. Surface-initiated atom transfer radical polymerization of oligo(ethylene glycol) methyl methacrylate from a mixed self-assembled monolayer on gold. *Adv. Funct. Mater.* **16**, 640–648 (2006).
36. Ma, H., Hyun, J., Stiller, P. & Chilkoti, A. 'Non-fouling' oligo(ethylene glycol)-functionalized polymer brushes synthesized by surface-initiated atom transfer radical polymerization. *Adv. Mater.* **16**, 338–341 (2004).
37. Magnusson, J. P., Bersani, S., Salmaso, S., Alexander, C. & Caliceti, P. *In situ* growth of side-chain peg polymers from functionalized human growth hormone—a new technique for preparation of enhanced protein – polymer conjugates. *Bioconjug. Chem.* **21**, 671–678 (2010).
38. Gao, W. P., Liu, W. G., Christensen, T., Zalutsky, M. R. & Chilkoti, A. *In situ* growth of a PEG-like polymer from the C terminus of an intein fusion protein improves pharmacokinetics and tumor accumulation. *Proc. Natl Acad. Sci. USA* **107**, 16432–16437 (2010).
39. Gao, W. P. *et al.* *In situ* growth of a stoichiometric PEG-like conjugate at a protein's N-terminus with significantly improved pharmacokinetics. *Proc. Natl Acad. Sci. USA* **106**, 15231–15236 (2009).
40. Ryan, S. M. *et al.* Conjugation of salmon calcitonin to a combed-shaped end functionalized poly(poly(ethylene glycol) methyl ether methacrylate) yields a bioactive stable conjugate. *J. Control. Release* **135**, 51–59 (2009).
41. Werner, A., Röhm, K.-H. & Müller, H.-J. Mapping of B-cell epitopes in *E. coli* asparaginase II, an enzyme used in leukemia treatment. In: *Biol. Chem.* **386**, 535–540 (2005).
42. Patel, N. *et al.* A dyad of lymphoblastic lysosomal cysteine proteases degrades the antileukemic drug l-asparaginase. *J. Clin. Invest.* **119**, 1964–1973 (2009).
43. Shaunak, S. *et al.* Site-specific PEGylation of native disulfide bonds in therapeutic proteins. *Nat. Chem. Biol.* **2**, 312–313 (2006).
44. Balan, S. *et al.* Site-specific PEGylation of protein disulfide bonds using a three-carbon bridge. *Bioconjug. Chem.* **18**, 61–76 (2006).
45. Tinberg, C. E. *et al.* Computational design of ligand-binding proteins with high affinity and selectivity. *Nature* **501**, 212–216 (2013).
46. Jayaram, H. N., Cooney, D. A., Jayaram, S. & Rosenblu, L. Simple and rapid method for estimation of L-asparaginase in chromatographic and electrophoretic effluents - comparison with other methods. *Anal. Biochem.* **59**, 327–346 (1974).
47. Bidlingmeyer, B. A., Cohen, S. A. & Tarvin, T. L. Rapid analysis of amino-acids using pre-column derivatization. *J. Chromatogr.* **336**, 93–104 (1984).

Acknowledgements

M.L. recognizes a doctoral scholarship from the Chinese Scholarship Council (CSC). Funding from the Sassella foundation (11/06) is gratefully acknowledged.

Author contributions

M.L., P.J., J.-C.L. and M.A.G. designed and conceived the study; M.L. synthesized and analysed all compounds. M.L. conducted all *in vivo* experiments with the help of F.Z. and P.J.; M.L., P.J., J.-C.L. and M.A.G. co-wrote the paper. All authors discussed the results and their implications, and commented on the manuscript at all stages.

Additional information

Competing financial interests: The authors declare no competing financial interests.

6

Externally controlled on-demand release of anti-HIV drug using magneto-electric nanoparticles as carriers

Madhavan Nair[1], Rakesh Guduru[1], Ping Liang[2], Jeongmin Hong[1], Vidya Sagar[1] & Sakhrat Khizroev[1,2]

Although highly active anti-retroviral therapy has resulted in remarkable decline in the morbidity and mortality in AIDS patients, inadequately low delivery of anti-retroviral drugs across the blood–brain barrier results in virus persistence. The capability of high-efficacy-targeted drug delivery and on-demand release remains a formidable task. Here we report an *in vitro* study to demonstrate the on-demand release of azidothymidine 5′-triphosphate, an anti-human immunodeficiency virus drug, from 30 nm $CoFe_2O_4$@$BaTiO_3$ magneto-electric nanoparticles by applying a low alternating current magnetic field. Magneto-electric nanoparticles as field-controlled drug carriers offer a unique capability of field-triggered release after crossing the blood–brain barrier. Owing to the intrinsic magnetoelectricity, these nanoparticles can couple external magnetic fields with the electric forces in drug–carrier bonds to enable remotely controlled delivery without exploiting heat. Functional and structural integrity of the drug after the release was confirmed in *in vitro* experiments with human immunodeficiency virus-infected cells and through atomic force microscopy, spectrophotometry, Fourier transform infrared and mass spectrometry studies.

[1] Department of Immunology, Center for Personalized Nanomedicine, Herbert Wertheim College of Medicine, Florida International University, Miami, Florida 33174, USA. [2] Department of Electrical Engineering, University of California, Riverside, California 92521, USA. Correspondence and requests for materials should be addressed to S.K. (email: khizroev@fiu.edu).

Although highly active anti-retroviral therapy has resulted in remarkable decline in the morbidity and mortality in AIDS patients, zero or inadequately low delivery of anti-retroviral drugs across the blood–brain barrier (BBB) and into the brain and other tissue organs results in virus persistence[1-3]. Hence, the elimination of human immunodeficiency virus-1 (HIV-1) reservoirs still remains a formidable task[4,5]. In recent years, use of nanotechnology in medicine has shown exciting prospect for the development of novel remotely controlled drug delivery systems[6,7]. Besides magnetic nanoparticles (MNs)[8-10], other delivery systems rely on using thermally responsive polymers, optically (ultraviolet (UV), visible wavelength and IR) and acoustically activated nanostructures, liposomes, electro-chemical processes and others. An extensive review of these and other active triggering approaches was presented in the article by Timko et al.[11]. The unique advantages of magnetically forced triggering place this approach in a class of its own. In this case, the speed of delivery is determined by the external magnetic field. For instance, as it is related to the delivery across the BBB, this approach provides a way to deliver drugs sufficiently fast to avoid their engulfing by the reticuloendothelial system. Nucleotide reverse transcriptase inhibitor 3′-azido-3′-deoxythymidine-5′-triphosphate (AZTTP) is among the most challenging anti-retroviral drugs to deliver across the BBB[12,13]. Previously we have shown that MNs tagged with AZTTP transmigrated across the BBB by the application of an external magnetic field without affecting the integrity of the BBB, and the transmigrated AZTTP demonstrated significant inhibition of HIV-1 p24 antigen production in an in vitro infection model system compared with the free AZTTP[14]. However, this MN-based delivery suffers from the lack of certainty of drug release from the carrier if and when the nano-carrier reaches the target. The current presumptive mechanisms of drug delivery depend on manually uncontrollable cellular phenomena such as exocytosis of drug containing intracellular vesicle, intracellular Ca^{2+} concentrations and pathology-specific responses (change in pH,

temperature, and so on)[15]. As a result, to obtain a relatively small physiologic change and to ensure the release of the drug, the binding force between the nano-carrier and the drug must be maintained relatively weak. Consequently, more than 99% of the drug/carriers are deposited in the liver, lungs and other lymphoid organs before they reach the target. Therefore, an approach for finely controlled and enhanced release of AZTTP in sufficient therapeutic levels in the brain or in other target organs is still sought after, as it is critical for the complete eradication of HIV.

We present a study to demonstrate that dissipation-free, energy-efficient and low-field on-demand drug release can be achieved if the conventional MN carriers are replaced by magneto-electric (ME) nanoparticles (MENs)[16]. ME materials represent a relatively recently introduced class of multi-functional nanostructures in which magnetic and electric fields can be strongly coupled at body temperature[17]. Similar to the MNs, MENs can be designed to have adequately high magnetic moments and, therefore, also can be used for targeted delivery by applying remote direct current (d.c.) magnetic fields. However, owing to their non-zero magneto-electricity, unlike the traditional MNs, MENs offer an additional feature that can enable a new dissipation-free mechanism to force a high-efficacy externally controlled drug release process at the sub-cellular level using remote low-energy d.c. and/or alternating current (a.c.) magnetic fields.

An exaggerated illustration in Fig. 1 explains the concept of the field-triggered on-demand drug release from MENs. To simplify the description, we use an example with a remote magnetic field in one specific direction, for example, along x axis, with respect to the MEN drug nano-complex. The original (zero field) ionic bond, with charge Q_{ionic} of the nanoparticle, is schematically shown in Fig. 1a. AZTTP molecules (typically interconnected in chains) surround each MEN in a symmetric manner. As shown in Fig. 1b, as a non-zero magnetic field is applied, a non-zero electric dipole moment is formed in the nanoparticle because of the non-zero ME effect. For simplicity assuming an isotropic model, the

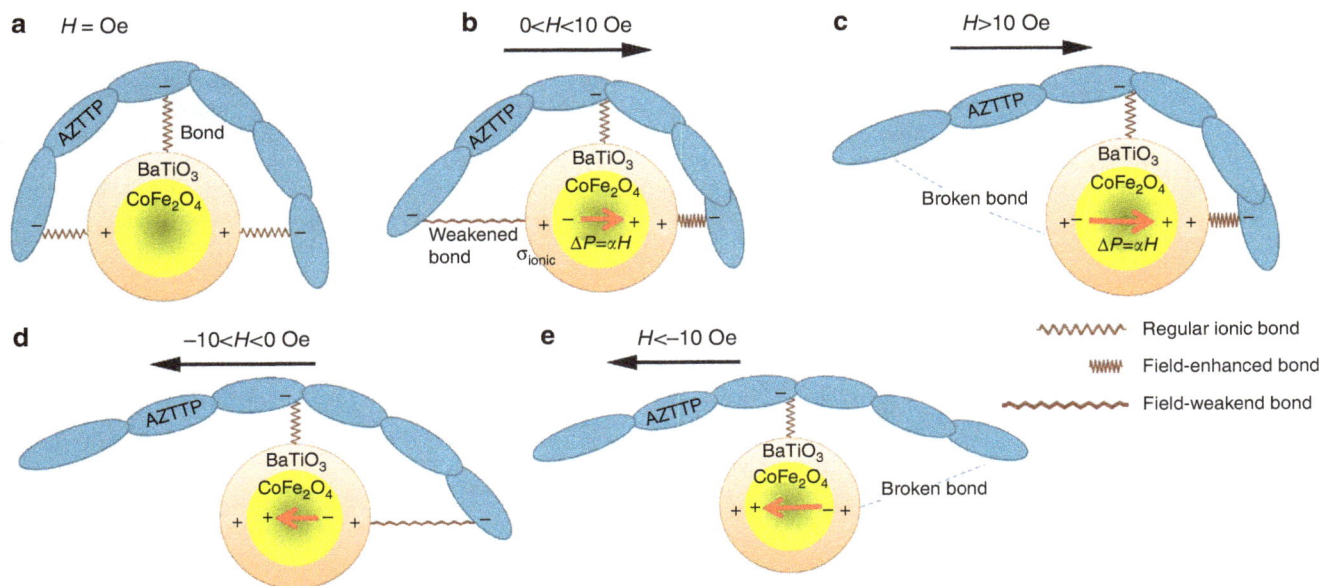

Figure 1 | Illustration of the underlying physics of the a.c.-field-triggered release. A simplified (one directional) illustration of the concept of on-demand drug (AZTTP) release by MENs stimulated by a uniform a.c. magnetic field in X direction. (**a**) At zero field, only the ionic charge is present in the MEN shell. (**b**) An additional dipole moment (proportional to the magnetic field) breaks the original symmetry of the charge distribution in the shell. (**c**) As the field is increased above the threshold value ($\sigma_{ionic} \sim \sigma_{ME}$), the bond on one side is broken. (**d,e**) The field is reversed to break the bond on the opposite side of the nanoparticle. The red arrows show the electric dipole due to the ME effect. In practice, owing to the random configurations of nanoformulations with respect to the field, the effect is present along every central bond orientation.

triggered dipole moment $\Delta P = \alpha H$, where α is the first order ME coefficient and H is the magnetic field. The amplitude of the dipole charge surface density on each side of the nanoparticle along the field would be of the order of $\sigma_{ME} \sim \pm \alpha H$, where 'positive' and 'negative' signs are applied to the opposite sides of the dipole, respectively. The dipole moment breaks the original symmetry of the charge in the MEN shell. Consequently, as the magnitude of the magnetic field is further increased above the threshold value at which the dipole charge density on the 'negative' side becomes comparable to the positive ionic charge density in the shell, $\sigma_{ME} \sim Q_{ionic}/\pi d^2$, that is, $H_{th} \sim Q_{ionic}/\pi d^2 \alpha$, where d is the diameter of the MEN, the bond in this direction along the x axis will be broken while the opposite bond will be further strengthened, as illustrated in Fig. 1c. By symmetry, to break the bond in the opposite direction, the field sequence should be repeated in the reverse direction, as illustrated in Fig. 1d,e. This simplified scenario doesn't take into account the randomness of the orientations of the nanoformulations. Ideally, applying an a.c. magnetic field that equivalently sweeps all bond orientations will create a more uniform and efficient bond-breaking process over the surface of the nanoformulation, and thus enhance the drug release efficacy. In the next generation of the technology, this goal can be achieved by using a spatially rotating field, which in turn can be accomplished, for example, by using an array of coils that generate a.c. fields with non-zero phase shifts with respect to each other.

In this study, we verified the hypothesis by demonstrating the on-demand release of AZTTP from 30-nm $CoFe_2O_4$@$BaTiO_3$ MENs by applying low a.c. and d.c. magnetic fields. We showed that a 44 Oe a.c. field at 1,000 Hz was sufficient to trigger over 89% release. Further, to support the dissipation-free release model, we could use a 66 Oe d.c. field to trigger a comparable release level.

Results

Design of the experiment. We used atomic force microscopy (AFM) in conjunction with UV spectrophotometry, Fourier transform infrared (FTIR) analysis and mass spectroscopy to directly trace the kinetics of the drug release process at different stages of the release under the influence of remote d.c. and a.c. magnetic fields. The three key stages included (i) the initial state with separate MEN carriers and AZTTP molecules, (ii) the loaded state in which MEN drug nanoformulations are formed and (iii) the final state after the a.c.-field-forced separation of AZTTP and MENs, that is, after the on-demand drug release. *In vitro* experiments on HIV-infected human cells were conducted to demonstrate the structural and functional integrity of AZTTP after this physical release process. Below we present the key

results of this experimental study. The experiments are described in more detail in the methods section.

Transmission electron microscopy study of MENs. In the experiments described below, for the role of MENs we used nanoparticles made of the popular core–shell composition $CoFe_2O_4$@$BaTiO_3$, in which the relatively high moment $CoFe_2O_4$ 1-nm shell was used to enhance the ME coefficient[18]. In general, nanoparticles as small as 5 nm in diameter can be fabricated with physical methods such as ion beam proximity lithography or imprint lithography[19]. In this study, considering the novelty of the approach, we focused on the main discovery of using MENs for on-demand drug release rather than on the development of scaling approaches. The default measurements were conducted with 30-nm MENs. A typical transmission electron microscopy image of the fabricated MENs, with clearly visible core–shell structures, is shown in Fig. 2a. The composition of the MENs was confirmed through energy-dispersive spectroscopy, as shown in Fig. 2b. The ME coefficient for the nanoparticles was measured via point I–V methods in the presence of a field to be the order of $100 \, V \, cm^{-1} \, Oe^{-1}$, using an approach described in our previous publication[20].

Spectrophotometry study of the release. The goal of the first experiment was to measure the amount of the drug (AZTTP) at different stages of the release process using the conventional approach of spectrophotometry by measuring the UV light absorption at the 267 nm maximum of the drug's absorption spectrum. We could bind ~24% of the drug to the nanoparticles by incubating AZTTP with the MENs in the Tris-EDTA (TE) buffer (pH 7.4) for 3 h. The amount of the bound drug was determined by estimating the concentration of AZTTP in the unbound fraction (supernatant) of the incubation mixture by spectrophotometry. To apply remote d.c. and a.c. magnetic fields, we used a low-energy low-field Helmholtz pair connected to a function generator. The chart in Fig. 3 summarizes the key results of this experiment, in which we measured the amount of the unbound drug depending on the external field strength and frequency. It can be seen that application of a 44 Oe field at 1,000 Hz results in 89.3% of the drug being released, while application of a d.c. field of the same amplitude releases only 16.4% of the drug. The data also confirm that with higher frequency, a lower magnetic field is needed to break the bonds because oscillation of the bonds caused by a higher frequency field facilitates the breaking of the bonds. However, when a strong enough d.c. field ($> \sim 65 \, Oe$) is applied, the bond-breaking side of the drug chain can gain enough momentum, causing the chain to break free from the MEN shell even at zero frequency. To fully exploit the

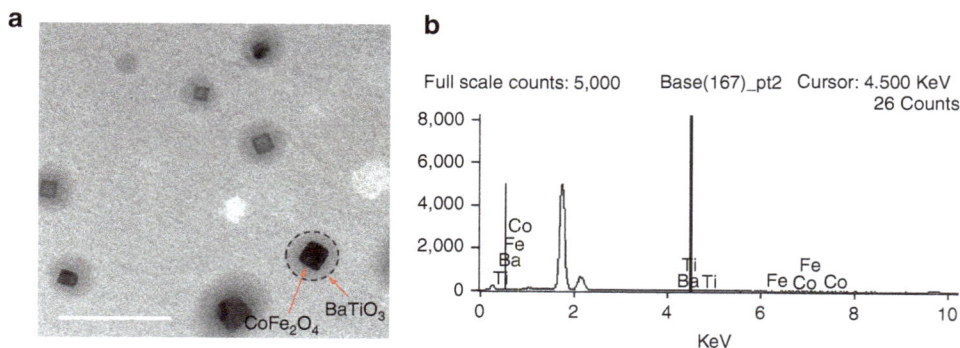

Figure 2 | Transmission electron microscopy (TEM) analysis of MENs. (**a**) A TEM image of MENs. The core–shell structure of a MEN is highlighted. Scale bar, 100 nm. (**b**) An energy-dispersive spectroscopy (EDS) analysis of MENs.

potential of the new controlled drug release nanotechnology, it is important to conduct a more detailed pharmacokinetics study.

Pharmacokinetics study. In this experiment, MENs loaded with AZTTP drug were exposed to an external magnetic field at different strengths (12, 44 and 66 Oe) and frequencies (0, 100, 1,000 Hz) for different treatment durations (1, 5, 10, 60 and 120 min) in order to understand the release kinetics. Results are summarized in the three-dimensional chart in Fig. 4. The quantitative values are also presented in Supplementary Table S1. For every field–frequency combination set we used a fresh solution with AZTTP-loaded MENs.

FTIR analysis. The concept of the drug release by a remote magnetic field was confirmed also through FTIR analysis, as shown for the three key stages of the process kinetics in Fig. 5: (top) free MENs and AZTTP before loading, (middle) loaded state: MEN–AZTTP nanoformulations and (bottom) MENs after the AZTTP release by a remote 44 Oe field at a 100 Hz frequency. Compared with the initial and final unbound states, the loaded state showed almost 30% weaker absorbance in general and a transformed spectrum in the wavenumber region from 1,750 to 1,250 cm^{-1}.

AFM study of the release kinetics. To observe the release process at the molecular level, we conducted the following AFM measurements. Figure 6 shows a sequence of AFM images that reflect the following four stages of the release process: free (a) MEN and (b) AZTTP chains, (c) loaded MEN–AZTTP nanoformulations, and (d) MENs and (e) AZTTP after the release by a 44-Oe a.c. field at 1,000 Hz. To obtain images c and d, the unloaded drug was washed away with the supernatant. One can observe that the MENs and AZTTP chains before the loading step and after the release process look similar.

Field-controlled delivery and drug release by MENs. Translocation experiments were performed on day 5 of BBB cell culture. In order to achieve the translocation of AZTTP across the BBB, AZTTP were loaded on MENs and subjected to an external magnetic field of 40 Oe (to avoid any unwanted drug release at higher fields) for 3 h and a gradient of ~22 Oe cm^{-1} (to pull the nanoparticles across the BBB) for 6 h of the incubation period. To apply a field normal to the BBB, the field coils were placed below the cell culture wells carrying the BBB model. Once the incubation was completed, the medium in the bottom chamber was isolated and subjected to the a.c. magnetic field (66 Oe at 100 Hz

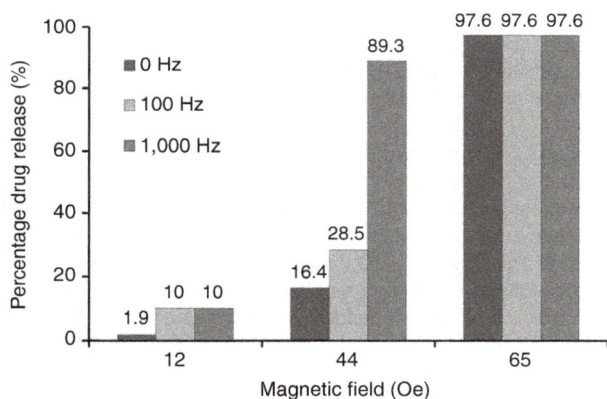

Figure 3 | Field strength and frequency dependence of the drug release. Chart showing the release efficacy of AZTTP drug bound to MENs by a remote magnetic field at different amplitudes and frequencies.

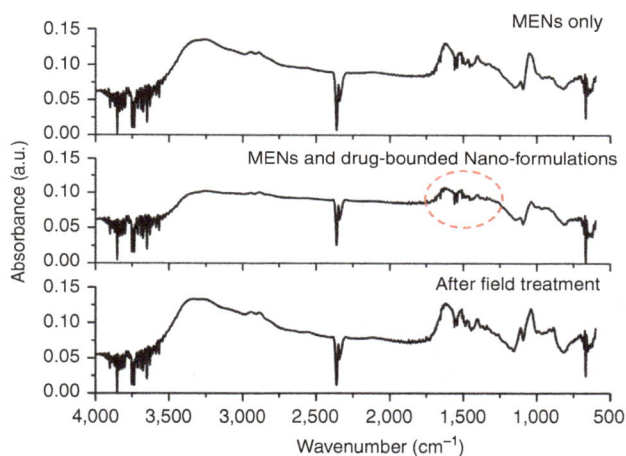

Figure 5 | FTIR measurements. FTIR measurements for MEN–AZTTP system at three different stages: (i) (top) MENs only, (ii) (middle) AZTTP-loaded MENs and (iii) MENs after the release by the a.c. field treatment (bottom).

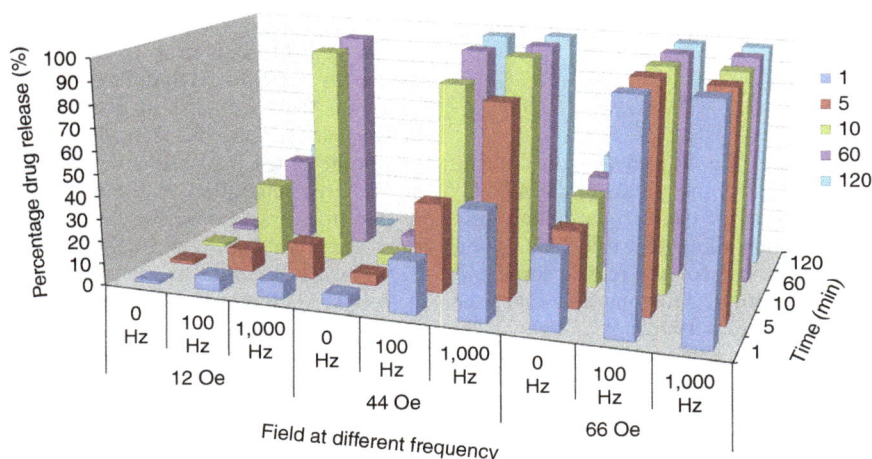

Figure 4 | Pharmacokinetics study. Pharmacokinetics study: three-dimensional chart representation of the drug release percentage at various combinations of the field strength (12, 44 and 66 Oe), the frequency (0, 100, and 1,000 Hz) and the treatment duration (1, 5, 10, 60 and 120 min).

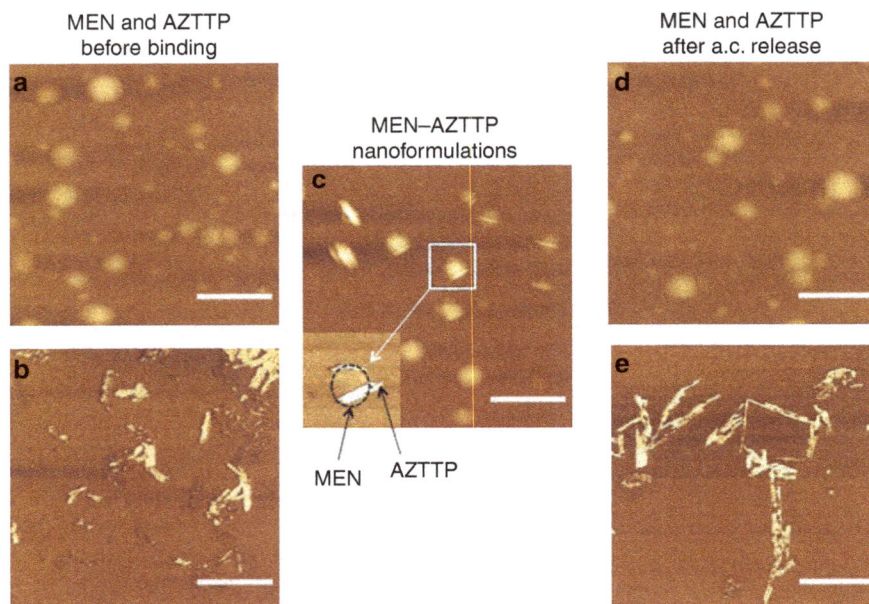

Figure 6 | Atomic force microscopy study of the drug release kinetics. AFM images at different stages of the release process: (**a**) MENs and (**b**) AZTTP chains before the loading (binding) step, (**c**) AZTTP–MEN nanoformulations after the loading process, (**d**) MENs and (**e**) AZTTP after the drug release by a 44-Oe a.c. field at 1,000 Hz. Scale bar, 100 nm.

field for 5 min) to increase the release percentage. After the field treatment, the MENs were isolated via a magnetic separation technique. Once separated, the supernatant was measured for the drug concentration via spectrophotometry. The results indicated that ∼40% of the drug was translocated across the BBB as a result of the process. These results are summarized in Supplementary Fig. S1.

To further confirm the structural and functional integrity of the drug after the a.c. release process, we conducted: (i) a mass spectrometry analysis of the drug before and after the release (Supplementary Fig. S2 and Supplementary Table S2), (ii) an *in vitro* experiment to study the p24 inhibition efficacy of the drug before and after the release (Supplementary Fig. S3). Finally, to understand the cytotoxicity of MENs ($CoFe_2O_4@BaTiO_3$), we performed an XTT (sodium 2,3,-bis(2-methoxy-4-nitro-5-sulfophenyl)-5-[(phenylamino)-carbonyl]-2H-tetrazolium inner salt) assay on human astrocyte (HA) cells for neural cytotoxicity and on human peripheral blood mononuclear cells (PBMCs) for peripheral cytotoxicity. The results indicated no significant toxicity at a concentration of $< 50 \,\mu g \,ml^{-1}$ (Supplementary Table S3).

Discussion

The spectrophotometry experiment (Fig. 3) indicates the threshold value, necessary for the field to start the release of the AZTTP drugs by the MENs, to be of the order of 10 Oe, even though only 10% of the drug was released at such a low field value. Using the simplified expression we derived above for the release threshold field ($H_{th} \sim Q_{ionic}/\pi d^2 \alpha$) and assuming the nanoparticle diameter ($d = 30$ nm) and the ME coefficient ($\alpha = 100 \,V \,cm^{-1} \,Oe^{-1}$), we can evaluate the value for the effective charge, Q_{ionic} (responsible for the ionic/covalent bond between the MEN and AZTTP cluster), to be $\sim 10^{-17} C$. The estimate seems reasonable and indicates that approximately a few hundred electrons are involved in the bond formation. Further, in agreement with the original hypothesis, the experiment also proves that the a.c. field provides a substantially more enhanced release compared with that of the

d.c. field. Indeed, at 12 Oe field amplitude, d.c. and a.c. (100 Hz) fields result in 1.9 and 10% released drug percentage, respectively. To achieve almost full (89.3%) drug release, a field of 44 Oe at a frequency of 1,000 Hz is required. The effect of the a.c. field control is significant in this case. For comparison, with a field of 44 Oe at the frequency of 100 Hz, the released amount was 28.5% while for the d.c. case at the same field amplitude was only 16.4%. The experiment indicates that such nanoformulations can be directed to the targeted cells via a d.c. magnetic field with a spatial gradient while the drug can be effectively released on demand via an external a.c. magnetic field at 1,000 Hz. Note that the highest applied field of 65 Oe immediately saturated the system, resulting in an almost full drug release even in the d.c. case. According to our hypothesis, the latter can be explained by the magnetic-field-triggered large electric force that gave enough momentum to break the bond. The results of the more detailed pharmacokinetics study (Fig. 4) also indicate the presence of a certain threshold field that needs to be applied to trigger the release. The threshold values at different frequencies reach their saturation value in about 60 min of the incubation process. Again, this threshold field exists even in the d.c. case (zero frequency) and can be further reduced in the a.c. case by increasing the frequency of an a.c. field. To separate the d.c. and a.c. functions for drug delivery and release, respectively, it is important to maintain the amplitude of the field below the saturation value, for example, at 44 Oe. This separation of the d.c.- and a.c.-driven delivery and release functions, respectively, was also confirmed in the *in vitro* experiment with a human BBB cell culture (Supplementary Fig. S2). The FTIR results are in agreement with spectrophotometry data (Fig. 5). Supporting the above release model, the initial state (before drug loading) and the final state (after the release) FTIR spectra look similar, while the altered intermediate state reflects the effect of binding between MENs and AZTTP molecules. The AFM measurements (Fig. 6) directly illustrate the physical difference between MEN–AZTTP nanoformulations and the free MENs before loading and after releasing the drugs. In agreement with the described spectrophotometry and FTIR measurements, the AFM analysis also indicates that the MENs return to their original unbound state after the drug release triggered by a.c. magnetic field. In addition, AFM also proves the nanoscale nature of the approach, with the potential to be applied at the sub-cellular level. The *in vitro* experiment using human PBMCs infected with HIV-1$_{Ba-L}$ proves the intact integrity of the drug after the a.c.-triggered release (Supplementary Fig. S3).

The fundamental difference between MNs and MENs is due to the presence in the latter of the quantum-mechanically caused ME effect that enables intrinsic coupling between the magnetic spin and the electric dipole. Consequently, energy-efficient and dissipation-free remote control of the intrinsic charge distribution in the MENs (and consequently, control of the bonding force between the MENs and the drug) can be enabled via application of an external magnetic field. Because of the intrinsic ME effect, even if the drug is strongly bonded to the MEN carriers (as required for high-efficacy delivery), it can be fully released at the target location via application of a local magnetic field with a strength above a certain threshold defined by the ME effect. For comparison, the drug release process using the conventional MNs is not controlled at the same fundamental level but instead is based on an irreversible energy dissipation process caused by an external a.c. magnetic field. In one MN implementation, super-paramagnetic nanoparticles and drug molecules are incorporated into temperature-sensitive synthetic polymers or other biomater-ials that release the drug as the nanoparticles are heated under the field exposure[21]. In other implementations, superparamagnetic nanoparticles can be coated with intermediate linkers (tailored to specific load molecules), embedded in a ferro-gel, or directly connected to the load molecules[22,23]. In either of these conventional cases, the release mechanism with MNs is based on extrinsic phenomena, that is, mechanical deformation and/or heat dissipation that affects the release kinetics, that are triggered by a relatively high frequency a.c. field (in the range of hundreds of kilohertz or above) and consume a substantial amount of power (in the kilowatt range). On the contrary, the MEN-triggered release process is achieved at the intrinsic level and does not require any intermediate materials. It is dissipation free and extremely energy efficient. The release with MENs can be triggered by an a.c. magnetic field at a relatively low frequency (below 100 Hz) and even at a d.c. field provided the field strength is above a certain threshold value, as described below in more detail, with power consumption in the sub-watt range.

One can argue that MENs may also experience the potential problem of having a relatively large fraction of the nanoparticles (together or without the drug) trapped in the reticuloendothelial system. One solution to this problem is to apply a 'zig–zag'-shaped time-varying field profile to move the nanoparticles through the system. Then, besides the force along the main delivery path, there is a significant 'jolting' force normal to this direction. This 'jolting' force ensures that the nanoparticles don't become trapped in the fibres of the reticular connective tissue. However, application of the strongly inertial 'zig–zag' force to the conventional MNs can also result in a significant loss of the drug. On the contrary, with MENs, the physical bond between the drug and the nanoparticle can be engineered to be adequately strong to avoid any loss until a command to release is given via an external field.

As a final remark, we would like to emphasize that although MENs indeed have a unique advantage of serving in both roles, (i) as regular MNs for drug delivery (via application of a d.c. remote field with a spatial gradient) and (ii) as drug release nanoscale sites, their capability of an on-demand drug release by application of a low remote magnetic field in an extremely low frequency range is unprecedented and therefore is a merit of its own (even without exploiting the drug delivery feature). In general, this physically controlled release method could be complementary to

any other drug delivery and tagging mechanism, whether it is physical or chemical. Although AZTTP is used in the experiment, the ability of on-demand drug release by a MEN nano-carrier discovered in this study is also relevant to the treatment of other diseases such as many CNS diseases, cancer and others, where deep-tissue high-efficacy drug delivery at the sub-cellular level is key[12].

Methods

Preparation of CoFe2O4-BaTiO3 core-shell MENs. CoFe$_2$O$_4$ nanoparticles were prepared by hydrothermal method. In this method, 15 ml of aqueous mixture of 0.058 g of Co(NO$_3$)$_2$.6H$_2$0, 0.16 g of Fe(NO$_3$)$_3$.9H$_2$0 and 0.2 g of poly-vinylpyrrolidone is dissolved in 5 ml of aqueous 0.9 g of sodium borohydride at 120 °C for 12 h. Next, precursor solution of BaTiO$_3$ was prepared by mixing 30 ml of aqueous 0.029 g of BaCO$_3$ and 0.1 g of citric acid with 30 ml of ethonalic solution of 0.048 ml titanium isopropoxide and 1 g of citric acid. CoFe$_2$O$_4$@BaTiO$_3$ core-shell MENs are prepared by dispersing 0.1 g of CoFe$_2$O$_4$ nanoparticles in the precursor solution. The mixture was sonicated for 2 h. Well-dispersed mixture was dried at 60 °C for overnight while stirring continuously. Later, the mixture was subjected to calcination at 780 °C for 5 h. By reducing the cooling rate (controlled by furnace CMF 1,100) from above 52 to below 14 °C min^{-1}, the average diameter of MENs could be controlled from below 25 nm to over 100 nm, respectively, with an adequate size distribution of <30%. The particle size distribution was measured by a Zetasizer Nano series via the standard dynamic light scattering approach. For the 25-nm process (14 °C min^{-1} cooling rate), the average size distribution ranged from ∼19 to 31 nm.

Nanoformulations of AZTTP-MEN. Ten microlitres of AZTTP drug (10 mM, concentration) was added to the solution of 190 μl of TE buffer and 50 μl of CoFe$_2$O$_4$BaTiO$_3$ core-shell MENs (5 mg ml^{-1}). Then, the solutions were incu-bated for 2and 3 h, respectively. After the incubation, the solution was subjected to the magnetic field in order to precipitate the MENs (conjugated with AZTTP). After the supernatant was isolated, its absorption was measured at 267 nm using spectrophotometer Agilent Cary 100.

Spectro-photometric analysis of drug loading. Drug loading percentage = (absorbance of total amount of drug used—absorbance of drug used in supernatant after incubating the drug and the MEN for a specific incubation time) × 100%.

After 2-h incubation, the percentage of the drug in the supernatant was ∼89%, which corresponded to ∼11% (100 − 89) of the drug bound to the MENs.

After 3-h incubation, the percentage of the drug in the supernatant was ∼76%, which corresponded to ∼24% (100 − 76) of the drug bound to the MENs.

Drug release percentage: drug release percentage = (absorbance of supernatant after magnetic field treatment)/(absorbance of supernatant after incubating the particles with drug) × 100%. The absorbance signal was measured at the maximum wavelength of 267 nm.

Magnetic field treatment. To eliminate any potential residual unbounded drug, after isolating the supernatant, the precipitate of the MENs conjugated with the drug was washed once with the TE buffer. Then, the drug-conjugated particles (AZTTP–MEN nanoformulations) were redispersed in 190 μl of the TE buffer, and subjected to a magnetic field of varying field strength and frequency. Finally, the solution was precipitated to pipette out the supernatant for further absorption measurements.

Surface charge of MENs and AZTTP molecules. Because of the triphosphate functional groups, in the chemical (covalent and/or ionic) bond between the MENs and the AZTTP molecular cluster chains, the CoFe$_2$O$_4$-BaTiO$_3$ MENs and the AZTTP chains were positively and negatively charged, respectively.

Mass spectrometry analysis of AZTTP molecules and AZTTP bound to MEN. To confirm the integrity of AZTTP (C$_{10}$H$_{16}$N$_5$O$_{13}$P$_3$; MW = 507) drug after the a.c.-triggered release by MENs, we conducted a mass spectrometry analysis. The analysis included a full scan qualitative identification of the target analyte, a chromatographic separation and an assessment of the presence of the drug in the composite material (AZTTP–MEN nanoformulations) using multiple reaction monitoring for appropriate transitions. Different mixes were contained in Eppendorf vials. Using a 100-μl micropipette, 100 μl of each vial was transferred to a new disposable polypropylene 96-well plate (part no. 5042-1386). The vials' contents were subjected to a flow injection analysis using electrospray ionization with Jet Stream Technology in both positive and negative mode to assess the presence of the AZTTP drug. The measurements were conducted with mass spectrometer Agilent LC/MS Triple quadruple G6460 LC-QQQ. The ionization conditions are presented in Supplementary Table S2. Supplementary Figure 2 shows the number of counts versus the mass-to-charge ratio for the three key stages of the release process: (top) standard AZTTP, (middle) AZTTP bound to

MENs, and (bottom) AZTTP and MEN after the a.c.-triggered release of the drug load. The molecular weight of the AZTTP molecule is ~ 507.

Preparation of samples for AFM and FTIR imaging. Ten microlitres of AZTTP drug (10 mM, concentration) was added to the solution of 190 μl of the TE buffer and 50 μl of $CoFe_2O_4$-$BaTiO_3$ core–shell MENs (5 mg ml^{-1}). Then, the solution was incubated for 3 h. After the incubation, one drop of solution was air dried on to a pre-cleaned Si wafer. Once dried AFM imaging (topography and phase contrast) was performed using Nanoscope IIIa Multimode.

For AZTTP the above solution without MENs was used and for MENs the above solution without AZTTP was used.

For FTIR measurements, the sample preparation procedures were similar to the one used for AFM.

***In vitro* BBB model**. *In vitro* BBB model was prepared according to the procedure described elsewhere[24]. The BBB model consisted of two compartments (upper and lower), which were separated by the polyethylene terephthalate membrane of a 3.0-μm pore size (Becton Dickinson Labware, NJ, USA). In a 24-well cell culture inserts, 2×10^5 human brain microvascular endothelial cells were grown to confluence on the upper side of the insert and the same amount of HAs were grown on the underside. BBB cell culture was incubated for 4 days in order to reach incubation confluence at 37 °C and 5% CO_2. Transendothelial electrical resistance was used to measure the intactness of the BBB. The average transendothelial electrical resistance value for individual BBB was about 150–200 ohms cm^{-2}, which is consistent with formation of BBB.

p24 Assay to confirm the integrity of AZTTP after field-controlled release. Normal PBMCs (10×10^6 cells) were infected with native HIV-1$_{Ba-L}$ (NIH AIDS Research and Reference Reagent Programme catalogue no. 510) at a concentration of 2 ng ml^{-1} cells for 2 h, washed with phosphate-buffered saline (GIBCO-BRL, Grand Island, NY) and returned to culture with and without fresh (new) or MEN-released AZTTP at equimolar concentrations (200 nM). The culture supernatants were quantitated for p24 antigen using a p24 ELISA kit (ZeptoMetrix, Buffalo, NY) on the 5th day of infection. While the control sample showed the p24 concentration of $\sim 33,050$ pg ml^{-1}, the use of fresh and MEN-released AZTTP drugs resulted in the concentration values of $\sim 1,300$ and 1,800 pg ml^{-1}, respectively (Supplementary Fig. S3). Therefore, considering the s.d. of ~ 300 pg ml^{-1}, the two drug forms demonstrated equal p24 inhibition efficacy.

***In vitro* cytotoxicity assay**. To understand the *in vitro* cytotoxicity of MENs ($CoFe_2O_4@BaTiO_3$), we performed XTT assay according to the manufacturer's protocol (ATCC). XTT is a quantitative colorimetric assay, which is based on the formation of an orange-coloured formazan dye by viable cells from the cleavage of XTT tetrazolium salts. The assay was performed on HA cells for neuronal cytotoxicity and on PBMCs for peripheral cytotoxicity. In this assay, desired cells were seeded in a 96-well cell culture plate at a 1×10^5 cells per well concentration and incubated for 48 h. (The cell concentration and incubation time were standardized by performing a pre-assay optimization protocol.) Following the incubation, the cell culture medium was replaced by a medium containing MENs at a differential concentration of 0–50 μg ml^{-1}. The cells were incubated in the MEN solution for 24 h. Once, the incubation period was completed the cells were washed with phosphate-buffered saline buffer and later supplemented with a fresh medium. Cell viability test was performed by XTT test kit as supplied by (ATCC) for 6 h. The experiments that were performed in triplicate indicated no significant toxicity at a concentration of <50 μg ml^{-1} (Supplementary Table S3).

References

1. Mocroft, A. & Lundgren, J. D. Starting highly active antiretroviral therapy: why, when and response to HAART. *J. Antimicrob. Chemother.* **54**, 10–13 (2004).
2. Wang, X., Chai, H., Lin, P. H., Yao, Q. & Chen, C. Roles and mechanisms of HIV protease inhibitor ritonavir and other anti-HIV drugs in endothelial dysfunction of porcine pulmonary arteries and human pulmonary artery endothelial cells. *Am. J. Pahol.* **174**, 771–781 (2009).
3. Saxena, S. K., Tiwari, S. & Nair, M. P. N. A global perspective on HIV/AIDS. *Science* **337**, 789 (2012).
4. Ayre, S. G. New approaches to the delivery of drugs to the brain. *Med. Hypothesis* **29**, 283–291 (1989).
5. Thomas, S. A. Anit-HIV drug distribution to the central nervous system. *Curr. Pharm. Des* **10**, 1313–1324 (2004).
6. Tong, R., Hemmati, H. D., Langer, R. & Kohane, D. S. Photoswitchable nanoparticles or triggered tissue penetration and drug delivery. *J. Am. Chem. Soc.* **134**, 8848–8855 (2012).
7. Cheong, I. *et al.* A bacterial protein enhances the release and efficacy of lipossamal cancer drugs. *Science* **314**, 1308–1311 (2006).
8. Senyei, A., Widder, K. & Czerlinski, C. Magnetic guidance of drug carrying microspheres. *J. Appl. Phys.* **49**, 3578–3583 (1978).
9. Derfus, A. M. *et al.* Remotely triggered release from magnetic nanoparticles. *Adv. Mater.* **19**, 3932–3936 (2007).
10. McBain, S. C., Yiu, H. P. & Dobson, J. Magnetic nanoparticles for gene and drug delivery. *Int. J. Nanomed.* **3**, 169–180 (2008).
11. Timko, B. P., Dvir, T. & Kohane, D. Remotely triggerabe drug delivery systems. *Adv. Mater.* **22**, 4925–4943 (2010).
12. Szebeni, J. *et al.* Inhibition of HIV-1 in monocyte/macrophage cultures by 2′, 3′-dideoxycytidine-5′-triphosphate, free and in liposomes. *AIDS Res. Hum. Retroviruses* **6**, 691–702 (1990).
13. Varatharajan, L. & Thomas, S. A. The transport of anti-HIV drugs across blood-CNS interfaces: summary of current knowledge and recommendations for further research. *Antiviral Res.* **82**, A99–A109 (2009).
14. Saiyed, Z. M., Gandhi, N. H. & Nair, M. P. Magnetic nanoformulation of azidothymidine 5′-triphosphate for targeted delivery across the blood-brain barrier. *Int. J. Nanomedicine* **5**, 157–166 (2010).
15. Batrakova, E. V., Gendelman, H. E. & Kabanov, A. V. Cell-mediated drugs delivery. *Expert. Opin. Deliv.* **8**, 415–433 (2011).
16. Xie, S., Ma, F., Liu, Y. & Li, J. Multiferroic CoFe2O4-Pb(Zr0.52Ti0.48)O3 core-shell nanofibers and their magnetoelectric coupling. *Nanoscale* **3**, 3152–3158 (2011).
17. Eerenstein, W., Mathur, N. D. & Scott, J. F. Multiferroic and magnetoelectric materials. *Nature* **442**, 759–765 (2006).
18. Corral-Flores, V., Bueno-Baqu, D. & Ziolo, R. F. Synthesis and characterization of novel CoFe2O4-BaTiO3 multiferroic core-shell-type nanostructures. *Acta Mater.* **8**, 764–769 (2010).
19. Litvinov, J., Nasrullah, A., Sherlock, T., Wang, Y., Ruchhoeft, P. & Wilson, R. C. High-throughput top-down fabrication of uniform magnetic particles. *PLOS ONE* **7**, e37440 (2012).
20. Hong, J., Bekyarova, E., Liang, P., de Heer, W., Haddon, R. & Khizroev, S. Room-temperature magnetic-order in functionalized graphene. *Sci. Rep.* **2**, 624 (2012).
21. Rovers, S. A., Hoogenboom, R., Kemmere, M. F. & Keurentjes, J. T. F. Repetitive on-demand drug release by magnetic heating of iron oxide containing polymeric implants. *Soft Matter* **8**, 1623–1627 (2012).
22. Hoare, T. *et al.* A Magnetically triggered composite membrane for on-demand drug delivery. *Nano Lett.* **9**, 3651–3657 (2009).
23. Torchilin, V. P. Recent advances with liposomes as pharmaceutical carriers. *Nat. Rev.* **4**, 145–160 (2005).
24. Persidsky, Y., Stins, M. & Way, D. *et al.* A model for monocytes migration through the blood brain barrier during HIV-1 encephalitis. *J. Immunol.* **158**, 3499–3510 (1997).

Acknowledgements

We acknowledge partial financial support from National Science Foundation award no. 005084-002, National Institute of Health DA no. 027049 and Department of Defense Defense Microelectronics Activity under contract no. H94003-09-2-0904. We thank Luis Arroyo for his help with NMR measurements.

Author contributions

S.K. designed, oversaw and supervised the entire project. R.G. conducted all the key measurements including AFM, FTIR, spectrophotometry, *in vitro* studies of the targeted delivery and release across BBB, and cytotoxicity measurements. M.N. designed and oversaw the p24 studies. P.L. helped engineer the magnetic field gradient sources. J.H. helped conduct AFM studies and V.S. conducted the p24 test.

Additional information

7

Photoswitchable fatty acids enable optical control of TRPV1

James Allen Frank[1], Mirko Moroni[2], Rabih Moshourab[2,3], Martin Sumser[1], Gary R. Lewin[2] & Dirk Trauner[1]

Fatty acids (FAs) are not only essential components of cellular energy storage and structure, but play crucial roles in signalling. Here we present a toolkit of photoswitchable FA analogues (FAAzos) that incorporate an azobenzene photoswitch along the FA chain. By modifying the FAAzos to resemble capsaicin, we prepare a series of photolipids targeting the Vanilloid Receptor 1 (TRPV1), a non-selective cation channel known for its role in nociception. Several azo-capsaicin derivatives (AzCAs) emerge as photoswitchable agonists of TRPV1 that are relatively inactive in the dark and become active on irradiation with ultraviolet-A light. This effect can be rapidly reversed by irradiation with blue light and permits the robust optical control of dorsal root ganglion neurons and C-fibre nociceptors with precision timing and kinetics not available with any other technique. More generally, we expect that photolipids will find many applications in controlling biological pathways that rely on protein–lipid interactions.

[1] Department of Chemistry and Center for Integrated Protein Science, Ludwig Maximilians University Munich, Butenandtstrasse 5–13, Munich 81377, Germany. [2] Molecular Physiology of Somatic Sensation, Max Delbrück Center for Molecular Medicine, Berlin 13125, Germany. [3] Department of Anesthesiology, Campus Charité Mitte und Virchow Klinikum, Charité Universitätsmedizin Berlin, Augustburgerplatz 1, Berlin 13353, Germany. Correspondence and requests for materials should be addressed to D.T. (email: dirk.trauner@lmu.de).

Lipids serve not only as sources of energy and integral components of membranes but are also involved in cellular communication through participation in a variety of signalling cascades and the modulation of transmembrane proteins[1]. Over the past several decades, interest in lipid chemistry has been overshadowed by advancements in proteomic and genomic technologies. However, recent developments in lipid research, including analysis of the lipidome[2], have shed new light on the roles of these molecules at all levels of biology. Many lipids consist of fatty acids (FAs). These ancient molecular building blocks typically feature a long linear carbon chain (up to 28 carbons)[3] that often contains one or several cis- double bonds.

The Vanilloid Receptor 1 (TRPV1) is the most studied of the transient receptor potential ion channels[4,5]. This family of non-selective cation channels is renowned for its ability to respond to a wide variety of chemical and physical inputs[6,7]. TRPV1 is involved in the regulation of body temperature[8] and the transduction of painful stimuli from the periphery towards the central nervous system[9]. It is expressed in sub-populations of sensory nerve fibres within the dorsal root and trigeminal ganglia[10], where it responds to temperatures greater than 43 °C[11], protons[12], as well as environmental toxins and poisons[13,14]. Importantly, TRPV1 is modulated by a plethora of FA amides, including the endogenous arachidonic acid derivatives anandamide[15] and N-arachidonoyl dopamine[16]. Its most famous exogenous agonist is the vanilloid capsaicin (CAP), the pungent component of chilli peppers[11]. Synthetic TRPV1 agonists include olvanil[17] and arvanil[18], which are FA-derived vanilloids developed as non-pungent CAP analogues.

TRPV1 is not only involved in responses to noxious stimuli, but is also believed to initiate the neurogenic inflammatory response[19], which has made it an attractive target for novel analgesics[11]. However, these attempts have proven more challenging than anticipated, as TRPV1 is involved in a variety of other biological pathways that can lead to unwanted side effects. An agonist or antagonist that could be applied globally but activated only locally could offer a solution to this problem. In addition to this, such a tool would be highly valuable for untangling the complex interactions that TRPV1 has with other proteins, such as the serotonin (5-HT), bradykinin (BK) and recently GABA$_B$ receptors[5,20,21].

Precision control can be achieved through photoswitchable small molecules that act as transducers between a light stimulus and protein function[22–24]. In 2013, our group was the first to place TRPV1 under reversible optical control when we developed a series of photoswitchable antagonists which could optically control TRPV1 in the presence of CAP to activate the channel[25]. Based on the structure of CAP and other TRPV1 agonists, we saw the opportunity to develop a photoswitchable TRPV1 agonist which would permit optical control over the ion channel without the use of a second factor.

In this study, we present a toolkit of photolipids that allow us to place lipid-modulated biological targets, such as TRPV1, under the precise spatial and temporal control of light. We show that AzCA4 permits optical control over TRPV1 in complex neural systems with a higher degree of spatiotemporal precision than is currently possible via other methods. More generally, this work represents the first example of the fusion of photopharmacology with lipid signalling and consequently sets the groundwork for future research in this field.

Results

Photolipid syntheses. In an effort to mimic FAs with a chain length of 18 carbons, we prepared a series of 8 photoswitchable

FA derivatives, FAAzo1–8. Each of these compounds contained an azobenzene photoswitch, which allowed for controllable cis/trans-isomerization along the length of the chain (Fig. 1a). FAAzo1–8 were prepared in between two and six steps in moderate yield (Supplementary Fig. 1)[26]. In their dark-adapted state, the FAAzos existed predominantly in the trans-configuration. Ultraviolet–visible spectroscopy showed that isomerization from trans- to cis- could be achieved by irradiation at $\lambda = 365$ nm and this process could be reversed by $\lambda = 460$ nm light.

Supported by structure–activity relationships and recent structural data[27], we envisioned a unique opportunity to create a series of photoswitchable vanilloids for the optical control of TRPV1. Our approach combined the vanilloid head group of CAP with the FAAzos, which would act as a photoswitchable tail mimicking that of N-arachidonoyl dopamine, anandamide, olvanil or arvanil (Fig. 1b). The preparation of these compounds (Fig. 1c and Supplementary Fig. 2) required only a peptide coupling between vanillamine and the appropriate FAAzo to afford eight photoswitchable vanilloids, AzCA1–8, in good yields (Fig. 1b). Photoswitching of AzCA1–8 was also achieved using $\lambda = 365/460$ nm and they showed similar photoswitching properties when compared with the FAAzos (Supplementary Fig. 3). As such, both FAAzos and AzCAs could be classified as 'regular' azobenzenes that require ultraviolet-A light for isomerization to their thermally unstable cis-form.

Optical control over TRPV1 in HEK293T cells. We evaluated the photopharmacology of AzCA1–8 using whole-cell electro-physiology in human embryonic kidney (HEK) 293T cells transiently expressing the yellow fluorescent protein (YFP)-tag-ged ion channel (TRPV1-YFP)[28]. Each compound (1 μM) was continuously applied while alternating between irradiation at $\lambda = 350$ nm and at $\lambda = 450$ nm, until a steady state of activity/desensitization was achieved on photoswitching. Their relative light-dependant activities were then assessed by performing voltage ramps (-100 to $+100$ mV over 5 s) under irradiation at both wavelengths (Fig. 2a and Supplementary Fig. 4a). Among the eight derivatives tested, three compounds—AzCA2, AzCA3 and AzCA4 (at 1 μM)—showed the most profound TRPV1 photoswitching effect (Fig. 2b and Supplementary Fig. 4b). For all three derivatives, larger currents were observed under irradiation at $\lambda = 350$ nm, indicating that these compounds had higher efficacies towards TRPV1 in their cis-configuration. At higher concentrations (>300 nM, bath application), smaller cellular currents were observed on application of the AzCAs in their dark-adapted states. This showed that in both configurations, the AzCAs were TRPV1 agonists; however, in all cases a larger current was observed under $\lambda = 350$ nm irradiation. Working at an optimized concentration (1 μM by puff pipette), the AzCAs could be applied to cells in the dark without any observable effect and this allowed immediate TRPV1 activation on irradiation with ultraviolet-A light (Supplementary Fig. 5). Photoswitching could be repeated over multiple cycles and only minor channel desensitization was observed (Fig. 2c).

The washout of AzCA4 with buffer was very slow and photoswitching currents persisted for minutes under constant perfusion. However, application of capsazepine (5 μM), a TRPV1 antagonist known to bind competitively against CAP, was capable of displacing AzCA4 and rapidly abolished inward currents on ultraviolet stimulation (Supplementary Fig. 6)[29,30]. In control experiments, no light-induced activity was observed in cells lacking TRPV1, before the application of an AzCA derivative (Supplementary Fig. 7a) or after the application of CAP (1 μM) (Supplementary Fig. 7b). The application of FAAzo2, FAAzo3

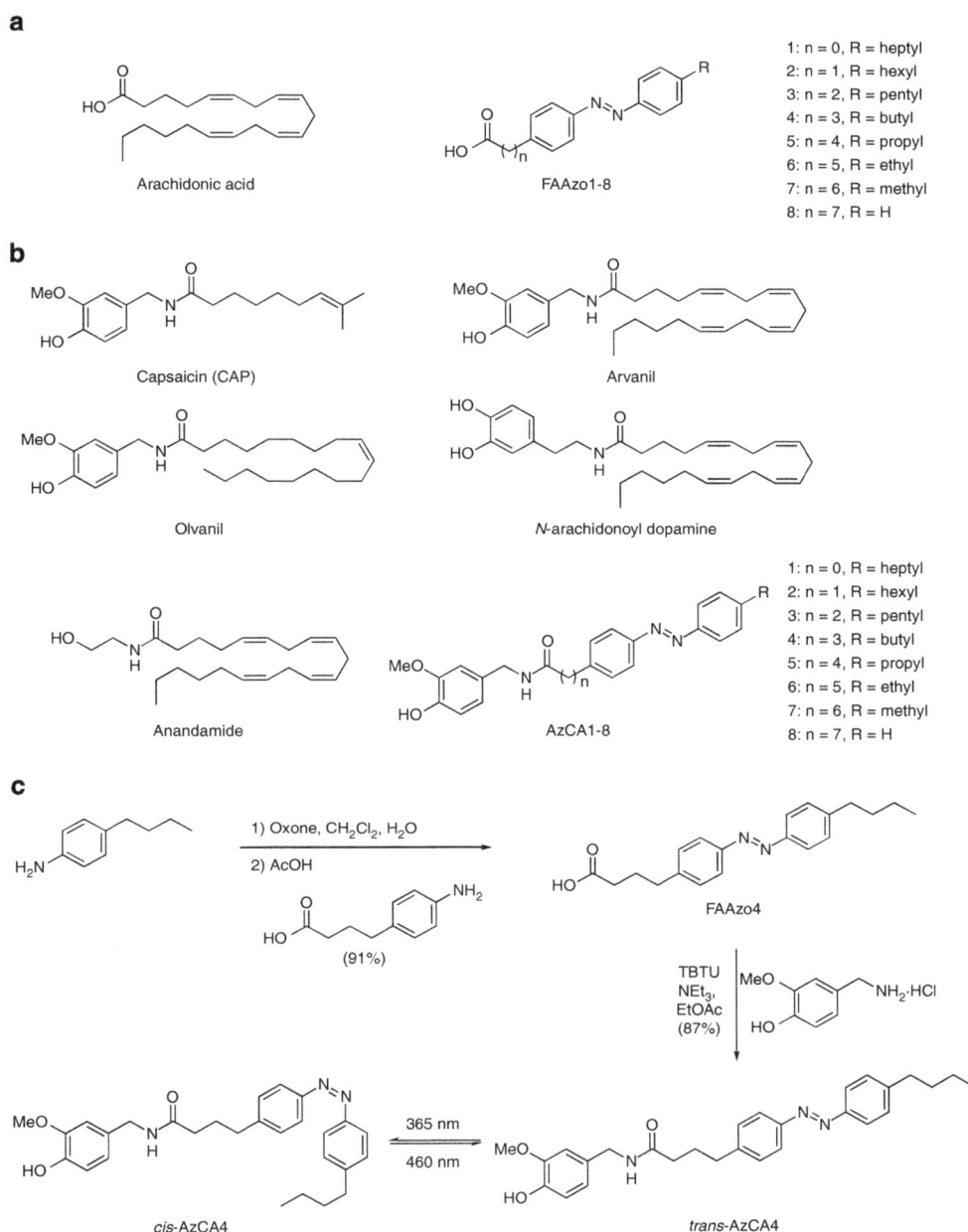

Figure 1 | Photolipids for the optical control of TRPV1. (a) Chemical structures of arachidonic acid and FAAzo1–8. **(b)** Chemical structures of TRPV1 agonists capsaicin (CAP), arvanil, olvanil, N-arachidonoyl dopamine and anandamide alongside photoswitchable vanilloids, AzCA1–8. **(c)** Chemical synthesis of AzCA4. Isomerization between cis- and trans-AzCA4 could be induced by irradiation with $\lambda = 365$ nm (trans to cis) and $\lambda = 460$ nm (cis to trans), respectively.

and FAAzo4 caused no effect (5 µM, $n \geq 3$ for each) in TRPV1-responding cells.

In voltage clamp experiments, the magnitude of the cellular currents could be controlled by adjusting the ON wavelength between $\lambda = 350$–390 nm. As shown by an action spectrum, the largest currents were observed under $\lambda = 350$ nm and they became smaller towards $\lambda = 390$ nm (Fig. 3a and Supplementary Fig. 8). Current clamp experiments revealed that the cellular membrane potential could be controlled in a similar manner, with $\lambda = 360$ nm yielding the largest depolarization (Fig. 3b). Through exponential curve fitting, we evaluated the effects of irradiation on the TRPV1 activation kinetics. The fastest ON response was observed at $\lambda = 360$ nm and all other τ_{on} values were normalized to this τ-value for comparison (Fig. 3c). At longer wavelengths, a slower response was observed. Taken together, these results indicate that the AzCAs permit precise, optical control over the activity of TRPV1 that cannot be achieved with other lipophilic agonists, such as CAP, alone. As AzCA4 could be prepared in high yield at low cost, we decided to focus our future investigations on this compound.

AzCA4 allowed optical control over cultured DRG neurons. Having demonstrated that AzCA4 acts as a photoswitchable TRPV1 agonist that is relatively inactive in the dark, we next evaluated its activity in isolated wild-type (wt) mouse dorsal root ganglia (DRG) neurons using both electrophysiology and intracellular Ca^{2+} imaging.

Whole-cell patch clamp electrophysiology showed that AzCA4 (200 nM) enabled reversible optical control over DRG neuronal

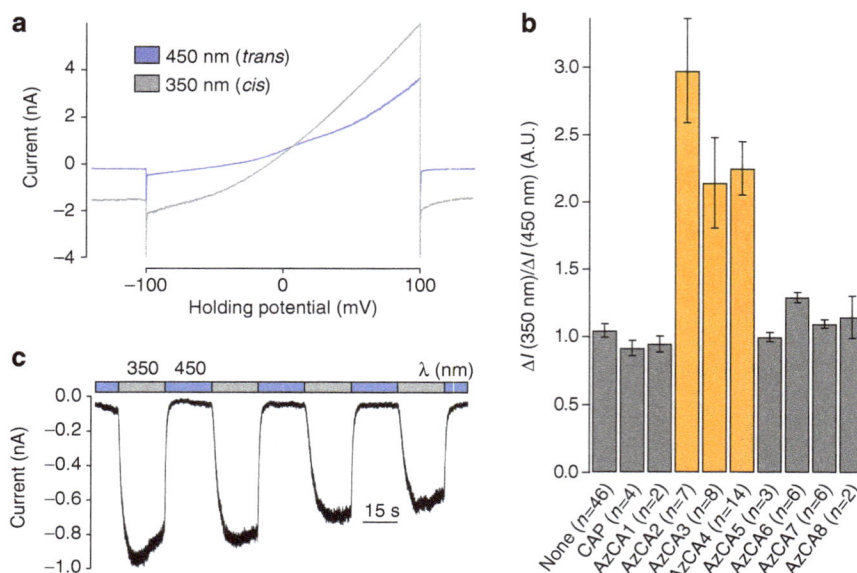

Figure 2 | AzCAs permit optical control of TRPV1 in HEK293T cells. HEK293T cells expressing TRPV1–YFP were observed using whole-cell patch clamp electrophysiology after the application of an AzCA derivative (1 μM). Error bars were calculated as s.e.m. (**a**) Voltage ramps were applied under both $\lambda = 350$ nm and $\lambda = 450$ nm irradiation. Larger currents were observed under $\lambda = 350$ nm irradiation (AzCA4). (**b**) AzCA2, AzCA3 and AzCA4 emerged as photoswitchable TRPV1 agonists. (**c**) When voltage clamped, photoswitching could be repeated over many cycles (AzCA3).

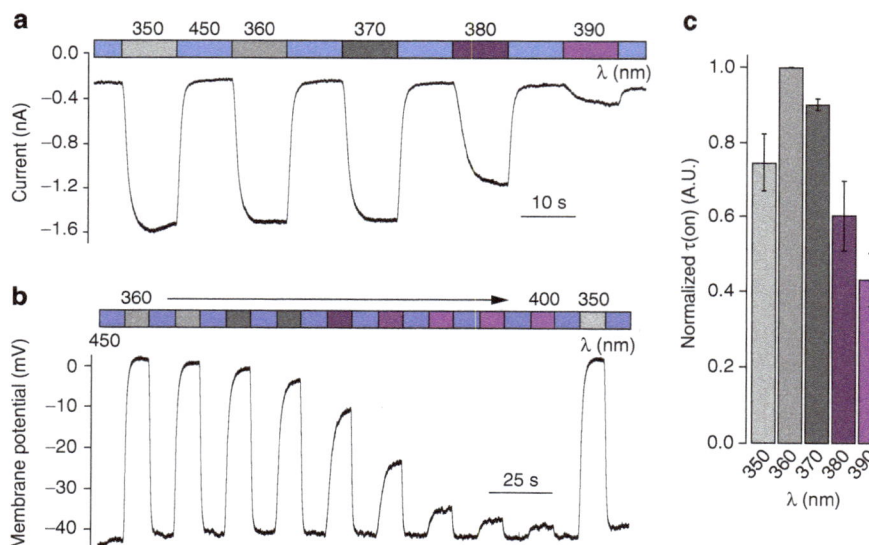

Figure 3 | TRPV1 activation can be precisely controlled with light. Cellular currents were observed using whole-cell patch clamp electrophysiology in HEK293T cells expressing TRPV1–YFP after the application of an AzCA derivative (1 μM). Error bars were calculated as s.e.m. (**a**) The current magnitude could be controlled by adjusting the ON wavelength between $\lambda = 350$ and 390 nm (AzCA3). (**b**) When current clamped, the membrane potential could be controlled by adjusting the ON wavelength between $\lambda = 350$ and 400 nm (AzCA4). (**c**) The activation rate could be controlled by adjusting the ON wavelength between $\lambda = 350$ and 390 nm (AzCA3, $n = 3$).

activity. Switching between $\lambda = 365$ nm and $\lambda = 460$ nm in the voltage clamp configuration at a holding potential of -60 mV resulted in reversible control over the transmembrane currents (Fig. 4a). Accordingly, the membrane potential and excitability of DRG neurons could be optically controlled as well. Action potential (AP) firing was reversibly switched ON and OFF by irradiation with $\lambda = 365$ nm and $\lambda = 460$ nm, respectively (Fig. 4b).

Bath application of AzCA4 (100 nM) and irradiation at $\lambda = 365$ nm (5 s) caused an increase in intracellular Ca^{2+} concentration in ~30% of DRG neurons cultured from 2- to

3-week-old mice (Fig. 4c and Supplementary Fig. 9). The remaining 70% of the DRG neurons did not respond to AzCA4 but still responded to a high potassium (Hi-K$^+$) solution (100 mM) (Fig. 4d). The percentage of AzCA4 responding neurons was consistent with the percentage of TRPV1 containing DRG neurons at this stage of mouse development ($33.6 \pm 1.3\%$ at P15, $30.5 \pm 3\%$ at P22)[31].

AzCA4 is selective for TRPV1-expressing neurons in the DRG. TRPV1 knockout mutant mice ($Trpv1^{-/-}$) have proven to be an

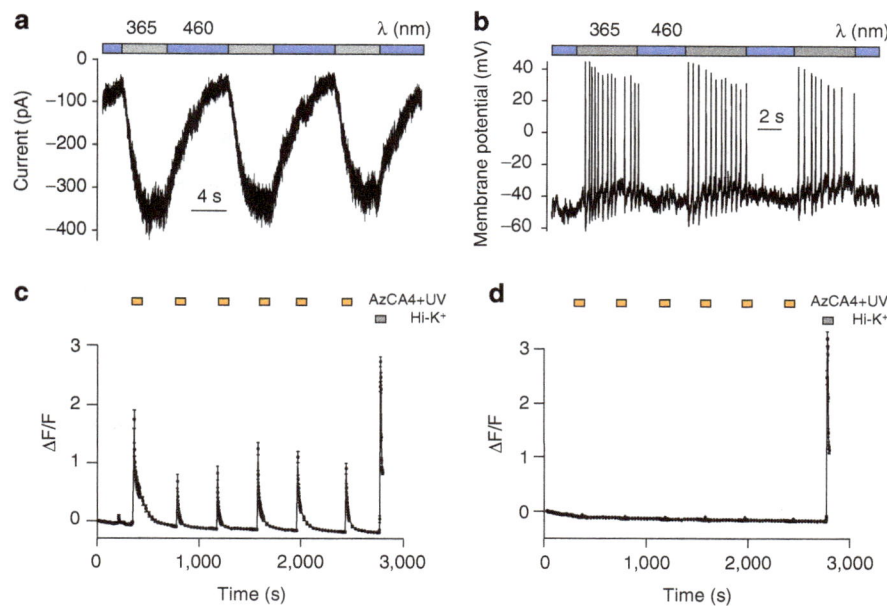

Figure 4 | AzCA4 enabled optical control over cultured wt DRG neurons. (**a**) After the bath application of AzCA4 (200 nM), neuronal currents could be modulated by monochromatic irradiation. When clamped at a holding potential of -60 mV, an inward current was observed on irradiation with $\lambda = 365$ nm and this effect could be reversed with irradiation at $\lambda = 460$ nm. (**b**) When clamped at a current of 0 pA and after the application of AzCA4 (200 nM), the neuronal membrane potential could be controlled. AP firing could be induced by irradiation at $\lambda = 365$ nm and halted with $\lambda = 460$ nm. This process could be repeated over many cycles. (**c**) Intracellular Ca^{2+} imaging showed that AzCA4 (100 nM) significantly increased the level of intracellular Ca^{2+} in TRPV1-positive neurons only after irradiation at $\lambda = 365$ nm (5 s). (**d**) Cells that did not respond to AzCA4 showed no increase in intracellular Ca^{2+} after the bath application of AzCA4 and an ultraviolet pulse (6 pulses, 100 nM, 5 s at $\lambda = 365$ nm). These cells still responded to a Hi-K$^+$ solution (100 mM), suggesting that they did not possess TRPV1. Error bars were calculated as s.e.m.

excellent negative control to study the functional aspects of TRPV1 and the role of CAP-sensitive afferent neurons in the mammalian nervous system[32]. We used this mouse line to assay the selectivity of AzCA4 in DRG neurons. As expected, Ca^{2+} imaging in $Trpv1^{-/-}$ mouse DRG neurons showed no neural activity in response to AzCA4 (300 nM) or CAP (300 nM). Control experiments showed that these neurons still responded to menthol (100 µM, data not shown), ATP (20 µM) and Hi-K$^+$ (100 mM) solutions (Supplementary Fig. 10). In combination, these results indicate that AzCA4 acted solely on TRPV1-positive neurons in the DRG.

Optical control of C-fibre nociceptors. We next evaluated the effects of AzCA4 on heat-sensitive C-fibre nociceptors (C-MH) in the *ex vivo* skin nerve preparation of the saphenous nerve. In wt mice, 19 out of 35 C-MH responded to AzCA4 photoswitching compared with none of the 11 C-MH examined in $Trpv1^{-/-}$ mice ($P < 0.001$, χ^2-test; Fig. 5a). We compared the activation of AzCA4 with that of CAP on C-MH in terms of the latency time to the first AP spike, as well as the AP discharge rates. Peak discharge rates during photostimulation with $\lambda = 365$ nm surged rapidly to 9.6 spikes per second and lasted on average 11.0 ± 6.9 s (Fig. 5b). The average peak discharge rates of C-MH due to AzCA4 photoswitching were not significantly different from CAP stimulation (Fig. 5c). However, the mean latency time to the first AP spike on irradiation with $\lambda = 365$ nm in the presence of AzCA4 was significantly shorter (1.9 ± 0.5 s; mean $\pm$ s.e.m.) when compared with the latencies to the first spike after CAP application (9.5 ± 3.5 s) (Fig. 5d, Mann–Whitney test, $P < 0.05$). The discharges of C-MH in response to AzCA4 were usually transient and adapted during the 20 s photostimulation period. These responses were completely reproducible after a 5 min recovery interval, during which AzCA4 was kept on the receptive field with

no signs of desensitization (Fig. 5e). Therefore, the photoswitching of AzCA4 could selectively activate TRPV1 receptors on the peripheral terminals of cutaneous C-MH to a similar magnitude as CAP. Advantageously, AzCA4 had the ability to trigger a more rapid neuronal response and did not require washout of the drug.

Serotonin and BK sensitized DRG neurons to AzCA4. TRPV1-mediated hyperalgesia is a complex process, which underlies inflammatory pain[19,33]. At sites of tissue injury, a number of chemical agents are released, which cause an inflammatory response resulting in an increased thermal pain sensation in response to normally non-painful stimuli. Several G protein-coupled receptors (GPCRs) mediate TRPV1 sensitization[33,34]. BK- and 5-HT-triggered GPCR cascades are able to decrease the threshold for TRPV1 activation and increase the number of receptors at the cell surface[5,33,35,36].

We used intracellular Ca^{2+} imaging in cultured wt mouse DRG neurons to determine whether these endogenous inflammatory agents still sensitized TRPV1 towards AzCA4. Our experiments showed that TRPV1 became sensitized to AzCA4 (200 nM) after the application of both BK (200 nM) and 5-HT (100 µM) (Fig. 6a,b). After 5 pulses of AzCA4 and ultraviolet irradiation, a steady state of TRPV1 desensitization was reached and the cells were washed with the sensitizing agent for 5 min (Fig. 6a). In both cases, a final pulse of AzCA4 and ultraviolet irradiation resulted in increased levels of intracellular Ca^{2+} when compared with the previous pulse. Experiments with both inflammatory agents produced similar results to those achieved when using CAP as the channel agonist (Fig. 6b and Supplementary Fig. 11). These results suggest that AzCA4 could be used as a tool to study the involvement of TRPV1 in inflammatory pain.

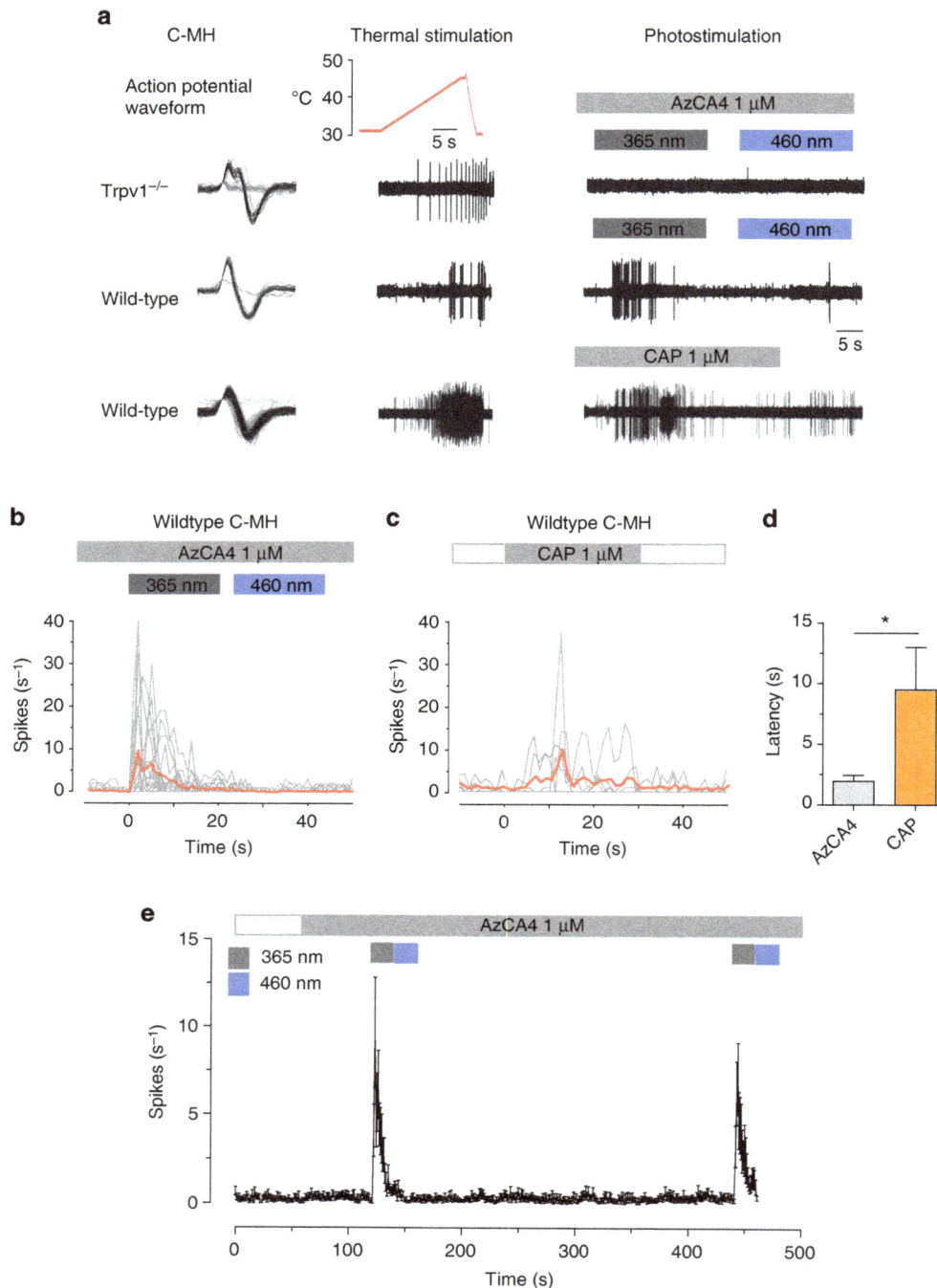

Figure 5 | Optical activation of TRPV1 in C-fibre nociceptors. (**a**) A typical sample trace showing the activation of a heat-sensitive C-fibre nociceptor (C-MH) by optical switching of AzCA4 (1 μM) with λ = 365 nm light and CAP (1 μM) application in wt mice. No photostimulation occurred in $Trpv1^{-/-}$ mice. (**b,c**) The average AP spiking rate (red) and the spiking rate for individual C-MHs (grey) in response to photostimulation in the presence of AzCA4 (1 μM, n = 19), and activation by CAP (1 μM, n = 6). (**d**) The latencies to the occurrence of the first AP spikes after photostimulation and after the application of CAP (*$P < 0.05$, Mann–Whitney test). (**e**) A second photostimulation in the presence of AzCA4 by λ = 365 nm light can be triggered 5 min after the first photostimulation; data are represented as the mean and s.d. of the number of spikes per 1 s bins of all activated C-MH.

AzCA4 is compatible with genetic tools. Genetically encoded Ca^{2+} indicators, such as GCaMP3 (ref. 37), have proven very useful for the study of neuronal activity *in vitro* and *in vivo*. We therefore tested the ability of AzCA4 to work in combination with this genetic tool. We crossed a mouse line that expresses the Cre recombinase under the promoter of TRPV1 (ref. 38), with a reporter mouse line that expresses GCaMP3 in a Cre-dependant manner ($Trpv1^{Cre/GCaMP3}$). As the majority of DRG neurons

express TRPV1 at embryonic stage E14.5 (ref. 31), we observed that 90% of the DRG neurons in culture showed a faint basal fluorescence, confirming that recombination had occurred in most neurons at an earlier developmental stage.

However, on application of CAP or AzCA4 alongside ultraviolet irradiation, only 30% of the neurons showed a Ca^{2+}-dependent increase in fluorescence. This confirmed not only the correct function and localization of GCaMP3 in

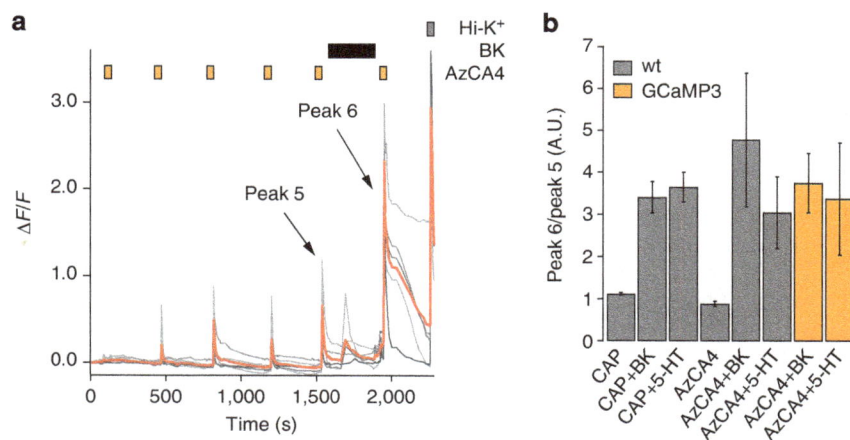

Figure 6 | Serotonin and BK sensitized TRPV1 to AzCA4. Intracellular Ca^{2+} imaging showed that both BK and 5-HT sensitized TRPV1 to CAP (100 nM) and AzCA4 (200 nM), with ultraviolet irradiation ($\lambda = 365$ nm, 5 s) in cultured wt DRG neurons. (**a**) After the application of BK (200 nM), an increased intensity and duration of Ca^{2+} influx was observed on application of AzCA-4 with ultraviolet irradiation when compared with the previous pulse. The neurons responded to a Hi-K$^+$ solution (100 mM). Shown here are five representative traces (grey) and average $\Delta F/F$ value (red). (**b**) TRPV1 sensitization experiments in wt mouse DRG neurons (grey) and the $Trpv1^{Cre/GCaMP3}$ mouse line (orange). The results were plotted as the ratio of peak heights for Peak 6/Peak 5 for the wt mouse as follows: CAP with no sensitization agent ($n = 520$); CAP with BK ($n = 210$); CAP with 5-HT ($n = 175$); AzCA4 with no sensitizing agent ($n = 36$); AzCA4 with BK ($n = 15$); and AzCA4 with 5-HT ($n = 12$). For the $Trpv1^{Cre/GCaMP3}$ mouse line, the results are plotted for the following: AzCA4 with BK ($n = 28$) and AzCA4 with 5-HT ($n = 10$). Error bars were calculated as s.e.m.

TRPV1-positive DRG neurons, but also that this small molecular photoswitch, AzCA4, can be used in combination with a genetic tool.

To further confirm the applicability of AzCA4 and the use of genetically encoded Ca^{2+} indicators to address physiologically relevant issues, we repeated the sensitization experiments on the $Trpv1^{Cre/GCaMP3}$ mouse line (Fig. 6b, orange). These results again confirmed that TRPV1 could be sensitized to AzCA4 by BK or 5-HT, even in the $Trpv1^{Cre/GCaMP3}$ mouse line.

QX-314 can be selectively transported into DRG neurons. QX-314 is a permanently charged lidocaine derivative that blocks Na$^+$ channels from the intracellular side but is unable to penetrate the plasma membrane due to its charged nature[39]. It has been shown that QX-314, and its photoswitchable derivative QAQ[40], could be shuttled into cells via TRPV1 when co-applied with CAP, to open the channel[41]. We hypothesized that intracellular Ca^{2+} build-up is not only caused by Ca^{2+} influx through TRPV1 but is a consequence of AP firing leading to Ca^{2+} release from intracellular stores. We showed AzCA4 (200 nM) in combination with $\lambda = 365$ nm irradiation, opened TRPV1 and allowed QX-314 to enter TRPV1-positive neurons in the DRG. The cells were first washed with a Hi-K$^+$ solution (40 mM) causing massive electrical activity. After the cells recovered, four pulses of AzCA4 (200 nM, 5 s at $\lambda = 365$ nm) reached a steady state of TRPV1 desensitization. Next, AzCA4 was co-applied with QX-314 (5 mM), followed by another pulse of AzCA4 and a final pulse of the Hi-K$^+$ solution. By comparing the peak heights of the first and final Hi-K$^+$ pulses (HK$_1$ and HK$_2$, respectively), we observed that the cells that were responsive to AzCA4 showed a lower HK$_2$/HK$_1$ ratio when compared with cells that did not respond to AzCA4 (Fig. 7). These results indicate that in combination with AzCA4, TRPV1 could be used as an import channel to localize a charged anaesthetic in TRPV1-positive cells, only.

Discussion

In this study, we present eight photoswitchable FAs, the FAAzos. We expect that these lipophilic modules will allow

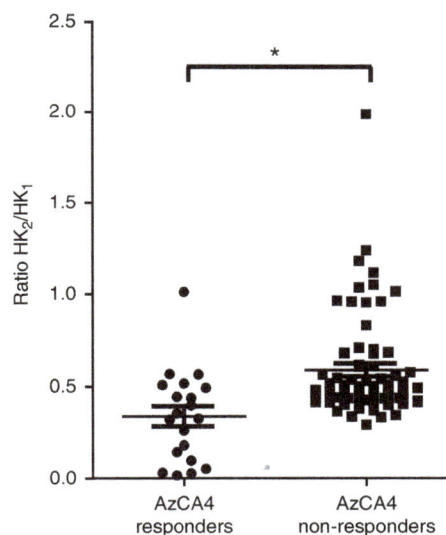

Figure 7 | QX-314 could be shuttled into TRPV1-positive DRG neurons using AzCA4. After the co-application of AzCA4 (200 nM) and QX-314 (5 mM), the peak heights of the Ca^{2+} signals of the Hi-K$^+$ (40 mM) pulses before (HK$_1$) and after (HK$_2$) drug application were compared. The results were plotted as the peak height ratio of two pulses, HK$_2$/HK$_1$, calculated for both AzCA4 responding and AzCA4 non-responding neurons. The error bars were calculated as s.e.m.

us to place a variety of lipid-modulated biological targets under photopharmacological control. The FAAzos are FAs mimetics, resembling in particular highly unsaturated FAs such as arachidonic acid. These compounds could be used as molecular building blocks for the construction of more complicated photolipids, which could facilitate the optical control of a wide range of ion channels, GPCRs and enzymes associated with FA signalling.

We hypothesized that an azobenzene photoswitch would be best suited towards integration into the FA backbone, as its hydrophobic nature may cause only a minimal disruption to the properties of a natural aliphatic chain. The FAAzos allow the position of the switch to be fine-tuned to complement structure–activity relationships between the ligand and its target. As a first installment illustrating this concept, we showed that the FAAzos could be incorporated into other photolipids through a simple amide coupling reaction. In HEK293T cells, three AzCAs stood out as the most promising candidates to enable the optical control of TRPV1 and showed significant, light-dependant efficacy at concentrations as low as 100 nM. All three compounds were more potent in their *cis*-configuration. Owing to the structural similarities between the AzCAs and other vanilloid TRPV1 agonists, we presume that the AzCAs act on the same vanilloid binding site as CAP, olvanil and arvanil. This is further supported by the requirement of the vanilloid headgroup, as was shown by the inactivity of FAAzo2–4. Channel activation by AzCA4 can also be completely blocked by the application of capsazepine, a known competitive antagonist for CAP, suggesting a common binding site and mode of activation.

We then demonstrated that AzCA4 was a powerful modulator of DRG neurons in wt mice and the $Trpv1^{Cre/GCaMP3}$ mouse line. Control experiments in untransfected HEK293T cells and $Trpv1^{-/-}$ mice showed no response to AzCA4, even on light stimulation. These results rule out the possibility of action through off-target mechanisms. This characteristic is essential for the study of signal transduction in the nociceptive neurons involved in inflammatory pain. To this end, we envision that AzCA4 could be used to study TRPV1-mediated hyperalgesia and the physiological processes involved with the inflammatory state that occurs at sites of tissue injury. We showed that application of components of the so-called 'inflammatory soup', such as BK or 5-HT, could sensitize TRPV1 to AzCA4 in DRG neurons. Furthermore, we proved that AzCA4 could be used in conjunction with genetic tools such as the GCaMP3 Ca^{2+} indicator selectively expressed in TRPV1-positive mouse neurons.

Importantly, AzCA4 allowed for greater temporal control over TRPV1 than that which can be achieved by other small-molecule agonists such as CAP, olvanil and arvanil. By working at an optimized concentration, AzCA4 showed no activity towards TRPV1 in its *trans*-configuration, but rapid TRPV1 activation was observed when it was isomerized to its *cis*-configuration. This ON and OFF effect became even more pronounced in neuronal systems when the nonlinear, 'all or nothing,' nature of the AP took effect. Previous studies have suggested that the rate of TRPV1 activation determines the balance between agonist potency and pungency[42–45]. Molecular weight and lipophilicity normally define the pharmacodynamics of TRPV1 agonists[42,43]. In the case of AzCAs, light provides another level of control. We showed that the magnitude and rate of cellular activation could be precisely tuned by adjusting the ON wavelength between $\lambda = 350$ and 390 nm. Therefore, AzCAs could provide a platform for the further understanding of hyperalgesia and could lead to the development of new anaesthetics.

When using CAP to stimulate C-fibres in the saphenous nerve, a relatively slow increase in AP firing was observed (Fig. 5b,c). This effect was probably caused by the time required for CAP to diffuse through the skin and plasma membrane to reach the vanilloid binding site[46–48]. We showed that AzCA4 could be applied to neurons as its dark-adapted, relatively inactive configuration. On isomerization, TRPV1 was activated and AP firing was immediately observed. It is this characteristic that makes AzCA4 a useful tool for the study of nociception, a process that relies on the rapid transmission of noxious stimuli from the periphery towards the coordinating centres of the central nervous system. AzCA4 also possesses significant advantages when

compared with other small molecules that have been used to place TRPV1 under the control of light. Caged CAP is a useful tool that has increased the level of control with which we are able to activate TRPV1 (ref. 49). However, compound uncaging and TRPV1 activation is a non-reversible, one-shot process. Repeated activation by uncaging relies on fast-acting transporters or deactivating enzymes to clear the synapse of the free ligand[50]. The fact that CAP and its analogues exhibit long-lasting effects suggests that they do not undergo transporter-mediated reuptake or significant enzymatic hydrolysis. These aspects are circumvented by the use of AzCA4, which allows for successive rounds of activation/inactivation without the requirement for washout of the drug. Previously, we showed that photoswitchable TRPV1 antagonists can optically control the activity of a constitutively active agonist on photoswitching[25]. In comparison, AzCA4 greatly simplifies this system and is capable of activating TRPV1 directly. This permits the optical control of neuronal excitability without the use of a second factor. Advantageously, AzCA4 is relatively inactive in the dark; therefore, a more rapid and reproducible initiation of activity can be achieved after it has distributed itself uniformly within more complex tissues.

In conclusion, this study provides the first application of photopharmacology to lipid signalling. Given the ubiquitous distribution of FA derivatives at all levels of nature, we envision that the FAAzos and their conjugates will emerge as broadly applicable tools for the optical control of biological functions which rely on protein–lipid interactions.

Methods

Whole-cell electrophysiology in HEK293T cells. HEK293T cells (obtained from the Leibniz-Institute DSMZ: 305) were incubated at 37 °C (10% CO_2) in DMEM medium + 10% fetal bovine serum and were split at 80%–90% confluency. For cell detachment, the medium was removed and the cells were washed with calcium-free PBS buffer and treated with trypsin for 2 min at 37 °C. The detached cells were diluted in growth medium and plated on acid-etched coverslips coated with poly-L-lysine in a 24-well plate. Cells (50,000) were added to each well in 500 µl standard growth medium along with the DNA (per coverslip: 500 ng TRPV1–YFP[28]) and JetPRIME transfection reagents, according to the manufacturer's instructions (per coverslip: 50 µl JetPRIME buffer, 0.5 µl JetPRIME transfection reagent). The transfection medium was exchanged for normal growth media 4 h after transfection and electrophysiological experiments were carried out 20–40 h later. Whole-cell patch clamp experiments were performed using a standard electrophysiology setup equipped with a HEKA Patch Clamp EPC10 USB amplifier and PatchMaster software (HEKA Electronik). Micropipettes were generated from 'Science Products GB200-F-8P with filament' pipettes using a Narishige PC-10 vertical puller. The patch pipette resistance varied between 5 and 9 MΩ. The bath solution contained the following: Solution A (in mM: 150 NaCl, 6.0 CsCl, 1.0 $MgCl_2$, 1.5 $CaCl_2$, 10 HEPES and 10 glucose (adjusted to pH 7.4 with 3 M NaOH))[51] or Solution B (in mM: 140 NaCl, 5 KCl, 5 HEPES, 1 MgCl and 5 glucose (adjusted to pH 7.4 with 3 M NaOH)). The pipette solution contained th following: Solution A' (in mM: 150 NaCl, 3 $MgCl_2$, 10 HEPES and 5 EGTA (adjusted to pH 7.2 with 3 M NaOH)) or solution B' (in mM: 100 K-gluconate, 40 KCl, 5 HEPES, 5 MgATP and 1 MgCl (adjusted to pH 7.2 with 1 M KOH)). The cells were first visualized to contain TRPV1–YFP by irradiation at $\lambda = 480$ nm using a Polychrome V (Till Photonics) monochromator. All cells had a leak current between −15 to −300 pA on breakin at −60 mV. All voltage clamp measurements were carried out at a holding potential of −60 mV. The cells were held at 0 pA for current clamp measurements. The compounds were applied by puff pipette using a 'Toohey Spritzer pressure system IIe' at 25 psi. The puff pipette resistance varied between 3 and 5 MΩ. All experiments were performed at room temperature.

Determination of AzCA photoswitching properties. The photoswitching properties of the prepared compounds were assessed using whole-cell voltage clamp electrophysiology in HEK293T cells transiently expressing TRPV1–YFP[28]. The compounds were dissolved as stock solutions in dimethylsulfoxide (DMSO; 2–6 mM) and then diluted into warmed extracellular solution at a concentration of 1 µM. The cell was held at −60 mV and voltage ramps (−100 to +100 mV over 5 s) were applied under both $\lambda = 450$ nm and $\lambda = 350$ nm irradiation. The AzCA derivative (1 µM) was then constantly applied (puff pipette application) while switching between the two wavelengths until a steady state of activity/ desensitization was observed on photoswitching (Supplementary Fig. 4a). The voltage ramps were applied again under each wavelength and the current change (ΔI) between the baseline ($-60\,mV$) and the ramp maximum ($+100\,mV$) was recorded (Supplementary Fig. 4b). $\Delta I(350\,nm)$ was normalized to $\Delta I(450\,nm)$ and this potentiation factor was averaged over multiple cells and plotted in Fig. 2b. TRPV1 activation and inactivation kinetics were determined by exponential curve fitting in Igor Pro.

Dorsal root ganglion neuronal culture. DRG were quickly dissected, collected in ice-cold DRG medium and digested in $1\,mg\,ml^{-1}$ Collagenase IV (Gibco) at $37\,°C$ for 50 min, to dissociate the tissue, followed by incubation in 0.05% trypsin (Gibco) in PBS at $37\,°C$ for 15 min. The trypsin was removed and cells were re-suspended in 1 ml of DRG medium. After gentle trituration, the DRGs were loaded onto a 2-ml BSA pillow and centrifuged at $250g$ for 10 min, to separate the myelin and debris. The resulting pellet was suspended in $50\,\mu l$ fresh DRG medium and plated onto poly-D-lysine ($100\,\mu g\,ml^{-1}$) and laminin ($10\,\mu g\,ml^{-1}$)-coated coverslips. The cells were flooded with medium 30 min after plating.

Whole-cell electrophysiology in cultured DRG neurons. Electrophysiological recordings of DRG neurons from 14- to 21-day-old mice were performed using a HEKA 10 amplifier (HEKA Instrument) and an ITC Analog Digital Converter (HEKA) in whole-cell voltage clamp or current clamp configuration. The currents were filtered with a built-in 5 kHz 8-pole Bessel filter and digitized at 50 kHz. The currents were analysed using Clampfit 10.3 (Molecular Devices) and graphs were plotted in Prism 5 (Graphpad). Experiments were performed 1–3 days after plating. The Trpv1^{Cre} and the GCaMP3 reporter mice were acquired from Jackson Laboratory. DRG neurons were prepared for imaging from 25-week-old Trpv1$^{Cre/GCaMP3}$ mice.

The extracellular solution contained in mM: 150 NaCl, 5 KCl, 10 HEPES, 10 glucose, 2 $CaCl_2$, 1 $MgCl_2$. The intracellular solution contained (values in mM): 130 KCl, 10 HEPES, 10 EGTA, 1 $CaCl_2$, 1 $MgCl_2$, 2 MgATP, 1 NaGTP, 4 NaCl and 4 PhosphoCreatine.

Thick-walled electrodes (Harvard Apparatus, $1.17 \times 0.87\,mm$, external and internal diameter, respectively) were pulled with a Sutter P-197 puller to a final resistance of $3–5\,M\Omega$. After the breakthrough, the intracellular solution was allowed to dialyse the intracellular medium for at least 1 min before the beginning of the recordings. Series resistance compensation reached values between 70 and 90%. Neurons were selected to have a leak current $< -100\,pA$ on breakin at $-60\,mV$. All experimental procedures were carried out in accordance with the State of Berlin Animal Welfare requirements and were approved by this authority.

Intracellular calcium imaging. DRG neurons plated on a 5-mm glass coverslip were placed in a recording chamber of $300\,\mu l$ volume (Harvard Apparatus) and were continuously perfused with extracellular solution at a rate of $2\,ml\,min^{-1}$. The wt neuron cells were loaded with Cal-520 ($5\,\mu M$, AAT-Bioquest) calcium dye for 1 h at $37\,°C$ in the presence of 0.02% pluronic acid dissolved in Ringer's solution (values in mM): 140 NaCl, 5 KCl, 2 $CaCl_2$, 2 $MgCl_2$, 10 HEPES, 10 glucose, adjusted to pH 7.4. CAP (100 nM, Tocris) was dissolved in extracellular solution from a stock concentration of 10 mM in ethanol. Fluorescent images were acquired with Metafluor Software (Molecular Devices) and analysed in Clampfit. All experiments were performed at room temperature. The dye excitation was performed at $\lambda = 480\,nm$. The results were plotted as the change in fluorescence over baseline fluorescence ($\Delta F/F$) as a function of time (s).

Ex-vivo skin nerve preparation. The skin-nerve preparation was used as previously described, to record from single primary afferents[52]. Mice were killed with CO_2 inhalation for 2–4 min, followed by cervical dislocation. The saphenous nerve and the shaved skin of the hind limb were dissected free and placed in an organ bath at $32\,°C$. The chamber was perfused with a synthetic interstitial fluid (SIF buffer) composed of (in mM): 123 NaCl, 3.5 KCl, 0.7 $MgSO_4$, 1.7 NaH_2PO_4, 2.0 $CaCl_2$, 9.5 Na-gluconate, 5.5 glucose, 7.5 sucrose and 10 HEPES at a pH of 7.4. The skin was placed with the corium side up in the organ bath for pharmacological application to the receptive fields of single sensory units. The saphenous nerve was placed in an adjacent chamber on a mirror, and under microscopy fine filaments were teased from the nerve and placed on the recording electrode. Electrical isolation was achieved with mineral oil. Signals from the filaments were amplified (Neurolog System, Digitimer Ltd) and sampled using a data acquisition system (PowerLab 4.0, ADInstruments). The receptive fields of individual mechanically sensitive C-fibre units were identified by manually probing the skin with the blunted tip of a glass probe. Their conduction velocities (calculated by dividing conduction distance over electrical latency for the first spike) were determined using an electrical stimulator ($1\,M\Omega$). All C-fibres studied were identified by mechanical probing and were heat sensitive (C-MH). The conduction velocities were in the C-fibre range ($<1\,m\,s^{-1}$). The thermal sensitivity of identified C-fibres was tested with a computer-controlled peltier device ($3 \times 5\,mm$, Yale University Medical School, Medical Instruments, New Haven, USA). A heat ramp was delivered from 32 to $48\,°C$ at a rate of $1\,°C\,s^{-1}$ to the mechanically localized receptive fields of single C-fibres. The receptive fields of heat-sensitive C-fibres were isolated with a metal cylinder ring (5 mm inner diameter, 10 mm in height and 1.44 g weight) for the administration of the drugs (AzCA4 or CAP). The metal

ring was tested for leakage before drug application. A stock solution of AzCA4 was prepared in DMSO and diluted in SIF buffer. One hundred microlitres of a 1-μM AzCA4 solution dissolved in SIF buffer was applied into the ring. The pharmacological testing protocol with AzCA4 had four distinct successive phases: (1) 60 s recording time before the application of AzCA4; (2) 60 s recording after application of AzCA4; (3) 20 s of recording during photostimulation of AzCA4 with light-emitting diode (LED) light, $\lambda = 365\,nm$ (Mic-LED-365, Prizmatix); (4) 20 s of recording during photoinhibition of AzCA4 with LED light, $\lambda = 460\,nm$ (UHP-LED-460, Prizmatix). AzCA4 was kept in the ring for 300 s and a second photostimulation with LED light 360 nm for 20 s was applied to test the reproducibility of the initial responses. One hundred microlitres of CAP ($1\,\mu M$, Sigma) was administered onto the receptive field of another set of heat-sensitive C-fibres for 20 s before washout. Recordings were obtained for 1 min before and 2 min after CAP administration. Spikes were discriminated offline, with the spike histogram extension of the software. Data were obtained from six skin-nerve preparations (2 Trpv1$^{-/-}$ and 4 wt C57Bl/6 N mice). All experimental procedures were carried out in accordance with the State of Berlin Animal Welfare requirements and were approved by this authority.

Compound switching. Compound switching for electrophysiology in HEK293T cells was achieved using a Polychrome V (Till Photonics) monochromator (intensity versus wavelength screen Supplementary Fig. 12) and the light beam was guided via a fibre-optic cable through the microscope objective and operated by the amplifier and PatchMaster software (HEKA Electronik).

Compound switching for electrophysiology in DRG neurons was achieved using a Prizmatix Mic-LED-365 high-power ultraviolet LED light source for illumination at $\lambda = 365\,nm$ and the Prizmatix UHP-Mic-LED-460 ultra-high-power LED light source for illumination at $\lambda = 460\,nm$. The light beam was guided by a fibre-optic cable and pointed directly towards the cells from above at an angle of about 45° from the side. The distance between the end of the cable and the cells was no greater than 2 cm. Ultraviolet illumination during intracellular calcium imaging was also performed using this light source.

Compound synthesis and characterization. All reagents and solvents were purchased from commercial sources (Sigma-Aldrich, TCI Europe N.V., Strem Chemicals and so on) and were used without further purification unless otherwise noted. Tetrahydrofuran was distilled under a N_2 atmosphere from Na/benzophenone before use. Triethylamine was distilled under a N_2 atmosphere from CaH_2 before use. Further dry solvents such as ethyl acetate, benzene, dichloromethane, toluene, ethanol and methanol were purchased from Acros Organics as 'extra dry' reagents and used as received. Solvents were degassed by sparging the freshly distilled solvent with argon gas in a Schlenk flask under ultrasonication using a Bandelin Sonorex RK510H ultrasonic bath for 20 min before use. Reactions were monitored by thin-layer chromatography on pre-coated, Merck Silica gel 60 F_{254} glass-backed plates and the chromatograms were first visualized by ultraviolet irradiation at 254 nm, followed by staining with aqueous ninhydrin, anisaldehyde or ceric ammonium molybdate solution and finally gentle heating with a heat gun. Flash silica gel chromatography was performed using silica gel (SiO_2, particle size 40-63 μm) purchased from Merck.

Ultraviolet visible spectra were recorded using a Varian Cary 50 Bio UV-Visible Spectrophotometer with Helma SUPRASIL precision cuvettes (10 mm light path). All compounds were dissolved at a concentration of $25\,\mu M$ in DMSO. Switching was achieved using a Polychrome V (Till Photonics) monochromator (intensity versus wavelength screen Supplementary Fig. 12). The illumination was controlled using PolyCon3.1 software and the light was guided through a fibre optic cable with the tip pointed directly into the top of the sample cuvette.

All NMR spectra were measured on a BRUKER Avance III HD 400 (equipped with a CryoProbe). Multiplicities in the following experimental procedures are abbreviated as follows: s, singlet; d, doublet; t, triplet; q, quartet; quint, quintet; sext, sextet; hept, heptet; br, broad; m, multiplet. Proton chemical shifts are expressed in parts per million (p.p.m., δ scale) and are referenced to the residual protium in the NMR solvent (CDCl$_3$: $\delta = 7.26$, D$_6$-DMSO: $\delta_H = 2.50$). Carbon chemical shifts are expressed in p.p.m. (δ scale) and are referenced to the carbon resonance of the NMR solvent (CDCl$_3$: $\delta = 77.16$, D$_6$-DMSO: $\delta = 39.52$). Note: owing to the trans/cis isomerization of some compounds containing an azobenzene functionality, more signals were observed in the ^1H and ^{13}C spectra than would be expected for the pure trans-isomer. Only signals for the major trans-isomer are reported; however, the identities of the remaining peaks were verified by two-dimensional correlation spectroscopy, heteronuclear single quantum coherence and heteronuclear multiple bond correlation experiments. The atom-numbering system is defined as depicted in Supplementary Fig. 13. All relevant synthetic details and NMR spectra can be found in Supplementary Figs 14–46 and the Supplementary Methods.

Infrared spectra were recorded as neat materials on a PERKIN ELMER Spectrum BX-59343 instrument. For detection, a SMITHS DETECTION DuraSam-pIIR II Diamond ATR sensor was used. The measured wave numbers are reported in cm^{-1}.

Low- and high-resolution electron ionization mass spectra were obtained on a MAT CH7A mass spectrometer. Low- and high-resolution electrospray ionization mass spectra were obtained on a Varian MAT 711 MS instrument operating in either positive or negative ionization modes.

References

1. Wang, X. Lipid signaling. *Curr. Opin. Plant Biol.* **7**, 329–336 (2004).
2. Shevchenko, A. & Simons, K. Lipidomics: coming to grips with lipid diversity. *Nat. Rev.* **11**, 593–598 (2010).
3. *IUPAC Gold Book—Fatty Acids* 1307 (Blackwell Scientific Publications, 1997).
4. Szallasi, A., Cortright, D. N., Blum, C. A. & Eid, S. R. The vanilloid receptor TRPV1: 10 years from channel cloning to antagonist proof-of-concept. *Nat. Rev. Drug Discov.* **6**, 357–372 (2007).
5. Chuang, H. H. *et al.* Bradykinin and nerve growth factor release the capsaicin receptor from PtdIns(4,5)P2-mediated inhibition. *Nature* **411**, 957–962 (2001).
6. Clapham, D. E. TRP channels as cellular sensors. *Nature* **426**, 517–524 (2003).
7. Venkatachalam, K. & Montell, C. TRP channels. *Annu. Rev. Biochem.* **76**, 387–417 (2007).
8. Gavva, N. R. Body-temperature maintenance as the predominant function of the vanilloid receptor TRPV1. *Trends Pharmacol. Sci.* **29**, 550–557 (2008).
9. Tominaga, M. *et al.* The cloned capsaicin receptor integrates multiple pain-producing stimuli. *Neuron* **21**, 531–543 (1998).
10. Holzer, P. Local effector functions of capsaicin-sensitive sensory nerve endings: involvement of tachykinins, calcitonin gene-related peptide and other neuropeptides. *Neuroscience* **24**, 739–768 (1988).
11. Caterina, M. J. *et al.* The capsaicin receptor: a heat-activated ion channel in the pain pathway. *Nature* **389**, 816–824 (1997).
12. Jordt, S. E., Tominaga, M. & Julius, D. Acid potentiation of the capsaicin receptor determined by a key extracellular site. *Proc. Natl Acad. Sci. USA* **97**, 8134–8139 (2000).
13. Cuypers, E., Yanagihara, A., Karlsson, E. & Tytgat, J. Jellyfish and other cnidarian envenomations cause pain by affecting TRPV1 channels. *FEBS Lett.* **580**, 5728–5732 (2006).
14. Siemens, J. *et al.* Spider toxins activate the capsaicin receptor to produce inflammatory pain. *Nature* **444**, 208–212 (2006).
15. Ross, R. Anandamide and vanilloid TRPV1 receptors. *Br. J. Pharmacol.* **140**, 790–801 (2003).
16. Huang, S. M. *et al.* An endogenous capsaicin-like substance with high potency at recombinant and native vanilloid VR1 receptors. *Proc. Natl Acad. Sci. USA* **99**, 8400–8405 (2002).
17. Brand, L. *et al.* NE-19550: a novel, orally active anti-inflammatory analgesic. *Drugs Exp. Clin. Res.* **13**, 259–265 (1987).
18. Melck, D. *et al.* Unsaturated long-chain N-acyl-vanillyl-amides (N-AVAMs): vanilloid receptor ligands that inhibit anandamide-facilitated transport and bind to CB1 cannabinoid receptors. *Biochem. Biophys. Res. Commun.* **262**, 275–284 (1999).
19. Davis, J. B. *et al.* Vanilloid receptor-1 is essential for inflammatory thermal hyperalgesia. *Nature* **405**, 183–187 (2000).
20. Hu, W. P., Guan, B. C., Ru, L. Q., Chen, J. G. & Li, Z. W. Potentiation of 5-HT3 receptor function by the activation of coexistent 5-HT2 receptors in trigeminal ganglion neurons of rats. *Neuropharmacology* **47**, 833–840 (2004).
21. Hanack, C. *et al.* GABA blocks pathological but not acute TRPV1 pain signals. *Cell* **160**, 759–770 (2015).
22. Velema, W. A., Szymanski, W. & Feringa, B. L. Photopharmacology: beyond proof of principle. *J. Am. Chem. Soc.* **136**, 2178–2191 (2014).
23. Mourot, A., Tochitsky, I. & Kramer, R. H. Light at the end of the channel: optical manipulation of intrinsic neuronal excitability with chemical photoswitches. *Front. Mol. Neurosci.* **6**, 5 (2013).
24. Fehrentz, T., Schönberger, M. & Trauner, D. Optochemical genetics. *Angew. Chem. Int. Ed. Engl.* **50**, 12156–12182 (2011).
25. Stein, M., Breit, A., Fehrentz, T., Gudermann, T. & Trauner, D. Optical control of TRPV1 channels. *Angew. Chem. Int. Ed. Engl.* **52**, 9845–9848 (2013).
26. Morgan, C. G., Thomas, E. W., Yianni, Y. P. & Sandhu, S. S. Incorporation of a novel photochromic phospholipid molecule into vesicles of dipalmitoyl-phosphatidylcholine. *Biochim. Biophys. Acta Biomembr.* **820**, 107–114 (1985).
27. Cao, E., Liao, M., Cheng, Y. & Julius, D. TRPV1 structures in distinct conformations reveal activation mechanisms. *Nature* **504**, 113–118 (2013).
28. Hellwig, N., Albrecht, N., Harteneck, C., Schultz, G. & Schaefer, M. Homo- and heteromeric assembly of TRPV channel subunits. *J. Cell Sci.* **118**, 917–928 (2005).
29. Bevan, S. *et al.* Capsazepine: a competitive antagonist of the sensory neurone excitant capsaicin. *Br. J. Pharmacol.* **107**, 544–552 (1992).
30. Walpole, C. S. *et al.* The discovery of capsazepine, the first competitive antagonist of the sensory neuron excitants capsaicin and resiniferatoxin. *J. Med. Chem.* **37**, 1942–1954 (1994).
31. Cavanaugh, D. J., Chesler, A. T., Bráz, J. M., Shah, N. M. & Basbaum, A. I. Restriction of TRPV1 to the peptidergic subset of primary afferent neurons follows its developmental downregulation in nonpeptidergic neurons. *J. Neurosci.* **31**, 10119–10127 (2011).
32. Bölcskei, K. *et al.* Investigation of the role of TRPV1 receptors in acute and chronic nociceptive processes using gene-deficient mice. *Pain* **117**, 368–376 (2005).
33. Huang, J., Zhang, X. & McNaughton, P. Inflammatory pain: the cellular basis of heat hyperalgesia. *Curr. Neuropharmacol.* **4**, 197–206 (2006).
34. Sugiuar, T., Bielefeldt, K. & Gebhart, G. F. TRPV1 function in mouse colon sensory neurons is enhanced by metabotropic 5-hydroxytryptamine receptor activation. *J. Neurosci.* **24**, 9521–9530 (2004).
35. Moriyama, T. *et al.* Sensitization of TRPV1 by EP1 and IP reveals peripheral nociceptive mechanism of prostaglandins. *Mol. Pain* **1**, 3 (2005).
36. Ohta, T. *et al.* Potentiation of transient receptor potential V1 functions by the activation of metabotropic 5-HT receptors in rat primary sensory neurons. *J. Physiol.* **576**, 809–822 (2006).
37. Zariwala, H. A. *et al.* A Cre-dependent GCaMP3 reporter mouse for neuronal imaging *in vivo*. *J. Neurosci.* **32**, 3131–3141 (2012).
38. Cavanaugh, D. J. *et al.* Trpv1 reporter mice reveal highly restricted brain distribution and functional expression in arteriolar smooth muscle cells. *J. Neurosci.* **31**, 5067–5077 (2011).
39. Yeh, J. Z. Sodium inactivation mechanism modulates QX-314 block of sodium channels in squid axons. *Biophys. J.* **24**, 569–574 (1978).
40. Mourot, A. *et al.* Rapid optical control of nociception with an ion-channel photoswitch. *Nat. Methods* **9**, 396–402 (2012).
41. Binshtok, A. M., Bean, B. P. & Woolf, C. J. Inhibition of nociceptors by TRPV1-mediated entry of impermeant sodium channel blockers. *Nature* **449**, 607–610 (2007).
42. Iida, T. *et al.* TRPV1 activation and induction of nociceptive response by a non-pungent capsaicin-like compound, capsiate. *Neuropharmacology* **44**, 958–967 (2003).
43. Wang, Y. *et al.* Kinetics of penetration influence the apparent potency of vanilloids on TRPV1. *Mol. Pharmacol.* **69**, 1166–1173 (2006).
44. Ursu, D., Knopp, K., Beattie, R. E., Liu, B. & Sher, E. Pungency of TRPV1 agonists is directly correlated with kinetics of receptor activation and lipophilicity. *Eur. J. Pharmacol.* **641**, 114–122 (2010).
45. Liu, L., Lo, Y., Chen, I. & Simon, S. a. The responses of rat trigeminal ganglion neurons to capsaicin and two nonpungent vanilloid receptor agonists, olvanil and glyceryl nonamide. *J. Neurosci.* **17**, 4101–4111 (1997).
46. Chou, M. Z., Mtui, T., Gao, Y. D., Kohler, M. & Middleton, R. E. Resiniferatoxin binds to the capsaicin receptor (TRPV1) near the extracellular side of the S4 transmembrane domain. *Biochemistry* **43**, 2501–2511 (2004).
47. Jung, J. *et al.* Capsaicin binds to the intracellular domain of the capsaicin-activated ion channel. *J. Neurosci.* **19**, 529–538 (1999).
48. Vyklický, L., Lyfenko, A., Kuffler, D. P. & Vlachová, V. Vanilloid receptor TRPV1 is not activated by vanilloids applied intracellularly. *Neuroreport* **14**, 1061–1065 (2003).
49. Zemelman, B. V., Nesnas, N., Lee, G. A. & Miesenbo, G. Photochemical gating of heterologous ion channels: Remote control over genetically designated populations of neurons. *Proc. Natl Acad. Sci. USA* **100**, 1352–1357 (2003).
50. Höglinger, D., Nadler, A. & Schultz, C. Caged lipids as tools for investigating cellular signaling. *Biochim. Biophys. Acta Mol. Cell Biol. Lipids* **1841**, 1085–1096 (2014).
51. Voets, T. *et al.* The principle of temperature-dependent gating in cold- and heat-sensitive TRP channels. *Nature* **430**, 748–754 (2004).
52. Moshourab, R. A., Wetzel, C., Martinez-Salgado, C. & Lewin, G. R. Stomatin-domain protein interactions with acid-sensing ion channels modulate nociceptor mechanosensitivity. *J. Physiol.* **591**, 5555–5574 (2013).

Acknowledgements

D.T. and J.A.F. gratefully acknowledge the Deutsche Forschungsgemeinschaft (SFB 1032) and the European Research Council (ERC Advanced Grant 268795 to D.T.) for financial support. Additional funds were obtained from grants from the Alexander von Humboldt foundation (stipend to M.M.) and a senior ERC Advanced grant (294678 to G.R.L). R.M. was supported by a fellowship from the clinical scientist programme of the MDC/Charité. We thank Dr Johannes Broichhagen, Arunas Damijonaitis, Dr David Barber, Cedric Hugelshofer and Dr Matthias Schönberger for insightful discussions leading to the preparation of the manuscript.

Author contributions

D.T. and G.R.L. coordinated and supervised the study. J.A.F. designed and synthesized the compounds, and carried out electrophysiological and imaging experiments in collaboration with M.M. and M.S. R.M. carried out experiments with C-fibres. J.A.F., D.T., M.M. and R.M. wrote the paper with input from all other co-authors.

Additional information

8

Pyrazoleamide compounds are potent antimalarials that target Na$^+$ homeostasis in intraerythrocytic *Plasmodium falciparum*

Akhil B. Vaidya[1], Joanne M. Morrisey[1], Zhongsheng Zhang[2], Sudipta Das[1], Thomas M. Daly[1], Thomas D. Otto[3], Natalie J. Spillman[4], Matthew Wyvratt[5], Peter Siegl[5], Jutta Marfurt[6], Grennady Wirjanata[6], Boni F. Sebayang[7], Ric N. Price[6,8], Arnab Chatterjee[9], Advait Nagle[9], Marcin Stasiak[2], Susan A. Charman[10], Iñigo Angulo-Barturen[11], Santiago Ferrer[11], María Belén Jiménez-Díaz[11], María Santos Martínez[11], Francisco Javier Gamo[11], Vicky M. Avery[12], Andrea Ruecker[13], Michael Delves[13], Kiaran Kirk[4], Matthew Berriman[3], Sandhya Kortagere[1], Jeremy Burrows[5], Erkang Fan[2] & Lawrence W. Bergman[1]

The quest for new antimalarial drugs, especially those with novel modes of action, is essential in the face of emerging drug-resistant parasites. Here we describe a new chemical class of molecules, pyrazoleamides, with potent activity against human malaria parasites and showing remarkably rapid parasite clearance in an *in vivo* model. Investigations involving pyrazoleamide-resistant parasites, whole-genome sequencing and gene transfers reveal that mutations in two proteins, a calcium-dependent protein kinase (PfCDPK5) and a P-type cation-ATPase (PfATP4), are necessary to impart full resistance to these compounds. A pyrazoleamide compound causes a rapid disruption of Na$^+$ regulation in blood-stage *Plasmodium falciparum* parasites. Similar effect on Na$^+$ homeostasis was recently reported for spiroindolones, which are antimalarials of a chemical class quite distinct from pyrazoleamides. Our results reveal that disruption of Na$^+$ homeostasis in malaria parasites is a promising mode of antimalarial action mediated by at least two distinct chemical classes.

[1] Department of Microbiology and Immunology, Center for Molecular Parasitology, Drexel University College of Medicine, 2900 Queen Lane, Philadelphia, Pennsylvania 190129, USA. [2] Department of Biochemistry, University of Washington, Box 357350, Seattle, Washington 98195, USA. [3] Wellcome Trust Sanger Institute, Hinxton, Cambridge CB101SA, UK. [4] Research School of Biology, The Australian National University, Canberra, Australian Capital Territory 0200, Australia. [5] Medicines for Malaria Venture, PO Box 1826, 20Rt de Pr-Bois, Geneva 15 1215, Switzerland. [6] Division of Global and Tropical Health, Menzies School of Health Research and Charles Darwin University, PO Box 41096, Casuarina, Northern Territory 0811, Australia. [7] Eijkman Institute for Molecular Biology, Jl. Diponegoro 69, Jakarta 10430, Indonesia. [8] Nuffield Department of Clinical Medicine, Centre for Tropical Medicine, University of Oxford, Oxford OX3 7LJ, UK. [9] Genomics Institute of the Novartis Research Foundation, 10675 John Jay Hopkins Drive, San Diego, California 92121, USA. [10] Center for Drug Candidate Optimisation, Monash University, 381 Royal Parade, Parkville, Victoria 3052, Australia. [11] GlaxoSmithKline, Malaria Support Group, Calle Severo Ochoa 2, Tres Cantos 28760, Spain. [12] Eskitis Institute, Griffith University, Don Young Road, Nathan, Queensland 4111, Australia. [13] Department of Life Sciences, South Kensington Campus, Imperial College, London SW7 2AZ, UK. Correspondence and requests for materials should be addressed to A.B.V. (email: avaidya@drexelmed.edu).

It is a well-established fact that microbial pathogens subjected to drug pressure tend to develop resistance to the drug. The probability of resistance emergence increases in proportion to the size of the population exposed to the antimicrobials. With hundreds of millions of malaria cases being treated with antimalarial drugs each year and with each individual patient bearing hundreds of billions of malaria parasites[1], it is necessary to continue to feed the antimalarial pipeline with new drugs to counter the likely emergence of resistance. The emergence and spread of chloroquine-resistant *Plasmodium falciparum* has been a major contributing factor for the resurgence in malaria morbidity and mortality during the 1980s and 1990s (ref. 2), which only now seems to be abating with the advent of artemisinin combination therapy and other interventions[3,4]. Reports of delayed clinical response to artemisinin derivatives in Southeast Asia as a harbinger of resistance emergence[5–7] provide further impetus for the need to have an available robust antimalarial pipeline. Over the past decade, the Medicines for Malaria Venture (MMV) has spearheaded efforts of academic and industrial partners to discover and develop antimalarial drugs. Several new compounds at various stages of development have been identified through these efforts[8].

We describe here our investigations of a new chemical class of antimalarial compounds with highly potent activity against *P. falciparum* and *P. vivax*, the most prevalent species causing human malaria. These compounds are active against parasites resistant to currently used antimalarials and are also inhibitory to the onward development of the sexual stages of *P. falciparum* indicating their potential to be an effective means for treating malaria and for its transmission. Genetic and biochemical studies indicate that the pyrazoleamides are likely to affect a cation-pumping P-type ATPase, resulting in rapid disruption of Na^+ homeostasis in intraerythrocytic *P. falciparum*. This mode of action is similar to a recent demonstration that NITD609 (ref. 9), an antimalarial spiroindolone under development with a very different chemical structure, also disrupts Na^+ homeostasis in malaria parasites[10].

Results

Pyrazoleamides as potent inhibitors of human *Plasmodium* spp. The initial hit compounds C416, a pyrazoleurea derivative, and C2-1, a pyrazoleamide derivative, (Fig. 1a) were identified through a structure-based *in silico* screening of a compound library[11] and showed growth inhibitory activity with effective concentration for 50% growth inhibition (EC_{50}) of 150 and 50 nM, respectively, against *P. falciparum*. An extensive medicinal chemistry campaign (to be described in detail elsewhere) was conducted by synthesizing variants of pyrazoleamide compound C2-1 and leading to a series of compounds with low nanomolar activity against *P. falciparum*. Structures of three of the late lead compounds, PA21A050 (EC_{50}: 0.7 nM), PA21A092 (EC_{50}: 5 nM) and PA21A102 (EC_{50}: 8 nM), are shown in Fig. 1a. On the basis of its biological, pharmaceutical and toxicological profiles, compound PA21A092 was designated as a preclinical drug candidate to be developed for first-in-human studies. Relatively equal activity of PA21A092 was observed over a 48-h period against *P. falciparum*, regardless of the stage of parasites used in the assay, with EC_{50} values ranging from 5 to 13 nM (Fig. 1b). The functional viability of *P. falciparum* mature Stage V male and

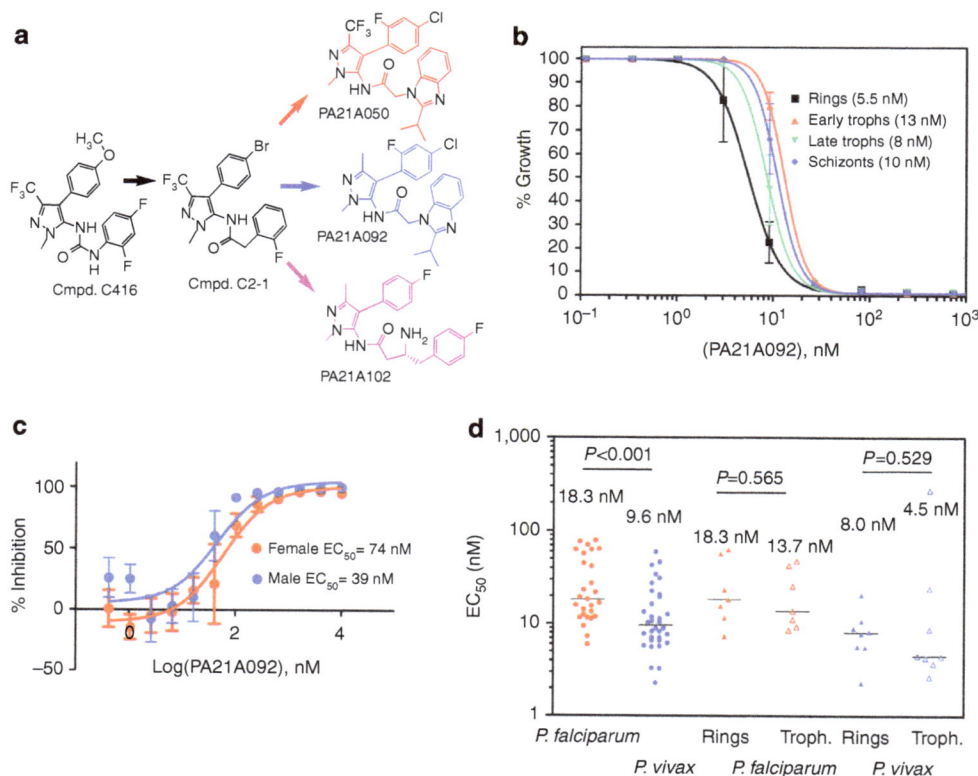

Figure 1 | Structure and antimalarial activities of pyrazoleamide compounds. (**a**) Structures of the hit and lead compounds. (**b**) Growth inhibition assays of PA21A092 against the indicated stages of Dd2 line of *P. falciparum*. (**c**) PA21A092 inhibits male (blue) and female (red) gamete production by mature gametocytes. EC_{50} values are estimated to be 39 and 74 nM for male and female gamete production, respectively; methylene blue as a positive control had EC_{50} values of 39 and 43 nM, respectively, in these assays. (**d**) PA21A092 is active against clinical field isolates of *P. falciparum* (red circles) and *P. vivax* (blue circles) in *ex vivo* growth inhibition assays with equal potency against ring (closed triangles) and trophozoite (open triangles) stages in both species.

female gametocytes as manifested by their ability to form male and female gametes, respectively, was inhibited when exposed to PA21A092 with an EC_{50} of 39 and 74 nM, respectively (Fig. 1c), indicating its potential to act also as a transmission-blocking drug. A panel of eight *P. falciparum* lines resistant to a number of currently used antimalarial drugs were susceptible to compound 21A092 (Supplementary Table 1), suggesting a mode of action different from currently used antimalarials. Furthermore, PA21A092 was tested against clinical isolates of *P. falciparum* and *P. vivax* infecting patients living in an area with high prevalence of multiple drug resistance. Using an *ex vivo* assay[12], we found that both species were highly susceptible to PA21A092, with a median EC_{50} of 18 nM against *P. falciparum* from 32 patients and 10 nM against *P. vivax* from 35 patients (Fig. 1d).

In vivo efficacy of pyrazoleamides against P. falciparum.

We used nonobese/severe combined immunodeficiency/IL2Rγ^{null} (NOD/SCID/IL2Rγ^{null}) mice engrafted with human erythrocytes and infected with an adapted line of *P. falciparum* as a model to assess *in vivo* efficacy of the pyrazoleamide compounds[13,14]. This model has been used previously for examining many different antimalarials for their *in vivo* activity against the human malaria parasite *P. falciparum*[15]. Groups of three mice each were treated once a day for 4 consecutive days, beginning on day 3 post infection, with four oral dose levels of PA21A092. As shown in Fig. 2a, PA21A092 was highly effective when administered orally with effective dose for 90% parasitemia reduction (ED$_{90}$) of 2.5 mg kg^{-1}. Compound PA21A050 had ED$_{90}$ of 0.9 mg kg^{-1} (Supplementary Fig. 1), whereas PA21A102 had an ED$_{90}$ of 4 mg kg^{-1} (Supplementary Fig. 2). The pharmacokinetics of PA21A092 in the mice employed in the therapeutic efficacy study

was studied by taking 25 µl serial blood samples up to 23 h after the first dose. As shown in Fig. 2b and Supplementary Table 2, oral pharmacokinetics were approximately linear in the dose range used. Assuming no significant accumulation during treatment, the estimated drug exposure necessary to inhibit *P. falciparum* parasitemia on day 7 post infection by 90% with respect to control mice (area under the curve at 90% effective dose, AUC$_{ED90}$) was 0.24 µg h ml^{-1} per day (Fig. 2c). In this *in vivo* assay, the AUC$_{ED90}$ is the average daily exposure necessary to achieve no net parasite growth on day 7. The maximum parasite clearance was achieved at PA21A092 blood exposure of above 1 µg h ml^{-1} per day and was comparable, in this model, to that seen with artesunate, which is thus far the fastest-acting antimalarial in use. Erythrocytes with only remnants of parasite nuclei were seen following 2-day treatments with the pyrazole compounds (Fig. 2d,e).

Investigating P. falciparum resistant to pyrazoleamides.

The lack of cross-resistance to the pyrazoleamides in parasites resistant to currently used antimalarial drugs suggests a potentially novel mode of action for this new chemical class. To gain mechanistic insight into the action of the pyrazoleamides, we derived *P. falciparum* lines resistant to the initial hit compound C2-1. Our assessment of resistance frequency for compounds PA21A050 and PA21A092 indicated a rate of $< 3 \times 10^{-9}$ under a standard protocol[16] of continuous exposure to $10 \times EC_{50}$ concentration of the compounds, suggesting a low propensity for parasite resistance development against these compounds. Therefore, resistant parasite lines were derived by exposure of the Dd2 line of *P. falciparum* to $3 \times EC_{50}$ concentration of the compound C2-1. Three lines resistant to compound C2-1 with an

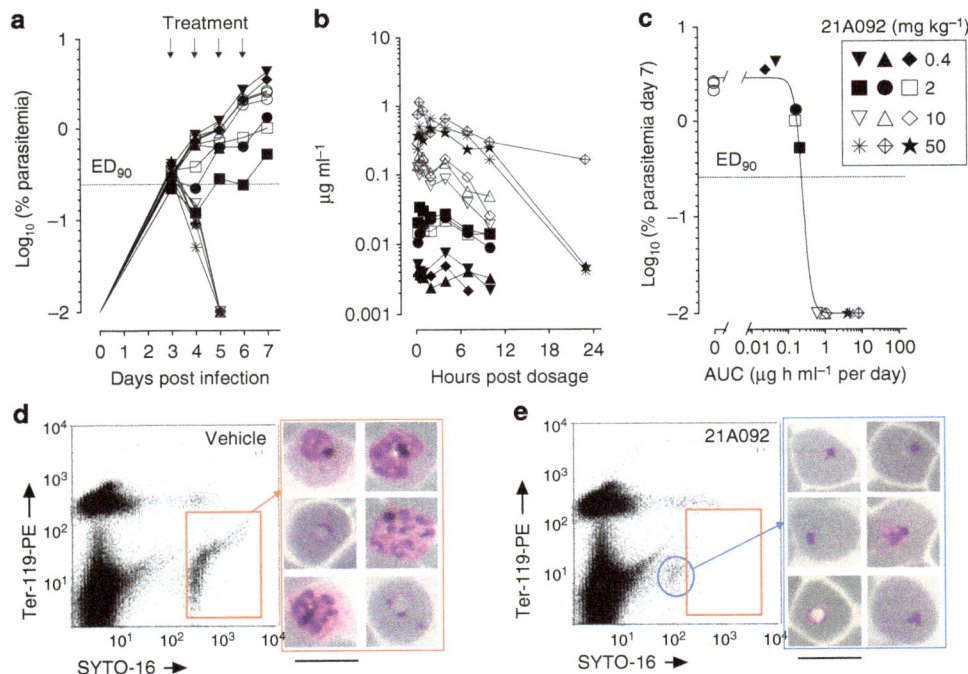

Figure 2 | *In vivo* efficacy of PA21A092 against *P. falciparum*. Four indicated doses of PA21A092 were administered orally to groups of three NOD/scid/ IL2Rγ^{null} mice each engrafted with human erythrocytes and infected with *P. falciparum*. The compound was administered starting on day 3 post infection for 4 consecutive days. Parasitemia was assessed each day from day 3 post infection up to 7 days (**a**). Concentrations of PA21A092 were measured by LC/MS in each mouse at 0.25, 0.5, 1, 2, 4, 7, 10 and 23 h after the first dose (**b**). The estimated drug exposure necessary to inhibit *P. falciparum* parasitemia on day 7 post infection by 90% (AUC$_{ED90}$) was 0.24 µg h ml^{-1} per day^{-1} (**c**). Comparison of morphology of parasitized human RBC (as observed in Giemsa-stained thin blood smears prepared on day 7 after infection) in vehicle-treated (**d**) and PA21A092-treated (**e**) mice revealed normal stages of parasites in control but erythrocytes with only highly pyknotic staining nuclei fragments in treated mice (scale bars, 10 µm). In **a–c**, each symbol represents individual mouse with the dose of compound indicated in the inset on the right. Open circles in **a** are mice treated with the vehicle only.

EC_{50} of $\sim$20-fold higher than the wild-type parasites were derived through this process of exposure to a reduced level of the compound (Supplementary Fig. 3). These resistant parasites were cross-resistant to all active pyrazoleamide compounds, including the late lead and candidate compounds (Supplementary Table 3), suggesting a common mode of action for the pyrazoleamide series.

To gain insight into the mode of action for and resistance to the pyrazoleamides, genomes of the Dd2 parental line and the three pyrazoleamide-resistant lines were sequenced using 'next-generation' sequencing technology[17]. Custom-designed bioinformatics for *P. falciparum* genome-sequence comparison[18] revealed non-synonymous single-nucleotide polymorphism (SNP) in five genes: PF3D7_0411900, DNA polymerase alpha (mutation D133Y); PF3D7_0630900, DEAD/DEAH box ATP-dependent RNA helicase (N142K, a polymorphic site); PF3D7_1034300, thioredoxin-like associated protein 2, (K465E); PF3D7_1211900, non-SERCA calcium ATPase (V178I); and PF3D7_1337800, calcium-dependent protein kinase 5 (T392A). These mutations were common to all three resistant lines compared with the parental Dd2 parasites. An assessment of potential effects of these mutations as well as expression patterns of these genes led us to focus initial attention on two proteins: the calcium-dependent protein kinase 5 (PfCDPK5; PF3D7_1337800) and a P-type cation ATPase annotated as a non-SERCA calcium ATPase, PfATP4 (PF3D7_1211900). Dvorin *et al.*[19] have shown PfCDPK5 to be essential for egress of progeny merozoites at the last step of erythrocytic schizogony by *P. falciparum*, and thus deemed an attractive drug target. The resistance-associated mutation, T392A, in PfCDPK5 was predicted to be in the junction region of the enzyme that links the kinase domain to the calmodulin-like EF-hand domains, and acts as a regulatory loop of the enzyme (Fig. 3a). PfATP4 was first described as a Ca^{2+} pump[20,21] and recently found to bear mutations in *P. falciparum* parasites resistant to a new class of antimalarials, the spiroindolones[9]. Spillman *et al.*[10] have provided evidence consistent with the hypothesis that PfATP4 is a P-type Na^+ ATPase and a target for the spiroindolones. The resistance-associated mutation in PfATP4, a conservative V178I change, was localized to the predicted first transmembrane domain of the protein (Fig. 3b), and was different from the mutations

observed by Rottmann *et al.*[9] in spiroindolone-resistant parasites. The pyrazoleamide-resistant lines described here were not cross-resistant to a spiroindolone (Supplementary Fig. 3b).

Mutations necessary for full resistance to pyrazoleamides. To assess the effects of expressing the mutated version of the enzyme (PfCDPK5^{T392A}), a transgenic Dd2 line of *P. falciparum* was constructed in which the PfCDPK5^{wt} allele was replaced by PfCDPK5^{T392A} allele via single crossover allelic exchange recombination (Supplementary Fig. 4). When this transgenic parasite line (Dd2::PfCDPK5^{T392A}) was examined for its response to pyrazoleamide compounds, it was found to have a slightly higher EC_{50} value compared with its parental line (Table 1 and Supplementary Fig. 5), showing that the PfCDPK5^{T392A} allele by itself appeared to result in a rather modest level of resistance to the pyrazoleamide compounds. We also derived transgenic Dd2 lines expressing either the PfATP4^{wt} or PfATP4^{V178I} allele from an ectopic site using a Mycobacteriophage recombination system[22]. Western blot analysis of transgenic parasites indicated relatively equal expression of the PfATP4 transgene (Supplementary Fig. 6). As shown in Table 1 and Supplementary Fig. 5, Dd2 parasites expressing PfATP4^{wt} responded to compound PA21A050 with an EC_{50} similar to the parental Dd2 line, whereas transgenic Dd2 line expressing PfATP4^{V178I} allele showed EC_{50} about twofold higher than the parental line. This indicated a slight gain of resistance by the transgenic parasites expressing PfATP4^{V178I} allele in a merodiploid state; however, the degree of resistance was much lower than that observed in the original resistant line. At this point, we used the Dd2::PfCDPK5^{T392A} line as the recipient of the wild-type or the mutant alleles of PfATP4 through transfection. Whereas there was no change in the EC_{50} value for the compound PA21A050 in the Dd2::PfCDPK5^{T392A} line expressing PfATP4^{wt} allele, a resistance level similar to the original resistant line was observed in the Dd2::PfCDPK5^{T392A} line expressing the PfATP4^{V178I} allele (Table 1 and Supplementary Fig. 5). The transgenic parasites bearing double mutations were also resistant to several different pyrazoleamide compounds (Table 1 and Supplementary Fig. 5). These results strongly support the contention that a combined activity of mutated alleles of both PfCDPK5 and PfATP4 is necessary to impart full resistance to pyrazoleamide compounds in *P. falciparum*.

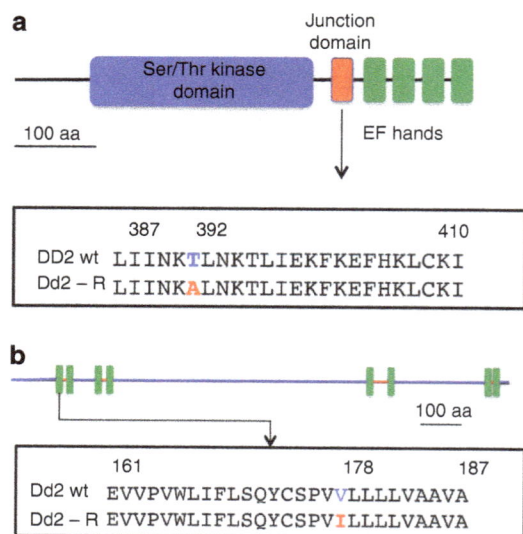

Figure 3 | Mutations in compound C2-1-resistant parasites. A Thr to Ala mutation at position 392 in *PfCDPK5* is in its predicted junction domain (**a**), and a Val to Ile mutation at position 178 in *PfATP4* (**b**) is in the first predicted transmembrane domain.

A pyrazoleamide disrupts Na^+ homeostasis in *P. falciparum*. As highlighted in a recent study[10], PfATP4 bears a close resemblance to the closely related ENA (**e**xitus **na**trum) Na^+ ATPases that extrude Na^+ ions from the cells of fungi and lower plants[23]. In the same study it was shown that antimalarial spiroindolones at therapeutic doses rapidly disrupt Na^+ homeostasis in blood-stage *P. falciparum* parasites, and that spiroindolone-resistant parasites with mutations in PfATP4 (ref. 9) had reduced sensitivity to disruption of Na^+ homeostasis by a spiroindolone[10]. As shown in Fig. 4a, the pyrazoleamide PA21A050 treatment of saponin-isolated parasites led to rapid increase in intracellular Na^+ concentration ($[Na^+]_i$), doing so in a dose-dependent manner. Remarkably, a maximum initial Na^+ influx rate of $\sim$0.07 mM s^{-1} was reached with the addition of just 1 nM PA21A050 (Fig. 4b). The increase in $[Na]_i$ was accompanied by an increase in intracellular pH (pH$_i$, Fig. 4c), whereas there was no significant change in intracellular Ca^{2+} ($[Ca^{2+}]_i$) on addition of PA21A050 (Fig. 4d). These results are similar to those reported for the spiroindolones[10] except that PA21A050 was more potent in its

Table 1 | Efficacy of pyrazoleamides and a spiroindolone in transgenic *P. falciparum*.

Parasite line	In vitro EC$_{50}$, nM ($\pm$ s.e.m.)			
	PA21A050	PA21A092	PA27-X41	NITD246
Dd2	0.7 ($\pm$0.2)	12.9 ($\pm$2.0)	0.7 ($\pm$0.15)	0.15 ($\pm$0.01)
Dd2-R21	16 ($\pm$0.5)	133 ($\pm$8.0)	122 ($\pm$10)	0.21 ($\pm$0.04)
Dd2::PfCDPK5^{T392A}	1.5 ($\pm$0.1)	23 ($\pm$3.0)	ND	0.17 ($\pm$0.04)
Dd2attB + PfATP4^{wt}	0.5 ($\pm$0.1)	22 ($\pm$9.0)	2 ($\pm$0.4)	0.34 ($\pm$0.08)
Dd2attB + PfATP4^{V178I}	2 ($\pm$0.3)	34 ($\pm$2.6)	17.4 ($\pm$4.0)	0.19 ($\pm$0.04)
Dd2::PfCDPK5^{T392A} + PfATP4^{wt}	0.8 ($\pm$0.07)	31 ($\pm$3.5)	2 ($\pm$0.01)	0.36 ($\pm$0.09)
Dd2::PfCDPK5^{T392A} + PfATP4^{V178I}	11 ($\pm$0.5)	176 ($\pm$8.0)	274 ($\pm$17)	0.62 ($\pm$0.07)

EC$_{50}$, effective concentration for 50% growth inhibition; ND, not done.
EC$_{50}$ values for three pyrazoleamides and a spiroindolone (NITD246) were derived from growth inhibition assays for Dd2 and a compound C2-1-resistant line, as well as five other transgenic lines derived from Dd2 parent. Growth inhibition curves are shown in Supplementary Fig. 5.

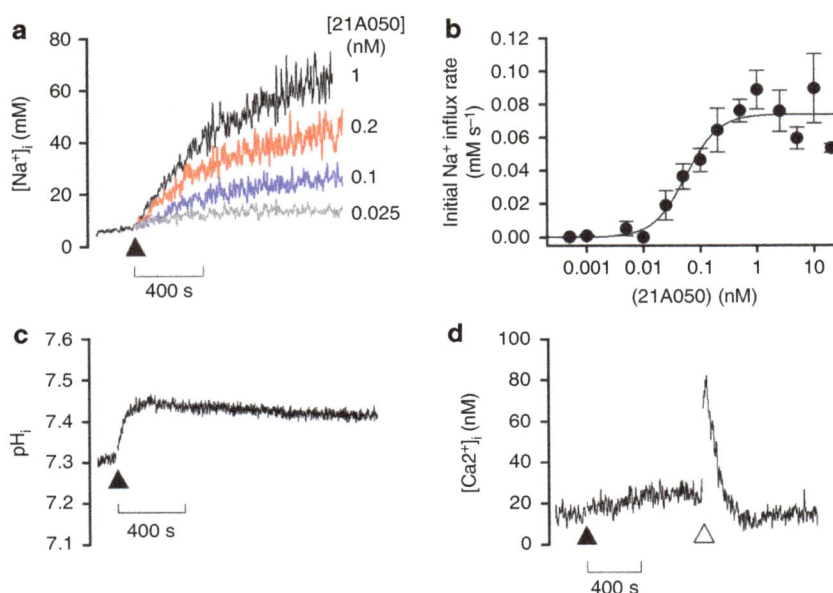

Figure 4 | Rapid influx of Na$^+$ in *P. falciparum* trophozoites following exposure to PA21A050. Intracellular concentrations of Na$^+$, Ca^{2+} and pH in saponin-isolated parasites loaded with appropriate fluorescent probes were determined by ratiometric methods as described in ref. 10. In **a,c,d**, the pyrazoleamide was added at the time point indicated by the closed triangle. The traces and influx rates shown are, in each case, representative of those obtained from at least three independent cell preparations. In control experiments it was shown that there was no direct effect of the pyrazoleamide on the fluorescence signals of any of the three fluorescent ion indicators used (not shown). (**a**) Concentration-dependent increase in [Na$^+$]$_i$ in response to PA21A050. (**b**) Initial Na$^+$ influx rate ($\pm$ s.e.m.; calculated as described in ref. 10) plotted as function of [21A050]. The estimated IC$_{50}$ for this effect was 0.08 nM. (**c**) PA21A050 at 1 nM caused a rapid rise in pH$_i$ from 7.3 to 7.45, consistent with a lifting of the 'acid-load' proposed to be imposed by the action of the (H$^+$ counter-transporting) Na$^+$ ATPase[10,33]. (**d**) PA21A050, at 1 nM, had no significant effect on [Ca^{2+}]$_i$ in parasites suspended in an EGTA-buffered medium containing 1 μM free Ca^{2+}. Addition of the endoplasmic reticulum Ca^{2+} pump inhibitor cyclopiazonic acid (unfilled triangle) resulted in a transient spike in [Ca^{2+}]$_i$.

activity in this assay. Antimalarials such as artesunate and chloroquine have no effect on [Na$^+$]$_i$ in this assay[10].

As *P. falciparum* matures from the ring stage to the trophozoite stage, new permeability pathways (also called *Plasmodial*-surface anion channels, or PSAC) are established in the erythrocyte membrane resulting in an increased permeability to a diverse range of low molecular weight solutes[24,25]. One consequence of this is an increase in [Na$^+$] inside the erythrocyte cytosol[26] and, hence, an inward [Na$^+$] gradient across the plasma membrane of the intraerythrocytic trophozoite.

We examined the effect of PA21A050 on *P. falciparum* development by time-lapse live cell imaging in erythrocytes starting from ring-stage parasites (Supplementary Movies 1 and 2). Ring-stage parasites progressed to develop into trophozoites while

being exposed to PA21A050. At the late trophozoite stage there was visible increase in volume of the parasite, which was followed by dramatic apparent bursting; schizogony or merozoites were not observed (Supplementary Movie 2; notice swelling and bursting from 2,400 to 2,600 min time frames). These observations are consistent with the proposition that pyrazoleamides disrupt Na$^+$ homeostasis, the effect of which becomes apparent coincident with the rise in [Na$^+$] within the infected erythrocyte cytoplasm at the trophozoite stage. An increase in [Na$^+$] in the parasite cytoplasm is predicted to give rise to an associated osmotic uptake of water and an associated swelling. To assess the extent of swelling, we measured the diameter of trophozoite-stage parasites in intact infected erythrocytes after 2 h of exposure to PA21A050 in still images of a number of parasites.

As shown in Fig. 5, the average diameter of the treated trophozoite stage increased to 4.6 µm in 2 h compared with 2.5 µm in untreated control trophozoites from the same culture, consistent with the parasite having undergone significant swelling.

Reduced sensitivity of parasites in low [Na$^+$] medium. The results described above suggest that a contributing factor for antimalarial properties of these compounds could be toxicity associated with high [Na$^+$]$_i$. Recently, Pillai et al.[27] have elegantly demonstrated that P. falciparum can tolerate a broad range of [Na$^+$] in growth medium as long as appropriate osmotic conditions are maintained by KCl and sucrose. We took advantage of the low [Na$^+$] growth medium used by Pillai et al.[27] to ask whether parasites grown under low [Na$^+$] condition had altered responses to antimalarial compounds that disrupt Na$^+$ homeostasis. As shown in Table 2, Dd2 line of P. falciparum showed three- to fivefold reduced susceptibility to both the pyrazoleamide and spiroindolone compounds when grown in low [Na$^+$] medium. It was interesting to note that the reduced susceptibility was more pronounced in a Dd2-21R line that was derived as resistant to a pyrazoleamide compound. These results further support the notion that Na$^+$ homeostasis disruption is a

key component of antimalarial action of these two chemically distinct classes of compounds.

Discussion

We have described a multinational collaborative effort that has delivered a new chemical entity as a candidate antimalarial drug worthy of being developed for clinical investigations. Potent inhibitory activity of pyrazoleamides against multiple isolates of P. falciparum as well as P. vivax suggests the potential of deploying these compounds as part of a malaria control and elimination strategy. An added attractive feature of these compounds is their activity against the mature sexual stages of P. falciparum, a property not common to most of the currently used antimalarial drugs. Inhibition of gamete production by these compounds would prevent parasite mating and transmission by mosquitoes, a goal that has to be part of a malaria elimination programme. Results from in vivo efficacy studies described here demonstrate rapid clearance of P. falciparum when exposed to orally administered pyrazoleamides. This rate of clearance is reminiscent of clearance by artemisinin derivatives, which are the fastest-acting antimalarials in clinical use.

We provide evidence suggesting rapid disruption of Na$^+$ homeostasis in intraerythrocytic parasites as a consequence of exposure to pyrazoleamides at pharmacologically relevant concentrations. It has been shown previously that the induction by the parasite of new permeability pathway/Plasmodial-surface anion channel in erythrocyte plasma membrane occurs as the ring-stage parasite transitions to the metabolically more active trophozoite stage[24,25]. As a consequence, [Na$^+$] inside the erythrocyte cytoplasm increases[24,25], yet [Na$^+$] inside the parasite remains physiologically low. Spillman et al.[10] have suggested that the maintenance of low [Na$^+$]$_i$ inside the parasite is mediated by a P-type Na$^+$ ATPase pump encoded by the parasite, and that the new antimalarial spiroindolone, NITD246, interferes with the activity of this pump leading to a rapid net uptake of Na$^+$. We show here that a pyrazoleamide has a similar effect to the spiroindolones on Na$^+$ influx in saponin-isolated parasites. Furthermore, we show that just a 2-h exposure to a pyrazoleamide results in a significant increase in the volume of intact intraerythrocytic trophozoite-stage parasites, followed by a dramatic bursting of the parasite. These results, in combination with our observation of reduced efficacy of the pyrazoleamide and spiroindolone against P. falciparum parasites growing under low [Na$^+$] conditions, provide strong evidence that these two chemically distinct classes of compounds share a common mode of action through disruption of Na$^+$ homeostasis.

The finding that mutations in PfATP4 are associated with acquisition of resistance to spiroindolone and pyrazoleamide compounds is consistent with the hypothesis that this P-type ATPase is a direct target of these compounds. However, some caution is warranted. A mutation in PfCDPK5, which by itself imparts minimal resistance to pyrazoleamides, greatly enhances

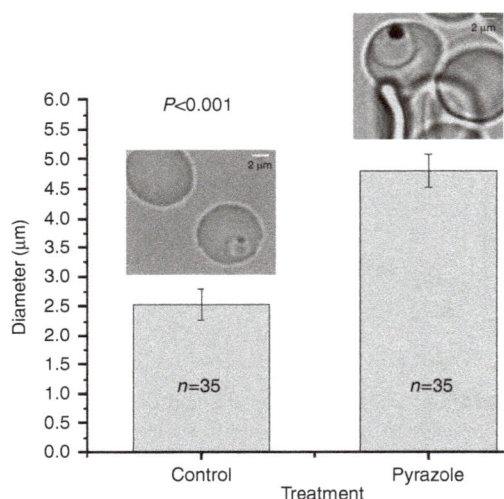

Figure 5 | PA21A050 causes swelling of intraerythrocytic P. falciparum. Live cell images of trophozoite stages were obtained at 2 h from untreated and PA21A050-treated parasites attached to a glass-bottom Petri plate by a Nikon microscope equipped with an incubation chamber for regulating temperature and gas mixture. The diameter of the indicated number of parasites were measured from the images using the ImageJ software. Error bars indicate s.d.

Table 2 | Efficacy of antimalarials on P. falciparum grown in low [Na$^+$] medium.

Compound	P. falciparum line	EC$_{50}$ in normal [Na$^+$] medium, nM ($\pm$ s.e.m.)	EC$_{50}$ in low [Na$^+$] medium, nM ($\pm$ s.e.m.)
PA21A050	Dd2	0.5 ($\pm$ 0.01)	2.7 ($\pm$ 0.3)
PA21A085	Dd2	5.7 ($\pm$ 0.3)	19 ($\pm$ 0.9)
PA21A085	Dd2-21R	221 ($\pm$ 20)	>5,000
NITD246	Dd2	0.5 ($\pm$ 0.03)	1.8 ($\pm$ 0.1)
NITD246	Dd2-21R	0.7 ($\pm$ 0.02)	3.3 ($\pm$ 0.15)
Artemisinin	Dd2	11 ($\pm$ 0.4)	7 ($\pm$ 0.13)

EC$_{50}$, effective concentration for 50% growth inhibition.
Growth inhibition assays were carried out for Dd2 and a compound 2-1 resistant line (Dd2-21R) using the indicated pyrazoleamide and a spiroindolone. The assays were carried out either in the normal growth medium or in a low [Na$^+$] medium described in ref. 27.

the level of resistance in combination with mutated *PfATP4*. *PfCDPK5* has been shown to be essential in the very last step of schizogony before merozoites egress[19]. It has also been shown that mature schizont-stage parasites undergo swelling just before merozoite egress, and this is thought to facilitate the egress process[28]. The finding in this study of an association between *PfATP4* and *PfCDPK5* raises the possibility that the swelling is the result of increased Na$^+$ influx, perhaps because of inhibition of PfATP4 activity, resulting from a cascade of events in which PfCDPK5 plays a regulatory function. Under this scenario, it might be envisioned that pyrazoleamides (and possibly spiroindolones) act as premature signals to initiate an egress-like cascade resulting in Na$^+$ influx and swelling.

Further experiments are needed to understand details of events that lead to the demise of the parasites exposed to these new antimalarials. It is clear, however, that observations reported here are hinting at a hitherto unknown pathway in malaria parasites, which can be interfered with by at least two different classes of chemicals. Recent observations from our and other laboratories suggest additional compounds of unrelated chemical structures may also target this pathway. We look forward to unravelling mechanistic details of this pathway with a view to discovering other new antimalarial drugs.

Methods

Synthesis schemes for pyrazoleamides. All reagents and starting materials described in the procedures are commercially available and were used without further purification. Synthetic route for N-(4-(4-chloro-2-fluorophenyl)-3-(tri-fluoromethyl)-1-methyl-1H-pyrazol-5-yl)-2-(2-isopropyl-1H-benzo[d]imidazol-1-yl)acetamide (Compound **PA21A050**) is illustrated in Fig. 6. To a mixture of 2-(2-

isopropyl-1H-benzo[d]imidazol-1-yl)acetic acid (0.16 mmol) and Mukaiyama's reagent (2-chloro-1-methylpyridinium iodide, 0.38 mmol) in 1.5 ml anhydrous dichloromethane (DCM), 4-(4-chloro-2-fluorophenyl)-3-(trifluoromethyl)-1-methyl-1H-pyrazol-5-amine (0.12 mmol), triethylamine (0.40 mmol) and 0.5 ml of anhydrous tetrahydrofuran were added. The mixture was vortexed and subjected to microwave irradiation for 30 min at 75 °C to give a deep-green clear solution. Then 80 ml of ethyl acetate was added and the solution was washed with 80 ml of saturated NaHCO$_3$ twice, and with brine, and then dried over MgSO$_4$. After solvent removal and purification on a flash silica gel column using ethyl acetate and hexane as eluent, a slightly brown-coloured solid was obtained. After recrystallization in ethyl acetate/hexane, 45 mg of Compound **PA21A050** was obtained as a white powder. Yield: 76%. Purity: >95% by HPLC (UV at 220 nm). ^{1}H NMR (500 MHz, MeOD) δ 7.81–7.83 (m, 1H), 7.60–7.70 (m, 3H), 7.26–7.36 (m, 3H), 5.54 (s, 2H), 3.92 (s, 3H), 3.50–3.55 (m, 1H), 1.50 (d, J = 6.9 Hz, 6H). ^{13}C-NMR (126 MHz, MeOD) δ 169.30, 162.35, 162.02, 160.36, 142.93, 136.64, 136.55, 136.24, 134.19, 125.84, 123.87, 123.59, 119.31, 117.68, 117.60, 117.56, 117.39, 110.42, 46.39, 37.06, 27.47, 21.81. high-resolution mass spectrometry, electrospray ionisation (HRMS(ESI)): M/Z calculated for C$_{23}$H$_{20}$ClF$_4$N$_5$O + H$^+$ [M + H$^+$]: 494.1365. Found: 494.1358. Traces of liquid chromatography/mass spectrometry (LC/MS), ^{1}H NMR and ^{13}C-NMR of **PA21A050** are shown in Supplementary Figs 7 and 8.

Synthetic route for N-(4-(4-chloro-2-fluorophenyl)-1,3-dimethyl-1H-pyrazol-5-yl)-2-(2-isopropyl-1H-benzo[d]imidazol-1-yl)acetamide (Compound **PA21A092**) is illustrated in Fig. 6. The synthesis followed the route for **PA21A050** described above using 4-(4-chloro-2-fluorophenyl)-1,3-dimethyl-1H-pyrazol-5-amine (0.12 mmol) as starting material. After silica gel chromatography using ethyl acetate and hexane as eluent, 42 mg of Compound **PA21A092** was obtained as a white powder. Yield: 80%, purity: >95% by HPLC (UV at 220 nm). ^{1}H NMR (500 MHz, MeOD) δ 7.62–7.64 (m, 1H), 7.23–7.33 (m, 6H), 5.15 (s, 2H), 3.73 (s, 3H), 3.18–3.21 (m, 1H), 2.17 (s, 3H), 1.39 (d, J = 6.8 Hz, 6H). ^{13}C-NMR (126 MHz, MeOD) δ 169.25, 162.16, 162.04, 160.18, 147.16, 142.89, 136.24, 134.90, 133.76, 125.92, 123.80, 123.56, 119.25, 117.67, 117.67, 116.51, 110.51, 110.31, 46.39, 35.59, 27.46, 21.82 and 12.67. HRMS (ESI): M/Z calculated for C$_{23}$H$_{23}$ClFN$_5$O + H$^+$ [M + H$^+$]: 440.1648. Found: 440.1641. Traces of LC/MS, ^{1}H NMR and ^{13}C-NMR of **PA21A092** are shown in Supplementary Figs 9 and 10.

Synthetic route for (*R*)-3-amino-4-(4-fluorophenyl)-N-(4-(4-fluorophenyl)-1,3-dimethyl-1H-pyrazol-5-yl)butanamide (Compound **PA21A102**) is illustrated in Fig. 6. To a solution of Fmoc-(*R*)-3-amino-4-(4-fluorophenyl)butanoyl chloride (43 mg, 0.20 mmol) produced from Fmoc-(*R*)-3-amino-4-(4-fluorophenyl)butanoic acid and thionyl chloride in 10 ml of anhydrous DCM were slowly added 4-(4-fluorophenyl)-1,3-dimethyl-1H-pyrazol-5-amine (31 mg, 0.15 mmol) in 5 ml of anhydrous DCM. The reaction mixture was stirred at room temperature overnight. The reaction mixture was quenched with methanol and solvents were removed. The residue was purified via silica gel with MeOH/DCM to obtain Fmoc-protected product. Fmoc-protected product was dissolved in 10 ml of ethyl acetate and 0.20 mmol of 1,8-diazabicyclo[5.4.0]undec-7-ene) in ethyl acetate was added. After 20 min, 20 ml of ethyl acetate was added and the mixture was washed with 20 ml of water. The organic layer was collected and solvent was removed. The residue was dissolved in MeOH and acidified with 0.2 N HCl. The solution was purified via preparatory RP-HPLC, eluting with H$_2$O/CH$_3$CN gradient (+0.05% trifluoroacetic acid, TFA). Product fractions were collected and concentrated. The residue was dissolved in a small amount of 2 M HCl in methanol and, after concentration *in vacuo*, 48 mg of Compound **PA21A102** was obtained as an HCl salt. Yield: 76%. Purity: >95% by HPLC (UV at 220 nm). To prepare the compound as free base, the salt form was dissolved in saturated Na$_2$CO$_3$ solution and extracted with ethyl acetate followed by removal of solvent. ^{1}H NMR of free base form (500 MHz, MeOD) δ 7.30–7.32 (m, 2H), 7.20–7.22 (m, 2H), 7.11–7.15 (m, 2H), 7.03–7.07 (m, 2H), 3.68 (s, 3H), 3.38–3.44 (m, 1H), 2.72–2.76 (m, 1H), 2.62–2.66 (m, 1H), 2.51–2.55 (m, 1H), 2.37–2.42 (m, 1H), 2.24 (s, 3H). ^{13}C-NMR (126 MHz, MeOD) δ 174.60, 164.17, 162.23, 146.13, 135.61, 135.58, 134.56, 132.06, 131.99, 131.90, 131.84, 129.70, 116.44, 116.31, 116.27, 116.14, 51.07, 43.28, 42.56, 35.57 and 12.78. HRMS (ESI): M/Z calculated for C$_{21}$H$_{22}$F$_2$N$_4$O + H$^+$ [M + H$^+$]: 385.1834. Found: 385.1832. Traces of LC/MS, ^{1}H NMR and ^{13}C-NMR of **PA21A102** are shown in Supplementary Figs 11 and 12.

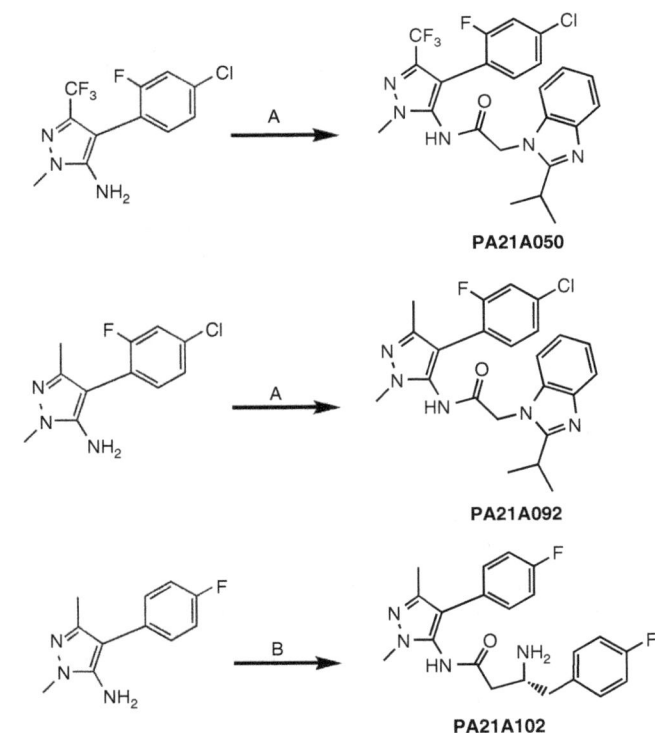

Figure 6 | Synthetic schemes and reaction conditions for pyrazoleamides. (a) For **PA21A050** and **PA21A092**: 2-(2-isopropyl-1H-benzo[d]imidazol-1-yl)acetic acid, Mukaiyama's reagent (2-chloro-1-methylpyridinium iodide), triethylamine, in dichloromethane/tetrahydrofuran, microwave, 75 °C, 30 min. **(b)** For **PA21A102**: (i) Fmoc-(R)-3-amino-4-(4-fluorophenyl)butanoyl chloride in dichloromethane, (ii) DBU (1,8-diazabicyclo[5.4.0]undec-7-ene) in ethyl acetate.

Parasites and growth inhibition assays. *P. falciparum* lines (obtained from Malaria Research and Reference Reagent Resource Center, http://www.mr4.org) were cultured under standard conditions in RPMI1640 medium supplemented with 0.5% Albumax in 90% N$_2$, 5% O$_2$ and 5% CO$_2$. Parasite growth inhibition was assessed by a modified version of the method originally described in ref. 29. The method assessed parasite growth as reflected by incorporation of ^{3}H-hypoxanthine by parasites. *P. falciparum* parasites in culture were exposed to graded dilutions of test compounds for 48 h and incorporation of ^{3}H-hypoxanthine over the last 24 h into parasite nucleic acids was determined by liquid scintillation spectroscopy. The dose–response data were analysed using nonlinear regression analysis (Prism GraphPad), and the EC$_{50}$ was derived using an inhibitory sigmoid maximum effect (E_{max}) model. For assessing parasite growth inhibition under low [Na$^+$] conditions, we used the medium composition designated 4suc:6 KCl as described in ref. 27. Briefly, the medium contained all ingredients specified for RPMI16040 except that NaCl, NaHCO$_3$ and Na$_2$HPO$_4$ were replaced by 64.8 mM KCl, 28.6 mM KCO$_3$ and 5.64 mM K$_2$HPO$_4$. In addition, 84.3 mM sucrose was included in the medium.

Addition of 10% human serum to the 4suc:6 KCl medium was estimated to result in ~ 7 mM Na^+ concentration in this medium. Efficacy of compounds to inhibit parasite growth in the low $[Na^+]$ 4suc:6 KCl + 10% human serum medium was assessed in parallel with that in standard RPMI1640 medium by ^{3}H-hypoxanthine incorporation as described above.

Dual *P. falciparum* male and female gamete formation assays. A recently reported assay was used to assess effects of various doses of PA21A092 on gamete production by the NF54 line of *P. falciparum*[30]. *P. falciparum* NF54 strain gametocytes were produced by standard methods. Briefly, asexual parasites in the log phase of growth were passaged to 1% parasitemia/4% haematocrit and cultured in RPMI medium + 25 mM HEPES + 50 mg l^{-1} hypoxanthine + 2 g l^{-1} sodium bicarbonate + 10% human serum with daily medium changes while maintaining 37 °C and 3% O_2/5% CO_2/92% N_2 at all times. Under these conditions, gamete formation is maximal by 14 days in culture and the assay performed. Cultures were divided into 200-μl microcultures containing test compound dilutions with no more than 0.5% dimethylsulphoxide. After 24 h incubation with the test compounds, gamete formation was stimulated by addition of 2.5 μM xanthurenic acid. At 20 min, exflagellation was recorded by time-lapse microscopy using × 10 objective and quantified using a custom algorithm. At 24 h post addition of xanthurenic acid, a Cy3-labelled anti-Pf25 antibody was added at 1:2,000 dilution to the cultures that specifically stains female gametes that were then recorded by fluorescence microscope using a × 20 objective and quantified using a custom algorithm.

Percent inhibition of male or female gamete formation was calculated with respect to the positive (10 μM methylene blue) and negative (DMSO) controls and the whole assay was repeated four times using independent cultures.

Assessing *in vivo* efficacy. Efficacy of pyrazoleamides was examined in 10- to 12-week-old female NOD/scid/IL2R$_\gamma^{null}$ mice engrafted with human erythrocytes and infected with an adapted *P. falciparum* line as described previously[13,14]. Briefly, three mice per group were inoculated intravenously with 2×10^7 parasitized erythrocytes (*P. falciparum* strain 3D7$^{0087/N9}$ adapted for *in vivo* growth). Beginning from day 3 after the inoculation, mice were administered the stated doses of the compound orally for 4 consecutive days. Chloroquine at 2.5, 5 and 10 mg kg^{-1} was used as a positive control. A group of infected mice given oral dosing of the vehicle serves as the control. Parasitemia was measured from days 3 to 7 after infection by flow cytometry, counting 10^6 events. SYTO-16 was used for staining parasite nucleic acids, and non-cytolytic antimouse erythrocyte monoclonal antibody Ter-119 conjugated with phycoerythrine was used for differentiating mouse and human erythrocytes. Thin smears of blood stained with Giemsa were examined and representative infected erythrocytes photographed on days 5 and 7 after infection in each mouse. Animal experiments were performed at the Association for Assessment and Accreditation of Laboratory Animal Care International-accredited GlaxoSmithKline Laboratory Animal Science facility in Tres Cantos (Madrid, Spain). All the experiments were approved by the GlaxoSmithKline Diseases of the Developing World Group Ethical Committee.

Pharmacokinetics of PA21A092 in NOD/SCID/IL2Rγ^{null} mice. The levels of PA21A092 in blood upon oral administration were measured for all the mice and dosing levels included in the efficacy study. Serial samples of peripheral blood (25 μl) were taken at 0.25, 0.5, 1, 2, 4, 7, 10 and 23 h after the first administration of PA21A092, mixed with 25 μl of water for erythrocyte lysis and immediately frozen and stored at − 80 °C until analysis. Protein precipitation by liquid–liquid extraction was performed in a 96-well plate with filter system (MultiScreen Solvinert 0.45 μm Hydrophobic PTFE; Millipore). Briefly, 120 μl of AcN:MeOH (80:20; v-v) with added internal standard were added to 10 μl of blood/saponin lysate sample per well. The plates were vortexed for 10 min, filtrated and the filtrates were analysed using LC-MS/MS in positive ion mode with electrospray (Sciex API 4000 Triple Quadrupole Mass Spectrometer, Sciex, Division of MDS Inc., Toronto, Canada). Noncompartmental analysis was performed using Phoenix, version 6.3. (Phoenix WinNonlin Copyright 1998–2012, Certara L.P.) and the main pharmacokinetic parameters were estimated. Additional statistical analysis of the data was performed with GraphPad Prism Version 5.01 (GraphPad Software Inc., San Diego CA).

Testing in field isolates of *P. falciparum* and *P. vivax*. *Plasmodium spp.* isolates were collected from patients with malaria attending outpatient clinics in Timika (Papua Province, Indonesia), a region highly prevalent for multidrug-resistant strains of *P. vivax* and *P. falciparum*. Patients with symptomatic malaria were recruited into the study if singly infected with *P. falciparum* or *P. vivax* and a parasitaemia of between 2,000 and 80,000 μl^{-1}. After written informed consent was obtained, venous blood (5 ml) was collected by venepuncture. Ethical approval for this project was obtained from the Human Research Ethics Committee of the Northern Territory Department of Health & Families and Menzies School of Health Research (HREC 2010-1396), Darwin (Australia) and the Eijkman Institute Research Ethics Commission (EIREC-47), Jakarta (Indonesia). *Plasmodium* drug susceptibility was measured using a protocol modified from the World Health Organization microtest as described previously[12]. Two hundred microlitres of a 2% haematocrit blood medium mixture, consisting of RPMI1640 medium plus 10%

AB^+ human serum (*P. falciparum*) or McCoy's 5A medium plus 20% AB^+ human serum (*P. vivax*), were added to each well of predosed drug plates containing 11 serial concentrations (twofold dilutions) of the compound PA21A092. A candle jar was used to mature the parasites at 37.0 °C for 32–56 h. Incubation was stopped when > 40% of ring-stage parasites had reached the mature schizont stage (that is, four or more distinct nuclei per parasite) in the drug-free control well.

Thick blood films made from each well were stained with 5% Giemsa solution for 30 min and examined microscopically. The number of schizonts per 200 asexual stage parasites was determined for each drug concentration and normalized to that of the control well. The dose–response data were analysed using nonlinear regression analysis (WinNonLn 4.1; Pharsight Corporation), and the EC$_{50}$ was derived using an E_{max} model.

Derivation of resistant parasites. *P. falciparum* line Dd2 was used to derive parasite lines resistant to the initial hit pyrazoleamide compound C2-1. Three flasks each containing 10^8 parasitized erythrocytes were continuously exposed to $3 \times$ EC$_{50}$ concentration of the compound with medium changes each day and fresh provision of human red blood cell (RBC) once a week. Emergence of parasites was monitored by examining stained thin smears. Each of the flasks yielded resistant parasites, which were confirmed to be resistant to pyrazoleamides.

Whole-genome sequencing and analysis. Parental Dd2 *P. falciparum* line and the three pyrazoleamide-resistant lines were sequenced using the Illumina GAII and the amplification-free methodology[17]. From each clone, 300-bp fragments of genomic DNA were prepared by focused sonication. An individual sequencing lane was used to produce 33–40 million paired 76-base reads for each sample. Between 55 and 71% of sequencing reads for each sample mapped uniquely to the *P. falciparum* clone 3D7 reference genome, with read-spacing accurately reflecting the expected fragment size.

Dd2 reads were aligned to the 3D7 genome and any single-base differences or small indels were identified by iCORN[18] to iteratively change the 3D7 sequence into the one that more closely resembled the actual sequence for Dd2 (hereafter termed Dd2′). Only sequence differences within regions of 10–15 × read coverage were accepted to minimize the possibility of using incorrectly mapped sequences, and iCORN was run for 17 iterations (until no further sequence differences could be found between the gene sequences of 3D7 and Dd2). In all, 41,841 base substitutions were made and 16,638 indels corrected.

Reads from each derived line were mapped to the Dd2′ reference to identify SNPs and indels, using three iterations of iCORN so that SNPs or indel could be identified even within polymorphic loci. Sequence variants were only identified within regions of at least × 40 coverage on Dd2′. Using a custom Perl script, genes were identified where a variant was found within the reads for all three derived clones. Five SNPs were found at the same base position in each of the three derived clones. These were the only differences observed when compared with Dd2′.

Approaches to generate transgenic parasites. A DNA fragment corresponding to nucleotides 9–1,704 of the coding region of *PfCDPK5* (PlasmoDB ID PF3D7_1337800) and having a 5′-*SpeI* site and an in-frame BsiWI site was amplified using Vent DNA polymerase (New England Biolabs) and cloned into pCR-Blunt (Invitrogen). The DNA sequence of the amplified fragment was confirmed. The *PfCDPK5^{T392A}* mutation was introduced into the plasmid using the QuikChange Site-Directed Mutagenesis Kit (Stratagene). The resulting SpeI-BsiWI DNA fragments were cloned into the *P. falciparum* vector pCC1-3HA and used to transform parasite strain Dd2. WR99210-resistant parasites were obtained, subjected to one drug-off/drug-on cycle to select for transgene insertion. The site-specific integration was confirmed with PCR using both gene-specific and integration-specific primers, as illustrated in Supplementary Fig. 4. The primers correspond to the following DNA regions: 5′-primer (− 425 to − 401 nucleotides upstream of the ATG codon); 3′-primer (+ 96 to + 123 nucleotides downstream of the Stop codon); C primer (nucleotides 1,671–1,704 of the coding sequence); 3HA primer corresponds to the influenza virus hemagglutination antigen epitope.

Full-length *PfATP4* gene was amplified by PCR using genomic DNA from either the wild-type Dd2 parasite (to produce *PfATP4^{wt}*), or Dd2-R21 parasites resistant to compound C2-1 (to produce *PfATP4^{T392A}*). DNA sequences were confirmed and the genes were cloned into the pLN plasmid[22] to be expressed under the calmodulin promoter[22]. Transfections of *P. falciparum* parasites were carried out as described elsewhere[31,32]. Briefly, ring-stage parasites at 5% parasitemia were electroporated with 50 μg plasmid DNA isolated using the Qiagen Plasmid Maxi Kit. Electroporation was conducted using a Bio-Rad GenePulser set at 0.31 kV and 960 μF. Two aliquots of DNA were electroporated for each transgene. Transfected parasites were maintained under drug pressure: 5 nM WR99210 for hdhfr (human dihydrofolate reductase), 2.5 μg ml^{-1} blasticidin for blasticidin deaminase and 125 μg ml^{-1} G418 for the neomycin selectable markers.

The following transgenic parasites were used in this study:

- Dd2::PfCDPK5^{T392A}—The Dd2 line with *PfCDPK5* allele bearing T392A mutation seen in Dd2-21R-resistant line. The wild-type allele is replaced with the mutated allele that also bears a 3 × HA tag at the C terminus.

- *Dd2attB + PfATP4^{wt}*–The Dd2attB line with the wild-type *PfATP4* gene inserted at the attB site. This line is a merodiploid with two copies of the wild-type *PfATP4*.
- *Dd2attB + PfATP6^{V178I}*—The Dd2attB line with PfATP4 bearing V178I mutation inserted at the attB site. This line is a meroheterozygote expressing both the wild-type and V178I alleles of *PfATP4*.
- *Dd2::PfCDPK5^{T392A} + PfATP4^{wt}*—Transgenic Dd2 line bearing T32A mutation in its *PfCDPK5* gene transfected with the same plasmid used to generate *Dd2attB + PfATP4^{wt}* line. The plasmid replicates as an episome.
- *Dd2::PfCDPK5^{T392A} + PfATP4^{V178I}*—Transgenic Dd2 line bearing T392A mutation in its *PfCDPK5* gene transfected with the same plasmid used to generate the *Dd2attB + PfATP4^{V178I}* line. The plasmid replicates as an episome.

Spectrofluorometer measurements of $[Na^+]_i$, $[Ca^{2+}]_i$ and pH_i. Trophozoite-stage, 3D7 *P. falciparum* parasites (36–40 h post invasion) were functionally isolated from their host erythrocytes by treatment with saponin (0.05% w/v, equating to 0.005% w/v of the active agent sapogenin) and then loaded with the appropriate fluorescent probe (Sodium-binding BenzoFuran Isophthalate for $[Na^+]_i$; BCECF-AM, 2′,7′-bis-(2-carboxyethyl)-5,6-carboxyfluorescein, acetoxymethyl ester for pH_i; Fura-2, 2-(6-(bis(2-((acetyloxy)methoxy)-2-oxoethyl)amino)-5-(2-(bis(2-((acetyloxy)methoxy)-2-oxoethyl)amino)-5-methylphenoxy)ethoxy)-2-benzofuranyl) for $[Ca^{2+}]_i$) and suspended in a medium containing 125 mM NaCl, 5 mM KCl, 25 mM HEPES, 20 mM glucose and 1 mM $MgCl_2$; pH 7.10. For the Fura-2/$[Ca^{2+}]_i$ experiments, this solution was supplemented with 1 mM EGTA and sufficient $CaCl_2$ to result in a final free extracellular Ca^{2+} concentration of 1 µM. Detailed methods for dye-loading, cell concentrations, calibration, rate calculations and appropriate ratiometric measurement using a spectrofluorometer were as described in ref. 10. Calibrations were performed for each experiment and are shown in Supplementary Fig. 13 along with the equations used for assessing ion concentrations.

Live cell imaging. *P. falciparum* line 3D7 parasites were synchronized through osmotic lysis of late-stage parasites incubated with 500 mM alanine. Parasitized erythrocytes in phenol red-free medium were attached to a glass-bottom Petri dish coated with concanavalin A. Images were obtained in an inverted Nikon Eclipse microscope equipped with a chamber stage in which temperature (37 °C) and gas mixture (5% O_2, 5% CO_2 and 95% N_2) were maintained. For time-lapse movies, images were collected every 30 min for 45 h using autofocus setting by a ×100 objective lens in phase contrast. Images were processed and assembled into videos using the ImageJ software. Static phase-contrast images of trophozoite-stage parasites either untreated or treated with 10 nM PA21A050 were obtained after 2-h incubation under the inverted Nikon microscope. The ImageJ software was used to measure diameters of untreated and treated parasite images assuming the erythrocyte diameter to be 8 µm.

References

1. Hay, S. I. *et al.* Estimating the global clinical burden of Plasmodium falciparum Malaria in 2007. *PLoS Med.* **7,** e1000290 (2010).
2. Wellems, T. E. & Plowe, C. V. Chloroquine-resistant malaria. *J. Infect. Dis.* **184,** 770–776 (2001).
3. Ashley, E. A. & White, N. J. Artemisinin-based combinations. *Curr. Opin. Infect. Dis.* **18,** 531–536 (2005).
4. Nosten, F. & White, N. J. Artemisinin-based combination treatment of falciparum malaria. *Am. J. Trop. Med. Hyg.* **77,** 181–192 (2007).
5. Muller, O., Sie, A., Meissner, P., Schirmer, R. H. & Kouyate, B. Artemisinin resistance on the Thai-Cambodian border. *Lancet* **374,** 1419 (2009).
6. White, N. J. Artemisinin resistance--the clock is ticking. *Lancet* **376,** 2051–2052 (2010).
7. Dondorp, A. M. *et al.* Artemisinin resistance in *Plasmodium falciparum* malaria. *New. Engl. J. Med.* **361,** 455–467 (2009).
8. Burrows, J. N., Chibale, K. & Wells, T. N. The state of the art in anti-malarial drug discovery and development. *Curr. Top. Med. Chem.* **11,** 1226–1254 (2010).
9. Rottmann, M. *et al.* Spiroindolones, a potent compound class for the treatment of malaria. *Science* **329,** 1175–1180 (2010).
10. Spillman, N. J. *et al.* Na(+) regulation in the malaria parasite *Plasmodium falciparum* involves the cation ATPase PfATP4 and is a target of the spiroindolone antimalarials. *Cell Host Microbe* **13,** 227–237 (2013).
11. Kortagere, S. *et al.* Structure-based design of novel small-molecule inhibitors of *Plasmodium falciparum*. *J. Chem. Inf. Model* **50,** 840–849 (2010).
12. Marfurt, J. *et al.* Comparative *ex vivo* activity of novel endoperoxides in multidrug-resistant *Plasmodium falciparum* and *P. vivax*. *Antimicrob. Chemother.* **56,** 5258–5263 (2012).
13. Angulo-Barturen, I. *et al.* A murine model of falciparum-malaria by in vivo selection of competent strains in non-myelodepleted mice engrafted with human erythrocytes. *PLoS ONE* **3,** e2252 (2008).
14. Jimenez-Diaz, M. B. *et al.* Improved murine model of malaria using Plasmodium falciparum competent strains and non-myelodepleted NOD-scid

IL2Rgammanull mice engrafted with human erythrocytes. *Antimicrob. Agents Chemother.* **53,** 4533–4536 (2009).
15. Jimenez-Diaz, M. B., Viera, S., Fernandez-Alvaro, E. & Angulo-Barturen, I. Animal models of efficacy to accelerate drug discovery in malaria. *Parasitology* **141,** 93–103 (2013).
16. Rathod, P. K., McErlean, T. & Lee, P. C. Variations in frequencies of drug resistance in *Plasmodium falciparum*. *Proc. Natl Acad. Sci. USA* **94,** 9389–9393 (1997).
17. Kozarewa, I. *et al.* Amplification-free Illumina sequencing-library preparation facilitates improved mapping and assembly of (G + C)-biased genomes. *Nat. Methods* **6,** 291–295 (2009).
18. Otto, T. D., Sanders, M., Berriman, M. & Newbold, C. Iterative Correction of Reference Nucleotides (iCORN) using second generation sequencing technology. *Bioinformatics* **26,** 1704–1707 (2010).
19. Dvorin, J. D. *et al.* A plant-like kinase in *Plasmodium falciparum* regulates parasite egress from erythrocytes. *Science* **328,** 910–912 (2010).
20. Krishna, S. *et al.* Expression and functional characterization of a *Plasmodium falciparum* Ca2 + -ATPase (PfATP4) belonging to a subclass unique to apicomplexan organisms. *J. Biol. Chem.* **276,** 10782–10787 (2001).
21. Dyer, M., Jackson, M., McWhinney, C., Zhao, G. & Mikkelsen, R. Analysis of a cation-transporting ATPase of *Plasmodium falciparum*. *Mol. Biochem. Parasitol.* **78,** 1–12 (1996).
22. Nkrumah, L. J. *et al.* Efficient site-specific integration in *Plasmodium falciparum* chromosomes mediated by mycobacteriophage Bxb1 integrase. *Nat. Methods* **3,** 615–621 (2006).
23. Rodriguez-Navarro, A. & Benito, B. Sodium or potassium efflux ATPase a fungal, bryophyte, and protozoal ATPase. *Biochim. Biophys. Acta* **1798,** 1841–1853 (2010).
24. Kirk, K. Membrane transport in the malaria-infected erythrocyte. *Physiol. Rev.* **81,** 495–537 (2001).
25. Desai, S. A. Ion and nutrient uptake by malaria parasite-infected erythrocytes. *Cell Microbiol.* **14,** 1003–1009 (2012).
26. Staines, H. M., Ellory, J. C. & Kirk, K. Perturbation of the pump-leak balance for Na(+) and K(+) in malaria-infected erythrocytes. *Am. J. Physiol. Cell Physiol.* **280,** C1576–C1587 (2001).
27. Pillai, A. D. *et al.* Malaria parasites tolerate a broad range of ionic environments and do not require host cation remodelling. *Mol. Microbiol.* **88,** 20–34 (2013).
28. Gruring, C. *et al.* Development and host cell modifications of *Plasmodium falciparum* blood stages in four dimensions. *Nat. Commun.* **2,** 165 (2011).
29. Desjardins, R. E., Canfield, C. J., Haynes, J. D. & Chulay, J. D. Quantitative assessment of antimalarial activity in vitro by a semiautomated microdilution technique. *Antimicrob. Agents Chemother.* **16,** 710–718 (1979).
30. Delves, M. J. *et al.* Male and female *Plasmodium falciparum* mature gametocytes show different responses to antimalarial drugs. *Antimicrob. Agents Chemother.* **57,** 3268–3274 (2013).
31. Fidock, D. A. & Wellems, T. E. Transformation with human dihydrofolate reductase renders malaria parasites insensitive to WR99210 but does not affect the intrinsic activity of proguanil. *Proc. Natl Acad. Sci. USA* **94,** 10931–10936 (1997).
32. Ke, H. *et al.* Variation among *Plasmodium falciparum* strains in their reliance on mitochondrial electron transport chain function. *Eukaryot. Cell* **10,** 1053–1061 (2011).
33. Spillman, N. J., Allen, R. J. & Kirk, K. Na + extrusion imposes an acid load on the intraerythrocytic malaria parasite. *Mol. Biochem. Parasitol.* **189,** 1–4 (2013).

Acknowledgements

This work was supported by grants from Medicines for Malaria Venture (MMV/08/0027) and US National Institutes of Health (R01 AI098413) to A.B.V. We thank Bryan Yeung and Thierry Diagana for providing reagents and sharing data for spiroindolones. K.K. and N.J.S. acknowledge support from the Australian National Health and Medical Research Council (Project Grants 585473 and 1042272 to K.K. and Overseas Biomedical Fellowship 1072217 to N.J.S.). Early phase of this work was also supported by the CURE Fund from Drexel University College of Medicine. L.W.B. acknowledges the support of NIH grant R01 AI068137. We also thank Therapeutic Efficacy, Pharmacology and Laboratory Animal Science groups at GSK, Tres Cantos Medicines Development Campus for assistance. We thank L.D. Shultz and The Jackson Laboratory for providing access to NOD/SCID/IL2Rγ^null mice through their collaboration with GSK Tres Cantos Medicines Development Campus. Genomic sequencing was supported by the Wellcome Trust (grant WT 098051). T.D.O. was funded by the European Community's Seventh Framework Programme (FP7/2007-2013) under grant agreement No. 242095 ('EVIMalaR'). The *in vitro* studies on field isolates were supported by a Senior Research Fellowship in Clinical Science (091625) to R.N.P. from the Wellcome Trust.

Author contributions

A.B.V. designed and directed biological studies, provided input into medicinal chemistry, analysed the data and wrote the manuscript; J.M.M. carried out parasitological studies, derived resistant parasites, carried out transfections and generated genetic data; Z.Z. carried out organic synthesis of compounds and conducted their chemical characterization with assistance from M.S.; S.D. carried out live cell imaging and videography; T.M.D. assisted in characterization of transfected parasites; T.D.O. and M.B. carried out whole-genome sequencing and bioinformatics; N.J.S. and K.K. designed and conducted ion homeostasis experiments, and wrote parts of the manuscript; M.W., P.S., S.A.C., A.C., A.N. and J.B. provided input into medicinal chemistry and pharmacology of compounds; J.M., G.W., B.F.S. and R.N.P. conducted and analysed *in vitro* tests on field isolates; I.A.-B., S.F., M.B.J.-D., M.S.M. and F.J.G. designed, directed, conducted and analysed all experiments involving the NOD/scid/IL2R$_\gamma^{null}$ mice; V.M.A., A.R. and M.D. designed, conducted and analysed experiments involving sexual stages of parasites; S.K. provided input into medicinal chemistry and molecular dynamics; E.F. directed organic synthesis of compounds and provided input into medicinal chemistry and characterization of compounds; and L.W.B. carried out construction of transfection plasmids and assisted with analysis of genetic data.

Additional information

Accession codes: Raw sequence reads from the whole-genome sequencing are deposited in the European Nucleotide Archive under study ERP000325 (http://www.ebi.ac.uk/ena/data/view/ERP000325) with sample ID numbers ERS005005 for the Dd2 parent, and ERS005006, ERS005007 and ERS005008 for the three resistant clones.

Competing financial interests: A.B.V., J.B., E.F., S.K., M.W., A.C. and A.N. are listed as inventors in a patent application covering compounds described here. The remaining co-authors declare no competing financial interests.

9

New peptide architectures through C–H activation stapling between tryptophan–phenylalanine/tyrosine residues

Lorena Mendive-Tapia[1,2,3], Sara Preciado[2], Jesús García[1], Rosario Ramón[4], Nicola Kielland[4], Fernando Albericio[1,2,3,5] & Rodolfo Lavilla[4,6]

Natural peptides show high degrees of specificity in their biological action. However, their therapeutical profile is severely limited by their conformational freedom and metabolic instability. Stapled peptides constitute a solution to these problems and access to these structures lies on a limited number of reactions involving the use of non-natural amino acids. Here, we describe a synthetic strategy for the preparation of unique constrained peptides featuring a covalent bond between tryptophan and phenylalanine or tyrosine residues. The preparation of such peptides is achieved in solution and on solid phase directly from the corresponding sequences having an iodo-aryl amino acid through an intramolecular palladium-catalysed C–H activation process. Moreover, complex topologies arise from the internal stapling of cyclopeptides and double intramolecular arylations within a linear peptide. Finally, as a proof of principle, we report the application to this new stapling method to relevant biologically active compounds.

[1] Institute for Research in Biomedicine, Barcelona Science Park, Baldiri Reixac 10-12, 08028 Barcelona, Spain. [2] Department of Organic Chemistry, University of Barcelona, Martí i Franqués 1-11, 08028 Barcelona, Spain. [3] CIBER-BBN, Networking Centre on Bioengineering, Biomaterials and Nanomedicine. [4] Barcelona Science Park, Baldiri Reixac 10-12, 08028 Barcelona, Spain. [5] School of Chemistry, Yachay Tech, Yachay City of Knowledge, 100119 Urcuqui, Ecuador. [6] Laboratory of Organic Chemistry, Faculty of Pharmacy, University of Barcelona, Avda. Joan XXII s.n., 08028 Barcelona, Spain. Correspondence and requests for materials should be addressed to F.A. (email: albericio@irbbarcelona.org) or to R.L. (email: rlavilla@pcb.ub.es).

Peptides are attracting great attention as therapeutics since they combine the high selectivity, potency and low toxicity of biologics with advantages such as the conformational restrictions and the reduced costs characteristic of small molecular entities[1,2]. In addition to the large number of commercialized peptides, many others are also found in clinical phases, thereby demonstrating their validity and application as active pharmaceutical ingredients[3]. However, the general use of peptides as drugs is severely hampered by their poor pharmacokinetic features. In this regard, it is widely believed that the characterization of protein–protein interactions, a fundamental issue in deciphering biological pathways, is better tackled through structurally defined small peptides with specific sequences. Therefore, there is a need for peptides with new topological architectures; however, these are difficult to obtain even using modern synthetic procedures[4,5]. To address these problems, general strategies for peptide macrocyclization have been developed to improve the properties (cell penetration, stability, selectivity and so on) and enhance the potential of peptides as therapeutics and bioprobes, with a special focus on poorly tractable targets[6-8]. In this context, peptides constrained via a non-amide sidechain-to-sidechain linkage (stapled peptides) provide a new structural paradigm because the conformational stabilized species display remarkably stronger biological activity. In this regard, the pioneering work of Verdine et al.[9,10] on the basis of all-hydrocarbon staples through olefin metathesis represents a breakthrough in the field.

So far, stapled peptides are generated through a variety of strategies[11], the main being the use of cysteine side chains to form disulfide bridges[12] and thioether formation (crosslinking with α,α'-dibromo-m-xylene[13] or aromatic nucleophilic substitutions with perfluoroaromatic reactants[14]); or with functionalized non-natural amino acids by means of biaryl linkages involving the borylated phenylalanine derivatives[15-18], ring-closing metathesis[19] and azide–alkyne cycloadditions (click chemistry)[20], and so on, usually in expensive and long stepwise syntheses. A comparative table summarizes the major strengths and weaknesses of the main conventional stapling strategies (Fig. 1a). Owing to the increasing interest in stapled peptides and other conformationally restricted structures, many efforts have been made to develop new practical and general preparative methods for their generation.

There is a considerable concern regarding the efficiency of synthetic aspects with respect to the preparation of complex bioactive compounds. In this context, the function-oriented synthesis approach to target simplified, although biologically meaningful, fragments of complex chemical entities is relevant, as it leads to practical syntheses of new specific drugs and probes, also in the field of peptides[21].

Tryptophan (Trp) has a low relative abundance in peptide and protein sequences ($\approx 1\%$ of the amino acids); however, its presence is critical for the activity of these biomolecules. Therefore, the development of new synthetic methods for the selective and straightforward chemical modification of Trp is highly significant[22].

Recently, metal-catalysed C–C coupling through direct C–H activation[23-29] has become a fundamental process in modern organic syntheses, allowing the straightforward preparation of a plethora of new structural types. In this respect, the functionalization of indoles using this approach has been extensively examined[30,31], including studies described in (refs 28, 32–35) among others. Particularly relevant to our research was the methodology of Larrosa for indole arylation using Pd(OAc)$_2$ in acidic media[36]. In particular, although the Pd-mediated C-2 arylation of Trp has been reported[37-39], it has not yet been applied to staple true peptides. We recently disclosed the direct C-2 arylation of indoles in Trp-containing peptidic sequences in an intermolecular manner, without additional requierements[37]. Although the alternative N-arylation processes are conceivable, such Ullmann-type reactions take place normally with Cu and Pd catalysts, in the latter case usually requiring strong bases[40]. No experimental evidence of these transformations have been recorded in our systems. The main restriction is that lower conversions are obtained for sequences that comprise methionine, cysteine or histidine residues, presumably because of selective hydrolysis of the peptide bond catalysed by bidentate palladium coordination; on-going experiments along this line show that working in nonaqueous solvents allows reasonable arylations (unpublished results). Later we reported on the arylation of Trp-diketopiperazines[41] and related transformations of Trp derivatives, leading to the generation of Fmoc-protected arylated Trps that are amenable to direct incorporation in solid-phase peptide synthesis (SPPS)[42]. These processes work well with N-protected peptides in dimethylformamide (DMF) or in aqueous environments.

In this work, we present a new stapling methodology involving Trp and Phe(Tyr) through a Pd-catalysed C–H activation process. The method is versatile, allowing the formation of constrained peptides of different ring sizes, amenable to solution- and solid-phase synthesis and can lead to the direct preparation of biologically meaningful peptide derivatives.

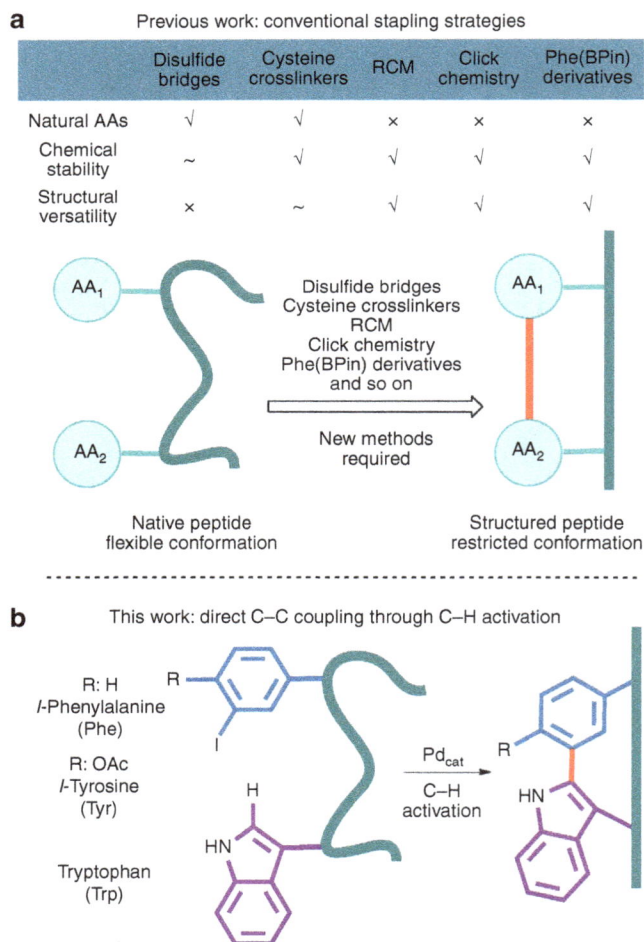

a Previous work: conventional stapling strategies

	Disulfide bridges	Cysteine crosslinkers	RCM	Click chemistry	Phe(BPin) derivatives
Natural AAs	√	√	×	×	×
Chemical stability	~	√	√	√	√
Structural versatility	×	~	√	√	√

b This work: direct C–C coupling through C–H activation

Figure 1 | Formation of stapled peptides. (a) Conventional stapling methods. **(b)** Phe/Tyr-Trp stapling via a selective Pd-catalysed C-H arylation process.

Table 1 | Results for the stapled bond formation of peptides 1 under microwave irradiation.

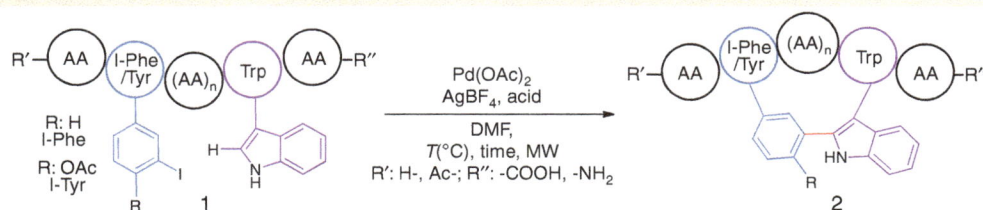

Entry	n	Linear peptide (1)	Coupling conditions*	Stapled peptide	Conv (%)†
1	1	Ac-Ala-*m*-I-**Phe**-Ala-**Trp**-Ala-OH (**1a**)	A	**2a**	38
2	2	Ac-Ala-*m*-I-**Phe**-Ala-Ala-**Trp**-Ala-OH (**1b**)	A	**2b**	100
3	3	Ac-Ala-*m*-I-**Phe**-Ala-Ala-Ala-**Trp**-Ala-OH (**1c**)	A	**2c**	100
4	1	Ac-Ala-*m*-I-**Tyr**-Ala-**Trp**-Ala-OH (**1d**)	A	**2d**	100
5	2	Ac-Ala-*m*-I-**Tyr**-Ala-Ala-**Trp**-Ala-OH (**1e**)	A	**2e**	100
6	3	Ac-Ala-*m*-I-**Tyr**-Ala-Ala-Ala-**Trp**-Ala-OH (**1f**)	A	**2f**	100
7	3	Ac-*m*-I-**Phe**-Asn-Gly-Arg-**Trp**-NH₂ (**1g**)	B	**2g**	77
8	3	Ac-*m*-I-**Phe**-Arg-Gly-Asp-**Trp**-NH₂ (**1h**)	B	**2h**	70
9	2	H-Ala-*m*-I-**Phe**-Ser-Ala-**Trp**-Ala-OH (**1i**)	B	**2i**	39‡
10	1	Ac-Ala-*m*-I-**Phe**-Val-**Trp**-Ala-OH (**1j**)	B	**2j**	71
11	0	Ac-Ala-*p*-I-**Phe**-**Trp**-Ala-OH (**1k**)	B	**2k**§	60

Conv, conversion; HPLC-MS, high-performance liquid chromatography-mass spectrometry; MW, microwave.
*Coupling conditions (A): 5 mol % Pd(OAc)₂, 1.0 eq. of AgBF₄, 1.5 eq. of 2-NO₂BzOH in DMF:PBS (1:1), MW 80 °C, 15 min. (B) 5 mol % Pd(OAc)₂, 2.0 eq. of AgBF₄, 1.0 eq. of TFA in DMF, MW 90 °C, 20 min.
†Conversion: estimated yield (HPLC-MS).
‡Additional MW irradiation cycles were necessary to obtain the desired product as the main compound (HPLC-MS).
§Cyclodimer **2k** was obtained in place of the putative monomeric structure **2k′**.

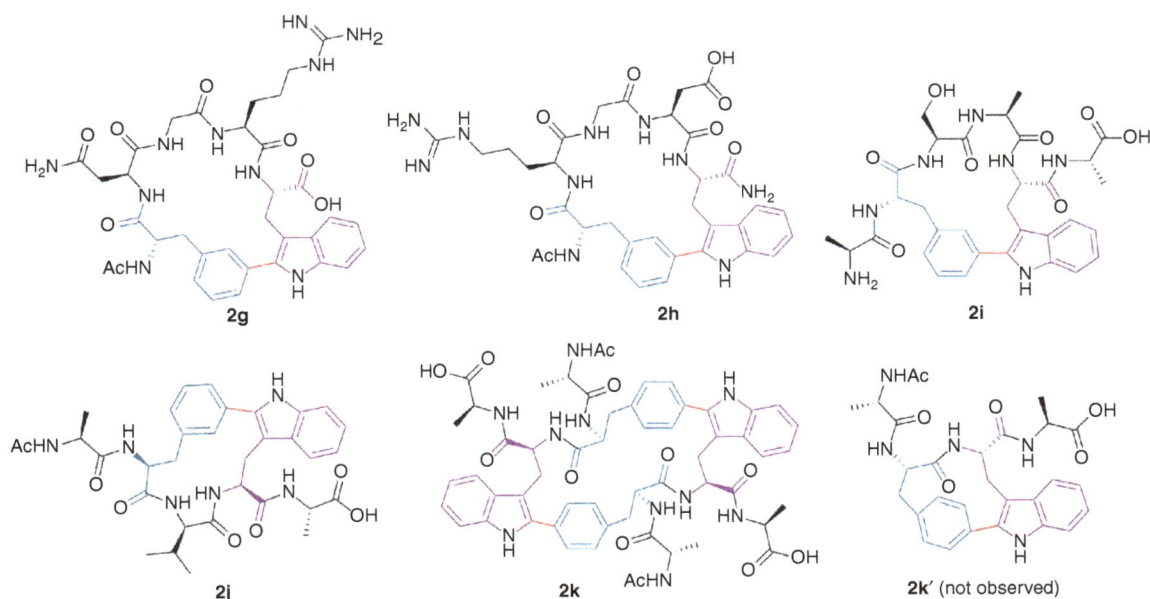

Figure 2 | Structure of isolated locked peptides 2g–2k. Schematic representation: Phe (blue), Trp (purple) and staple bond (red).

Results

Preliminary studies. Here we present a one-step process for the synthesis of Trp–Phe(Tyr)-stapled peptides directly from commercially available precursors. The method is based on an intramolecular Pd-catalysed C–H activation reaction between a Trp residue and an iodo-phenylalanine (or tyrosine) unit (Fig. 1b).

After a preliminary modelling study, we established the structural features for the intramolecular C–H arylation, placing the iodo-substituent for Phe or Tyr amino acids in the *meta* position. The preferential distances between these latter residues and Trp ranged from one to three amino acids in a series of linear *N*-terminal-acetylated sequences.

The initial experiments were carried out using the conditions previously applied in the arylation of the Trp diketopiperazine:[41] Overall, 5 mol% Pd(OAc)₂, AgBF₄ (1.0 eq.) and *o*-nitrobenzoic acid (2-NO₂BzOH) (1.5 eq.) in PBS:DMF (1:1) under microwave (MW) irradiation at 80 °C for 15 min (Table 1, entries 1–6). These preliminary observations suggested that these arrangements are suitable for stapled peptide formation, affording good to excellent conversions for Trp–Phe(Tyr) staples located at i–i+2, i–i+3 and i–i+4 positions (Table 1, entries 1–6). Furthermore, a series of representative sequences displaying from one to three amino acids between Trp and *m*-iodinated Phe were constrained in useful yields (Table 1, entries 7–10; Fig. 2; see Supplementary Fig. 1), in an

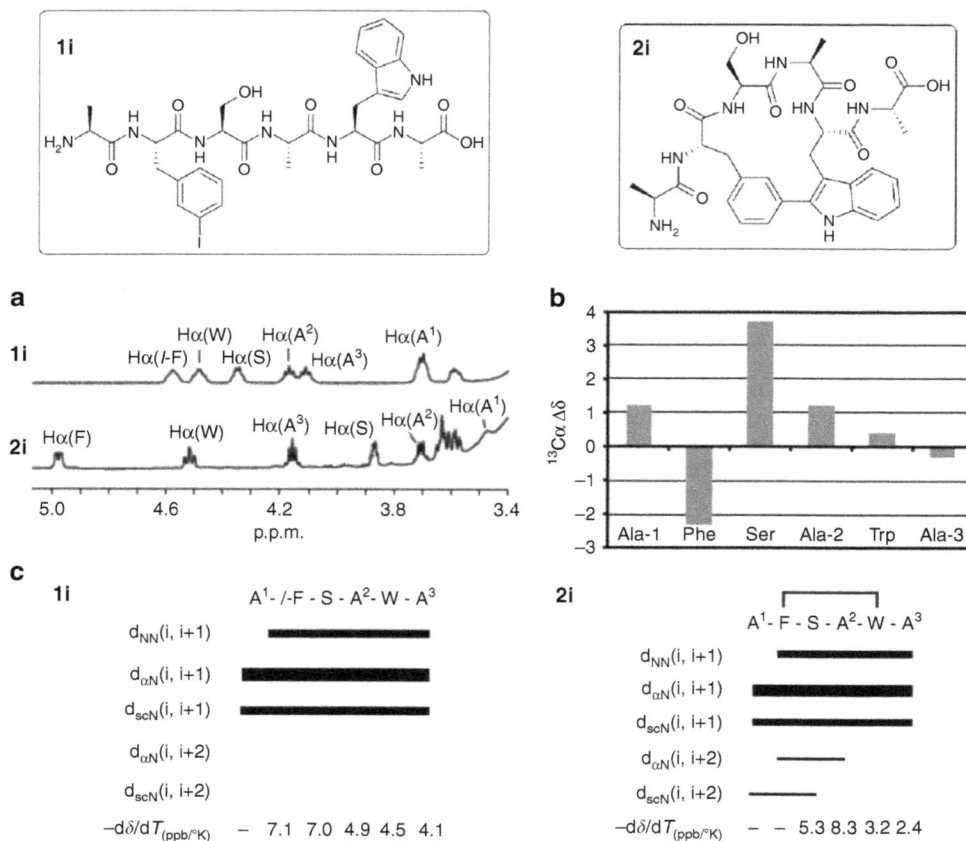

Figure 3 | Peptide NMR spectra comparison between stapled peptide 2i and its linear counterpart 1i. (a) NMR H_α region of peptide **2i** and its linear precursor **1i**. (b) Plot of the $^{13}C_\alpha$ chemical shift differences ($^{13}C_\alpha \Delta\delta_{cyclic-linear}$) between stapled peptide **2i** and its linear counterpart **1i**. (c) Summary of NOE connectivity and temperature coefficients of the NH amide protons ($\Delta\delta/\Delta T$) of peptide **1i** (bottom left) and **2i** (bottom right). The thickness of the bars reflects the intensity of the NOEs, that is, weak ($-$), medium ($\blacksquare$) and strong ($\blacksquare$). *I*-F: *m*-iodophenylalanine.

anhydrous medium using trifluoroacetic acid (TFA) as the acid, applying the optimized conditions previously reported for the preparation of Fmoc-protected arylated Trps[42]. Although these transformations may lead to atropoisomeric diastereomers, only one stereochemically defined structure was observed in each case. Of note is the successful application of this technique to stapled peptides containing the Asn-Gly-Arg (-NGR-) and Arg-Gly-Asp (-RGD-) tumour-homing signalling sequences (**2g** and **2h**, Table 1, entries 7 and 8, respectively).

Preliminary studies on the capacity of the RGD-containing compound **2h** and its linear precursor **1h** to inhibit cellular adhesion showed that these substances act selectively as antagonists for the $\alpha v \beta 3$ in front of $\alpha v \beta 5$ integrin receptors; compound **2h** showing a moderate EC$_{50}$ (6 μM) is more active than its linear precursor (**1h**, 26 μM, see Biochemical and Cellular Studies in Supplementary Methods). Compound **2h** is considerably less potent than cilengitide, not surprisingly as this drug has been thoroughly optimized. However, it has to be considered that even linear analogues display a much lower potency (10–10^3 times, depending on the targeted integrin) than the parent cilengitide[43,44]. These preliminary results clearly show that this stapling technique preserves the activity of the natural sequence, while improving its potency, in line with pioneering experiments in macrocyclization techniques for medchem peptide development[45,46].

We next tackled the preparation of the more challenging locked peptide i − i + 1. Three sequences with adjacent Trp— (*ortho*-, *meta*- or *para*)-I-Phe were synthesized. A constrained C–C linked structure was obtained for the *meta*-derivative (60%),

although it could not be properly characterized. With respect to the *ortho* analogue, only the reduced peptide was detected. Interestingly, the *para*-I-Phe peptide **1k** was successfully reacted under the usual conditions to yield cyclodimer **2k** (60%, Table 1, entry 11; see Supplementary Figs 2 and 3). Presumably, the putative monomeric structure **2k'** would be highly strained (molecular models display a nonplanar phenyl ring, see Supplementary Fig. 4) and the process evolves through a ditopic pathway, in a remarkable demonstration of the process versatility.

A detailed nuclear magnetic resonance (NMR) study was performed on dimethylsulphoxide to analyse the conformational behaviour of the peptides synthesized. The NMR spectra of linear sequences **1g–1j** were indicative of flexible, unstructured peptides. H_α and $^{13}C_\alpha$ chemical shifts displayed values typical for random coil, and the NH temperature coefficients and $^3J(H_\alpha NH)$ couplings were within the range expected for unstructured peptides[47].

Staple bond formation caused a substantial modification of the peptide NMR spectra. Compared with their linear precursors, peptides **2g–2j** showed larger H_α chemical shift dispersion (Fig. 3a and Supplementary Figs 5–7), indicating less conformational flexibility. However, broad resonances were observed at 25 °C for some backbone NH protons, suggesting that peptides **2g–2j** show some flexibility. Significant differences in $^{13}C_\alpha$ chemical shifts were observed between stapled peptides **2g–2j** and their linear counterparts **1g–1j** (Fig. 3b and Supplementary Figs 5–7). The temperature dependence of the amide NH groups was also significantly affected by staple formation (Fig. 3c and Supplementary Figs 5–7). Stapled peptides showed a wider distribution of $\Delta\delta/\Delta T$ values within the amino-acid sequence and

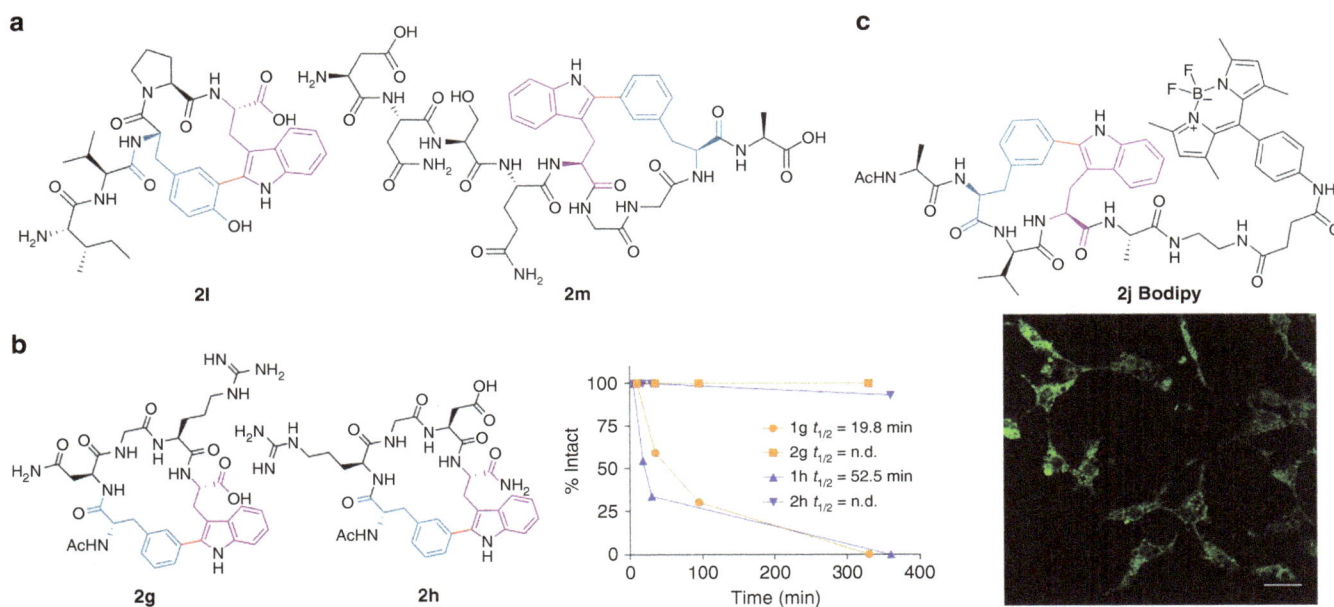

Figure 4 | Bioactive stapled peptides, biochemical and cellular studies. (a) Structure of stapled peptides **2l** (valorphin analogue) and **2m** (baratin analogue). **(b)** Proteolytic degradation assay of stapled peptides **2g** and **2h** and their linear precursors **1g** and **1h**. **(c)** Structure of labelled-stapled peptide **2j Bodipy** (left) and the corresponding confocal microscopy image of SH-SY5Y cells treated with compound **2j Bodipy** (750 nM). Scale bar, 25 μm (right).

also featured values characteristic of solvent-shielded NH groups (lower than -3 ppb/K). NOE connectivity was also affected by staple formation. In the case of peptides **2h**, **2i** and **2j**, several nonsequential NOEs indicated that the peptides were constrained by intramolecular cyclization (Fig. 3c and Supplementary Figs 6 and 7). Incidentally, we detect all N_{indole}–H atoms, and also we find the corresponding indole Cα positions consequently substituted, therefore ruling out any interference by N-arylation processes. The aryl–aryl moieties show NOE correlations consistent with a defined single configuration in each case, which matches with the arrangement predicted from molecular modelling.

Moreover, circular dichroism measurements of stapled peptides **2g** and **2h** were performed in order to detect evidence of secondary structure and were then compared with their linear precursors **1g** and **1h**, respectively (See Supplementary Figs 8–11). Stapled peptides **2** show a positive maximum at ∼190 nm and minimum peaks at 206 nm, which indicate some levels of structuring. In contrast, linear peptides exhibit a more flattened profile typical of a flexible unfolded structure.

Extension to biologically relevant peptides. To further explore the potential of the methodology, we planned to make the stapled analogues of known linear bioactive peptides, and at the same time test the influence of new features, such as the presence of proline (Pro) in the sequence, the overall length of the chain (up to nine amino acids) and the possibility of performing the C–H arylation on the solid phase, which enables the transformation of unprotected N-terminal peptides. In this way, we prepared the stapled version of an active valorphin analogue[48], which is a potent dipeptidyl peptidase III inhibitor, displaying Pro in a five amino-acid sequence containing also Trp and Tyr (see Supplementary Fig. 12). Interestingly, this peptide is closely related to spinorphin, an endogenous antinociceptive peptide, a potent and noncompetitive antagonist at the ATP-activated human P2X3 receptor[49]. The SPPS method was used to synthesize the Fmoc-protected sequence, which was intramolecularly arylated on resin. Subsequent N-terminal

deprotection and cleavage, successfully afforded the stapled peptide **2l** (Fig. 4a). This solid-phase protocol is fully compatible with the Pd chemistry involved and, interestingly, allows the preparation of arylated sequences having unprotected terminal amino groups. Futhermore, baratin[50], a neuro-stimulating peptide, was stapled following a related procedure. In this way, the standard SPPS protocol was interrupted to perform the on-resin C–H activation step, to be continued with the incorporation of the final four amino acids. Afterwards, deprotection and cleavage afforded the desired derivative **2m** (Fig. 4a, see Supplementary Methods and Supplementary Fig. 12).

Next, we determined the proteolytic stability of a couple of meaningful stapled peptides, in comparison with their respective linear counterparts. We followed a chymotrypsin-based protocol, previously used to evaluate stapled peptides[51]. Plotting the HPLC-MS profiles of the couples **2g/1g** and **2h/1h** (Fig. 4b, also Supplementary Figs 13–15) clearly shows an almost total protection of the stapled peptides towards enzymatic degradation, after 5–6 h, whereas the linear precursors suffered a rapid hydrolytic cleavage to remove the N-terminal amino acid, and completely disappeared after this time lapse.

Finally, we studied the controlled labelling of the stapled peptides. The goal was to selectively attach a fluorophore to the C-terminal amino acid to trace cellular permeabilization and localization. Thus, we linked a Bodipy residue to cyclopeptide **2j** through an amino spacer (the novel Bodipy construct was designed and prepared for this purpose, see Supplementary Fig. 16 and Supplementary Methods), to get the desired labelled-stapled peptide **2j Bodipy** (Fig. 4c) in a convenient manner. This compound exhibits low cytotoxicity at 750 nM after 24 h of incubation in SH-SY5Y cells (MTT assay; see Supplementary Fig. 17), and this concentration was used for the cell penetration studies. In a preliminary flow cytometry experiment (fluorescence-activated cell sorting assay), SH-SY5Y cells resulted in brightly stained sections on incubation for 30 min (see Supplementary Fig. 18). The cells treated in this manner were analysed using confocal microscopy. The stapled peptide **2j Bodipy** was localized both in the membrane and in the cytoplasmatic region (Fig. 4c). Incidentally, the Bodipy-labelled

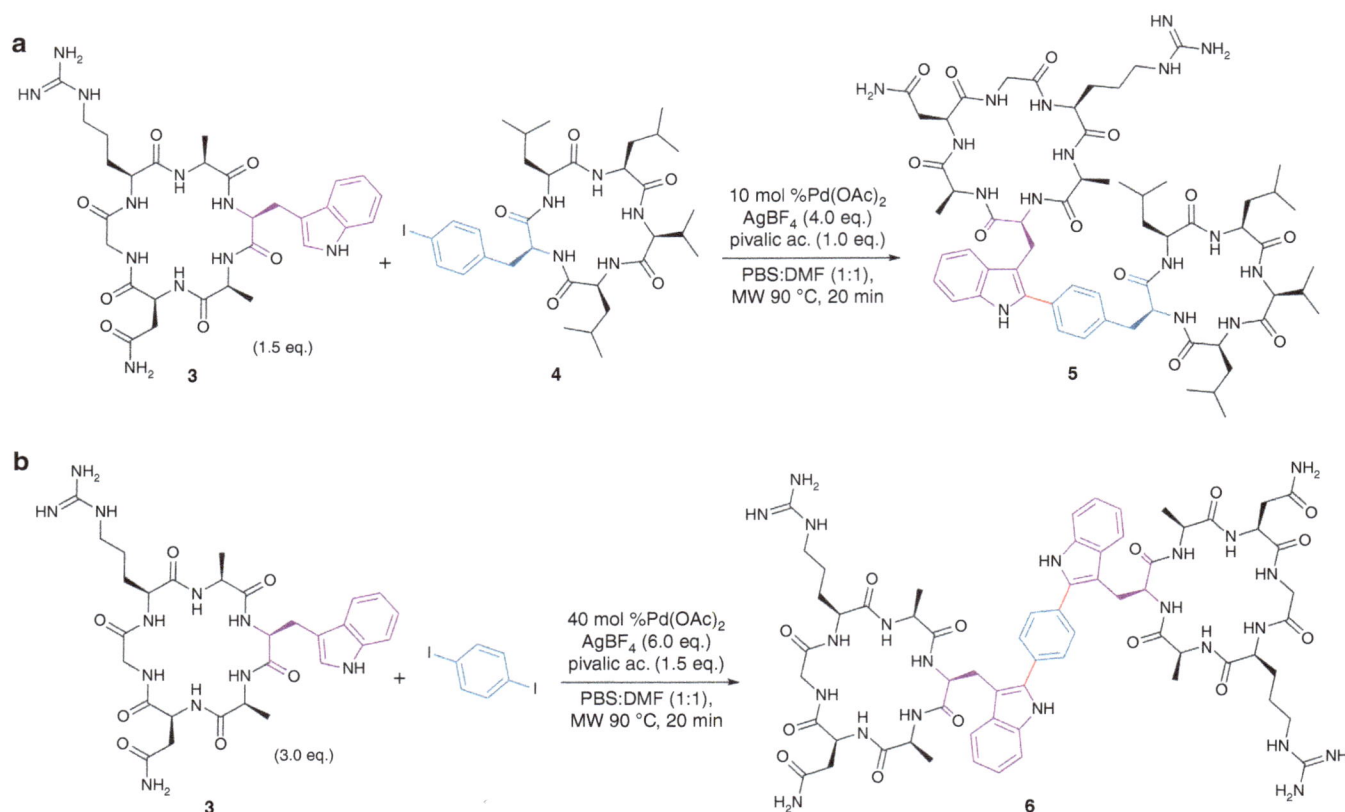

Figure 5 | Macrocyclic conjugation via C–H activation. (**a**) Intermolecular conjugation of NGR cyclopeptide **3** with the sansalvamide derivative **4** via C–H activation. (**b**) Double conjugation of the NGR cyclopeptide **3** with 1,4-diiodobenzene.

linear precursor **1j** Bodipy also penetrates into cells in a comparable extent; however, there are appreciable differences in toxicity and cell permeability with respect to the stapled analogue (see Supplementary Figs 19 and 20). Overall, these results enable the performance of systematic bioimaging studies on these compounds.

Intermolecular peptide conjugation through C–H activation. Chemical conjugation can effectively link drugs to carriers, and this technique is routinely used to modify biologics, especially antibodies with therapeutic indications[52]. We next explored peptide–peptide conjugation via C–H activation to achieve bismacrocyclic peptide constructs linked through a nonhydrolysable bond.

Peptides that inhibit the new blood vessel growth (angiogenesis) have become a promising tool for treating cancer. In this context, it has been reported that cyclic forms of NGR-containing sequences (tumour-homing peptides) lead to an improvement of the anticancer activity of an associated drug[53]. We selected the previously studied Asn-Gly-Arg (NGR) array and synthesized the corresponding Trp-containing macrocycle **3** to be conjugated to a synthetic p-I-Phe-cyclopeptide derivative of the cyclic depsipeptide sansalvamide A (**4**, Fig. 5a), a natural product whose synthetic analogues have demonstrated significant anticancer activity[54]. Using a standard Pd-catalysed reaction in an aqueous medium of PBS–DMF, the two partners were successfully coupled to yield the C–C conjugate **5** (Fig. 5a).

In a second example, the conjugation of two units of the NGR Trp-containing cyclopeptide **3** with a 1,4-diiodobenzene connector via a double C–H arylation was achieved. Again, the process yielded the expected bis-NGR-adduct **6** in a single step (Fig. 5b).

To evaluate the effects of macrocyclic conjugation, the NMR spectra of conjugated peptide **5** and its cyclic precursors **3** and **4** were compared (see Supplementary Fig. 21). After conjugation, small shifts were observed in the H_α resonances of the sansalvamide A analogue **4**. In contrast, the H_α chemical shifts of the NGR-containing cycle were almost identical in peptides **5** and **3**. Comparison of $^{13}C_\alpha$ chemical shifts showed that in both cycles the larger $^{13}C_\alpha$ chemical shift change corresponded to the residue involved in the intermolecular bond formation: Trp (1.2 p.p.m.) in the NGR-containing cycle and Phe (0.6 p.p.m.) in the sansalvamide A derivative. More modest changes were observed in the $^{13}C_\alpha$ of the remaining amino acids. The resemblance of the H_α and $^{13}C_\alpha$ chemical shifts, which are highly sensitive to conformational changes, suggests that conjugation provided a minimal perturbation of the overall structures of peptides **3** and **4**. The NMR analysis was extended to peptide **6** and its precursor **3**. The effects of conjugation in the H_α and C_α resonances are shown in Supplementary Fig. 22.

Unfortunately, in preliminary biological studies evaluating the conjugated peptide **5** and its macrocycle precursors **3** and **4** against several cancer cell lines, only the cyclopeptide **4** showed activity ($IC_{50} < 10\,\mu M$). Nevertheless, the protocol seems general and offers new possibilities for peptide-based conjugation.

Stapled cyclopeptides. We then explored access to complex topologies, focusing on the synthesis of bicyclic peptide chemotypes. In a first approach, the synthesis of a stapled cyclopeptide was attempted by promoting the usual C–H arylation through an intramolecular Trp-I-Phe interaction. Preliminary studies showed that alanine (Ala) hexapeptides containing a m-I-Phe and Trp units, respectively, placed at positions i − i + 2 and i − i + 3 afforded the corresponding macrocycles after routine amide

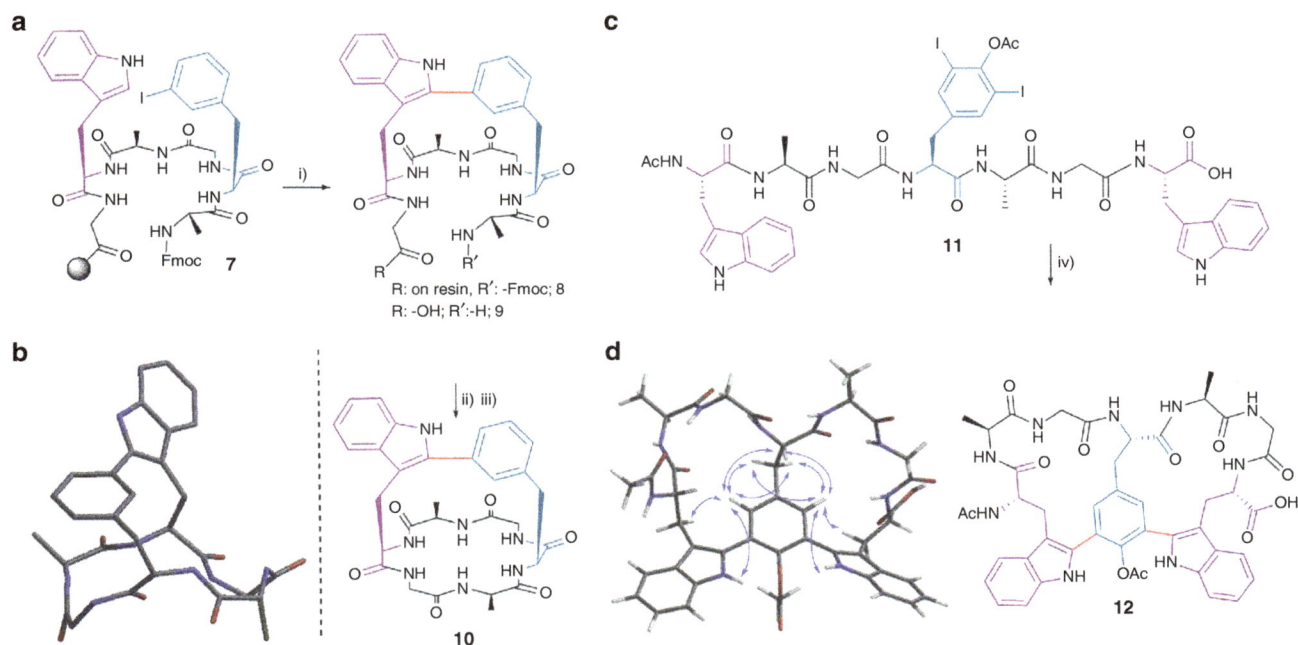

Figure 6 | Synthesis of macrobicyclic peptides 10 and 12. (**a**) Synthesis of macrobicyclic peptide **10** through solid-phase stapling. Reaction conditions: (i) Pd(OAc)$_2$ (0.05 eq.), AgBF$_4$ (1.0 eq.), 2-NO$_2$BzOH (1.5 eq.), DMF, MW 90 °C, 20 min; (ii) (1) 1% sodium diethyldithiocarbamate (DDC) in DMF. (2) Piperidine–DMF (1:4; 1 × 1 min, 2 × 5 min). (3) TFA-TIS-H$_2$O (95:2.5:2.5), r.t, 1 h; (iii) PyAOP (2.0 eq.), DIEA (6.0 eq.), DMF, r.t, 1.5 h. (**b**) Minimized geometry of compound **10** generated by the Spartan '14 suite. Hydrogens omitted for clarity. (**c**) Double C–H arylation to cyclic biaryl **12** (25% conversion, estimated by HPLC). Reaction conditions: (iv) 40 mol %Pd(OAc)$_2$, AgBF$_4$ (6.0 eq.), pivalic ac. (1.5 eq.), DMF, MW 90 °C, 20 min. (**d**) Minimized geometry of compound **12** generated by Spartan '14 suite showing the diagnostic NOE correlations (blue arrows).

coupling in quantitative yields; however, the subsequent intramolecular C–H arylations did not take place under the standard conditions, probably because of a highly restricted conformation. Remarkably, when the stapling on the linear sequence anchored to the resin **7** was carried out first on the solid phase, we obtained the corresponding NH-free amino terminal-stapled peptide **9** after cleavage from resin. Finally, we isolated the desired bicyclic compound **10** by amide cyclization (Fig. 6a,b). Furthermore, in this way, we overcame the relative limitation of irreversible protection of the *N*-terminal amino group, as previously reported[37]. Incidentally, preliminary results showed that increasing the Pd(OAc)$_2$ amount up to 0.2 eq. gave acceptable intermolecular arylations for NH-free amino terminal sequences (data not shown). The stapled cyclopeptide **10** was prepared in a suitable manner, involving a solid-phase arylation, thus facilitating the purification step, followed by a routine peptide coupling. This protocol may enable the synthesis of further derivatives of this attractive and unexplored structural class.

The ^{1}H NMR spectrum of the linear stapled peptide **9** was characterized by a large chemical shift dispersion of the NH and H$_\alpha$ resonances. Bicyclopeptide **10** showed a slightly larger chemical shift range for the H$_\alpha$ protons, as expected for a more rigid and structured peptide. Backbone cyclization was also reflected in a large splitting of the methylene H$_\alpha$ atoms of Gly-1 and H$_\beta$ atoms of Phe. In the case of peptide **9**, the chemical shift difference between the two geminal protons was <0.2 (H$_\alpha$, Gly-1) and 0.1 (H$_\beta$, Phe) p.p.m., whereas for peptide **10** this difference increased to >0.9 (H$_\alpha$, Gly-1) and >0.7 (H$_\beta$, Phe) p.p.m. Backbone cyclization was further evidenced by significant changes in ^{13}C$_\alpha$ chemical shifts and in the temperature coefficients of amide NH (Supplementary Fig. 23).

Double stapling of linear peptides. Biaryl bismacrocyclic peptide-derived natural products such as vancomycin[55] and complestatin[56] display very interesting bioactivity profiles and

as synthetic targets they are extremely difficult to prepare[57]. Thus, the development of new methodologies to access simplified scaffolds is crucial to enable structural diversification, thereby allowing practical medicinal chemistry and biological studies. Hence, it was envisioned that intramolecular double C–H arylation of a sequence containing a diiodinated Tyr (commercially available) flanked by two Trp units would give raise to bicyclic peptide topologies with adjacent biaryl moieties in a straightforward manner. In order to establish the conditions for this transformation, we performed some preliminary experiments where the intermolecular C–H activation of a Ac-*m,m'*-I,I-Tyr(OAc)-OH unit with 2.0 eq. of Ac-Trp-OH was tested. An increase in the amount of the Pd catalyst (40%) and AgBF$_4$ (6.0 eq.)[58] and use of a mild excess of pivalic acid resulted in a productive reaction (see Supplementary Methods). Next, we designed the linear peptide sequence **11** (Fig. 6c), which was synthesized in a straightforward manner on the solid phase. Using the previous C–H activation conditions for the diodoTyr, we successfully obtained the double stapled peptide **12** directly from the corresponding linear precursor in one step in a 25% HPLC conversion, together with monoarylated cycles and dehalogenated derivatives, which were probably produced in competitive processes (Fig. 6c). This remarkable result is the proof of principle that even these complex peptidic topologies are accessible through the present methodology. The ^{1}H NMR spectrum of the double stapled peptide **12** is characterized by a wide chemical shift range for the NH and H$_\alpha$ protons (see Supplementary Fig. 134). The observed pattern of NOEs, summarized in Fig. 6d, indicates that each side of the Tyr aromatic ring faces a distinct Trp-Ala-Gly motif.

As an optimization of this methodology, we have developed the exclusive use of standard proteinogenic amino acids (Tyr), which, once coupled, are modified *in situ*, thus simplifying the protocol and rendering it considerably more affordable. In this way, the corresponding linear precursor of peptide **11** can be obtained through routine amide couplings followed by on-resin iodination of the Tyr residue to yield derivative **11** (41% conversion, unoptimized, see Supplementary Fig. 24)[59]. This remarkable result enables the direct synthesis of bicyclopeptide **12** to be performed on solid-phase from commercially available reagents in a single sequence.

Discussion

Metal-catalysed arylations through C–H activation are suitable processes to gain access to minimalistic staples (two-electron) in relevant Trp-containing peptide sequences directly from Trp and iodo-phenylalanine (-tyrosine) precursors. The validation of the methodology includes the analysis of the scope of the transformation, compatibility with other amino acids and the applicability to SPPS. This approach has also been applied to constrain biologically active signalling sequences. In an intermolecular mode, the process efficiently links two Trp peptides to a benzene connector and is also useful to conjugate peptides through a C–C bond. All compounds showed a structured nature, as revealed by spectroscopic characterization. Finally, we have developed a simple protocol for the straightforward access to novel peptide topologies such as dimeric macrocycles, stapled bicyclopeptides and biaryl–biaryl species (see Supplementary Figs 4 and 25) from the corresponding linear precursors in only one step. These findings open up general access to a variety of novel constrained peptidic chemotypes, and we believe that this breakthrough will make a significant contribution to the development of a broad range of applications for peptides in biological and medicinal chemistry.

Methods

General. For abbreviations and detailed experimental procedures see Supplementary Methods. For NMR analysis of the compounds, see Supplementary Figs 26–148 and Supplementary Tables 1–40.

Peptide synthesis. All peptides were manually synthesized on a 2-Chlorotrityl, H-Rink-Amide Chemmatrix or TentaGel S NH$_2$ resin using standard Fmoc chemistry for SPPS.

Linear peptide cyclization. The free-amine free-acid linear peptide (1.0 eq.) was dissolved in ACN/DMF or DMF (0.001–0.003 M) and N,N-diisopropylethylamine (DIEA) (6.0 eq.) and the corresponding coupling agents (1.5–3.0 eq.), benzotriazol-1-yl-oxytripyrrolidinophosphonium hexafluorophosphate (PyBOP) with hydroxybenzotriazole (HOBt) or 1-[Bis(dimethylamino)methylene]-1H-1,2,3-triazolo[4,5-b]pyridinium 3-oxid hexafluorophosphate (HATU) and O-(benzotriazol-1-yl)-N,N,N′,N′-tetramethyluronium tetrafluoroborate (TBTU) or (7-azabenzotriazol-1-yloxy)tripyrrolidinophosphonium hexafluorophosphate (PyAOP)) were added. The solution was stirred at r.t until the cyclization was complete (1–3 h). Workup was performed by extraction with aqueous solutions of NH$_4$Cl$_{sat}$ and NaHCO$_{3sat}$. Organic layers were combined, dried over anhydrous sodium sulfate, filtered and concentrated under vacuum. When remaining protecting groups were present, the macrocycle was treated with a 95% TFA, 2.5% triisopropylsilane (TIS) and 2.5% H$_2$O cocktail (3 h), washed with Et$_2$O, dissolved in ACN:H$_2$O and lyophilized to furnish the corresponding deprotected peptide. When necessary, the macrocycle was purified by flash column chromatography on silica gel or semipreparative RP-HPLC.

General protocol for the stapled bond formation in solution. The linear peptide (50 mg), AgBF$_4$ (2.0 eq.), trifluoroacetic acid (1.0 eq.) and Pd(OAc)$_2$ (0.05 eq.) were placed in a MW reactor vessel in DMF (1.2 ml). The mixture was heated under MW irradiation (250 W) at 90 °C for 20 min. The residue was filtered and purified using semipreparative RP-HPLC. This process was scaled up to 0.907 mmol of peptide, affording the stapled/locked peptides **2g–2k** in isolated yields ranging from 1 to 32%.

Procedure for the single macrocycle conjugation. Cyclopeptide **4** (40.0 mg, 0.056 mmol), cyclopeptide **3** (55.3 mg, 0.084 mmol, 1.5 eq.), AgBF$_4$ (43.8 mg, 0.225 mmol, 4.0 eq.), pivalic acid (5.7 mg, 0.056 mmol, 1.0 eq.) and Pd(OAc)$_2$ (1.4 mg, 0.077 mmol, 0.1 eq.) were placed in a MW reactor vessel in 1 ml of PBS:DMF (1:1). The mixture was heated under MW irradiation (250 W) at 90 °C for 20 min. The irradiation cycle was repeated after adding a new portion of Pd(OAc)$_2$ and AgBF$_4$. The residue was filtered and partially purified in a PoraPak Rxn reverse phase column (1.63 mg, 2% estimated using HPLC-MS). A pure fraction was obtained using analytic RP-HPLC to yield pure conjugate **5**.

Procedure for the double macrocycle conjugation. 1,4-diiodobenzene (35 mg, 0.106 mmol), macrocycle **3** (209 mg, 0.318 mmol, 3.0 eq.), AgBF$_4$ (124 mg, 0.637 mmol, 6.0 eq.), pivalic acid (16.3 mg, 0.159 mmol, 1.5 eq.) and Pd(OAc)$_2$ (9.5 mg, 0.042 mmol, 0.4 eq.) were placed in a MW reactor vessel in 2 ml of PBS:DMF (1:1). The mixture was heated under MW irradiation (250 W) at 90 °C for 20 min. The crude product was filtered, and the workup was carried out by washing with AcOEt and then precipitating by adding ACN to the aqueous phase. The resulting precipitate was washed with ACN, decanted and dried, obtaining 159 mg of crude product (pale solid, 42% estimated using HPLC-MS). A pure fraction was obtained with semipreparative RP-HPLC to yield pure conjugate **6**.

Typical procedure for the stapled cyclopeptide formation on the solid phase. Once sequence **7** was synthesized on a TentaGel S NH$_2$ resin via an AB linker, the peptide anchored to the resin (139 mg, 0.145 mmol), AgBF$_4$ (28 mg, 0.144 mmol, 1.0 eq.), 2-nitrobenzoic acid (36 mg, 0.215 mmol, 1.5 eq.) and Pd(OAc)$_2$ (1.6 mg, 7.1 µmol, 0.05 eq.) in DMF (2 ml) was placed in a MW reactor vessel. The mixture was heated under MW irradiation (250 W) at 90 °C for 20 min. Eight more batches were carried out following the same procedure and were then combined. The resin was treated with 1% DDC in DMF and the Fmoc group was removed. The peptide was cleaved from the resin with a 95% TFA, 2.5% TIS and 2.5% H$_2$O cocktail (1 h), yielding the stapled sequence **9** (85% purity, estimated using HPLC-MS). Finally, the stapled peptide **9** was cyclized (see above for standard cyclization procedure) and the crude product was purified using semipreparative RP-HPLC to yield bicyclopeptide **10** (pale solid, 18% unoptimized).

One-step double arylation to biaryl–biaryl stapled peptide. Linear peptide **11** (50 mg, 0.044 mmol), AgBF$_4$ (51 mg, 0.262 mmol, 6.0 eq.), pivalic acid (6.7 mg, 0.066 mmol, 1.5 eq.) and Pd(OAc)$_2$ (3.9 mg, 0.018 mmol, 0.4 eq.) were placed in a MW reactor vessel in DMF (500 µl). The mixture was heated under MW irradiation (250 W) at 90 °C for 20 min. Three more batches were carried out following the same procedure and then filtered and combined (25% conversion, estimated using HPLC-MS). A pure fraction of bicyclopeptide **12** was isolated using semipreparative RP-HPLC.

References

1. Ramakers, B. E. I., van Hest, J. C. M. & Löwik, D. W. P. M. Molecular tools for the construction of peptide-based materials. *Chem. Soc. Rev.* **43**, 2743–2756 (2014).
2. Craik, D. J., Fairlie, D. P., Liras, S. & Price, D. The future of peptide-based drugs. *Chem. Biol. Drug Des.* **81**, 136–147 (2013).
3. Albericio, F. & Kruger, H. G. Therapeutic peptides. *Future Med. Chem.* **4**, 1527–1531 (2012).
4. Lawson, K. V., Rose, T. E. & Harran, P. G. Template-constrained macrocyclic peptides prepared from native, unprotected precursors. *Proc. Natl Acad. Sci. USA* **110**, E3753–E3760 (2013).
5. Marsault, E. *et al.* Efficient parallel synthesis of macrocyclic peptidomimetics. *Bioorg. Med. Chem. Lett.* **18**, 4731–4735 (2008).
6. Royo-Gracia, S., Gaus, K. & Sewald, N. Synthesis of chemically modified bioactive peptides: recent advances, challenges and developments for medicinal chemistry. *Future Med. Chem.* **1**, 1289–1310 (2009).
7. White, C. J. & Yudin, A. K. Contemporary strategies for peptide macrocyclization. *Nat. Chem.* **3**, 509–524 (2011).
8. Heinis, C. Tools and rules for macrocycles. *Nat. Chem. Biol.* **10**, 696–698 (2014).
9. Verdine, G. L. & Hilinski, G. J. Stapled peptides for intracellular drug targets. *Methods Enzymol.* **503**, 3–33, 2012).
10. Walensky, L. D. & Bird, G. H. Hydrocarbon-stapled peptides: principles, practice, and progress. *J. Med. Chem.* **57**, 6275–6288 (2014).
11. Lau, Y. H., de Andrade, P., Wu, Y. & Spring, D. R. Peptide stapling techniques based on different macrocyclisation chemistries. *Chem. Soc. Rev.* **44**, 91–102 (2015).
12. Góngora-Benítez, M., Tulla-Puche, J. & Albericio, F. Multifaceted roles of disulfide bonds. Peptides as therapeutics. *Chem. Rev.* **114**, 901–926 (2014).
13. Jo, H. *et al.* Development of α-helical calpain probes by mimicking a natural protein-protein interaction. *J. Am. Chem. Soc.* **134**, 17704–17713 (2012).
14. Spokoyny, A. M. *et al.* A perfluoroaryl-cysteine SNAr chemistry approach to unprotected peptide stapling. *J. Am. Chem. Soc.* **135**, 5946–5949 (2013).
15. Bois-Choussy, M., Cristau, P. & Zhu, J. Total synthesis of an atropdiastereomer of RP-66453 and determination of its absolute configuration. *Angew. Chem. Int. Ed.* **42**, 4238–4241 (2003).
16. Carbonnelle, A.-C. & Zhu, J. A novel synthesis of biaryl-containing macrocycles by a domino miyaura arylboronate formation: intramolecular suzuki reaction. *Org. Lett.* **2**, 3477–3480 (2000).
17. Afonso, A., Feliu, L. & Planas, M. Solid-phase synthesis of biaryl cyclic peptides by borylation and microwave-assisted intramolecular Suzuki–Miyaura reaction. *Tetrahedron* **67**, 2238–2245 (2011).

18. Meyer, F.-M. *et al.* Biaryl-bridged macrocyclic peptides: conformational constraint via carbogenic fusion of natural amino acid side chains. *J. Org. Chem.* **77,** 3099–3114 (2012).

19. Blackwell, H. E. & Grubbs, R. H. Highly efficient synthesis of covalently cross-linked peptide helices by ring-closing metathesis. *Angew. Chem. Int. Ed.* **37,** 3281–3284 (1998).

20. Dharanipragada, R. New modalities in conformationally constrained peptides for potency, selectivity and cell permeation. *Future Med. Chem.* **5,** 831–849 (2013).

21. Wender, P. A. Toward the ideal synthesis and molecular function through synthesis-informed design. *Nat. Prod. Rep.* **31,** 433–440 (2014).

22. Sletten, E. M. & Bertozzi, C. R. Bioorthogonal chemistry: fishing for selectivity in a sea of functionality. *Angew. Chem. Int. Ed.* **48,** 6974–6998 (2009).

23. Yu, J.-Q. & Shi, Z. *Topics in Current Chemistry* 384 (Springer, 2010).

24. Seechurn, C. C. C. J., Kitching, M. O., Colacot, T. J. & Snieckus, V. Palladium-catalyzed cross-coupling: a historical contextual perspective to the 2010 Nobel Prize. *Angew. Chem. Int. Ed.* **51,** 5062–5086 (2012).

25. Ackermann, L. Carboxylate-assisted transition-metal-catalyzed C-H bond functionalizations: mechanism and scope. *Chem. Rev.* **111,** 1315–1345 (2011).

26. McMurray, L., O'Hara, F. & Gaunt, M. J. Recent developments in natural product synthesis using metal-catalysed C-H bond functionalisation. *Chem. Soc. Rev.* **40,** 1885–1898 (2011).

27. Wencel-Delord, J., Dröge, T., Liu, F. & Glorius, F. Towards mild metal-catalyzed C-H bond activation. *Chem. Soc. Rev.* **40,** 4740–4761 (2011).

28. Daugulis, O., Do, H. & Shabashov, D. Palladium- and copper-catalyzed arylation of carbon-hydrogen bonds. *Acc. Chem. Res.* **42,** 1074–1086 (2009).

29. Noisier, F. M. & Brimble, M. A. C − H functionalization in the synthesis of amino acids and peptides. *Chem. Rev.* **114,** 8775–8806 (2014).

30. Rossi, R., Bellina, F., Lessi, M. & Manzini, C. Cross-Coupling of heteroarenes by C-H functionalization: recent progress towards direct arylation and heteroarylation reactions involving heteroarenes containing one heteroatom. *Adv. Synth. Catal.* **356,** 17–117 (2014).

31. Lebrasseur, N. & Larrosa, I. Recent advances in the C2 and C3 regioselective direct arylation of indoles. *Adv. Heterocycl. Chem.* **105,** 309–351 (2012).

32. Liégault, B., Petrov, I., Gorelsky, S. I. & Fagnou, K. Modulating reactivity and diverting selectivity in palladium-catalyzed heteroaromatic direct arylation through the use of a chloride activating/blocking group. *J. Org. Chem.* **75,** 1047–1060 (2010).

33. Wang, X., Gribkov, D. V. & Sames, D. Phosphine-free palladium-catalyzed C-H bond arylation of free (N-H)-indoles and pyrroles. *J. Org. Chem.* **72,** 1476–1479 (2007).

34. Phipps, R. J., Grimster, N. P. & Gaunt, M. J. Cu(II)-catalyzed direct and site-selective arylation of indoles under mild conditions. *J. Am. Chem. Soc.* **130,** 8172–8174 (2008).

35. Islam, S. & Larrosa, I. "On water", phosphine-free palladium-catalyzed room temperature C-H arylation of indoles. *Chem. Eur. J.* **19,** 15093–15096 (2013).

36. Lebrasseur, N. & Larrosa, I. Room temperature and phosphine free palladium catalyzed direct C-2 arylation of indoles. *J. Am. Chem. Soc.* **130,** 2926–2927 (2008).

37. Ruiz-Rodríguez, J., Albericio, F. & Lavilla, R. Postsynthetic modification of peptides: chemoselective C-arylation of tryptophan residues. *Chem. Eur. J.* **16,** 1124–1127 (2010).

38. Williams, T. J., Reay, A. J., Whitwood, A. C. & Fairlamb, I. J. S. A mild and selective Pd-mediated methodology for the synthesis of highly fluorescent 2-arylated tryptophans and tryptophan-containing peptides: a catalytic role for Pd(0) nanoparticles? *Chem. Commun.* **50,** 3052–3054 (2014).

39. Dong, H., Limberakis, C., Liras, S., Price, D. & James, K. Peptidic macrocyclization via palladium-catalyzed chemoselective indole C-2 arylation. *Chem. Commun.* **48,** 11644–11646 (2012).

40. Monguchi, Y., Marumoto, T., Takamatsu, H., Sawama, Y. & Sajiki, H. Palladium on carbon-catalyzed one-pot N-arylindole synthesis: intramolecular aromatic amination, aromatization, and intermolecular aromatic amination. *Adv. Synth. Catal.* **356,** 1866–1872 (2014).

41. Preciado, S. *et al.* Synthesis and biological evaluation of a post-synthetically modified Trp-based diketopiperazine. *Med. Chem. Comm.* **4,** 1171–1174 (2013).

42. Preciado, S., Mendive-Tapia, L., Albericio, F. & Lavilla, R. Synthesis of C-2 arylated tryptophan amino acids and related compounds through palladium-catalyzed C-H activation. *J. Org. Chem.* **78,** 8129–8135 (2013).

43. Mas-moruno, C., Rechenmacher, F. & Kessler, H. Cilengitide: the first anti-angiogenic small molecule drug candidate. Design, synthesis and clinical evaluation. *Anticancer Agents Med. Chem.* **10,** 753–768 (2010).

44. Weide, T., Modlinger, A. & Kessler, H. Spatial screening for the identification of the bioactive conformation of integrin ligands. *Top. Curr. Chem.* **272,** 1–50 (2007).

45. Boger, D. L. & Myers, J. B. Design and synthesis of a conformational analogue of deoxybouvardin. *J. Org. Chem.* **56,** 5385–5390 (1991).

46. Jackson, S. *et al.* Template-constrained cyclic peptides: design of high-affinity ligands for GPIIb/IIIa. *J. Am. Chem. Soc.* **116,** 3220–3230 (1994).

47. Dyson, H. J. & Wright, P. E. Nuclear Magnetic Resonance methods for elucidation of structure and dynamics in disordered states. *Methods Enzymol.* **339,** 258–270 (2001).

48. Chiba, T. *et al.* Inhibition of recombinant dipeptidyl peptidase III by synthetic hemorphin-like peptides. *Peptides* **24,** 773–778 (2003).

49. Jung, K.-Y. *et al.* Structure - activity relationship studies of spinorphin as a potent and selective human P2X3 receptor antagonist. *J. Med. Chem.* **50,** 4543–4547 (2007).

50. Nässel, D. R., Persson, M. G. S. & Muren, J. E. Baratin, a nonamidated neurostimulating neuropeptide, isolated from cockroach brain: distribution and actions in the cockroach and locust nervous systems. *J. Comp. Neurol.* **286,** 267–286 (2000).

51. Bird, G. H. *et al.* Hydrocarbon double-stapling remedies the proteolytic instability of a lengthy peptide therapeutic. *Proc. Natl Acad. Sci. USA* **107,** 14093–14098 (2010).

52. Du, A. W. & Stenzel, M. H. Drug carriers for the delivery of therapeutic peptides. *Biomacromolecules* **15,** 1097–1114 (2014).

53. Colombo, G. *et al.* Structure-activity relationships of linear and cyclic peptides containing the NGR tumor-homing motif. *J. Biol. Chem.* **277,** 47891–47897 (2002).

54. Pan, P.-S. *et al.* A comprehensive study of Sansalvamide A derivatives: the structure-activity relationships of 78 derivatives in two pancreatic cancer cell lines. *Bioorg. Med. Chem.* **17,** 5806–5825 (2009).

55. Boger, D. L. *et al.* Total synthesis of the vancomycin aglycon. *J. Am. Chem. Soc.* **121,** 10004–10011 (1999).

56. Wang, Z., Bois-Choussy, M., Jia, Y. & Zhu, J. Total synthesis of complestatin (chloropeptin II). *Angew. Chem. Int. Ed.* **49,** 2018–2022 (2010).

57. Feliu, L. & Planas, M. Cyclic peptides containing biaryl and biaryl ether linkages. *Int. J. Pept. Res. Ther.* **11,** 53–97 (2005).

58. Arroniz, C., Denis, J. G., Ironmonger, A., Rassias, G. & Larrosa, I. An organic cation as a silver(i) analogue for the arylation of sp2 and sp3 C–H bonds with iodoarenes. *Chem. Sci.* **5,** 3509–3514 (2014).

59. Arsequell, G. *et al.* First aromatic electrophilic iodination reaction on the solid-phase: iodination of bioactive peptides. *Tetrahedron Lett.* **39,** 7393–7396 (1998).

Acknowledgements

This work was supported by DGICYT—Spain (project BQU-CTQ2012-30930), Generalitat de Cataluña (2014 SGR 137) and Institute for Research in Biomedicine Barcelona (Spain). We acknowledge an FPU fellowship for L.M.-T. from the Ministerio de Educación, Cultura y Deporte–Spain (MECD). NMR instruments were made available by the Scientific and Technological Centre of the University of Barcelona (CCiT UB). Dr M. J. Macias, Dr M. Vilaseca, Dr M. Teixidó and J. Garcia (IRB Barcelona), Dr F. Mitjans (BioLeitat), Dr M. Royo (Barcelona Science Park) and Professors R. Pérez-Tomás and V. Soto-Cerrato (U. Barcelona) are gratefully acknowledged for useful suggestions and for the biological assays.

Author contributions

L.M.-T., F.A. and R.L. wrote the manuscript. L.M.-T., S.P., N.K. and R.R. performed the experiments, compound characterization and data analysis. J.G. performed the NMR studies. R.L. and F.A. supervised the research and evaluated all the data.

Additional information

10

4'-O-substitutions determine selectivity of aminoglycoside antibiotics

Déborah Perez-Fernandez[1,*], Dmitri Shcherbakov[2,*], Tanja Matt[2], Ng Chyan Leong[3,4,*], Iwona Kudyba[1], Stefan Duscha[2], Heithem Boukari[2], Rashmi Patak[1], Srinivas Reddy Dubbaka[1], Kathrin Lang[3], Martin Meyer[2], Rashid Akbergenov[2], Pietro Freihofer[2], Swapna Vaddi[5], Pia Thommes[5], V. Ramakrishnan[3], Andrea Vasella[1] & Erik C. Böttger[2]

Clinical use of 2-deoxystreptamine aminoglycoside antibiotics, which target the bacterial ribosome, is compromised by adverse effects related to limited drug selectivity. Here we present a series of 4',6'-O-acetal and 4'-O-ether modifications on glucopyranosyl ring I of aminoglycosides. Chemical modifications were guided by measuring interactions between the compounds synthesized and ribosomes harbouring single point mutations in the drug-binding site, resulting in aminoglycosides that interact poorly with the drug-binding pocket of eukaryotic mitochondrial or cytosolic ribosomes. Yet, these compounds largely retain their inhibitory activity for bacterial ribosomes and show antibacterial activity. Our data indicate that 4'-O-substituted aminoglycosides possess increased selectivity towards bacterial ribosomes and little activity for any of the human drug-binding pockets.

[1] Laboratorium für Organische Chemie, ETH Zürich, Wolfgang-Pauli-Strasse 10, 8093 Zürich, Switzerland. [2] Institut für Medizinische Mikrobiologie, Universität Zürich, Gloriastrasse 30/32, 8006 Zürich, Switzerland. [3] MRC Laboratory of Molecular Biology, Francis Crick Avenue, Cambridge Biomedical Campus, Cambridge CB2 0QH, UK. [4] Institute of Systems Biology, Universiti Kebangsaan Malaysia, 43600, Bangi, Selangor, Malaysia. [5] Euprotec Limited, Unit 12 Williams House, Manchester Science Park, Lloyd Street North, Manchester M15 6SE, UK. * These authors contributed equally to this work. Correspondence and requests for materials should be addressed to A.V. (email: vasella@org.chem.ethz.ch) or to E.C.B. (email: boettger@imm.uzh.ch).

Selectivity is of particular concern for ribosomal antibiotics[1,2] as the ribosome is present in all three domains of life and is a relatively conserved structure. Among this class, aminoglycosides are listed by the WHO as critically important antimicrobials for human therapy[3]. Their high efficacy, broad-spectrum antibacterial potency and lack of drug-related allergy are well-known features and make aminoglycosides a common choice for the treatment of serious infections including multidrug-resistant tuberculosis[4]. A major drawback of amino-glycosides relates to their adverse effects. Aminoglycoside-induced ototoxicity, that is, the compounds' ability to cause irreversible hearing loss due to destruction of inner ear sensory hair cells[5], occurs in a sporadic, dose-dependent manner. In addition, inherited forms of hypersensitivity to aminoglycoside ototoxicity exist, which are linked to point mutations in mitochondrial rRNA, such as A1555G and C1494U[6,7]. Recent evidence converges on mitochondrial function as a key element in aminoglycoside-induced ototoxicity, as experimental evidence was provided for both aminoglycoside-induced dysfunction of the mitochondrial ribosome and A1555G/C1494U-linked mito-chondrial hypersusceptibility to aminoglycoside antibiotics[8,9]. These findings suggest that aminoglycoside ototoxicity is directly related to the drugs' mechanism of action on the eukaryotic ribosome.

The 2-deoxystreptamine aminoglycoside antibiotics bind to helix 44 (h44) of 16S rRNA, which is part of the decoding site of the bacterial 30S ribosomal subunit[10,11], thereby decreasing translational fidelity and inhibiting translocation[12-15]. The interaction core formed by rings I and II is mainly responsible for drug binding. Ring I intercalates into the internal loop formed by A1408, A1492, A1493 and the base pair C1409–G1491. Here ring I becomes properly positioned by stacking interaction with G1491 and the formation of hydrogen bonds with A1408 (Fig. 1). Despite variations in chemical composition, ring I always binds in the same orientation and forms a pseudo base-pair interaction with the Watson–Crick edge of adenine 1408. The ring oxygen of ring I accepts a hydrogen bond from the N6 of adenine, and the amino- or hydroxyl-group at position 6′ donates a hydrogen bond to the N1 of adenine[10,11]. Additional hydrogen bonds link the hydroxyl groups at positions 3′ and 4′ of ring I to the phosphate groups of the two bulged adenine bases 1492 and 1493, further stabilizing the position of ring I.

The use of 2-deoxystreptamine aminoglycosides as antimicrobial agents builds upon the compounds' preferential activity for the prokaryotic versus the eukaryotic ribosome[1,2]. At the structural level, the selectivity of these compounds rests upon two residues in the drug-binding pocket—residues 1408 and 1491 (refs 16-19). Residue 1408 is an adenine in bacterial and mitochondrial ribosomes as compared with a guanine in cytosolic ribosomes. Residue 1491 is a guanine in bacterial ribosomes, but a cytosine in mitochondrial and an adenine in cytosolic ribosomes. Both these changes disrupt the bacterial C1409–G1491 base-pair interaction (see Supplementary Fig. 1 for a comparison of bacterial and eukaryotic drug-binding pockets). A guanine at residue 1408 mainly affects 2-deoxystreptamines with a 6′NH$_2$ as it would preclude the proper insertion of a corresponding ring I into the binding pocket, that is, the 6′ ammonium group cannot accept hydrogen bonds from the Watson–Crick sites of the guanine residue, and additionally its positive charge would create repulsion against the N1 and N2 amino groups[20]. In contrast, 2-deoxystreptamines with a 6′OH group are less affected by a 1408G as the 6′ hydroxyl group could still become an acceptor of a hydrogen bond from N1 or N2 (ref. 20; Fig. 1). A C1409–C1491 opposition mainly affects 2-deoxystreptamines with a 6′OH but much less so compounds with a 6′NH$_2$. Possibly, the 6′OH–N1 A1408 interaction is less stable as compared with the 6′NH$_2$–N1

A1408 interaction, making 6′OH 2-deoxystreptamines highly dependent on proper stacking interaction with residue 1491 (refs 21,22).

Here we address the question of whether the specificity of the 2-deoxystreptamine aminoglycosides can be modified to increase selectivity at the drug-target level in spite of the constraints imposed by the high conservation of the drug-binding pocket. We focus on ring I, as it interacts with phylogenetically variable 16S rRNA residues 1408 and 1491. As we expected, structural modifications on ring I affect drug selectivity. In addition, our results reveal the unanticipated finding that well-known synthetic intermediates can show promising biological properties.

Results

Synthesis of compounds and assessment of specificity. Paromomycin and neomycin are closely related 4,5-disubstituted aminoglycosides, their structure differing by the ring I 6′ sub-stituent (6′OH versus 6′NH$_2$, see Fig. 1c,d). Ring I of paromomycin was modified by substitutions of the 4′ hydroxyl position. We first synthesized 4′,6-O-acetals, starting with ben-zylidene derivatives (Fig. 1e). The 4′,6′-O-benzylidene acetal 1 was synthesized and tested for growth inhibition activity (mini-mal inhibitory concentration, MIC) of bacterial cells using wild type and recombinant strains of *Mycobacterium smegmatis* with single point mutations in the drug-binding pocket. The point mutations were chosen to reflect the phylogenetically variable 16S rRNA residues, namely positions 1408 (A bacterial/mitochon-drial, G cytosolic) and 1491 (G bacterial, A cytosolic, C mito-chondrial). We subsequently synthesized acetals 2–36 (for a complete list of chemical structures synthesized see Supplementary Fig. 2) to investigate structure–activity relations (SAR) and compared their growth inhibition activity with those of neomycin and paromomycin. As previously noted[21], the interaction of neomycin and paromomycin with the A site shows varying degrees of specificity for A1408 and G1491. Thus, the MIC activities (Table 1) demonstrate that interaction of the 6′ amino neomycin is dependent on an adenine at residue 1408 (MIC for A1408 is 0.8 µM, MIC for G1408 is >720 µM), while mutational alterations of G1491 have less of an effect (MIC G1491 0.8 µM versus MIC C1491 27 µM). In comparison, interaction of the 6′ hydroxyl paromomycin with the ribosome is less affected by a G1408 alteration (MIC A1408 1.6 µM versus MIC G1408 102 µM) as compared with mutational alteration of residue G1491 (MIC G1491 1.6 µM versus MIC C1491 >720 µM). Surprisingly, the interaction of the 4′,6′-O-acetals with the A site was observed to be largely dependent on both rRNA residues 1408 and 1491. Thus, high MIC values are associated with each single nucleotide alteration affecting rRNA residue A1408 or G1491 (MIC G1408 ≥720 µM, MIC C/A1491 ≥720 µM). MIC activities for selected acetals 1–3, 9 and 30 are summarized in Table 1.

SAR studies based on >30 acetals (see Supplementary Table 1 for a summary of MIC activities) revealed that the nature, position and number of substituents at the equatorial hydro-phobic residue at C(2) of the acetal 1,3-dioxane ring have a modest effect on compound activity in general, for example, replacement of the phenyl group in 1 by a 3- or 4-chlorophenyl substituent (10, 2), a 4-fluorophenyl substituent (6), a 3,5-dichlorophenyl analogue (16), a 3- or 4-methoxyphenyl analogue (11, 3), a 2,5-dimethoxyphenyl analogue (18), a 4-dimethylami-nophenyl (4), a 3- or 4-hydroxyphenyl (12, 5), a 4-trifluor-omethylphenyl (9), a 2-, 3- or 4-nitrophenyl analogue (15, 13, and 7) all have relatively little effect. Together with the lower activity of the cyclohexyl analogue 25 of 1 this suggests that both hydrophobic and stacking interactions are relevant to the

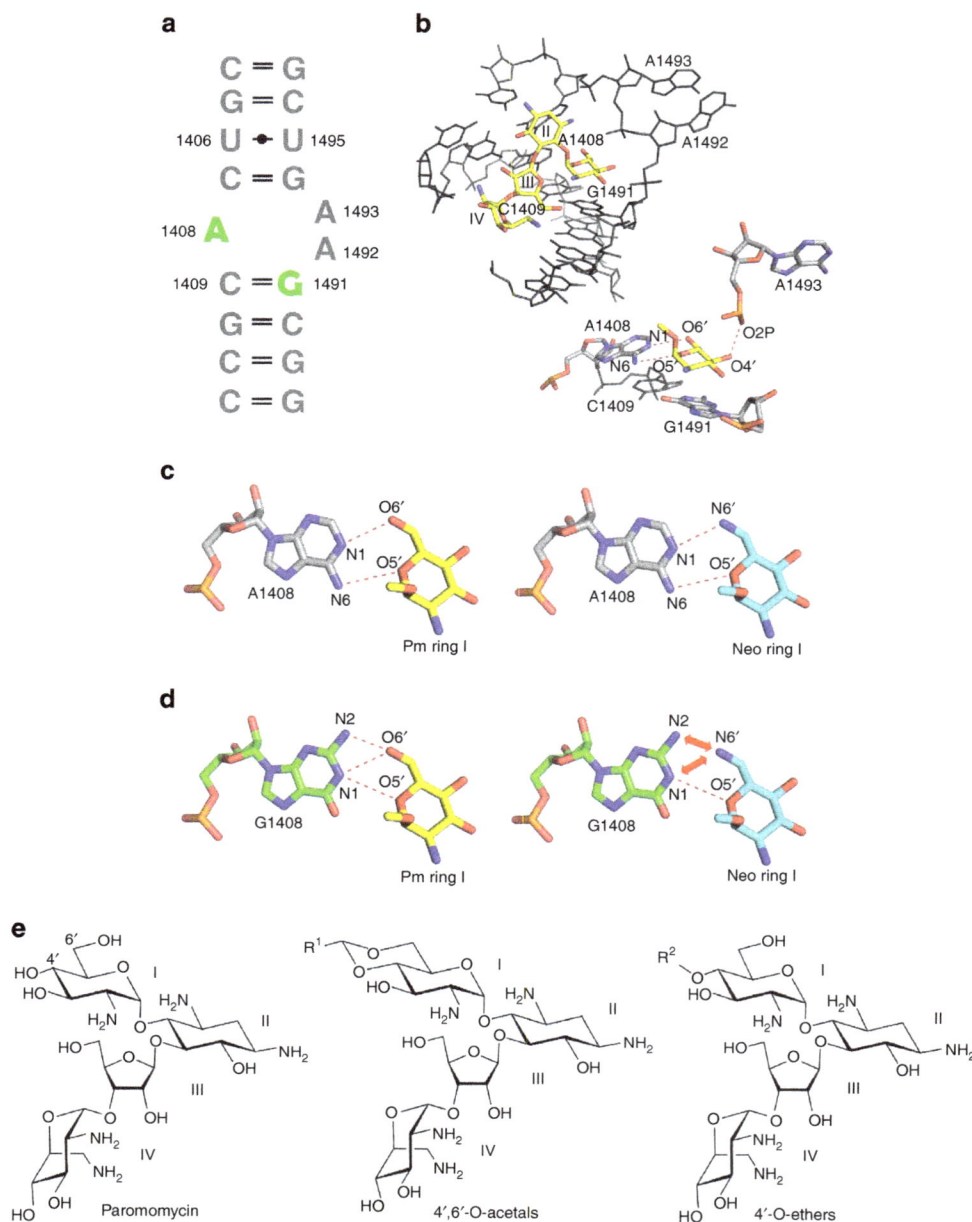

Figure 1 | Interaction of ring I with residues in the A site loop of 16S rRNA. (a) Secondary structure of the aminoglycoside-binding pocket in helix 44 of 16S rRNA. Key polymorphic residues determining the selectivity of aminoglycosides are residues 1408 and 1491, highlighted in bold green. **(b)** Overview of paromomycin bound to the bacterial A site. Detailed view of the 6'OH paromomycin ring-I stacking interaction with G1491 and hydrogen bonding with A1408 and A1493 (ref. 10). Hydrogen bonds between aminoglycoside ring I and A1408 are shown as red dotted lines, as is hydrogen bonding between 4'OH and O2P of A1493. **(c)** Ring I interaction with A1408. Left paromomycin (Pm), right neomycin (Neo). Hydrogen bond interaction between the 6'-substituent (6'OH, 6'NH$_2$) and the N1 of A1408 is indicated by a red dotted line, as is hydrogen bond interaction between O5' and N6 of A1408. **(d)** Ring I interaction with G1408 (model)[20]. Left paromomycin, right neomycin. Possible hydrogen bond interactions are indicated by red dotted lines. The positive charge of neomycin's 6'-ammonium group would create repulsion against the N1 and N2 amino groups of G1408, indicated by red arrows. **(e)** General chemical structure of 4',6'-O-acetals and 4'-O-ethers in comparison to paromomycin, the 6' and 4' positions that were target for substitution are indicated.

drug–ribosome interaction. This interpretation is in agreement with the activities of **23** and **24**, where the phenyl substituent has been replaced by an electron-rich 2-furyl or 2-thiophenyl ring, and with the activities of **26** and **27**, possessing larger aromatic moieties. Introducing a linker between the phenyl ring and C(2) of the 1,3-dioxane ring had a marked effect on the properties of the acetals: a two-carbon chain between the aromatic moiety and C(2) of the 1,3-dioxane ring being optimal (**1, 29–34**). Disruption of ring I of the benzylidene acetals abolishes activity (**35** and **36** versus **1**).

We next synthesized the C(4')O-substituted ethers **37** and **39–42**, the linear acetal **43** and the C(6')O-substituted ether **38**. The MIC data (Table 2) demonstrate a similar selectivity profile for the C(4')O-substituted ethers **37** and **39–42** as for the corresponding 4',6'-O-acetal analogues **1–3, 9** and **30**, respectively. The acetal **1** and the C(4')-O-benzyl ether **37** show significantly higher antibacterial activity than the corresponding C(6')-O-benzyl ether **38**, and the linear acetal **43** is noticeably less active than the corresponding cyclic acetal **30** (see summarized MIC data in Supplementary Table 1). Altogether, this indicates

Table 1 | Minimal inhibitory concentrations (MIC, μM) of 4',6'-O-benzylidene acetals.

Bacterial A site	Neomycin Ring I	Paromomycin Ring I	1	2	3	9	30
WT	0.8	1.6	5.6	5.6	5.6	2.8–5.6	2.8
1491C	27	>720	>720	>720	>720	720	≥720
1491A	3.2	51-102	720	>720	>720	720	≥720
1408G	>720	51-102	720	>720	>720	>720	720

Table 2 | Minimal inhibitory concentrations (MIC, μM) of C(4')-O-ethers.

Bacterial A site	37	39	40	41	42
WT	5.6	2.8	11	11	5.6
1491C	>720	≥720	>720	≥720	≥720
1491A	≥720	≥720	>720	>720	≥720
1408G	>720	≥720	>720	>680	≥720

Table 3 | Compound interaction with polymorphic residues in the drug-binding pocket (IC$_{50}$, μM).

Bacterial A site	Paromomycin	Neomycin	37 4'-O-ether	1 4',6'-O-acetal	39 4'-O-ether	2 4',6'-O-acetal	42 4'-O-ether	30 4',6'-O-acetal
Wild type	0.03	0.03	0.14	0.28	0.14	0.14	0.28	0.14
G1491C	19.2	1.1	122.0	131.0	83.3	80.4	255.5	163.5
G1491A	1.1	0.08	38.4	79.3	29.0	43.0	87.4	66.4
A1408G	0.5	31.4	17.5	19.0	5.9	10.5	16.1	9.5

that proper orientation and location of the aromatic residue rather than just hydrophobic effects are relevant for selectivity.

Drug–target interaction in cell-free translation assays. To study drug–target interaction and the contribution of the polymorphic residues 1408 and 1491 to drug binding more directly, we assessed compound activity in cell-free ribosomal translation assays for selected pairs of 4',6'-O-acetals and corresponding 4'-O-ethers, that is, compounds 1, 2, 30, 37, 39 and 42. Compound activity in the *in vitro* translation assay is defined as the drug concentration that inhibits the *in vitro* translation reaction by 50% (inhibitory concentration, IC$_{50}$). Corroborating the MIC data, the ribosomal activity of the 4',6'-O-acetals and 4'-O-ethers was found to be highly dependent on both specific nucleobases present at 16S rRNA positions 1408 and 1491, with little difference between corresponding acetals and ethers (Table 3). To address the question of how these compounds affect the eukaryotic A site we assessed drug susceptibility of recombinant

bacterial hybrid ribosomes. The hybrid ribosomes were engineered to carry the cytoplasmic A site, the mitochondrial wild-type A site or the mitochondrial mutant deafness A (A1555G, C1494U)[8,9,18]. Neomycin and paromomycin each showed a characteristic pattern of interaction with the eukaryotic drug-binding pockets. In addition, both aminoglycosides interact preferentially with the mitochondrial deafness A1555G, C1494U mutant A site (Table 4). In contrast, the series of 4',6'-O-acetals and 4'-O-ethers did not show a preferential activity for any of the eukaryotic drug-binding pockets—these compounds are poor inhibitors of mitochondrial, mitochondrial mutant deafness and cytosolic hybrid ribosomes.

We compared the target specificity and drug–target interaction of the present series of compounds with that of paromomycin, neomycin, gentamicin, tobramycin, amikacin and kanamycin. Aminoglycoside activity against 1491C and 1491A mutant bacterial ribosomes correlates well ($R^2 = 0.97$), yet no such correlation exists between the activity against 1491C and 1408G mutant ribosomes (Supplementary Fig. 3). Compared with

Table 4 | Compound interaction with hybrid ribosomes—selectivity profile (IC$_{50}$, µM).

Eukaryotic A site	Paromomycin	Neomycin	37 4'-O-ether	1 4',6'-O-acetal	39 4'-O-ether	2 4',6'-O-acetal	42 4'-O-ether	30 4',6'-O-acetal
Mitochondrial wild type	81.5	2.9	93.7	127.5	120.7	115.1	85.0	259.7
Mitochondrial mutant A1555G	6.7	0.3	67.9	61.3	71.5	65.8	118.6	161.8
Mitochondrial mutant C1494U	5.1	0.3	69.3	53.3	53.3	51.1	121.2	168.7
Cytosolic wild type	14.4	29.4	87.8	66.8	94.1	93.7	225.1	203.7

available 4,5 and 4,6 2-deoxystreptamines and as per interaction with the eukaryotic ribosome the present series of compounds have retained aminoglycoside selectivity for the cytosolic ribosome, but show decreased interaction with mitochondrial wild type and, in particular, mitochondrial mutant deafness hybrid ribosomes (Fig. 2).

Aminoglycoside-mediated dysfunction of the eukaryotic ribosome has been connected to drug cytotoxicity in mammalian cells[9,18,23,24]. To assess the potential cytotoxicity of the 4',6'-O-acetals and the 4'-O-ethers we determined cell toxicity of compounds 1, 30, 37 and 39 in HEK293 cells. Cytotoxicity of the compounds was significantly lower than that of geneticin, an aminoglycoside known to be cytotoxic to mammalian cells (see Supplementary Fig. 4).

Determination of antibacterial activity. To assess antimicrobial activity, we determined the MIC values of compounds 1, 2, 30, 37, 39 and 42 against clinical isolates of *Escherichia coli* and *Staphylococcus aureus* in comparison to those of paromomycin and aminoglycosides used in the clinic for the treatment of infectious diseases, that is, gentamicin, tobramycin, kanamycin and amikacin (Table 5). The acetals and ethers—in particular the arylalkyl ethers 39 and 42—showed antimicrobial activity that was comparable to that of the parental paromomycin.

To investigate whether the *in vitro* activity of our compounds translates to activity *in vivo*, we determined the antibacterial *in vivo* activity in neutropenic murine models of septicaemia[25,26]. Efficacy of compounds 30, 37 and 39 was compared with amikacin and the parental paromomycin. In animals infected with methicillin-resistant *S. aureus*, treatment with 30, 37 and 39 reduced the bacterial burden both in blood and in kidney and was as effective as the comparator amikacin and the parental paromomycin. Compared with the vehicle-treated mice, drug treatment reduced bacterial burden in the kidney between 3 to 6 log$_{10}$ and in blood between 2 to 3 log$_{10}$ in a dose-dependent manner. Among all drugs studied, the greatest efficacy in reducing *S. aureus* burden in the blood was following treatment with 30 and 37, which both reduced the bacterial burden below detectable limits (Fig. 3).

Crystal structure analysis. The distinct ribosomal activity profile of the acetal and ether derivatives differentiates them from available 4,5- and 4,6-disubstituted aminoglycosides. To study the structural basis of drug-target interaction we determined the three-dimensional (3D) structure of a number of the acetals and ethers in complex with the small ribosomal subunit of *Thermus thermophilus*. Two acetals, the parental phenyl derivative 1 and the most active phenethyl analogue 30, and two ethers, the 4'-O-benzyl ether 37 and the closely related 4-(chlorophenyl) methyl ether 39 were chosen for analysis.

The overall structures of the 30S subunit in complex with all four compounds were globally similar to previous 30S ribosomal subunit structures (with RNA phosphate root mean-squared

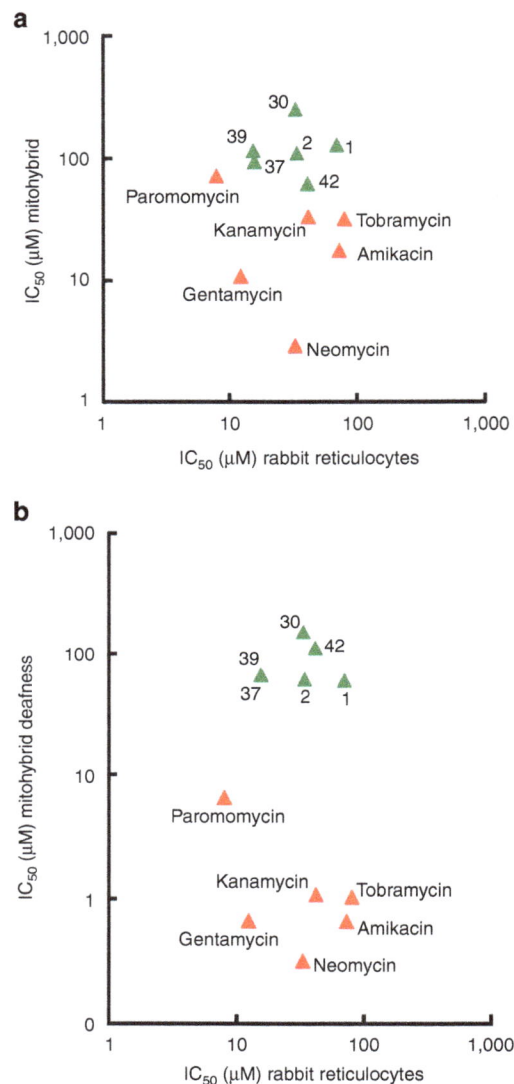

Figure 2 | Drug-induced inhibition of protein synthesis in ribosomes. Inhibition of protein synthesis depicted as IC$_{50}$ (µM); IC$_{50}$ values represent the drug concentrations required to inhibit *in vitro* synthesis of firefly luciferase to 50%. (**a**) y axis: IC$_{50}$ mitohybrid ribosomes, x axis: IC$_{50}$ rabbit reticulocyte ribosomes; (**b**) y axis: IC$_{50}$ mitohybrid deafness ribosomes, x axis: IC$_{50}$ rabbit reticulocyte ribosomes.

deviation of ~0.6 Å). Both acetals (1, 30) and ethers (37, 39) were found inserted in the major groove of helix 44 of 16S rRNA in a manner that resembles the structures of 30S–apramycin[27] and 30S–paromomycin[10] complexes (Fig. 4 and Supplementary Figs 5 and 6). Similar to paromomycin, rings II, III and IV of all four derivatives maintained their interactions with residues in helix 44, showing that neither the acetal nor the ether

Table 5 | Minimal inhibitory concentrations (MIC, μM) of clinical isolates.

	Gentamicin	Tobramycin	Kanamycin	Amikacin	Paromomycin	37 4′-O-ether	1 4′,6′-O-acetal	39 4′-O-ether	2 4′,6′-O-acetal	42 4′-O-ether	30 4′,6′-O-acetal
Staphylococcus aureus (MRSA)											
AG 042	70–140	≥538	538	27	>415	22	22	5.6–11	5.6–11	5.6	5.6–11
AG 043	70–140	67	269–538	14–27	6.5–13	11–22	11–22	5.6	11	5.6–11	5.6
AG 044	35	17	134	6.8	6.5–13	22	22–45	11–22	22	11	22
AG 045	35	17	134	6.8	6.5	22	22–45	11	11–22	5.6–11	22
AG 053	70–140	34–67	538	14	6.5	11	22	5.6	11	5.6–11	5.6–11
Escherichia coli											
AG 001	8.8–18	8.4–17	34	n.d.	26–52	45–90	45–90	11–22	22–45	22	45–90
AG 002	4.4	4.2	8.4–17	n.d.	13–26	45–90	45–90	22	22–45	22	45–90
AG 003	560–1120	67	34–67	n.d.	13–26	45–90	45	11–22	22–45	11–22	45
AG 004	1120	134	67–134	n.d.	52	45–90	90	11–22	22–45	22	22–45

modifications alter the fundamental binding mode to the ribosome. However, the orientations of A1492 and A1493 that are extruded from helix 44 were tilted relative to the paromomycin structure (Fig. 4c,d). The synthetically added substituents of compounds 1 and 30, which result in a ring system mimicking apramycin's bicyclic moiety, stacked perfectly with the nucleobase of G1491. Unlike all other aminoglycosides that form a pseudo basepair interaction between ring I and A1408 consisting of two hydrogen bonds, no pseudobase interaction was observed for the acetal series as a consequence of the absence of hydrogen bonding with N1 of A1408. The loss of this interaction constitutes the main structural difference between the benzylidene and benzyl compounds examined (37, 39). For both the benzyl and benzylidene compounds (1, 30, 37 and 39), the 4′-O-substituent prevents hydrogen bonding with O2P of A1493 (Fig. 4e). The aromatic substituent is positioned in the minor groove of the 1409–1491 basepair in proximity to the backbone and ribose of A1492. It mainly points out into the solvent and does not show stacking interaction to ribosomal moieties.

The 3D structure of the drug–ribosome interaction and the benzylidene acetal's chemical structure resemble that of apramycin, while the IC_{50} values for mutant ribosomes indicate important differences. Compared with the 4′,6′-O-acetals and their susceptibility to mutational alteration of residue 1491, the antiribosomal activity (IC_{50}) of apramycin is strongly affected by the A1408G alteration (see Supplementary Table 2 and compare to Table 3). To challenge these disparate findings we synthesized 44 by removing rings 3 and 4 from the 4′,6′-O-benzylidene acetal 1 (for a comparison of the structure of 44 and apramycin both isolated and in complex with the ribosome, see Supplementary Fig. 7). In contrast to apramycin, compound 44 had virtually no activity on any of the bacterial ribosomes tested (Supplementary Table 2). Further evidence for a distinct mode of interaction of the 4′,6′-O-benzylidene acetals with the ribosome as compared with apramycin was found in their ability to induce misreading. The effects were studied on bacterial ribosomes and on eukaryotic cytosolic ribosomes, using acetal 1 as representative in comparison to apramycin and paromomycin. Acetal 1 induced pronounced misreading on bacterial ribosomes but little if any misreading on eukaryotic ribosomes (Fig. 5). This unique pattern of misreading induction differentiates acetal 1 from both the parental paromomycin (misreading on both bacterial and eukaryotic ribosomes) and the comparator apramycin (no misreading on bacterial or eukaryotic ribosomes).

Discussion

Here we addressed the question of whether it is possible to modify 4,5-disubstituted 2-deoxystreptamine aminoglycosides

that show a preference for either the cytoplasmic ribosome (paromomycin) or the mitochondrial ribosome (neomycin), but which have comparable activities for the bacterial ribosome. With a view to develop aminoglycoside derivatives that are more selective at the ribosomal target level, chemical synthesis was guided by a collection of mutant bacterial ribosomes with single point mutations in h44. Previous work has established the important role of this mutant model system in understanding the SAR of aminoglycosides and mechanisms of antibiotic action[20,21]. A selective response of aminoglycosides to alterations of rRNA residues 1408 or 1491 (*E. coli* numbering) can potentially overcome drug ototoxicity[8,9,17,27].

We succeeded in the synthesis of a series of compounds that exploit the polymorphic residues present in the drug-binding pocket. Phylogenetic selectivity in aminoglycoside binding involves rRNA residue 1491C for mitoribosomes and rRNA residues 1491A and 1408G for cytoribosomes[9,17,18]. Compared with the parental scaffolds paromomycin and neomycin the 4′,6′-O-acetals and 4′-O-ethers are highly susceptible to any alteration of residues 1408 or 1491 (Table 3). Hybrid ribosomes carrying the cytoplasmic A site, the mitochondrial wild-type A site or the mitochondrial deafness A site (A1555G, C1494U) were used to study compound interaction with the eukaryotic drug-binding pockets. These bacterial hybrid ribosomes have been shown to faithfully reflect drug susceptibility of eukaryotic ribosomes[8,9,18,27]. In contrast to paromomycin or neomycin, the series of 4′,6′-O-acetals and 4′-O-ethers have lost most, if not all of the preferential activity for any of the eukaryotic drug-binding pockets—these compounds bind poorly to mitochondrial wild-type and cytosolic hybrid ribosomes (Table 4) and have also lost the aminoglycosides' characteristic activity for the mitochondrial mutant deafness A site[9]. However, these compounds retain to a large extent their activity for bacterial ribosomes and show good antibacterial activity *in vitro* and *in vivo* (Table 5, Fig. 3). These results identify C(4′) and its substituents as promising sites through which the drug–target interaction can be manipulated for increased selectivity.

By crystal structure analysis an additional aminoglycoside-binding site at helix 69 of the 23S rRNA has been postulated in bacterial ribosomes[28,29]. Although single-molecule measurements point to an involvement of H69 in aminoglycoside-mediated inhibition of translocation and ribosome recycling[30], the implications of this suggested additional binding site for aminoglycoside action are as yet unclear, as mutations in H69 reportedly have not been associated with aminoglycoside resistance. In contrast, single point mutations in the A site at 16S rRNA positions 1408 and 1491 are both necessary and sufficient to confer non-responsiveness to aminoglycoside action in bacteria[16,20,21].

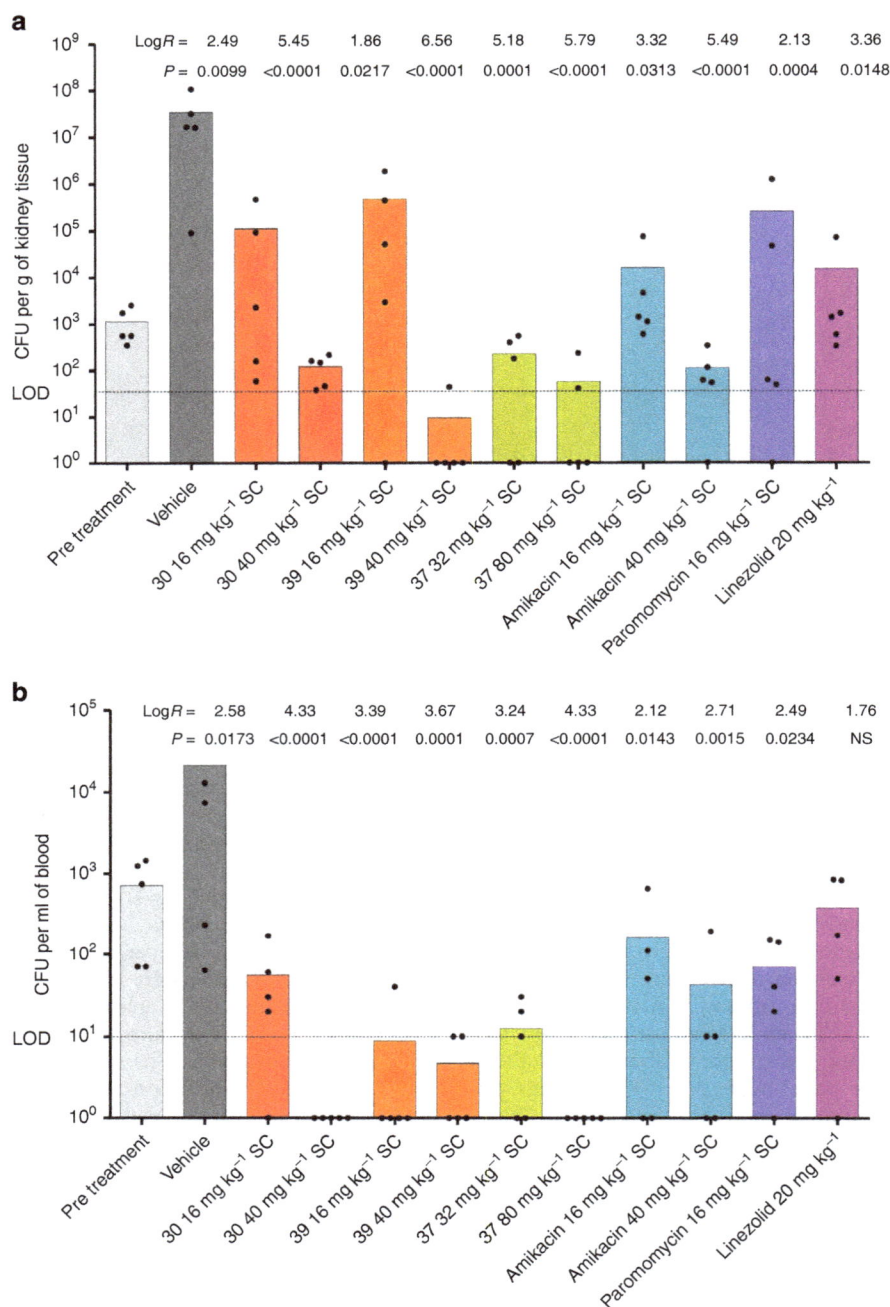

Figure 3 | *In vivo* activity of aminoglycoside compounds and comparators in a murine septicaemia model. (a) Bacterial burden in kidney, CFU per g tissue. **(b)** Bacterial burden in blood, CFU ml^{-1}. The CFU values for the individual animals are indicated by dots, the mean of the group (five mice per treatment group) by the bar. The log reduction compared with the vehicle control as well as the *P*-values (non-parametric Kruskal–Wallis using pairwise comparisons) are indicated as numbers above each group. Colour coding—pre-treatment: light grey; vehicle control: dark grey; **30**: red; **39**: orange; **37**: green; amikacin: light blue; paromomycin: dark blue; linezolid: violet. LOD, limit of detection.

The molecular basis for the compounds' increased selectivity was revealed by the observation that it is possible to separate compound interaction with residue 1408 (main denominator of cytosolic selectivity) from compound interaction with residue 1491 (main denominator of mitochondrial selectivity), that is, aminoglycoside activity for A1408G mutant ribosomes does not go hand-in-hand with activity for G1491C mutant ribosomes. This separation of ribosomal activities has provided the basis for the synthesis of more selective aminoglycosides, that is,

compounds with a selective decrease in activity for mito-ribosomes (mitochondrial wild type, mitochondrial mutant deafness) but not at the expense of increased activity for the cytoribosome (Fig. 2).

The structural basis for the altered specificity of the series of modified aminoglycosides is unclear. Globally, the crystal structures of the bacterial 30S subunit in complex with compounds **1**, **30**, **37** and **39** resemble the structures of available 30S–aminoglycoside complexes[10,11], in particular the

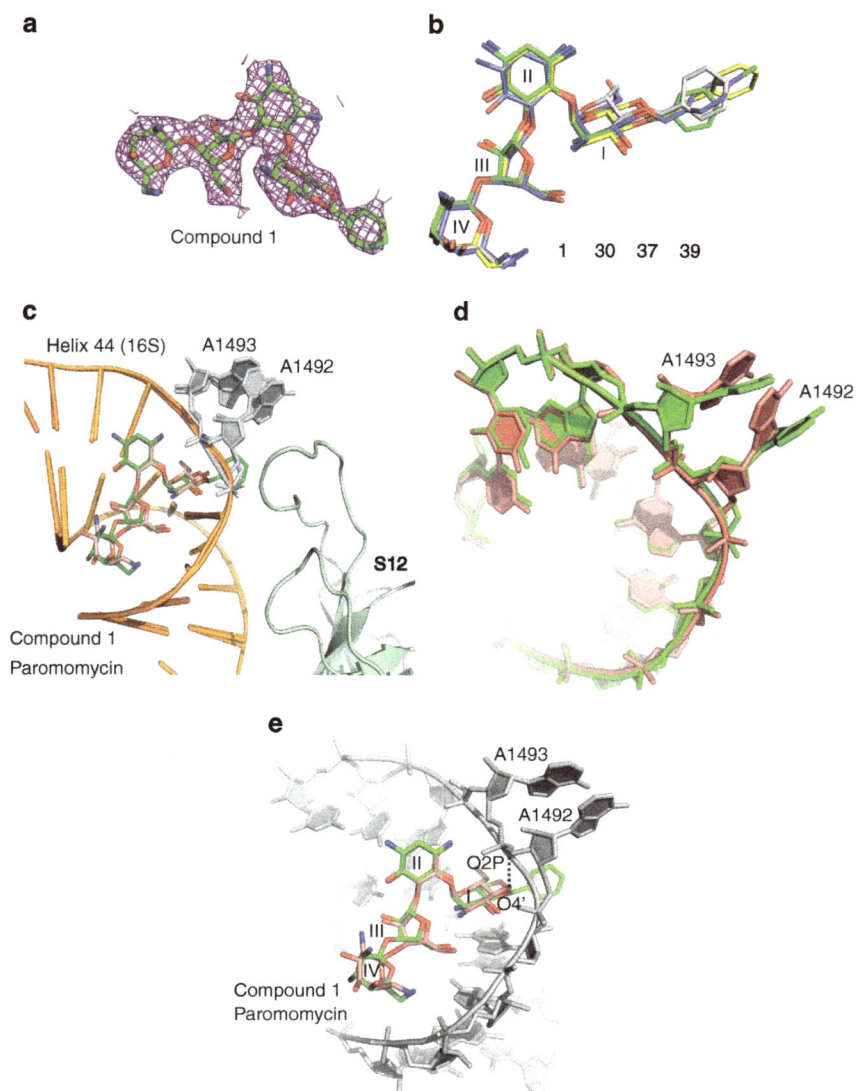

Figure 4 | Structures of antibiotics bound to the decoding center of the 30S ribosomal subunit. (**a**) $3F_o-2F_c$ difference Fourier density around compound **1** (green) contoured at 1.0σ. (**b**) Superposition of antibiotics in the decoding center, colour coding as indicated by the numbering. (**c**) Decoding center of the 30S subunit (helix 44 of 16S RNA, orange; protein S12, light green), showing compound **1** in green. The conformation of A1492 and A1493 (grey) is shown. The benzyl ring is in proximity to the nucleobase of the flipped-out A1492. Also shown is a superposition with paromomycin (Par, salmon). (**d**) Superposition of helix 44 of 16S RNA for structures of 30S-compound **1** (green) and 30S-paromomycin (salmon, Protein Data Bank ID code 1FJG); the orientations of A1492 and A1493 that are flipped-out from helix 44 are tilted relative to the paromomycin structure. (**e**) View of compound **1** and loss of a hydrogen bond with O2P of A1493 compared with paromomycin. The benzyl ring is in proximity to the nucleobase of the flipped-out A1492.

30S–apramycin complex[27], even if subtle differences are present (see Results and Fig. 4). This work exemplifies the difficulty of predicting specificity at the typical resolutions of $\sim 3\,\text{Å}$ as for current ribosomal crystal structures. Such specificity may arise as the result of subtle energetics that cannot easily be deduced from the structures. A more thorough understanding of the structural basis for the compounds' selectivity will require a careful comparison with structures of both higher eukaryotic cytosolic and mitochondrial ribosomes in complex with 2-deoxystreptamine aminoglycosides, preferably at higher resolutions than possible to date. Such structures are currently not feasible because the appropriate experimental conditions have not been established. At the functional level, misreading-inducing activity on bacterial ribosomes but not on eukaryotic ribosomes (Fig. 5) and the compounds' unique structure–activity profiles of drug–mutant ribosome interaction (Table 3) differentiates them from available aminoglycosides, and establishes the series of 4′

modifications as a novel chemotype with a unique mode of interaction with h44.

Interest in aminoglycosides has recently seen a revival not least because structural details of drug–target interactions and aminoglycoside-modifying enzymes have provided a wealth of knowledge[31–33], facilitating hypothesis-driven approaches to developing aminoglycosides recalcitrant to resistance determinants[34–36]. The description of aminoglycoside–ribosome complexes at atomic resolution[10,11] has greatly stimulated efforts at structure-based design of new bioactive derivatives[37–42]. However, rational design of specificity using these structures is limited by the current resolution of crystallographic analysis and an incomplete understanding of the thermodynamic and kinetic factors involved in antibiotic binding[43,44]. These limitations in understanding small molecule–RNA interactions and the constraints imposed by the limited sequence polymorphism in the drug-binding pocket make it a formidable challenge to

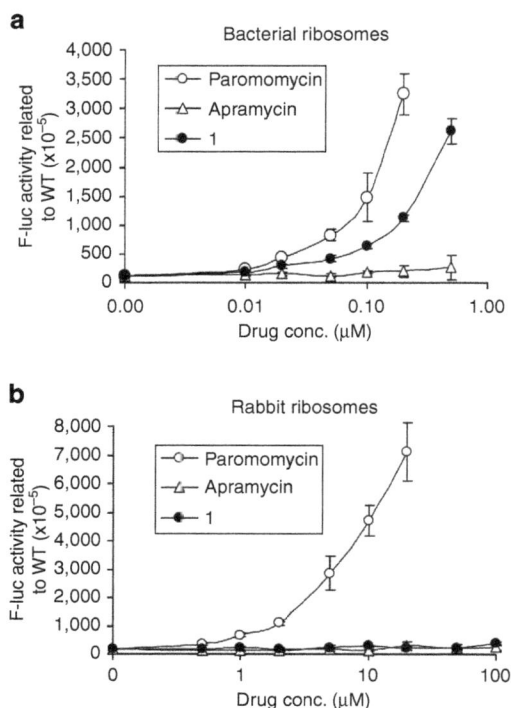

Figure 5 | Aminoglycoside-induced misreading. Dose–response curves of aminoglycoside-induced misincorporation of amino acids using the H245R near-cognate mutant F-luc mRNA as template. Shown is luciferase activity upon translation of mutant template relative to wild-type F-luc mRNA (mean ± s.d.; n = 3). (**a**) Bacterial ribosomes; (**b**) rabbit reticulocyte ribosomes. **1** (filled circles), paromomycin (open circles) and apramycin (open triangles).

synthesize aminoglycosides that are more selective at the drug-target level. The combined chemical synthesis, structural analysis, genetics and functional studies employed here have enabled us to manipulate a complex biological system of drug–target interaction. By introducing defined substitutions we have identified a new chemotype of aminoglycosides with increased selectivity and little activity for any of the human drug-binding pockets, an important step towards the development of less toxic aminoglycosides.

Methods

Antibiotics. Paromomycin, neomycin, gentamicin, tobramycin, kanamycin, amikacin and apramycin were obtained from Sigma.

Compound synthesis. Chemical synthesis procedures are detailed in the Supplementary Methods.

Strains harbouring mutant ribosomes. The construction of these strains, which are derived from single rRNA allelic *M. smegmatis ΔrrnB*, has been described previously[8,18]. They consist of recombinant mutant strains with single point mutations in the small ribosomal subunit A site (16S rRNA positions 1408A→G, 1491G→A and 1491G→C) and mutant strains with hybrid ribosomes where the bacterial A site had been replaced by various eukaryotic homologues (cytoribosome, mitoribosome and deafness mitoribosome).

Bacterial strains. Clinical isolates of *E. coli* and *S. aureus* were obtained from the Diagnostic Department, Institute of Medical Microbiology, University Zurich. MIC values were determined by broth microdilution assays. Microtitre plates were incubated overnight for *E. coli* and *S. aureus*, and 72 h for *M. smegmatis*.

***In vivo* infection experiments.** All animal experiments were performed under UK Home Office Licenses with clearance by the ethical review committee at the

University of Manchester. Male mice aged 7–8 weeks were used in this study. Mice were supplied by Charles River UK and were specific pathogen-free. The strain of mouse used was Hsd:ICR (CD-1), which is a well-characterized outbred strain. Mice weights at the start of the experiment were 22–25 g. Mice were housed in sterile individual ventilated cages with free access to sterile food and water and were exposed to 12 h light/dark cycles with dawn/dusk phases. Five mice were used in each group.

Mice were rendered temporarily neutropenic by immunosuppression with cyclophosphamide at 200 mg kg^{-1} 4 days before infection and 150 mg kg^{-1} 1 day before infection by intraperitoneal injection. The immunosuppression regime leads to neutropenia starting 24 h post administration, which continues throughout the study. For *in vivo* infection a methicillin-resistant strain of *Staphylococcus aureus*, clinical isolate MRSA AG041, was used. Twenty four hours post the second round of immunosuppression mice were infected with *S. aureus* MRSA AG041 by intravenous injection into the lateral tail vein using ~1 × 10^7 CFU per mouse. This strain had the following MIC values (μM given in brackets)—amikacin 4.0 mg l^{-1} (7.0), paromomycin 4.0 mg l^{-1} (6.5), **30** 4.0 mg l^{-1} (5.6), **37** 8.0 mg l^{-1} (11.2), **39** 4.0 mg l^{-1} (5.6) and linezolid 1.0 mg l^{-1}. Compounds **30**, **37**, **39** and comparator amikacin were administered at 4 times and at 10 times the MIC value in mg kg^{-1}, the parental paromomycin at four times the MIC value in mg kg^{-1}. Linezolid (20 mg kg^{-1}) was used as positive control. Test articles and comparators were reconstituted and diluted in 0.9% saline. Dosing solutions were prepared immediately prior to administration of the first dose and stored at 4 °C between treatments. Antibacterial treatment was initiated 1 h post infection and delivered subcutaneously at 10 ml kg^{-1} (linezolid was given by intravenous bolus injection). All drugs were administered at 1, 9 and 17 h post infection.

At 1 h (pre-treatment group) or 24 h post infection blood samples were collected by cardiac puncture under isoflurane anaesthesia and mice were humanely killed using pentobarbitone overdose. Both kidneys were removed and homogenized in 2 ml ice cold sterile phosphate-buffered saline. Kidney homogenates were quantitatively cultured onto mannitol salt agar (MSA) and incubated at 37 °C for 24 h before being counted. Individual blood samples were quantitatively cultured onto cysteine lactose electrolyte-deficient (CLED) agar and incubated at 37 °C for 24 h before being counted. Data were analysed, by StatsDirect software (version 2.7.8), using the non-parametric Kruskal–Wallis test (pairwise comparisons, Conover–Inman).

Isolation and purification of ribosomes. Ribosomes were purified from bacterial cell pellets as described previously[45]. In brief, ribosome particles were isolated by successive centrifugation and fractionated by sucrose gradient (10–40%) centrifugation. The 70S ribosome-enriched fraction was pelleted, resuspended in association buffer, incubated for 30 min at 4 °C, dispensed into aliquots and stored at − 80 °C following shock freezing in liquid nitrogen. Ribosome concentrations of 70S were determined by absorption measurements on the basis of 23 pmol ribosomes per A$_{260}$ unit. Integrity of purified 70S ribosomes was determined by analytical ultracentrifugation.

Cell-free luciferase translation assays. Purified 70S hybrid ribosomes were used in translation reactions of luciferase mRNA. Luciferase mRNA was produced *in vitro* using T7 RNA polymerase (Thermo Scientific) on templates of modified plasmids pGL4.14 (firefly luciferase) and pGL4.75 (renilla luciferase, both Promega), where the mammalian promoter driving transcription of luciferases was replaced by the T7 bacteriophage promoter. A typical translation reaction with a total volume of 30 μl contained 0.25 μM 70S ribosomes, 4 μg firefly (F-luc) mRNA, 0.4 μg renilla (R-luc) mRNA, 40% (vol/vol) *M. smegmatis* S100 extract, 200 μM amino acid mixture, 24 units of RiboLock (Thermo Scientific), 0.4 mg ml^{-1} tRNAs, and energy was supplied by addition of 12 μl of commercial S30 Premix without amino acids (Promega). In addition to ribosomes, rabbit reticulocyte lysate (Promega) was used for *in vitro* translation of F-luc mRNA. A standard 30 μl reaction contained 20 μl reticulocyte lysate, 4 μg F-luc mRNA, 0.4 μg R-luc mRNA, amino-acid mixture (200 μM each) and 24 units RiboLock. Following addition of serially diluted aminoglycosides, the reaction mixture was incubated at 37 °C for 35 min and stopped on ice. Thirty microliter samples of the reaction mixture were assayed for luciferase activities using the Dual Luciferase Reporter Assay System (Promega). Luminescence was measured using a luminometer FLx800 (Bio-Tek Instruments).

Misreading was assessed in a gain-of-function assay as described previously[27]. In brief, we introduced Arg245 (CGC, near-cognate codon) into the firefly luciferase protein to replace residue His245 (CAC codon). Arg245 F-luc mRNA and wt F-luc mRNA were used in *in vitro* translation reactions; in addition, R-luc mRNA was used as internal control. We quantified misreading by calculating mutant firefly/renilla luciferase activity as compared with wild-type firefly/renilla luciferase activity.

Crystal structure analysis. Crystals obtained from purified *T. thermophilus* 30S ribosomes[46] were soaked for 4 days in cryoprotectant solution (100 mM MES-KOH (pH 6.5), 200 mM KCl, 75 mM NH$_4$Cl, 15 mM MgCl$_2$, 26% MPD and 100μM antibiotic) before being flash-frozen. Crystals were pre-screened and data sets were collected at the European Synchrotron Radiation Facility (ESRF). Data were integrated and scaled using XDS[47]. A starting model consisting of the empty 30S ribosome (without anticodon-stem loop, mRNA and ions) was used for initial refinement and phase calculation using CNS[48]. The anticodon-stem loop and mRNA were then fitted into the unbiased difference map ($mF_o–DF_c$ map) and the model was subjected to another round of refinement. Finally, ligands were placed manually into unbiased difference maps ($mF_o–DF_c$ map) using COOT[49], which were refined to resolutions between 2.9 and 3.5 Å. Data and refinement statistics are reported in Supplementary Table 3.

References

1. Poehlsgaard, J. & Douthwaite, S. The bacterial ribosome as a target for antibiotics. *Nat. Rev. Microbiol.* **3**, 870–881 (2005).
2. Wilson, D. N. The A-Z of bacterial translation inhibitors. *Crit. Rev. Biochem. Mol. Biol.* **44**, 393–433 (2009).
3. World Health Organisation, Report of the second WHO Expert Meeting, Copenhagen, Denmark (2007); Critically important antimicrobials for human health, http://www.who.int/foodborne_disease/resistance/antimicrobials_human.pdf (WHO, Geneva, Switzerland).
4. Chambers, H. F. Chemotherapy of microbial diseases. In: Goodmann & Gilman's, *The Pharmaceutical Basis of Therapeutics* 10th edn, (Eds Hardman, J. G. & Limbird, L. E.) 1103–1121 (The McGraw-Hill Companies, 1996).
5. Forge, A. & Schacht, J. Aminoglycoside antibiotics. *Audiol. Neurootol.* **5**, 3–22 (2000).
6. Prezant, T. R. *et al.* Mitochondrial ribosomal RNA mutation associated with both antibiotic-induced and non-syndromic deafness. *Nat. Genet.* **4**, 289–294 (1993).
7. Zhao, H. *et al.* Maternally inherited aminoglycoside-induced and nonsyndromic deafness is associated with the novel C1494T mutation in the mitochondrial 12S rRNA gene in a large Chinese family. *Am. J. Hum. Genet.* **74**, 139–152 (2004).
8. Hobbie, S. N. *et al.* Mitochondrial deafness alleles confer misreading of the genetic code. *Proc. Natl Acad. Sci. USA* **105**, 3244–3249 (2008).
9. Hobbie, S. N. *et al.* Genetic analysis of interactions with eukaryotic rRNA identify the mitoribosome as target in aminoglycoside ototoxicity. *Proc. Natl Acad. Sci. USA* **105**, 20888–20893 (2008).
10. Carter, A. P. *et al.* Functional insights from the structure of the 30S ribosomal subunit and its interactions with antibiotics. *Nature* **407**, 340–348 (2000).
11. François, B. *et al.* Crystal structures of complexes between aminoglycosides and decoding A site oligonucleotides: role of the number of rings and positive charges in the specific binding leading to miscoding. *Nucleic Acids Res.* **33**, 5677–5690 (2005).
12. Davies, J., Gorini, L. & Davis, B. D. Misreading of RNA codewords induced by aminoglycoside antibiotics. *Mol. Pharmacol.* **1**, 93–106 (1965).
13. Cabanas, M. J., Vazquez, D. & Modolell, J. Inhibition of ribosomal translocation by aminoglycoside antibiotics. *Biochem. Biophys. Res. Commun.* **83**, 991–997 (1978).
14. Peske, F., Savelsbergh, A., Katunin, V. I., Rodnina, M. V. & Wintermeyer, W. Conformational changes of the small ribosomal subunit during elongation factor G-dependent tRNA-mRNA translocation. *J. Mol. Biol.* **343**, 1183–1194 (2004).
15. Feldman, M. B., Terry, D. S., Altman, R. B. & Blanchard, S. C. Aminoglycoside activity observed on single pre-translocation ribosome complexes. *Nat. Chem. Biol.* **6**, 244 (2010).
16. Recht, M. I., Douthwaite, S. & Puglisi, J. D. Basis for prokaryotic specificity of action of aminoglycoside antibiotics. *EMBO J.* **18**, 3133–3138 (1999).
17. Böttger, E. C., Springer, B., Prammananan, T., Kidan, Y. & Sander, P. Structural basis for selectivity and toxicity of ribosomal antibiotics. *EMBO Rep.* **2**, 318–323 (2001).
18. Hobbie, S. N. *et al.* Engineering the rRNA decoding site of eukaryotic cytosolic ribosomes in bacteria. *Nucleic Acids Res.* **35**, 6086–6093 (2007).
19. Fan-Minogue, H. & Bedwell, D. M. Eukaryotic ribosomal RNA determinants of aminoglycoside resistance and their role in translational fidelity. *RNA* **14**, 148–157 (2008).
20. Pfister, P., Hobbie, S., Vicens, Q., Bottger, E. C. & Westhof, E. The molecular basis for A-site mutations conferring aminoglycoside resistance: relationship between ribosomal susceptibility and X-ray crystal structures. *Chembiochem.* **4**, 1078–1088 (2003).
21. Pfister, P. *et al.* Mutagenesis of 16S rRNA C1409-G1491 base-pair differentiates between 6'OH and 6'NH3 + aminoglycosides. *J. Mol. Biol.* **346**, 467–475 (2005).
22. Matt, T. *et al.* The ribosomal A-site: decoding, drug target and disease. *Isr. J. Chem.* **50**, 60–70 (2010).
23. Kandasamy, J. *et al.* Increased selectivity toward cytoplasmic versus mitochondrial ribosome confers improved efficiency of synthetic aminoglycosides in fixing damaged genes: a strategy for treatment of genetic diseases caused by nonsense mutations. *J. Med. Chem.* **55**, 10630–10643 (2012).
24. Hobbie, S. N. *et al.* Genetic reconstruction of protozoan rRNA decoding sites provides a rationale for paromomycin activity against Leishmania and Trypanosoma. *PLoS Negl. Trop. Dis.* **5**, e1161 (2011).
25. Kokai-Kun, J. F., Chanturiya, T. & Mond, J. J. Lysostaphin as a treatment for systemic *Staphylococcus aureus* infection in a mouse model. *J. Antimicrob. Chemother.* **60**, 1051–1059 (2007).
26. Majithiya, J., Sharp, A., Parmar, A., Denning, D. W. & Warn, P. A. Efficacy of isavuconazole, voriconazole and fluconazole in temporarily neutropenic murine models of disseminated *Candida tropicalis* and *Candida krusei. J. Antimicrob. Chemother.* **63**, 161–166 (2009).
27. Matt, T. *et al.* Dissociation of antibacterial activity and aminoglycoside ototoxicity in the 4-monosubstituted 2-deoxystreptamine apramycin. *Proc. Natl Acad. Sci. USA* **109**, 10984–10989 (2012).
28. Borovinskaya, M. A. *et al.* Structural basis for aminoglycoside inhibition of bacterial ribosome recycling. *Nat. Struct. Mol. Biol.* **14**, 727–732 (2007).
29. Scheunemann, A. E. *et al.* Binding of aminoglycoside antibiotics to helix 69 of 23S rRNA. *Nucleic Acids Res.* **38**, 3094–3105 (2010).
30. Wang, L. *et al.* Allosteric control of the ribosome by small-molecule antibiotics. *Nat. Struct. Mol. Biol.* **19**, 957–963 (2012).
31. Wright, G. D., Berghuis, A. M. & Mobashery, S. Aminoglycoside antibiotics—structure, function and resistance. In: *Resolving the antibiotic paradox (Eds Rosen, B. P. & Mobashery, S.)* pp 27–69 (Springer, 1998).
32. Magnet, S. & Blanchard, J. S. Molecular insights into aminoglycoside action and resistance. *Chem. Rev.* **105**, 477–498 (2005).
33. Hermann, T. & Tor, Y. RNA as a target for small-molecule therapeutics. *Expert Opin. Ther. Pat.* **15**, 49–62 (2005).
34. Sucheck, S. J. *et al.* Design of bifunctional antibiotics that target bacterial rRNA and inhibit resistance-causing enzymes. *J. Am. Chem. Soc.* **122**, 5230–5231 (2000).
35. Bastida, A. *et al.* Exploring the use of conformationally locked aminoglycosides as a new strategy to overcome bacterial resistance. *J. Am. Chem. Soc.* **128**, 100–116 (2006).
36. Aggen, J. B. *et al.* Synthesis and spectrum of the neoglycoside ACHN-490. *Antimicrob. Agents Chemother.* **54**, 4636–4642 (2010).
37. Greenberg, W. A. *et al.* Design and synthesis of new aminoglycoside antibiotics containing neamine as an optimal core structure: correlation of antibiotic activity with in vitro inhibition of translation. *J. Am. Chem. Soc.* **121**, 6527–6541 (1999).
38. Haddad, J. *et al.* Design of novel antibiotics that bind to the ribosomal acyltransfer site. *J. Am. Chem. Soc.* **124**, 3229–3237 (2002).
39. Francois, B. *et al.* Antibacterial aminoglycosides with a modified mode of binding to the ribosomal-RNA decoding site. *Angew. Chem. Int. Ed. Engl.* **43**, 6735–6738, 2004).
40. Zhao, F. *et al.* Molecular recognition of RNA by neomycin and a restricted neomycin derivative. *Angew. Chem. Int. Ed. Engl.* **44**, 5329–5334 (2005).
41. Vourloumis, D. *et al.* Aminoglycoside-hybrid ligands targeting the ribosomal decoding site. *Chembiochem.* **6**, 58–65 (2005).
42. Shaul, P. *et al.* Assessment of 6'- and 6'''-N-acylation of aminoglycosides as a strategy to overcome bacterial resistance. *Org. Biomol. Chem.* **9**, 4057–4063 (2011).
43. Barbieri, C. M., Srinivasan, A. R. & Pilch, D. S. Deciphering the origins of observed heat capacity changes for aminoglycoside binding to prokaryotic and eukaryotic ribosomal RNA a-sites: a calorimetric, computational, and osmotic stress study. *J. Am. Chem. Soc.* **126**, 14380–14388 (2004).
44. Kaul, M., Barbieri, C. M. & Pilch, D. S. Aminoglycoside-induced reduction in nucleotide mobility at the ribosomal RNA A-site as a potentially key determinant of antibacterial activity. *J. Am. Chem. Soc.* **128**, 1261–1271 (2006).
45. Bruell, C. M. *et al.* Conservation of bacterial protein synthesis machinery: initiation and elongation in *Mycobacterium smegmatis. Biochemistry* **47**, 8828–8839 (2008).
46. Clemons, Jr W. M. *et al.* Crystal structure of the 30 S ribosomal subunit from *Thermus thermophilus*: purification, crystallization and structure determination. *J. Mol. Biol.* **310**, 827–843 (2001).
47. Kabsch, W. Xds. *Acta Crystallogr. D. Biol. Crystallogr.* **66**, 125–132 (2010).
48. Brünger, A. T. *et al.* Crystallography & NMR system: A new software suite for macromolecular structure determination. *Acta Crystallogr. D. Biol. Crystallogr.* **54**, 905–921 (1998).
49. Emsley, P., Lohkamp, B., Scott, W. G. & Cowtan, K. Features and development of Coot. *Acta Crystallogr. D. Biol. Crystallogr.* **66**, 486–501 (2010).

Acknowledgements

We thank Tanja Janusic, Claudia Ritter and Sven Hobbie for help and expert technical assistance, Dr David Crich (Wayne State University, Detroit, USA) for critically reviewing the manuscript and valuable input, Takayuki Kato for help with NMR analysis of compounds, the members of the Böttger lab for stimulating discussions during the entire work and Susanna Salas for help with the manuscript preparation. E.C.B. was supported by the University of Zurich and the European Community, A.V. was supported by the ETH Zurich, V.R. was supported by the UK Medical Research Council (U105184332) and the Wellcome Trust.

Author contributions

E.C.B. and A.V. designed the study; D.P.-F., I.K., R.P. and S.R.D. performed chemical synthesis; D.S., T.M., M.M., S.D., R.A., H.B. and P.F. generated mutant strains, prepared ribosomes, conducted *in vitro* ribosomal assays and MIC determinations; N.C.L. and K.L. prepared drug–ribosome complexes and determined crystal structures; S.V. and P.T. performed the *in vivo* infection experiments; all authors analysed and discussed the results; E.C.B., A.V. and V.R. wrote and assembled the manuscript with input from all authors.

Additional information

Accession codes: Coordinates and structure factors for 30S-compound **1** complex, 30S-compound **30** complex, 30S-compound **37** complex and 30S-compound **39** complex have been deposited in the Protein Data Bank under accession codes 4b3m, 4b3r, 4b3s and 4b3t.

Competing financial interests: E.C.B, D.P.-F. and A.V. are co-inventors on a patent filed by the University of Zurich on 4′ modifications of disubstituted 2-deoxystreptamines (WO2008/092690A10). The remaining authors declare no competing financial interests. The University of Zurich has filed a patent application on 4′ modifications of disubstituted 2-deoxystreptamines (WO2008/092690A1).

11

Ca$_V$1.3-selective L-type calcium channel antagonists as potential new therapeutics for Parkinson's disease

Soosung Kang[1], Garry Cooper[1,2], Sara F. Dunne[3], Brendon Dusel[3], Chi-Hao Luan[3,4], D. James Surmeier[2] & Richard B. Silverman[1,4]

L-type calcium channels expressed in the brain are heterogeneous. The predominant class of L-type calcium channels has a Ca$_V$1.2 pore-forming subunit. L-type calcium channels with a Ca$_V$1.3 pore-forming subunit are much less abundant, but have been implicated in the generation of mitochondrial oxidant stress underlying pathogenesis in Parkinson's disease. Thus, selectively antagonizing Ca$_V$1.3 L-type calcium channels could provide a means of diminishing cell loss in Parkinson's disease without producing side effects accompanying general antagonism of L-type calcium channels. However, there are no known selective antagonists of Ca$_V$1.3 L-type calcium channel. Here we report high-throughput screening of commercial and 'in-house' chemical libraries and modification of promising hits. Pyrimidine-2,4,6-triones were identified as a potential scaffold; structure-activity relationship-based modification of this scaffold led to 1-(3-chlorophenethyl)-3-cyclopentylpyrimidine-2,4,6-(1H,3H,5H)-trione (**8**), a potent and highly selective Ca$_V$1.3 L-type calcium channel antagonist. The biological relevance was confirmed by whole-cell patch-clamp electrophysiology. These studies describe the first highly selective Ca$_V$1.3 L-type calcium channel antagonist and point to a novel therapeutic strategy for Parkinson's disease.

[1] Department of Chemistry, Chemistry of Life Processes Institute, and Center for Molecular Innovation and Drug Discovery, Northwestern University, Evanston, Illinois 60208, USA. [2] Department of Physiology, Feinberg School of Medicine, Northwestern University, Chicago, Illinois 60611, USA. [3] High-Throughput Analysis Laboratory, Chemistry of Life Processes Institute, Northwestern University, Evanston, Illinois 60208, USA. [4] Department of Molecular Biosciences, Chemistry of Life Processes Institute, and Center for Molecular Innovation and Drug Discovery, Northwestern University, Evanston, Illinois 60208, USA. Correspondence and requests for materials should be addressed to R.B.S. (email: Agman@chem.northwestern.edu).

Parkinson's disease (PD) is the most common neurodegenerative movement disorder, characterized by tremors, bradykinesia and rigidity[1]. PD has no cure, and nothing is known to slow its progression. The defining motor symptoms of PD result from the degeneration of dopaminergic neurons in the substantia nigra pars compacta (SNc)[2,3]. Recently, we reported that the engagement of L-type calcium channels[4] (LTCCs) during autonomous pacemaking renders adult SNc neurons vulnerable to toxins used to create models of PD[5]. More recently, we demonstrated that the activity-dependent engagement of LTCCs elevates mitochondrial oxidant stress in SNc dopaminergic neurons, providing a means by which LTCCs could increase toxin sensitivity[6]. Interestingly, LTCCs do not appear to be necessary for normal functioning of SNc dopaminergic neurons, making them viable therapeutic targets[7].

The involvement of LTCCs in determining neuronal vulnerability is based on the ability of 1,4-dihydropyridines[8] (DHP) to protect SNc dopaminergic neurons against toxins and to diminish their mitochondrial oxidant stress. DHPs are use-dependent antagonists of LTCCs that have a long history of success in the treatment of hypertension in humans[9]. In agreement with the propositions that LTCCs contribute to pathogenesis, retrospective epidemiological studies conducted in the United Kingdom[10] and Denmark[11] have revealed that the treatment of hypertension with DHPs that cross the blood–brain barrier diminish the observed risk of PD.

The problem with DHPs from a therapeutic perspective, however, is that they are not selective[12]. LTCCs are a heterogenous class of multi-subunit ion channels[13,14] that can be divided into four classes based on the identity of their pore-forming alpha 1 subunit, $Ca_V1.1-4$. This pore-forming subunit governs key features of the channel, including gating and pharmacology. The predominant (~90%) LTCC in the brain has a $Ca_V1.2$ subunit; this channel also is abundant in a variety of peripheral organ systems, including the cardiovascular system and is effectively antagonized by DHPs, accounting for their therapeutic efficacy in hypertension[15]. However, the LTCC responsible for mitochondrial oxidant stress and increased vulnerability in SNc dopaminergic neurons is largely attributable to expression of LTCCs with a $Ca_V1.3$ subunit[5,6]. Among the DHPs, isradipine has the highest relative affinity for $Ca_V1.3$ LTCCs, but it is still $Ca_V1.2$ LTCC selective[14]. This diminishes the therapeutic potential of DHPs in PD, as cardiovascular side effects limit the dosing and antagonism of $Ca_V1.3$ LTCCs. As there are no selective $Ca_V1.3$ LTCC antagonists known, there is a real translational need to develop a new therapeutic agent.

The antagonistic effects of well-known LTCC antagonists[16,17], like isradipine, verapamil and diltiazem (Fig. 1a), were investigated with

stably expressing $Ca_V1.3$ and $Ca_V1.2$ LTCCs in HEK293 cells. Using a fluorometric imaging plate reader (FLIPR)[18] assay with Fluo-8 calcium dye[19], we found that all three were weak antagonists of $Ca_V1.3$ LTCCs, and all were more potent antagonists of $Ca_V1.2$ LTCCs. Over 100 DHPs were screened in an attempt to identify a $Ca_V1.3$ channel selective antagonist[20]; however, none was selective for $Ca_V1.3$ LTCCs. As a consequence, a screen of novel small molecules was undertaken, and the $Ca_V1.3$-selective hits were modified. Here we report the identification of the first highly selective $Ca_V1.3$ LTCC antagonist (8).

Results

High-throughput screen setup and identification of hits. The biological assay utilized a preparation of HEK293 cells that stably expressed $Ca_V1.3$ and $Ca_V1.2$ LTCCs. A FLIPR-based high-throughput screen (HTS) for both $Ca_V1.2$ and $Ca_V1.3$ LTCCs was used to screen 60,480 commercial compounds (ADSI set of 6,800 compounds; ChemBridge diverse/lead like set of 20,000 compounds; ChemDiv diverse set of 30,000 compounds; NIH clinical trial set of 480 compounds and NCI/DTP set of 3,200 compounds (see the DTP website address http://dtp.cancer.gov (2012)). Testing of these commercial compounds for $Ca_V1.3$ LTCCs resulted in not a single hit. Subsequently, we screened a few hundred compounds from our (Silverman lab) non-commercial compound library. From that screen, the pyrimidine 2,4,6-trione (PYT) scaffold was identified as the first class of selective antagonists for $Ca_V1.3$ LTCCs. The initial symmetric PYT hit (Fig. 1b) displayed moderate potency and $Ca_V1.3$ channel selectivity (approximately eightfold from a comparison of the IC_{50} value with $Ca_V1.3$ to that with $Ca_V1.2$). The scaffold also was of interest because of its favourable pharmacological and absorption, distribution, metabolism and excretion (ADME) properties, as well as low toxicity, brain penetration and oral bioavailability, as previously determined[21].

Structure-activity relationship-based hit modification. About 120 PYT analogues were synthesized to develop insight into structure-activity relationships (SARs). The general approach taken to N,N-disubstituted PYT synthesis involved the use of the Wöhler[22] urea synthesis, the coupling of isocyanate with various amines, and Biltz and Wittek's[23] condensation of ureas with activated malonic acid (Fig. 2). Treatment of malonyl chloride with the ureas provided the condensation products in good yields. Further optimization of each step allowed a one-pot parallel synthesis, and sufficient sample purity was achieved by fractional filtration of the final reaction mixture through a silica gel plug (10 cm). This synthetic route permitted the construction of the majority of the PYT library members in

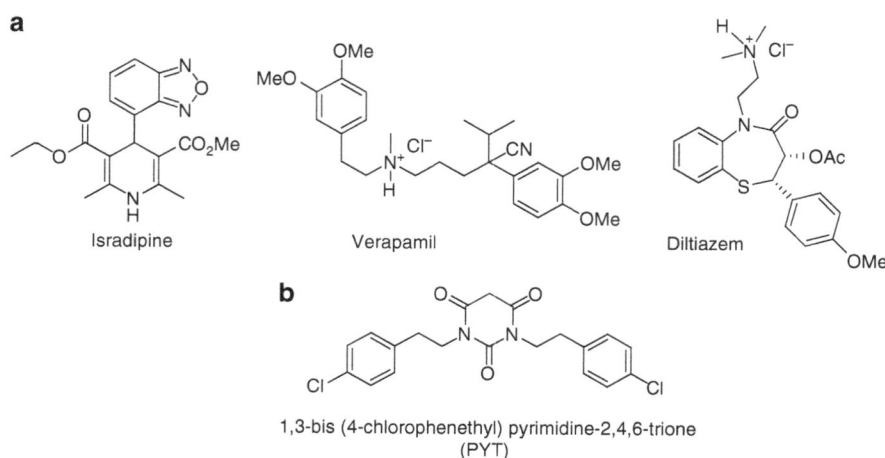

a

Isradipine   Verapamil   Diltiazem

b

1,3-bis (4-chlorophenethyl) pyrimidine-2,4,6-trione
(PYT)

Figure 1 | Various LTCC antagonists. (a) Antihypertensive drugs that non-selectively antagonize LTCCs **(b)** HTS initial hit compound PYT.

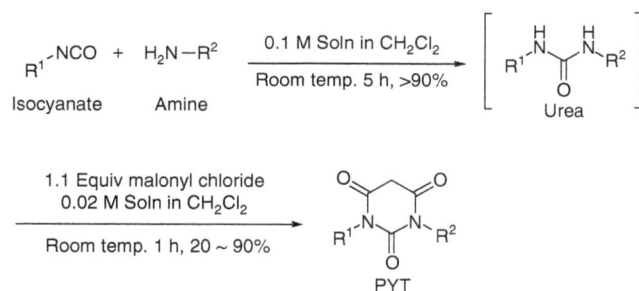

Figure 2 | Common synthetic route to the PYT scaffold. Procedures are described in detail in Methods and in Supplementary Methods, and characterization of the compounds is given in Supplementary Methods.

sufficient quantities and purity for assay against $Ca_V1.3$ and $Ca_V1.2$ LTCCs; promising compounds were purified further and retested.

Using this methodology three sets of PYT analogues were synthesized to probe different structural features of the initial hit PYTs, including substitutions on each of the nitrogens of the PYT core (Fig. 3). The results of the assay are shown in Table 1. The trend that emerged from this library was a steric effect of the lipophilic side chain. Among the cycloalkyl groups, the cyclopentyl derivatives (**7** and **8**) were the most highly selective antagonists for the $Ca_V1.3$ LTCCs; **8** (1-(3-chlorophenethyl)-3-cyclopentylpyrimidine-2,4,6-(1H,3H,5H)-trione) was the most isoform-selective $Ca_V1.3$ antagonist, inhibiting $Ca_V1.3$ LTCCs > 600-fold more potently than $Ca_V1.2$ LTCCs, (determined from the ratio of IC_{50} values) with an IC_{50} of $1.7\,\mu M$ (Fig. 4). Compounds **9** and **10** were the most potent antagonists of this series of molecules (800 nM and 600 nM, respectively), having moderate selectivity (~25-fold).

Pharmacophoric model. The crystallographic data of **8** are given in a .cif file (Supplementary Data 1) and are available from the Cambridge Crystallographic Data Centre (deposition number CCDC 899840). Crystal data for **8**: Monoclinic, Pn space group, $a = 6.9749(2)$ Å, $b = 30.6660(8)$ Å, $c = 7.3929(2)$ Å, $\beta = 92.0160(10)°$, $V = 1580.31(7)$ Å^3, $Z = 4$, $R_1 = 0.0329$, $wR_2 = 0.0861$, F.W. = 334.79, c.d. = $1.407\,g\,cm^{-3}$.

X-ray crystallographic analysis of compound **8** shows that the PYT ring is oriented perpendicularly to the plane of the cycloalkyl ring (Fig. 5). As the most selective PYTs have an N-substituted cycloalkyl group, it is possible that the $Ca_V1.3$ channel can accommodate a PYT ring twisted relative to the plane of the N-cycloalkyl group, but the $Ca_V1.2$ channel cannot.

Bioactivity and relevance confirmation. As IC_{50} values determined in our FLIPR assay depend strongly on assay conditions, the absolute values and selectivity patterns attained through this assay were confirmed using a technically different, yet relevant, measure. To that end, the inhibition of stably expressing $Ca_V1.3$ and $Ca_V1.2$ LTCCs by compound **8** was measured by voltage-clamp experiments (Fig. 6). Whole-cell voltage-clamp recordings (Fig. 6a,b) in the presence of compound **8** showed that **8** selectively (as determined by the ratio of $Ca_V1.3$ to $Ca_V1.2$ inhibition by **8** at a given concentration) inhibits $Ca_V1.3$ LTCCs over $Ca_V1.2$ LTCCs. Compound **8** at $5\,\mu M$ exhibited 31.2% and 4.4% inhibition for $Ca_V1.3$ and $Ca_V1.2$ channel current, respectively (Fig. 5c), which correlates with the results of the FLIPR assay (85.4% and 8.0% inhibition for $Ca_V1.3$ and $Ca_V1.2$ LTCCs, respectively, at $5.5\,\mu M$ concentration). The observed IC_{50} with **8** for $Ca_V1.3$ from the whole-cell patch clamp experiment was $24.3 \pm 0.7\,\mu M$, and because the potency of **8** was too small to generate a concentration–response curve for $Ca_V1.2$ channels, the IC_{50} with **8** for $Ca_V1.2$ was not computed.

Discussion

As $Ca_V1.3$ and $Ca_V1.2$ LTCC-expressing cells were used for comparative screens, it was necessary for each of these cell lines to have similar characteristics to allow ready comparison of compound activity. To this end, cell lines with roughly equivalent channel densities were grown, aliquoted and then cryopreserved, so that the cells used for the assay remained homogenous throughout the screening process. Compounds selected for this screen were not from libraries containing known ion channel antagonists because we wanted to identify novel molecules that were not only selective for $Ca_V1.3$ LTCCs, but also were unlikely to significantly antagonize other classes of ion channels.

The first library of PYTs (63 members) was synthesized to probe several different structural features based on results from our initial hit PYTs, including substitution on the side chain and substitution on the aryl ring (Fig. 3). Four R^2 substituents were used (4-chlorophenethyl, 3-phenylpropyl, 4-phenylbutyl and 2-naphthylethyl). To probe the electronic effects and steric demands on the R^1 aryl ring, electron-withdrawing (F, Cl, Br, CF_3 and NO_2) substituents and methyl were chosen. As electron-rich substituents in the original library did not exhibit good selectivity or potency with $Ca_V1.3$ LTCCs, electron-rich substituents (except methyl) were not considered at this stage. To probe the required distance between the PYT ring and the aryl ring of R^2, four different alkyl chains (C_1–C_4) were incorporated into the sidechain. To probe the steric requirements of R^1, cyclopentyl, cyclohexyl, 2-phenylpropyl, indanyl and tetralinyl substituents were used. From the first library of analogues assayed, three members (**1**, **2** and **3**) were shown to inhibit $Ca_V1.3$ LTCCs with excellent selectivity (> 28-fold from a comparison of the IC_{50} value with $Ca_V1.2$ to that with $Ca_V1.3$) compared with that of the initial hit (Table 1). This is the first class of antagonists that inhibits $Ca_V1.3$ considerably more potently than $Ca_V1.2$ LTCCs. The bulky R^1 cycloalkyl group may be involved in specific steric interactions with neighbouring residues in the $Ca_V1.2$ channel-binding site causing weak binding. All of the analogues assayed, and their associated activities, are shown in Supplementary Tables S1–S3.

The second library (22 members) was prepared to probe the electronic and steric demands on aryl ring R^2 using a cyclohexyl group for R^1. Electron-withdrawing substituents (F, Cl, Br, CF_3, CO_2H, CN and NO_2) and electron-donating substituents (MeO, Me) were used on the R^2 side (Fig. 3). When R^1 was cyclohexyl, the analogues with R^2 m-chlorophenethyl (**3**), m-methylphenethyl (**4**), m-bromophenethyl (**5**) and m-trifluoromethylphenethyl (**6**) were the most selective antagonists for $Ca_V1.3$ LTCCs (Table 1). The selectivity of the meta-substituted analogues results from the loss of antagonism to $Ca_V1.2$ LTCCs. This meta-substitution effect also prevailed when utilizing cyclopentyl as the R^1 substituent, encompassing the third library. However, hydrophilic functional groups on the arylalkyl R^2 diminished antagonism to both LTCCs; $-CO_2H$, $-NO_2$, $-CN$ or $-OMe$ substituted arylalkyl members mostly displayed IC_{50} values > $9\,\mu M$ for both $Ca_V1.3$ and $Ca_V1.2$ LTCCs.

The third library (32 members) was prepared to probe the steric demands on R^1, while maintaining the three best side chains (m-chlorophenethyl, p-chlorophenethyl and m-trifluoromethylphenylethyl) of previous libraries as R^2. Cycloalkyl substituents (cycloheptyl, cyclohexyl, cyclopentyl, cyclobutyl and cyclopropyl), bicycloalkyl substituents (($\pm$)-2-endo-norbonyl, ($\pm$)-2-exo-norbonyl), tricycloalkyl substituents (1-adamantyl, 2-adamantyl), and various other bulky substituents were used for R^1 (Fig. 3).

Three general pharmacophores can be drawn after analysing all of the trends. First, the most selective compounds for $Ca_V1.3$ LTCCs have a cyclohexyl or cyclopentyl substituent (R^1) on the PYT skeleton, implying that a perpendicularly arranged 5- or 6-membered alkyl ring is needed for selective antagonism of the $Ca_V1.3$ LTCCs. Second, a meta-substituted phenethyl moiety (R^2) improves selectivity for the $Ca_V1.3$ LTCCs. Third, $Ca_V1.3$

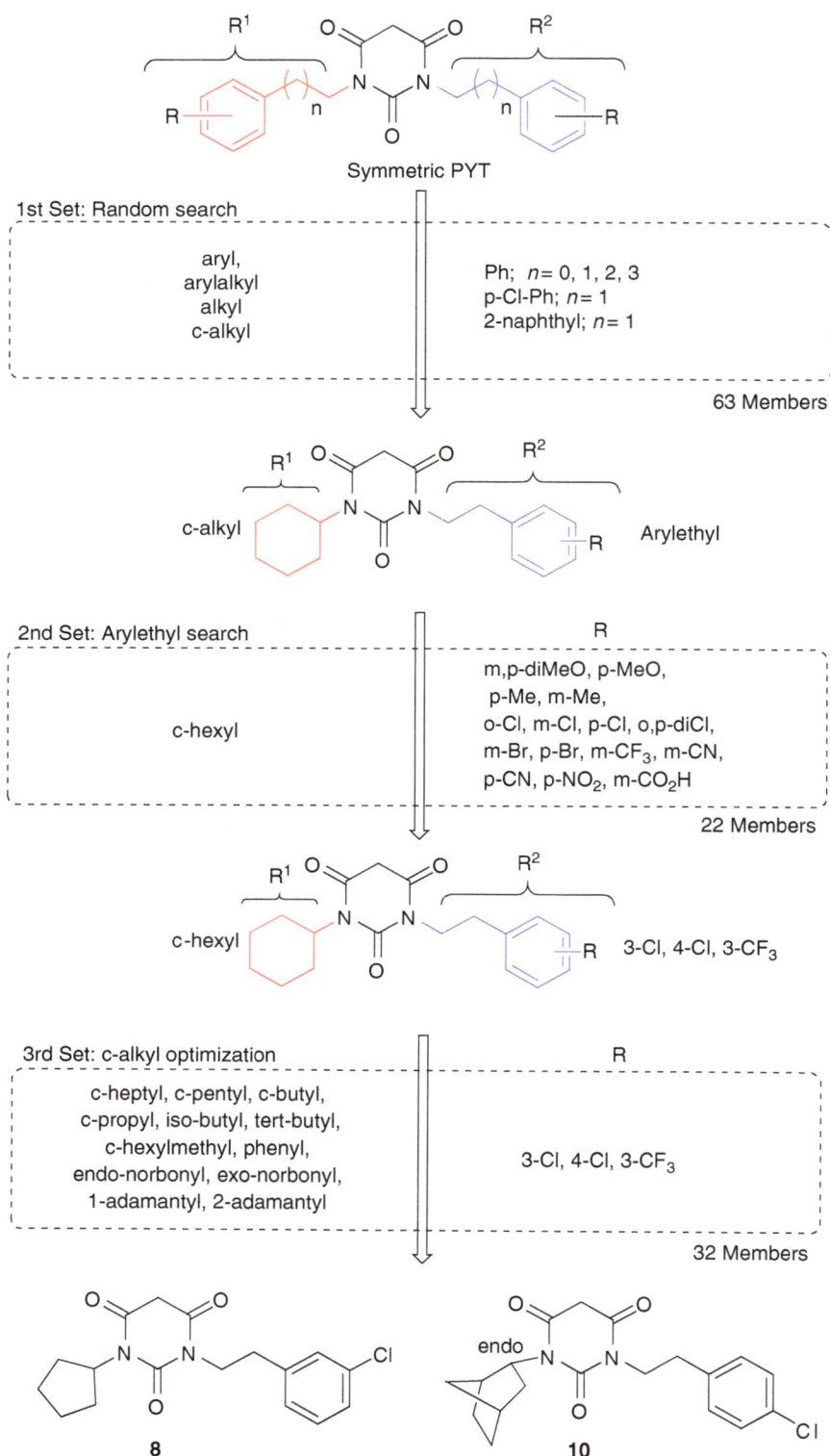

Figure 3 | General scheme for SAR-based modifications. Three regions of structural modifications are defined with the number of compounds prepared in each set to interrogate those regions.

LTCCs respond to a variety of bulky structures at the cycloalkyl binding site; however, substituents with exceptional steric demand antagonize non-selectively.

HEK293 cells that stably expressed $Ca_V1.3$ and $Ca_V1.2$ LTCCs using the FLIPR assay (Fig. 4) and whole-cell voltage-clamp recordings (Fig. 6) confirmed the $Ca_V1.3$ selectivity of **8**. Although the two

assay methods and relative magnitude of inhibition of **8** are different; the observed % of inhibition and IC_{50} values confirm that PYT is a viable selective antagonist scaffold, and compound **8** is a highly selective analogue.

In conclusion, $Ca_V1.3$ LTCCs have recently been implicated in the pathogenesis of PD; however, there are no known selective

Table 1 | IC$_{50}$ values and selectivity of select PYT analogues after lead modification.

Set	Number	Structure	IC$_{50}$ (μM)*,†		Selectivity‡ IC$_{50}$ Ca$_V$1.2/ IC$_{50}$ Ca$_V$1.3
			Ca$_V$1.3	Ca$_V$1.2	
1st	1		1.4 (±0.7)	38.8 (±4.0)	28 (17–61)
	2		1.3 (±0.5)	43.8 (±8.2)	34 (20–65)
	3		1.4 (±0.4)	53.1 (±4.5)	38 (27–58)
2nd	4		2.2 (±0.9)	77.1 (±40)	35 (12–90)
	5		1.3 (±0.4)	45.8 (±13)	34 (19–65)
	6		1.3 (±0.1)	25.8 (±8.5)	20 (12–29)
3rd	7		1.1 (±0.2)	>108§	>83
	8		1.7 (±0.2)	>1162§	>612
	9		0.8 (±0.1)	20.1 (±5.0)	25 (17–36)
	10		0.6 (±0.1)	13.5 (±3.1)	23 (15–33)

*IC$_{50}$ values, that is, the concentration of test compounds required to inhibit 50% of calcium-dependent fluorescence response in the FLIPR assay, were determined from 12-point dose-response curves (0.1 nM–100 μM) in triplicate. IC$_{50}$ values and associated s.d.'s were calcuated by curve fitting the percentage inhibition data from the FLIPR assay to a sigmoidal model for one-site compound target interaction using XLfit. The general method for IC$_{50}$ determination and the fluorescence readings for Ca$_V$1.3 and Ca$_V$1.2 LTCCs with **8** or isradipine are shown in Supplementary Method S1

†IC$_{50}$ values and associated s.d.'s of all library members are described in Supplementary Tables S1–3.

‡The selectivity of antagonism for Ca$_V$1.3 relative to Ca$_V$1.2 LTCCs was determined by the inverse of the ratio of the IC$_{50}$ value with Ca$_V$1.2 LTCCs to that with Ca$_V$1.3 LTCCs.

§IC$_{50}$ is not observed. Given number is the calculated value.

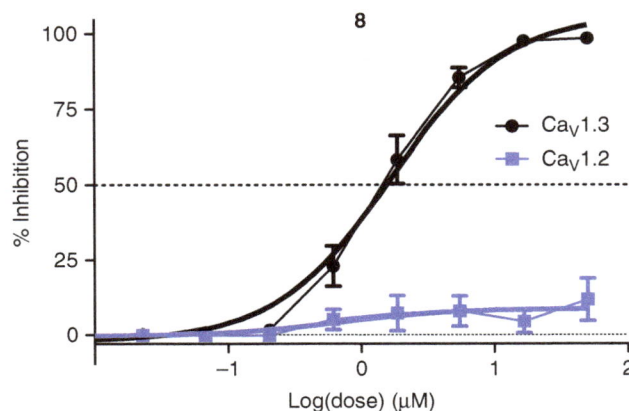

Figure 4 | Concentration-dependent LTCC antagonism by 8 in FLIPR assay. FLIPR assay concentration dependence of percentage inhibition for Ca$_V$1.3 LTCCs and Ca$_V$1.2 LTCCs with compound **8**. Curves are drawn with nonlinear regression (mean±s.e.m.) using Prism. Ca$_V$1.3: IC$_{50}$ = 1.7±0.2 μM; Ca$_V$1.2: IC$_{50}$ = not observed (calculated IC$_{50}$ = 1730±469 μM). Values are mean±s.d.; $n = 6$ for both Ca$_V$1.3 and Ca$_V$1.2. The values are measured by sigmoidal fit using XLfit.

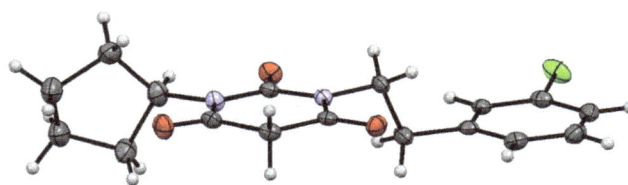

Figure 5 | X-ray crystal structure of compound 8. The cyclopentyl ring is perpendicular to the PYT ring (CCDC deposition number 899840).

antagonists for Ca$_V$1.3 LTCCs. To address this important medical need, a HTS using a FLIPR calcium assay was performed on diverse chemical libraries as an attempt to identify Ca$_V$1.3-selective antagonists. The PYT scaffold was identified, and further SAR based modifications led to 1-(3-chlorophenethyl)-3-cyclopentylpyrimidine-2,4,6-(1H,3H,5H)-trione (**8**), the first potent and highly selective Ca$_V$1.3 antagonist, confirmed by whole-cell voltage-clamp recordings of HEK293 cells expressing functional Ca$_V$1.3 and Ca$_V$1.2 LTCCs. This novel compound is undergoing preclinical evaluation.

Methods

Transfection of HEK293 cells with Ca$_V$1. 3 and Ca$_V$1.2.
Rat Ca$_V$1.3α1D (GenBank accession number: AF370010) containing all alternative splice sites, rat Ca$_V$β3 (GenBank accession number: M88751), rat Ca$_V$α2δ-1 (GenBank accession number: AF286488) and rabbit Ca$_V$1.2α1C (GenBank accession number: P15381) complementary DNAs were used. The potential difference in drug sensitivity caused by alternative splice isoforms of either Ca$_V$1.2 or Ca$_V$1.3 were not evaluated in these studies. All constructs were provided by Dr Diane Lipscombe (Brown University) and Dr Johannes Hell (University of Iowa). General methods for constructs development and transfection[14,20] of Ca$_V$1.2α1C or Ca$_V$1.3α1D, Ca$_V$β3 and Ca$_V$α2δ-1 into HEK293 cells for FLIPR screens were described in our earlier study[20].

General procedure for high-throughput screening. Ca$_V$1.3. or Ca$_V$1.2 LTCCs antagonism was determined using Screen Quest Fluo-8 NW Calcium Assay Kit (ABD Bioquest Inc., Sunnyvale, CA, USA) on a FLIPR tetra (Molecular Devices LLC, Sunnyvale, CA, USA) as follows: HEK293 cells (4×10^4 cells per well) expressing either Ca$_V$1.2 or Ca$_V$1.3 LTCCs were cultured in DMEM with 10% fetal bovine serum for 4 days on tissue culture-treated, 384-well plates, clear-bottom black plates (Greiner Bio-One North America Inc., Monroe, NC, USA). The assay plates were coated with BD Matrigel matrix to improve cell adherence. Dilution series of lead compounds were generated in separate 384-well plates using an Echo550 acoustic liquid transfer system (Labcyte Inc., Sunnyvale, CA, USA). Fluo-8 reagent was prepared in Hanks-buffered saline solution(+) (with 20 mM Hepes and 5 mM additional CaCl$_2$ added, pH 7.4). Then 100 μl of the Fluo-8 reagent was added to the compound dilution series and controls, and well mixed by pipetting using a Biomek FX liquid handler (Beckman Coulter Inc., Brea, CA, USA). The media was then removed from the cells and 45 μl of the compound/Fluo-8 mixture was transferred to assay plates of each cell line using the Biomek FX. The treated cells were incubated at 37 °C for 45 min and then removed from the incubator and placed at room temperature for an additional 30 min. The plates were placed in the FLIPR tetra, which was programmed to measure the fluorescence intensity before, during and for 2 min after adding 25 μl of KCl solution (450 mM KCl in Hanks-buffered saline solution(+) solution, pH 7.4). FLIPR tetra data acquisition parameters were as follows: excitation wavelength 470–495 nm, emission wavelength 515–575 nm, gain 80, exposure 0.4 s, excitation intensity 80.

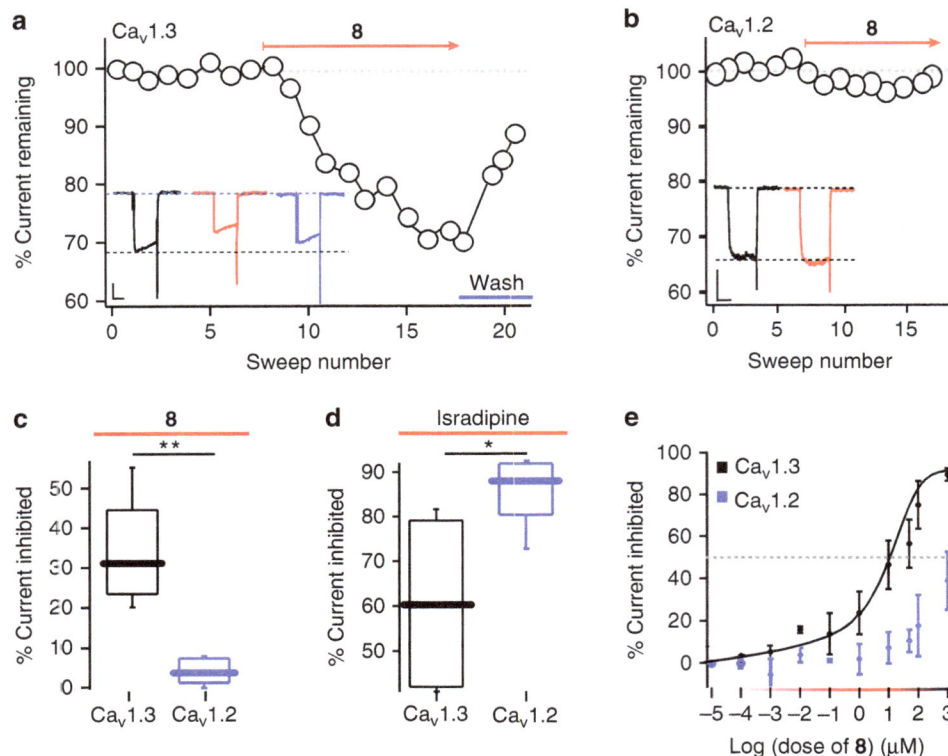

Figure 6 | Whole-cell patch-clamp experiments. Time course of effects of (**a**) $Ca_V1.3$ and (**b**) $Ca_V1.2$ calcium channel peak currents (○) for compound **8** (5 µM). Example of current traces from control (black), compound **8** (red), and wash (blue) are inserted. All vertical scale bars are 50 pA, and horizontal scale bars are 50 ms. Population data of the inhibition conferred by (**c**), compound **8** (5 µM) with $Ca_V1.3$ (black, $n = 17$, median = 0.312) and $Ca_V1.2$ (blue, $n = 10$, median = 0.0439), which was deemed signficant by the Mann–Whittney rank-sum Test (**$P < 0.001$); and (**d**), isradipine (300 nM) with $Ca_V1.3$ (black, $n = 5$, median = 0.604) and $Ca_V1.2$ (blue, $n = 5$, median = 0.881), which was deemed significant by the Mann–Whittney Ram-sum test (*$P < 0.05$). (**e**) Concentration–response curves for compound **8** inhibition of $Ca_V1.3$ and $Ca_V1.2$ LTCCs. Data were fit to the Hill equation: $(I_{control} - I_{compound\ 8})/I_{control} = 1/(1 + (IC_{50}/C_{compound\ 8})^h)$, where IC_{50} is the concentration of compound **8** required to inhibit 50% of peak current, and h is the Hill cofficient. $Ca_V1.3$: $IC_{50} = 24.3 \pm 0.7$ µM; $h = 0.42 \pm 0.04$; $Ca_V1.2$: $IC_{50} =$ not observed; $h =$ not observed.

General procedure for whole-cell patch-clamp assay. After 24–48 h of incubation at 37 °C on poly-D-lysine-treated coverslips, stably transfected HEK293 cells underwent whole-cell patch-clamp electrophysiology. The external solution contained the following (in mM): 140 NaCl, 1 MgCl₂, 10 BaCl₂, 10 HEPES, 10 dextrose, 10 sucrose and 20 CsCl at pH 7.4 and an osmolarity of ~320 mOsm l⁻¹. The test compound stock solutions in dimethylsulphoxide (100 mM or just dimethylsulphoxide) were diluted with the external solution to the desired concentration (10^{-9} to 10^{-3} M), which was perfused (2 ml per min) into the recording chamber while measuring the evoked barium currents. In experiments where concentration–response curves were obtained, local perfusion of the desired concentration was employed. Barium currents were measured from whole-cell voltage patch-clamp recordings using the Pulse 8.4 software data acquisition system (HEKA, Germany). Signals were low-pass filtered at 1 kHz, digitized (sampled) at 10 kHz, and were amplified with an Axopatch 200B patch-clamp amplifier (Axon Instruments). Barium currents were evoked by a depolarizing voltage step from a holding potential of −70 to 0 mV for 100 ms with a frequency of 0.05 Hz at room temperature (22–25 °C). Patch pipettes were pulled from thin-wall borosilicate glass coated with dental wax and maintained at a resistance of ~3–5 mΩ. Internal pipette solutions contained the following (in mM): 180 N-methyl-D-glucosamine, 40 HEPES, 4 MgCl₂, 12 phosphocreatine, 0.1 leupeptin, 2 Na₂ATP, 0.5 Na₃GTP, 5 BAPTA, pH 7.2–7.3 and an osmolarity of ~290 mOsm l⁻¹. Electrophysiological signals were analysed using Clampfit 9.2 (Axon Instruments) and IgorPro 6 software.

General synthetic procedure. To an isocyanate (1 mmol) in dry dichloromethane (10 ml) was added an amine (1 mmol), and the mixture was stirred at room temperature for 3–5 h. After dilution with dry dichloromethane (50 ml), malonyl chloride (1.1 mmol) was added dropwise under vigorous stirring at room temperature for 5 min. The resulting pale yellow solution was stirred for an additional 1 h and concentrated at reduced pressure to a small volume. The resultant reaction mixture was purified by flash chromatography on 50 g of silica gel in a column (20 mm internal diameter) using 20–33% ethyl acetate in hexanes to give analytically

pure compounds (20–90% yield). Compound characterization data are shown in Supplementary Method S3.

Crystal structure acquisition. A colourless plate crystal of **8** having approximate dimensions of 0.37×0.16×0.04 mm was mounted using oil (Infineum V8512) on a glass fibre. All measurements were made on a Bruker APEX-II CCD detector with MX optics monochromated CuK\α radiation and processed using SAINTPLUS from Bruker. The data were collected at a temperature of 100 K with a theta range for data collection of 6.16–67.32°. Data were collected in 0.5° oscillations with 5 s exposures. The crystal-to-detector distance was 40.00 mm.

References

1. Jankovic, J. Parkinson's disease: clinical features and diagnosis. *J. Neurol. Neurosurg. Psychiatry* **79**, 368–376 (2008).
2. Fearnley, J. M. & Lees, A. J. Ageing and Parkinson's disease: substantia nigra regional selectivity. *Brain* **114**, 2283–2301 (1991).
3. Riederer, P. & Wuketich, S. Time course of nigrostriatal degeneration in Parkinson's disease. A detailed study of influential factors in human brain amine analysis. *J. Neural. Transm.* **38**, 277–301 (1976).
4. Casamassima, F. *et al.* L-type calcium channels and psychiatric disorders: a brief review. *Am. J. Med. Genet. Part B* **153B**, 1373–1390 (2010).
5. Chan, C. S. *et al.* 'Rejuvenation' protects neurons in mouse models of Parkinson's disease. *Nature* **447**, 1081–1086 (2007).
6. Guzman, J. N. *et al.* Oxidant stress evoked by pacemaking in dopaminergic neurons is attenuated by DJ-1. *Nature* **468**, 696–700 (2010).
7. Guzman, J. N., Sánchez-Padilla, J., Chan, C. S. & Surmeier, D. J. Robust pacemaking in substantia nigra dopaminergic neurons. *J. Neurosci.* **29**, 11011–11009 (2009).
8. Triggle, D. J. 1,4-Dihydropyridines as calcium channel ligands and privileged structures. *Cell Mol. Neurobiol.* **23**, 293–303 (2003).
9. Epstein, M. Calcium antagonists: still appropriate as first line antihypertensive agents. *Am. J. Hypertens.* **9**, 110–121 (1996).

10. Becker, C., Jick, S. S. & Meier, C. R. Use of antihypertensives and the risk of Parkinson disease. *Neurology* **70**, 1438–1444 (2008).
11. Ritz, B. *et al.* L-type calcium channel blockers and Parkinson disease in Denmark. *Ann. Neurol.* **67**, 600–606 (2010).
12. Xu, W. & Lipscombe, D. Neuronal Ca$_V$1.3α_1 L-type channels activate at relatively hyperpolarized membrane potentials and are incompletely inhibited by dihydropyridines. *J. Neurosci.* **21**, 5944–5951 (2001).
13. Catterall, W. A., Perez-Reyes, E., Snutch, T. P. & Striessnig, J. International Union of Pharmacology. XLVIII. Nomenclature and structure-function relationships of voltage-gated calcium channels. *Pharmacol. Rev.* **57**, 411–425 (2005).
14. Lipscombe, D., Helton, T. D. & Xu, W. L-type calcium channels: the low down. *J. Neurophysiol.* **92**, 2633–2641 (2004).
15. Sinnegger-Brauns, M. J. *et al.* Expression and 1,4-dihydropyridine-binding properties of brain L-type calcium channel isoforms. *Mol. Pharmacol.* **75**, 407–414 (2009).
16. Triggle, D. J. *et al.* Synthetic organic ligands active at voltage-gated calcium channels. *Ann. N Y Acad. Sci.* **635**, 123–138 (1991).
17. Triggle, D. J. L-type calcium channels. *Curr. Pharmaceut. Des.* **12**, 443–457 (2006).
18. Sullivan, E., Tucker, E. M. & Dale, L. Measurement of [Ca2+] using the fluorometric imaging plate reader (FLIPR). *Meth. Mol. Biol.* **114**, 125–33 (1999).
19. Minta, A., Kao, J. P. Y. & Tsien, R. Y. Fluorescent indicators for cytosolic calcium based on rhodamine and fluorescein chromophores. *J. Biol. Chem.* **264**, 8171–8178 (1989).
20. Chang, C.- C. *et al.* Antagonism of 4-substituted 1,4-dihydropyridine-3,5-dicarboxylates toward voltage-dependent L-type Ca2+ channels Ca$_V$1.3 and Ca$_V$1.2. *Bioorg. Med. Chem.* **18**, 3147–3158 (2010).
21. Xia, G. *et al.* Pyrimidine-2,4,6-trione derivatives and their inhibition of mutant SOD1-dependent protein aggregation. Toward a treatment for amyotrophic lateral sclerosis. *J. Med. Chem.* **54**, 2409–2421 (2010).
22. Wöhler, F. On the artificial formation of urea. *Ann. Phys. Chem.* **88**, 253–256 (1828).
23. Biltz, H. & Wittek, H. Darstellug von Barbitursaure und N-Alkyl-barbitursauren. *Chem. Ber.* **54**, 1035–1058 (1921).

Acknowledgements

We are grateful to the Michael J. Fox Foundation (Therapeutics Development Initiative) and the RJG Foundation for financial support of this research. We thank Dr Diane Lipscombe for providing calcium channel clones.

Author contributions

S.K. synthesized all compounds and wrote the initial draft of the manuscript; G.C. performed all patch-clamp experiments and contributed to the initial draft of the manuscript; S.F.D. carried out the HTSs; B.D. carried out some of the HTSs; C.H.L. managed and interpreted the HTSs; D.J.S. directed the electrophysiology research and edited the manuscript; R.B.S. directed the chemical research and edited the manuscript.

Additional information

Accession codes: The X-ray crystallographic coordinates for structures reported in this Article have been deposited at the Cambridge Crystallographic Data Centre (CCDC), under deposition number CCDC 899840. These data can be obtained free of charge from The Cambridge Crystallographic Data Centre via http://www.ccdc.cam.ac.uk/data_request/cif.

Competing financial interests: The authors declare no competing financial interests.

12

Crystallographic structure of a small molecule SIRT1 activator-enzyme complex

Han Dai[1,2], April W. Case[1], Thomas V. Riera[1], Thomas Considine[1], Jessica E. Lee[3], Yoshitomo Hamuro[3], Huizhen Zhao[2], Yong Jiang[2], Sharon M. Sweitzer[2], Beth Pietrak[2], Benjamin Schwartz[2], Charles A. Blum[1], Jeremy S. Disch[1], Richard Caldwell[1], Bruce Szczepankiewicz[1], Christopher Oalmann[1], Pui Yee Ng[1], Brian H. White[1], Rebecca Casaubon[1], Radha Narayan[1], Karsten Koppetsch[1], Francis Bourbonais[1], Bo Wu[4], Junfeng Wang[4], Dongming Qian[5], Fan Jiang[5], Cheney Mao[5], Minghui Wang[2], Erding Hu[2], Joe C. Wu[1], Robert B. Perni[1], George P. Vlasuk[1] & James L. Ellis[1,2]

SIRT1, the founding member of the mammalian family of seven NAD^+-dependent sirtuins, is composed of 747 amino acids forming a catalytic domain and extended N- and C-terminal regions. We report the design and characterization of an engineered human SIRT1 construct (mini-hSIRT1) containing the minimal structural elements required for lysine deacetylation and catalytic activation by small molecule sirtuin-activating compounds (STACs). Using this construct, we solved the crystal structure of a mini-hSIRT1-STAC complex, which revealed the STAC-binding site within the N-terminal domain of hSIRT1. Together with hydrogen-deuterium exchange mass spectrometry (HDX-MS) and site-directed mutagenesis using full-length hSIRT1, these data establish a specific STAC-binding site and identify key inter-molecular interactions with hSIRT1. The determination of the interface governing the binding of STACs with human SIRT1 facilitates greater understanding of STAC activation of this enzyme, which holds significant promise as a therapeutic target for multiple human diseases.

[1]Sirtris, a GlaxoSmithKline Company, 200 Technology Square, Suite 300, Cambridge, Massachusetts 02139, USA. [2]GlaxoSmithKline, 1250S. Collegeville Road, Collegeville, Pennsylvania 19426, USA. [3]ExSAR Corporation, 11 Deer Park Drive, Suite 103, Monmouth Junction, New Jersey 08852, USA. [4]High Magnetic Field Laboratory, Hefei Institutes of Physical Science, Chinese Academy of Sciences, 350 Shushanhu Road, Hefei, Anhui Province 230031, China. [5]Viva Biotech, 334 Aidisheng Road, Zhangjiang High-tech Park, Shanghai 201203, China. Correspondence and requests for materials should be addressed to H.D. (email: Han.x.Dai@gsk.com).

Sirtuins are a family of highly conserved NAD^+-dependent deacylases that have been linked to a number of important biological processes across a broad span of diverse organisms such as *Saccharomyces cerevisiae*, *Caenorhabditis elegans*, *Drosophilla melanogaster* and *Mus musculus*, among others[1,2]. Sirtuins generally catalyze the deacylation of modified lysine residues in protein substrates coupled with the breakdown of NAD^+ into nicotinamide (NAM) and 2'-O-acyl-ADP-ribose. Of the seven sirtuins (SIRT1-7) that have been identified in mammals[3], human SIRT1 (hSIRT1) is the most studied isoform, and has been shown to be regulated by calorie restriction and to be involved in multiple biological processes[4–7]. The validated, protective role of increased mammalian SIRT1 activity in metabolic disorders[8], neurodegeneration[9] and inflammation[10,11] makes this enzyme an attractive therapeutic target. To this end, the development of pharmacological approaches to increase the enzymatic activity of hSIRT1 might lead to a new generation of therapeutic agents for a wide spectrum of diseases associated with aging. Small molecule sirtuin-activating compounds (STAC) have been developed which increase the catalytic deacetylation of specific Lys residues by hSIRT1 in multiple substrates, resulting in a variety of biological responses[12–14]. However, the molecular mechanism of hSIRT1 activation by STACs remains controversial. Questions as to whether STACs directly activate hSIRT1 persist[15] despite evidence of allosteric activation[13]. Recently, a single point mutation of the Glu^{230} residue of hSIRT1 has been shown to attenuate kinetic activation by STACs[16], further demonstrating a direct effect on hSIRT1. Structural characterizations of hSIRT1 fragments have shed light on the inhibitor binding and key regulatory element[17,18]. Similar to other sirtuins, hSIRT1 catalytic domain contains a Rossmann-fold large lobe and a zinc-binding small lobe and undergoes a significant conformational change of domain closure upon substrate/ligand occupying the active site[19–21]. However, the molecular details governing the binding of STACs to SIRT1 remain elusive, due to the difficulty in obtaining a detailed X-ray crystallographic structure of the full-length enzyme. To address this, we developed an engineered hSIRT1 (mini-hSIRT1) that is biochemically equivalent to the full-length enzyme with respect to basal catalytic activity and activation by STACs. X-ray crystallographic analysis of mini-hSIRT1 resulted in the first detailed structural determination of a fully functional human SIRT1 with a bound small molecule activator. The details of STAC binding to mini-hSIRT1 were translated to the full-length enzyme using structure-guided mutagenesis which corroborated the importance of key amino acids in the binding of STACs. These data are important in elucidating the molecular basis for STAC-mediated activation of hSIRT1 which will be critical for the development of future therapeutic agents.

Results

Mini-hSIRT1 design and characterization. To identify and characterize the key functional regions of hSIRT1, we performed hydrogen-deuterium exchange mass spectrometry (HDX-MS) on the full-length hSIRT1 protein. The rate of H–D exchange is highly dependent on the dynamic properties of the protein, with faster exchange occurring at solvent exposed and/or flexible regions and slower exchange occurring at the more buried and/or rigid regions[22]. Consistent with the previous study on hSIRT1(19–747)[16], full-length hSIRT1 contains three major structured regions: the catalytic core region; residues 229–516 (referred to as hSIRT1cd hereafter)[3,20]; the N-terminal region of 183–229 immediately preceding the catalytic core and a remote region following the catalytic core around 641–665, previously reported as human C-terminal regulatory segment (CTR)

peptide[18]; and murine essential for SIRT1 activity peptide[23]. (Fig. 1a and Supplementary Fig. 1a).

To probe the STAC-binding site on hSIRT1, HDX-MS was performed in the absence or presence of STAC **1** (Supplementary Fig. 2). Addition of **1** reduces the H–D exchange rate around residues 183–229 in the N-terminal region of hSIRT1, suggesting that this domain is involved in STAC binding. Hereafter, this domain is referred to as the STAC-binding domain (SBD) (Fig. 1a,b and Supplementary Fig. 1a). Addition of **1** to hSIRT1 in the presence of a p53-derived peptide substrate (Ac-p53(W5))[13] results in perturbation of the H–D exchange rates around the SBD and further protection at the substrate-binding site (residues 417–424) in the catalytic domain compared with the hSIRT1/Ac-p53(W5) complex, indicating that STAC binding in the N-terminal domain and substrate binding within the catalytic domain of hSIRT1 are coupled (Fig. 1b). This is consistent with the previous observation that STACs enhance substrate binding to hSIRT1, thereby increasing hSIRT1 catalytic efficiency[12].

In the absence of the CTR peptide, the catalytic core (hSIRT1cd) only shows ~15% of the activity of the full-length enzyme using deacetylation assay conditions previously reported (Supplementary Fig. 1b)[13]. The addition of the CTR peptide restores the catalytic activity of hSIRT1cd, to 80% of that of full-length hSIRT1, consistent with previous observations[23,24] (Supplementary Fig. 1b). Kinetic characterization reveals that the CTR peptide restores activity by lowering the K_M values for both peptide substrate and NAD^+ of hSIRT1cd by 4–5-fold (Supplementary Table 1).

Taken together, the above data suggest a tripartite architecture for a minimally functional hSIRT1 that includes: (1) the central domain constituting the basic catalytic machinery; (2) the N-terminal SBD that mediates STAC binding and activation; and (3) the C-terminal CTR peptide which stabilizes the catalytic domain resulting in more efficient deacetylase activity. Based on this, we designed several hSIRT1 constructs encompassing all three of the minimal structural elements covalently bound, which we termed mini-hSIRT1s. The constructs span 183–505 or 183–516, which are connected to the CTR peptide via a flexible poly-glycine/serine linker (GS, $(GGGS)_2$ or $(GGGS)_3$) (Fig. 1a)[25]. The K_M and k_{cat} values are comparable between mini-hSIRT1 constructs and the full-length enzyme, as are the IC_{50} values for the hSIRT1 inhibitors EX-527 (ref. 26) or NAM, confirming functional fidelity of mini-hSIRT1s (Supplementary Tables 2 and 3). In addition, there is an excellent correlation between mini-hSIRT1 and the full-length enzyme with respect to STAC-mediated activation across a broad set of chemotypes (Fig. 1c). Removal of the SBD completely abolishes STAC-mediated activation of mini-hSIRT1, confirming the critical importance of this domain for activation (Fig. 1d). In contrast, mini-hSIRT1 lacking the CTR retains a significant level of STAC activation (Fig. 1e) suggesting that CTR is not required for STAC-mediated activation. Finally, the E230K mutation also attenuates STAC-mediated activation in mini-hSIRT1 as in the full-length enzyme[16] (Fig. 1f). Collectively, these observations demonstrate that at half the molecular size, mini-hSIRT1 can serve as an active and activatable surrogate for full-length hSIRT1.

Structure of the mini-hSIRT1-STAC complex. Although the X-ray crystallographic structures of the hSIRT1 catalytic domain and complex of SIRT1cd/CTR have been reported[17,18], no structure of the full-length enzyme is available. Solving the structure of the full-length hSIRT1 has been challenging, likely due to the conformational flexibility of the extended N- and C-terminal domains[16,27]. The mini-hSIRT1 constructs, which contain only the functionally critical regions of the N and

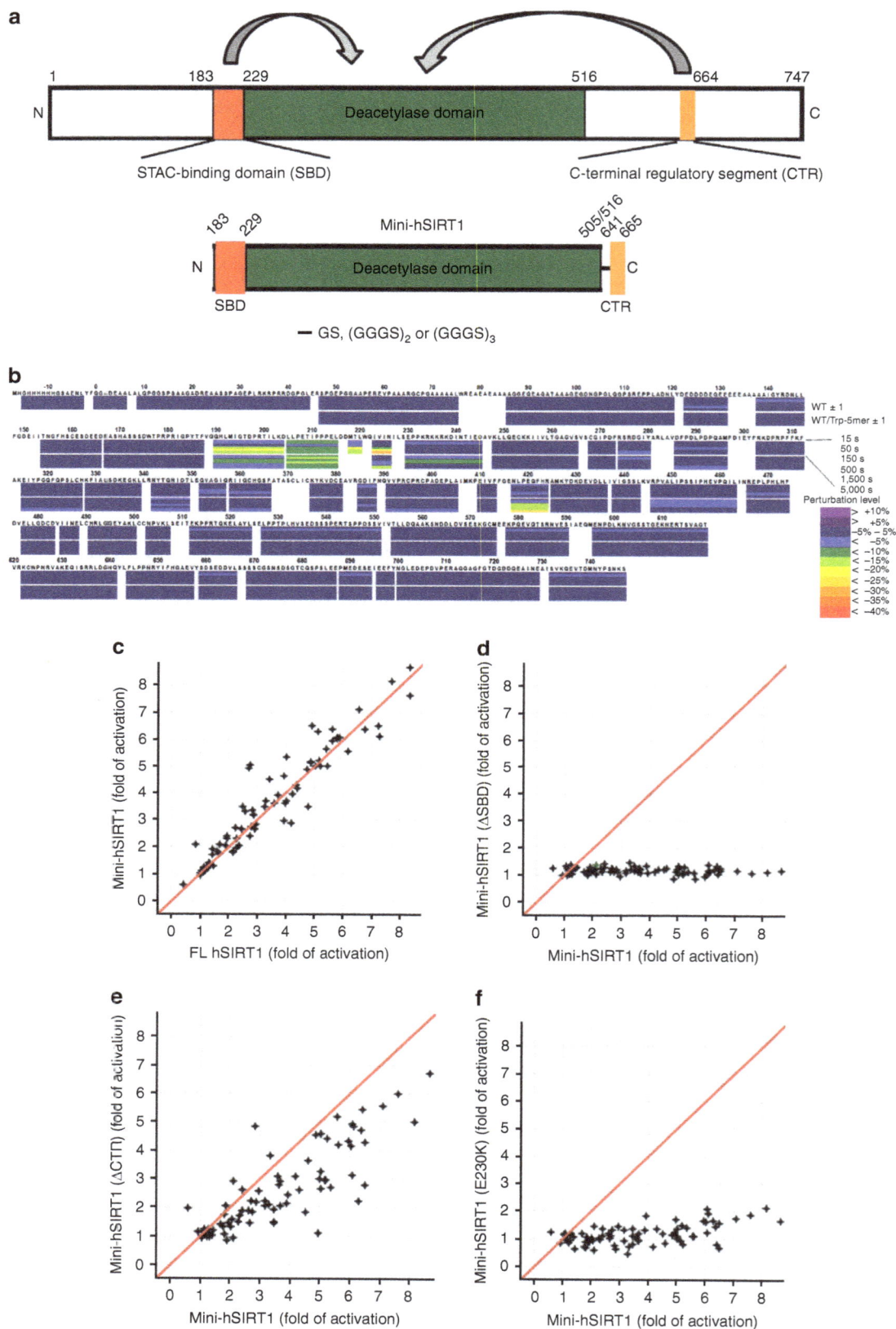

Figure 1 | Mini-hSIRT1 construct design and characterization. (**a**) Schematic diagram of human full-length hSIRT1 and Mini-hSIRT1 constructs. The N-terminal SBD, the central catalytic domain and the CTR are highlighted in red, green and orange. (**b**) Heat map of the HDX-MS perturbation of binding of **1** to hSIRT1 in the absence or presence of Ac-p53(W5) (Trp-5mer) at six different time points (15–5000 s). (**c**) Pivot plot of the activation by a chemically diverse STAC set using the Ac-p53(W5) substrate for mini-hSIRT1 versus full-length hSIRT1, as measured by OAcADPR assay. The red line represents $y = x$ correlation. (**d**) Pivot plot of the STAC activation of mini-hSIRT1(ΔSBD) versus mini-hSIRT1. (**e**) Pivot plot the STAC activation of mini-hSIRT1(ΔCTR) versus mini-hSIRT1. (**f**) Pivot plot of the STAC activation of mini-hSIRT1(E230K) versus mini-hSIRT1.

C-terminal domains, afforded us the opportunity to crystallize a functional surrogate of the full-length enzyme. We successfully crystallized mini-hSIRT1 (183–505-(GGGS)2-CTR) with STAC **1** used in the HDX-MS experiments and determined the structure of the complex (mini-hSIRT1/**1**) at 3.1 Å by molecular replacement using a search model based on the homologous model of SIRT3 (ref. 20).

Mini-hSIRT1 comprises a catalytic domain that assumes a Rossmann-fold large lobe and a zinc-binding small lobe common to all sirtuins[19], an N-terminal three-helical bundle encompassing the SBD and a C-terminal β-hairpin CTR peptide[18] (Fig. 2a). The CTR peptide mediates β-augmentation with the six-stranded β-sheet of the Rossmann-fold lobe of the catalytic domain

(Fig. 2a), in agreement with the HDX-MS results of hSIRT1cd perturbation upon CTR binding (Supplementary Fig. 3a,b). The CTR-mediated β-augmentation appears to stabilize the active site of the hSIRT1cd which restores the K_M values observed for both acetylated peptide and NAD$^+$ substrates[18]. The N-terminal SBD forms an independently folded, three-helix bundle with **1** binding to the helix-turn-helix (H2-T-H3) motif within the SBD, consistent with the HDX-MS and enzyme kinetic results (Fig. 2a). STAC **1** interacts extensively with the hydrophobic side chains of Leu[206], Thr[209] (methyl), Pro[211], Pro[212], Leu[215], Thr[219] (methyl), Ile[223] and Ile[227] from the H2-T-H3 motif with only one hydrophilic interaction: a hydrogen bond with Asn[226] (Fig. 2b). The major mini-hSIRT1/**1**-binding site is a shallow

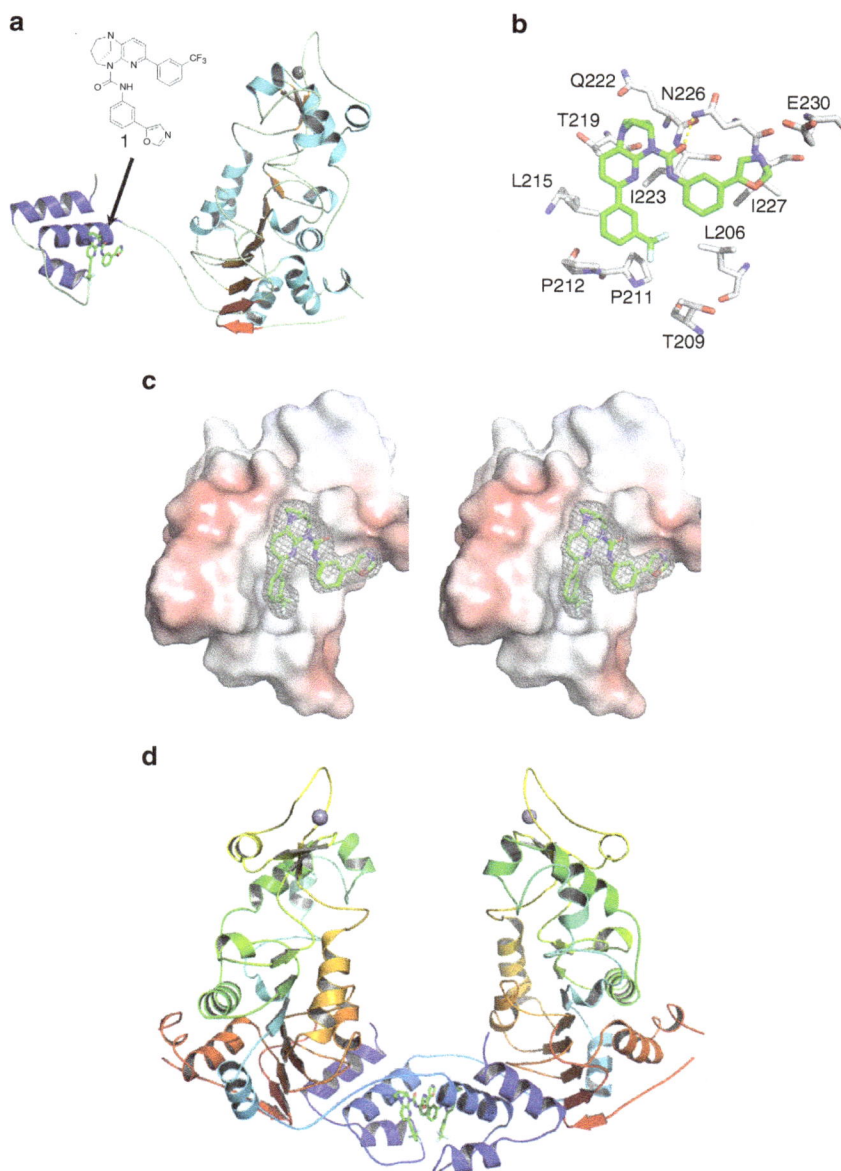

Figure 2 | Structure of Mini-hSIRT1/1 complex. (**a**) Structure of Mini-hSIRT1/**1** complex shown in ribbon diagram. The α-helices and β-strands in the catalytic domain are shown in cyan and orange, respectively. The α-helices in the N-terminal SBD are shown in blue. The β-strands in the C-terminal CTR are shown in red. All the loops are shown in light gray. The STAC **1** is shown in green, red and blue for carbon, oxygen and nitrogen atoms. The zinc ion is shown as a gray sphere. (**b**) hSIRT1-binding site of **1** with interacting residues shown in stick representation. Hydrogen bonds are shown as yellow dotted lines. (**c**) Stereo view of the electrostatic surface potential of the N-terminal SBD and electron density map of STAC **1**. The electrostatic potential is contoured at the 5 kT/e level, with red denoting negative potential and blue denoting positive potential. The 2Fo-Fc omit map of **1** is contoured at 1.0 σ level. (**d**) Crystallographic dimer of Mini-hSIRT1/**1** complex. The protein ribbon is rainbow-colored from blue at the N-terminus to red at the C-terminus.

hydrophobic surface depression with an off-center, deeper hydrophobic pocket, that the CF_3 group of **1** occupies (Fig. 2c). This is consistent with the observed structure-activity relationships developed across multiple STAC chemotypes, indicating the requirement of overall flatness of the core scaffold maintained by an intramolecular hydrogen bond[28]. A remarkable similarity in terms of domain configuration is observed between the mini-hSIRT1 structure and that of yeast Sir2 with both having an N-terminal helical bundle and the C-terminal β-augmentation by a β-hairpin beyond the typical Rossmann-fold large lobe[29] (Supplementary Fig. 3c). However, yeast Sir2 does not include the 130 amino acid insertion (510–640) observed in hSIRT1 and appears to be a natural 'mini-SIRT1' in yeast.

Interestingly, a STAC-mediated dimer of mini-hSIRT1 related by crystallographic symmetry was observed in the crystal lattices (Fig. 2d). Size exclusion chromatography (SEC) indicates that the apparent size of mini-hSIRT1 increases in the presence of STAC **1**, which is likely correspondent to the mini-hSIRT1 dimer species (Supplementary Fig. 4). We are currently attempting to determine if the observed crystallographic dimer has any relevance in the observed biology of STAC-mediated SIRT1 activation.

In addition to the mini-hSIRT1/**1** complex structure, we also determined a 2.73 Å structure of a quaternary complex of mini-hSIRT1, **1**, a seven amino acid peptide substrate derived from p53 (Ac-p53), and the nonhydrolyzable NAD^+ analog carbaNAD and a 2.74 Å structure mini-hSIRT1/**1** in complex with an active-site directed inhibitor **2** (ref. 30) that occupies the peptide and NAD^+-binding sites (Fig. 3a,b and Supplementary Fig. 2). In the quaternary complex structure, the Ac-p53 peptide and carbaNAD bind to the active site cleft between the large and small lobes. Ac-p53 adopts an extended conformation, similar to the backbone-mediated β-strand like interactions observed in many Sirtuin/Ac-peptide complexes[19,31]. The main chain amide groups of Ac-p53 form hydrogen bonds with those of the residues Gly[415] and Glu[416] from the small lobe and those of the residues Lys[444] and Arg[446] from the large lobe (Supplementary Fig. 5a). The hydrogen bonds between the amide of the peptide +1 position and that of Arg[446] render a potential interaction between the side chain and a bulky and hydrophobic +1 residue, which might be important in STAC-mediated hSIRT1 activation[13]. The acetyl-lysine side chain inserts into a hydrophobic cavity lined by Phe[414], Leu[418] and Val[445]. The acetyl group is sandwiched between His[363] and Phe[297], with the ε-N of the acetyl-lysine hydrogen bonded with the carbonyl oxygen of Val[412], which maintains the orientation and the extended conformation of the acetyl-lysine side chain. CarbaNAD also makes multipoint contacts with hSIRT1 (Supplementary Fig. 5b), most of which are similar to those observed in reported Sirtuin/NAD^+ structures[19,31]. Inhibitor **2** occupies both the acetyl-lysine-binding site and the NAM-binding C-pocket of mini-hSIRT1, similar to the recently reported structure of the SIRT3/**2** complex[30] (Supplementary Fig. 5c). Similar to SIRT3, binding of substrates or the active-site inhibitor leads to domain closure, bringing the small and large lobes together[20,21,30]. Comparison of the three structures shows that the locations of the N-terminal SBD domain relative to the catalytic core are divergent among the three structures, likely to be impacted by different crystal packings (Fig. 3c). The hinge residue, Arg[234], is located within the polybasic linker (residues 233–238, KRKKRK) and anchors the N-terminal SBD to the catalytic domain through a salt bridge formed between its guanidinium group and the carboxylate group of Asp[475] and hydrogen bonds to the carbonyl groups of His[473] and Val[459] (Supplementary Fig. 5d). In contrast, the SBD domain itself is relatively rigid, with a superimposable STAC-binding helix-turn-helix (H2-T-H3) motif with only the

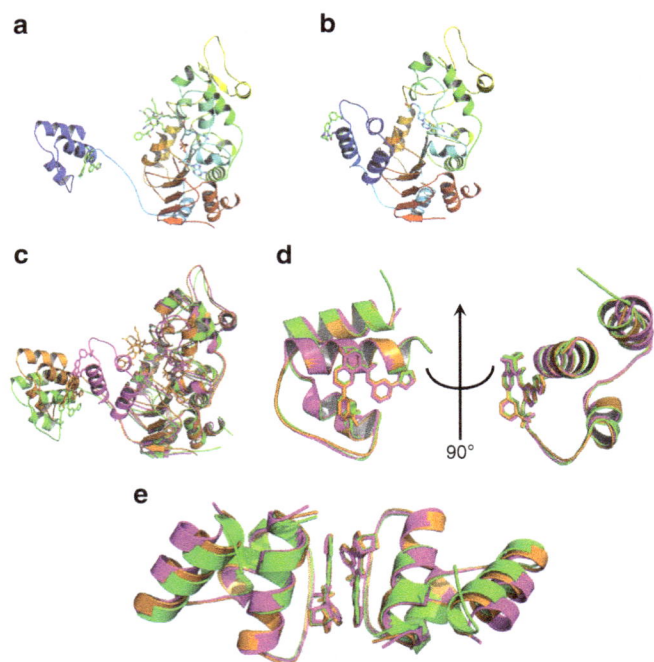

Figure 3 | Structures of Mini-hSIRT1-STAC/ligand complex. (**a**) Structure of mini-hSIRT1/**1**/Ac-p53 7-mer/CarbaNAD quaternary complex. The STAC **1** and Ac-p53 7-mer are shown in green, red and blue for carbon, oxygen and nitrogen atoms. The CarbaNAD is shown in cyan, red, blue and orange for carbon, oxygen, nitrogen and phosphate atoms. The protein ribbon is rainbow-colored from blue at the N-terminus to red at the C-terminus. (**b**) Structure of mini-hSIRT1/**1**/**2** complex. The mini-hSIRT1 shown in this complex is hSIRT1(183–516)-GS-CTR as the same complex containing hSIRT1(183–505)-(GGGS)₂-CTR diffracts to 3.5 Å even though the structures are almost identical. The STAC **1** is shown in green, red and blue for carbon, oxygen and nitrogen atoms. The Inhibitor **2** is shown in cyan, red, blue and yellow for carbon, oxygen, nitrogen and sulfur atoms. The protein ribbon is rainbow-colored from blue at the N-terminus to red at the C-terminus. (**c**) Structural comparison of mini-hSIRT1/**1** complex (green), mini-hSIRT1/**1**/Ac-p53 7-mer/CarbaNAD quaternary complex (orange) and mini-hSIRT1/**1**/**2** complex (magenta). (**d**) Superimposition of the SBD domains from mini-hSIRT1/**1** complex (green), mini-hSIRT1/**1**/Ac-p53 7-mer/CarbaNAD quaternary complex (orange) and mini-hSIRT1/**1**/**2** complex (magenta). (**e**) Comparison of the STAC-mediated dimer interface of mini-hSIRT1/**1** complex (green), mini-hSIRT1/**1**/Ac-p53 7-mer/CarbaNAD quaternary complex (orange) and mini-hSIRT1/**1**/**2** complex (magenta).

first helix tilting out slightly in the mini-hSIRT1/**1**/**2** complex structure (Fig. 3d). The STAC-mediated dimer interface also seems to be conserved among the three structures (Fig. 3e).

Site-directed mutagenesis of the STAC binding pocket. We used site-directed mutagenesis on the full-length hSIRT1 to confirm the key residues of the SBD that were identified by the mini-hSIRT1 structures. The following point mutants of full-length hSIRT1 were generated probing three classes of residues: (a) residues which appear to directly interact with STACs (T219A, I223A, N226A and I227A); (b) SBD residues with no apparent role in activator binding (Q222A and V224A); and (c) Glu[230], previously demonstrated to be important for SIRT1 activation[16] (E230K, E230A and E230Q) (Fig. 2b). None of the mutants significantly impaired the basal catalytic activity using the Ac-p53(W5) substrate or affected inhibition by EX-527, a

Trifluoroacetic acid (TFA)-p53 peptide (Ac-RHK-K^{TFA}-L-Nle-F-NH$_2$), or NAM (Supplementary Tables 4 and 5).

The impact of the mutations on activation was first assessed by comparing the fold-activation of wild-type versus mutant full-length SIRT1 using a structurally diverse set of 246 STACs tested at a fixed concentration of 25 μM. Additionally, we investigated the effect of the mutations on STAC binding versus activation by monitoring shifts in their EC$_{50}$ and maximum activation values respectively using a panel of eight compounds (STACs **1**, **3–9**, Supplementary Fig. 2, Supplementary Tables 6 and 7). T219A, I223A and I227A all exhibit broad impairment of activation with increases in EC$_{50}$ values compared with wild-type hSIRT1, suggesting impaired activator binding consistent with the mini-hSIRT1 structures (Fig. 4a and Supplementary Table 6). Interestingly, I223A was the most compound-dependent mutant, exhibiting both attenuated and enhanced activation, the latter particularly for STACs containing an ortho-CF$_3$ substituted phenyl ring (Fig. 4a and Supplementary Fig. 6a). In the crystal structure, Ile^{223} lies directly beneath the STAC and lines the pocket into which the meta-CF$_3$ of **1** inserts. The cavity created by mutation of Ile^{223} to Ala would be expected to better accommodate an ortho- versus a meta-substitution. This observation further validates the key molecular interactions governing STAC binding indicated in the structure and points to strategies for altering STAC interaction with the SBD.

Asn^{226} appears to form a hydrogen bond between its carboxamide nitrogen and the carbonyl oxygen of **1** on the surface of the protein (Fig. 2b). However, activation of N226A was only minimally impaired compared with the wild type (Fig. 4a). The small contribution from this H-bond is likely because of its high solvent exposure.

In contrast to the above mutants, Q222A and V224A displayed normal activation which is consistent with their positions away from the STAC in the mini-hSIRT1/**1** structure (Fig. 4a and Supplementary Fig. 6b,c). Importantly, all of these data obtained with full-length hSIRT1 are consistent with what the mini-SIRT1 crystal structures predict further validating the biochemical significance of these structures.

Despite the broad impact of the mutations described above, none of them completely abolished activation of hSIRT1 as seen with removal of the SBD. As Ile^{223} lies directly beneath the bound STAC and activation of I223A is highly compound-dependent, we reasoned that further mutating this residue, to incorporate a more disruptive interaction in hSIRT1, would result in a more highly activation-impaired full-length enzyme. To test this hypothesis, we prepared an I223R mutant to introduce steric bulk and charge into the hydrophobic STAC-binding site. Consistent with our hypothesis, activation is completely lost for all 246 activators using both the Ac-p53(W5) or FOXO-3a substrate peptides (Fig. 4b and Supplementary Fig. 6d), while the basal catalytic activity and inhibition by EX-527, TFA-p53 peptide or NAM is not impacted in the I223R mutant (Supplementary Tables 4, 5 and 8). SEC of the STAC-binding deficient mini-hSIRT1 I223R mutant remains the same in the presence of STAC **1**, confirming that the observed mini-hSIRT1 dimerization in solution is mediated by STAC **1**. (Supplementary Fig. 4).

Mutation of Glu^{230} to either Lys or Ala has been recently reported to broadly impair activation by STACs, although the mechanism by which this occurs is unclear[16]. We tested activation of E230K, E230A and E230Q full-length hSIRT1 proteins and found that the maximum activation is impaired with a minimal impact on the EC$_{50}$ (Supplementary Tables 6 and 7), suggesting a role for Glu^{230} in the formation or stabilization of the activated conformation of hSIRT1. Activation of E230Q is also broadly impaired indicating that the negative charge of

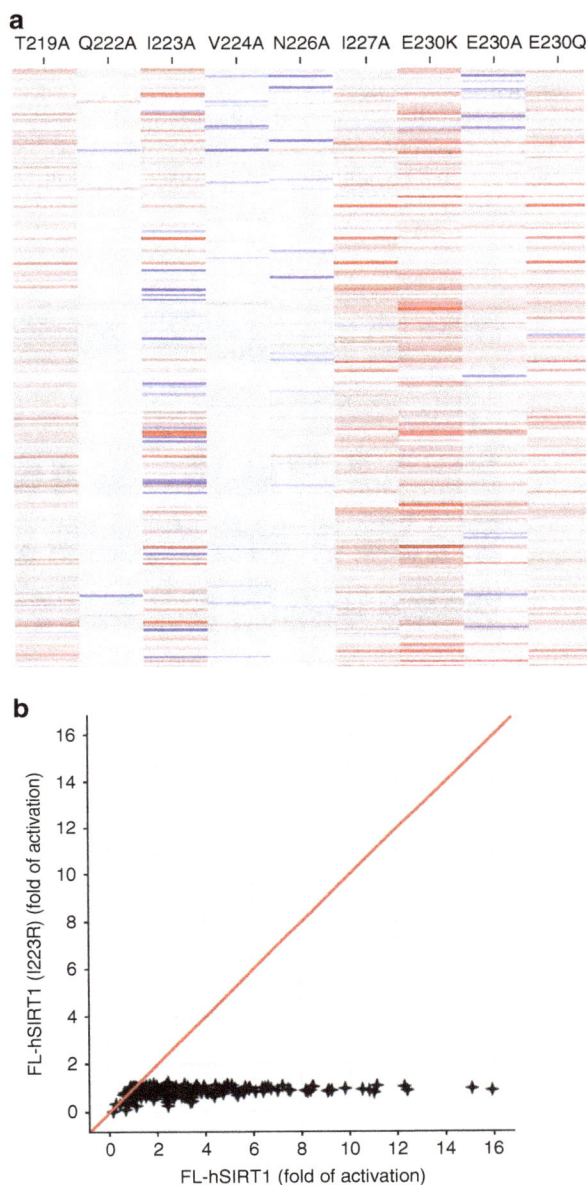

Figure 4 | Activation of full-length hSIRT1 mutants. (**a**) Heat map of the ratio of wild-type/mutant fold-activation for hSIRT1 mutants for each compound from a structurally diverse collection of 246 STACs. Ratios from 0.80 to 1.16 are colored gray. This range covers one s.d. of the mean for V224A (0.98 ± 0.18-fold, Supplementary Fig. 5b) which does not affect activation. Activation impairment denoted as a red gradient (ratios of 1.17/6.78). Activation enhancement is shown as a blue gradient (ratios of 0.78/0.24). (**b**) Comparison of the fold-activation of I223R versus wild-type hSIRT1 with a structurally diverse collection of STACs. All of the data were generated with the OAADPr assay using the Ac-p53(W5) substrate. A different compound set (~250 STACs) was used for the site-directed mutagenesis studies compared with that used for the initial characterization of mini-hSIRT1 (~80 STACs).

Glu^{230} is important for stabilizing the activated conformation of hSIRT1 and likely interacts with a positively charged residue in the activated state.

Allosteric coupling between STAC and substrate binding. We further probed the role of Glu^{230} in STAC-mediated activation using HDX-MS which revealed that, in contrast to wild-type hSIRT1, STAC binding to the E230K mutant no longer confers protection around the peptide-binding site in the E230K/1/Ac-p53(W5) complex (Fig. 5a and Supplementary Fig. 7). This indicates that the E230K mutation may negatively affect the coupling between the STAC and substrate-binding sites. The HDX-MS and activation data together suggest that Glu230 is not directly involved in STAC binding but is instead, a critical residue

mediating the coupling of STAC and substrate binding to promote activation.

The observation that regions outside STAC-binding site and substrate-binding site show minimal perturbation in HDX-MS in the presence of both ligands suggests the possibility that the two binding sites might be physically close to each other in the activated conformation. Given this observation and the

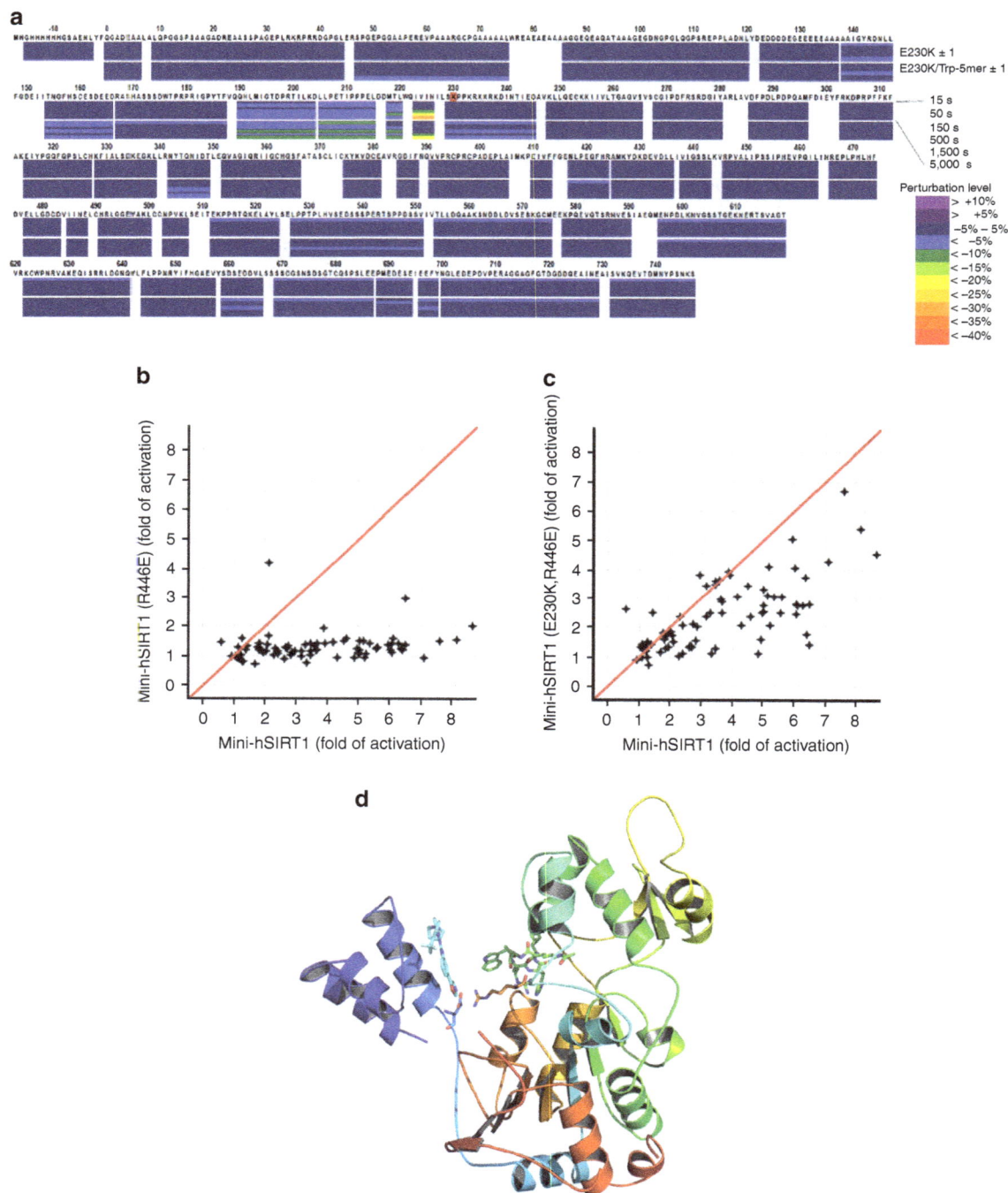

Figure 5 | E230K impairs the coupling between STAC and substrate binding and potential role of an electrostatic interaction between Glu230 and Arg446 in the activated conformation. (**a**) Heat map of the HDX-MS perturbation of binding of **1** to hSIRT1(E230K) in the absence or presence of Ac-p53(W5) at six different time points (15–5000 s). (**b**) Pivot plot of the STAC activation of mini-hSIRT1(R446E) versus mini-hSIRT1. (**c**) Pivot plot of the STAC activation of the double charge-reversal mutant mini-hSIRT1(R446E/E230K) versus mini-hSIRT1. (**d**) Speculative model of the activated conformation of SIRT1. Glu230 and Arg446 are shown in stick representation. The protein ribbon is rainbow-colored from blue at the N-terminus to red at the C-terminus. **1** and modeled Ac-p53(W5) are shown in cyan and green, respectively.

importance of the negative charge of Glu^{230} for activation, we postulated that Arg^{446} located at the active site might be a possible electrostatic partner for Glu^{230}, stabilizing the activated conformation of hSIRT1 and mediating the observed coupling. To this end, we made the mini-hSIRT1 R446E/E230K double mutant with E230K and R446E mini-hSIRT1 as controls. Mini-hSIRT1(E230K) mutant does not affect the basal catalytic activity using the Ac-p53(W5) substrate, as observed in full-length SIRT1 (Supplementary Table 2). Both mini-hSIRT1(R446E) mutant and mini-hSIRT1(E230K,R446E) mutant show higher K_M values for both peptide substrate and NAD$^+$, which might result from the potential hydrophobic interaction between the aliphatic part of Arg^{446} side chain and the substrate as R446F mutant does not affect the basal catalytic activity (Supplementary Table 2). Whereas either E230K or R446E results in significant attenuation of STAC activation of mini-hSIRT1, the E230K,R446E double mutant partially restores STAC-mediated activation of mini-hSIRT1 compared with E230K or R446E, supporting the importance of potential electrostatic interaction between Glu^{230} and Arg^{446} in the activated conformation (Fig. 5b,c).

Discussion

In this study, we describe the design and construction of a functional mini-hSIRT1 that recapitulates three key features of full-length hSIRT1: (1) the steady-state enzyme kinetics and inhibition; (2) the STAC activation profile across multiple chemotypes; and (3) STAC activation impairment by E230K mutation. We used this mini-hSIRT1 construct to obtain the first reported crystallographic structure of hSIRT1 with a bound STAC. The biochemical and structural characterization confirms the hSIRT1 intramolecular interactions between the CTR and catalytic domain, which enhance the basal deacetylation activity of hSIRT1. The structures of the mini-hSIRT1-STAC complex reveal the detailed architecture of the STAC-binding site, which was validated in full-length hSIRT1 by site-directed mutagenesis. The STAC-binding site appears to be a shallow hydrophobic surface depression, which matches the flat and hydrophobic nature of the STACs. Consequently, the mini-hSIRT1-STAC structure reported here provides important information for future structure-based drug design. In addition, we demonstrated the coupling between the STAC-binding site and the active site using HDX-MS, which is impaired by the previously reported E230K mutant. Structure-based mutagenesis suggested that the electrostatic interaction between Glu^{230} and Arg^{446} might stabilize the activated conformation. The exact nature of the activated conformation is still elusive. Apparently, Glu^{230} and Arg^{446} in the reported structure are too far to make electrostatic interactions. Modeling with the N-terminal SBD treated as a rigid body to rotate around the hinge point Arg^{234} suggests that rotating the SBD around Arg^{234} could bring Glu^{230} close to Arg^{446}, which interestingly also bring the STAC **1** close to the active site, esp. the hydrophobic side chain of the modeled Ac-p53(W5) (Fig. 5d). This model is highly speculative and needs to be tested experimentally, but does seem to be attractive as it might help to explain the requirement of some hydrophobic moiety on the peptide for SIRT1 activation by STACs, by participating in the composite activator-binding site and facilitating the formation of the activated conformation. However, some key questions remain to be answered with further investigation: (1) is the observed STAC induced SIRT1 dimer relevant for SIRT1 activation by STACs? (2) How does the STAC binding in the N-terminal SBD enhance the substrate binding at the active site, which is not obvious from the comparison of current structures of Mini-SIRT1/**1** and Mini-SIRT1/**1**/ p53 7-mer/CarbaNAD? (3) Does STAC binding itself induce conformational change of the N-terminal SBD, in other words, what does apo Mini-SIRT1 look like? The current structures served as a stepping stone to answer these important questions and elucidate the mechanism of activation of SIRT1 by STACs. In summary, the results presented here provide unambiguous visual and functional proof of direct allosteric activation of hSIRT1 by small molecules, and provide a basis for further elucidation of the mechanism of hSIRT1 activation by STACs.

Methods

Protein cloning, expression and purification. Mini-hSIRT1 constructs were cloned into a modified pET21b vector (Novagen). The protein was expressed in *Escherichia coli* BL21-Gold (DE3) cells (Stratagene) as an N-terminal fusion to a hexahistidine affinity tag with integrated Tobacco Etch Virus (TEV) protease site. A single colony was inoculated in LB media containing 100 μg ml^{-1} ampicillin at 37 °C, 250 r.p.m. until the A_{600} reached 0.3. The culture was then transferred to 16 °C, 250 r.p.m. until the A_{600} reached 0.6. Isopropyl 1-thio-β-D-galactopyranoside was added to a final concentration of 0.2 mM, and expression was continued at 16 °C, 250 r.p.m. overnight. Cells were collected by centrifugation, and the pellet was resuspended in lysis buffer (25 mM HEPES, pH 7.5, 200 mM NaCl, 5% glycerol and 5 mM 2-mercaptoethanol) and sonicated to break the cells. Supernatant was separated from cell debris by centrifugation at 10,000g for 40 min at 4 °C and loaded onto a Ni-NTA column (Qiagen) that equilibrated with the buffer containing 25 mM HEPES, pH 7.5, 200 mM NaCl, 5% glycerol, 5 mM 2-mercaptoethanol and 20 mM imidazole. The column was washed with five column volumes of the buffer containing 25 mM HEPES, pH 7.5, 200 mM NaCl, 5% glycerol, 5 mM 2-mercaptoethanol and 50 mM imidazole, and eluted with the buffer containing 25 mM HEPES, pH 7.5, 200 mM NaCl, 5% glycerol, 5 mM 2-mercaptoethanol and 250 mM imidazole. The eluted protein was dialyzed in lysis buffer and digested with TEV protease (Invitrogen) to remove the N-terminal His tag at 4 °C overnight. The protein was loaded on a second Ni-NTA column equilibrated with lysis buffer. The untagged protein was eluted by the buffer containing 25 mM HEPES, pH 7.5, 200 mM NaCl, 5% glycerol, 5 mM 2-mercaptoethanol and 5 mM imidazole. The purified protein was dialyzed against the dialyzing buffer containing 20 mM Tris-HCl, pH 8.0, 250 mM NaCl, 5% glycerol and 10 mM dithiothreitol, and concentrated. The protein was further purified by a S200 column (GE Healthcare) to 95% purity as assessed by SDS–polyacrylamide gel electrophoresis analysis stained by Coomassie Brilliant Blue R-250 and concentrated to 10–15 mg ml^{-1} in the dialyzing buffer.

Full-length human SIRT1 (hSIRT1) proteins were expressed with a N-terminal His$_6$ tag and purified as described in Hubbard *et al.*[16] except for Q222A, and I223R SIRT1 which were purified using an ÄKTAxpress (GE Lifesciences). Each cell paste was resuspended in buffer A (50 mM Tris-HCl pH 7.5, 250 mM NaCl, 25 mM imidazole and 0.1 mM TCEP) with 1,000 U Benzonase nuclease (Sigma-Aldrich, St Louis, MO, USA) supplemented with cOmplete, EDTA-free Protease Inhibitor Cocktail Tablets (Roche) on ice. Cells were disrupted by pulse sonication with 50% on and 50% off for 12 min total at 40 W. Insoluble debris was removed by centrifugation. Clarified supernatant was directly loaded onto a 1 ml HisTrap FF Crude column (GE Lifesciences). After washing with buffer A, SIRT1 was eluted with buffer B (50 mM Tris-HCl pH 7.5, 250 mM NaCl, 500 mM imidazole and 0.1 mM TCEP). Protein was further purified by SEC in buffer C (50 mM Tris-HCl pH 7.5, 300 mM NaCl and 0.1 mM TCEP) using a Hi-load Superdex 200 16/60 column (GE Lifesciences). Enzyme concentrations were determined by Bradford assay using bovine serum albumin (BSA) as a standard. Final protein purity was assessed by gel densitometry. Proteins were confirmed by liquid chromatography/ mass spectrometry. All proteins were greater than 90% pure except V224A and T219A (80%) and E230A (85%).

SIRT1 deacetylation reactions. SIRT1 deacetylation reactions were performed in reaction buffer (50 mM HEPES-NaOH, pH 7.5, 150 mM NaCl, 1 mM dithiothreitol and 1% dimethylsulfoxide (DMSO)) at 25 °C monitoring either NAM production using the continuous PNC1/GDH coupled assay[32] or O-acetyl ADP ribose (OAcADPr) production by mass spectrometry[16]. Final concentrations of the PNC1/GDH coupling system components used were 20 units per ml bovine GDH (Sigma-Aldrich), 1 μM yeast PNC1, 3.4 mM α-ketoglutarate and 220 μM NADH or NADPH. An extinction coefficient of 6.22 mM^{-1}cm^{-1} and a pathlength of 0.81 cm were used to convert the absorbance at 340 nm to product concentration for the 150 μl reactions used. Assays monitoring OAcADPr production were performed in reaction buffer with 0.05% BSA and time points were taken by quenching the deacetylation reaction with a stop solution which gave a final concentration of 1% formic acid and 5 mM NAM. Quenched reactions were diluted fivefold with 1:1 acetonitrile:methanol and spun at 5,000g for 10 min to precipitate protein before being analyzed with an Agilent RapidFire 200 High-Throughput Mass Spectrometry System (Agilent, Wakefield, MA) coupled to an ABSciex API 4000 mass spectrometer fitted with an electrospray ionization source. The p53-based Ac-p53(W5) (Ac-RHKKAcW-NH2) and FOXO-3a 21-mer (Ac-SADDSPSQLSKAcWPGSPTSRSS-NH2) peptides were obtained from Biopeptide. Deacetylation assays used the Ac-p53(W5) substrate unless otherwise noted.

Substrate K_M determinations were performed by varying one substrate concentration at a fixed, saturating concentration of the second substrate. SIRT1 activation and inhibition assays were run in reaction buffer with 0.05% BSA at 25 °C and analyzed using the OAcADPr assay. Enzyme and compound were preincubated for 20 min before addition of substrates. For the activation screen of full-length hSIRT1, a structurally diverse set of 246 compounds was tested in duplicate at a final concentration of 25 μM each. In order to be sensitive to K_M-modulating activators, substrate concentrations of approximately one-tenth their K_M values were used. The dose-dependence of eight compounds was tested and the fold-activation data were described by equation (1)

$$\frac{v_x}{v_o} = b + \frac{RV_{max} - b}{1 + \frac{EC_{50}}{[X]_o}} \quad (1)$$

where v_x/v_0 is the ratio of the reaction rate in the presence (v_x) versus absence (v_0) of activator (X), RV_{max} is the relative velocity at infinite activator concentration, EC_{50} is the concentration of activator required to produce one-half RV_{max} and b is the minimum value of v_x/v_0.

SEC assay. The assays were performed with a Superdex 75 10/300 GL column (GE healthcare) injecting 100 μl samples containing 10 μM mini-hSIRT1 in the absence or presence of 100 μM STAC, dissolved in 50 mM HEPES-NaOH, pH 7.5, 150 mM NaCl and 0.5 mM TCEP. Binding reactions were incubated for 1 h at room temperature before injection into the column.

HDX-MS. On-exchange experiment of SIRT1. H/D-exchange reactions followed by pepsin digestion, desalting, high-performance liquid chromatographic separation and mass spectrometric analysis were carried out using a fully automated system, described in detail elsewhere[22]. Particular to this set of experiments, on-exchange reactions were initiated by mixing 20 μl of a SIRT1 stock solution (0.77 mg ml^{-1} SIRT1, ± 3.88 mM Ac-p53(W5), ± 192 μM ligand, in 1.9% DMSO) and 20 μl of 100 mM phosphate, pH read 7.0 in D2O. The 50% D$_2$O mixture was incubated at 0 °C for 15, 50, 150, 500, 1,500 or 5,000 s. For SIRT1 (229–516), on-exchange reactions were initiated by mixing 4 μl of a SIRT1 stock solution (1.36 mg ml^{-1} SIRT1 (229–516), ± 1.67 mM CTR peptide) and 36 μl of 200 mM phosphate, pH read 7.0 in D2O. The 90% D2O mixture was incubated at 0 °C for 15, 50, 150, 500, 1,500, or 5,000 s. Addition of 20 μl of 1.6 M guanidine hydrochloride (GuHCl), 0.8% formic acid, pH 2.3, quenched the on-exchange reaction immediately prior to being analyzed.

General protein process for standard HDX sample. The quenched solution was passed through a pepsin column (104 μl bed volume) filled with porcine pepsin (Sigma) immobilized on Poros 20 AL media (Life Technologies, Carlsbad, CA, USA) per the manufacturer's instructions, with 0.05% aqueous TFA (200 μl min^{-1}) for 2 min. The digested fragments were temporarily collected onto a reverse phase trap column (4 μl bed volume) and desalted. The peptide fragments were then eluted from the trap column and separated by a C18 column (BioBasic-18; Thermo Scientific, San Jose, CA, USA) with a linear gradient of 13% solvent B to 40% solvent B over 23 min (solvent A, 0.05% TFA in water; solvent B, 95% acetonitrile, 5% buffer A; flow rate 10 μl min^{-1}). Mass spectrometric analyses were

carried out using a LTQ OrbiTrap XL mass spectrometer (Thermo Fisher Scientific) with capillary temperature at 200 °C.

Digestion/separation optimization and nondeuterated experiment of SIRT1. Before H/D-exchange experiment, digestion and separation conditions were optimized to yield high sequence coverage of SIRT1 by peptic fragments with high resolution under nondeuterated conditions. In this step, a mixture of 20 μl of 0.77 mg ml^{-1} (9.2 μM) SIRT1 and 20 μl of H2O was quenched by the addition of 20 μl of various acidic buffers. For SIRT1 (229–516), a mixture of 4 μl of a SIRT1 stock solution (1.36 mg ml^{-1} SIRT1 (229–516) and ± 1.67 mM CTR peptide) and 36 μl of H2O was quenched by the addition of 20 μl of various acidic buffers. The quenched mixtures were subjected to aforementioned general protein process. The nondeuterated peptic fragments were identified by Sequest in Proteome Discoverer 1.1 (Thermo Fisher Scientific).

Fully deuterated experiment of SIRT1. The fully deuterated sample was prepared by incubating a mixture of 45 μl of 0.77 mg ml^{-1} (9.2 μM) SIRT1 with 45 μl of 100 mM TCEP in D2O, pH 2.5 at 60 °C for 3 h. For SIRT1 (229–516), the fully deuterated sample was prepared by incubating a mixture of 9 μl of 1.36 mg ml^{-1} (41.7 μM) SIRT1 (229–516) with 81 μl of 100 mM TCEP in D2O, pH 2.5 at 60 °C for 3 h. After incubation, the sample was kept at 0 °C before being quenched identically to an on-exchanged solution and subjected to the general protein process.

Determination of deuteration level of each peptide after on-exchange reaction. The centroids of peptide isotopic envelopes were measured using the in-house-program developed in collaboration with Sierra Analytics (Modesto, CA, USA). Corrections for back-exchange during the protein processing step were made employing the following standard equation equation (2):

$$\text{Deuteration level}(\%) = \frac{m(P) - m(N)}{m(F) - m(N)} \times 100 \quad (2)$$

where $m(P)$, $m(N)$ and $m(F)$ are the centroid value of partially deuterated (on-exchanged) peptide, nondeuterated peptide and fully deuterated peptide, respectively.

Protein crystallization, data collection and structure determination. The crystals of mini-hSIRT1/1 binary complex were obtained by hanging drop vapor diffusion method at 18 °C. The crystals appeared overnight and grew to a final size of ~0.1 × 0.1 × 0.1 mm within 2 days. 10 mg ml^{-1} protein was incubated with compound 1 for ~1 h and the molar ratio of compound 1:protein is 5:1 with 1% DMSO. The drop was composed of 1 μl of protein/compound mixture and 1 μl crystallization buffer of 0.2 M Magnesium chloride, 0.1 M Tris pH 8.5, and 16% w/v PEG 4000. The crystals of mini-hSIRT1/1/2 were obtained by hanging drop vapor diffusion method at 18 °C. The crystals appeared overnight and grew to a final size of ~0.1 × 0.1 × 0.1 mm within 2 days. 10 mg ml^{-1} protein was incubated with compound 1 for about 1 h, then incubated with compound 2 for 2 h and the molar ratio of compound 1:compound 2:protein is 5:5:1 with 2% DMSO. The drop was composed of 1 μl of protein/compound mixture and 1 μl crystallization buffer of 0.55 M Sodium chloride, 0.1 M MES pH 6.5 and 20% w/v PEG 4000. The crystals of mini-hSIRT1/1/p53-7mer/carbaNAD complex were obtained by hanging drop vapor diffusion method at 18 °C. The crystals appeared overnight and grew to a

Table 1 | Data processing and refinement statistics.

	Mini-SIRT1/1	Mini-SIRT1/1/2	Mini-SIRT1/1/ p53 7-mer/CarbaNAD
Data collection			
Resolution (Å)*	45.67-3.10 (3.18-3.10)	39.98-2.73 (2.81-2.73)	91.36-2.74 (2.81-2.74)
Space group	I2₁2₁2₁	P6122	I4122
Unit-cell parameters			
a (Å)	99.19	122.15	94.51
b (Å)	111.64	122.15	94.51
c (Å)	132.52	104.92	356.84
Completeness (%)*	99.5 (99.8)	99.9 (100.0)	99.5 (99.4)
Redundancy*	4.8 (4.9)	17.6 (18.2)	9.6 (9.9)
Average I/σI*	17.4 (2.0)	38.8 (4.0)	20.7 (3.3)
Rmerge (%)*	6.7 (78.1)	5.3 (80.3)	8.2 (82.9)
Refinement			
Resolution (Å)*	45.67-3.10 (3.34-3.10)	39.98-2.73 (3.01-2.73)	45.68-2.74 (2.87-2.74)
R_{work} (%)*	18.7 (29.7)	19.1 (23.7)	18.3 (27.3)
R_{free} (%)*	23.8 (37.7)	23.5 (30.0)	22.1 (33.2)
r.m.s.d In bond lengths (Å)	0.006	0.004	0.005
r.m.s.d in bond angles (°)	1.039	0.898	0.938
Mean B factors (Å2)	103.3	92.0	71.9

*Values in parentheses are for the highest-resolution shell.

final size of ~0.1 × 0.1 × 0.1 mm within 2 days. 10 mg/ml protein was incubated with compound **1** for about 1 h, then incubated with p53-7mer and CarbaNAD for 2 h and the molar ratio of compound **1**:p53-7mer: CarbaNAD:protein is 5:5:10:1 with 1% DMSO. The drop was composed of 1 μl of the protein/compound/substrate mixture and 1 μl of the crystallization buffer of 5% v/v Tacsimate, pH.00.1 M HEPES pH 7.0 and 10% w/v PEG 5000 MME.

The crystals were cryo-protected in mother liquor containing 20% glycerol before being flash-frozen in liquid nitrogen. Diffraction data were collected at SSRF BL17U1, APS 21-ID-D or APS 21-ID-G beamlines at 100 K and processed using the Xia2 program[33]. The molecular replacement software Phaser[34] was used to solve the structure with a search model containing residues 242–494 based on the homolog model of SIRT3 (PDB code: 3GLU) initially and later also with a search model of SIRT1 (PDB code 4IG9) when available. Iterative structure refinement and model building were performed between Phenix.refine[35] and Coot[36]. Bulk solvent correction and Translation/Libration/Screw-motion (TLS) refinement were used during the refinement and model building. Detailed information regarding the diffraction data, refinement and structure statistics is listed in Table 1.

Details of the chemical compounds synthesismethods are provided in Supplementary Methods.

References

1. Finkel, T., Deng, C. X. & Mostoslavsky, R. Recent progress in the biology and physiology of sirtuins. *Nature* **460**, 587–591 (2009).
2. Baur, J. A., Ungvari, Z., Minor, R. K., Le Couteur, D. G. & de Cabo, R. Are sirtuins viable targets for improving healthspan and lifespan? *Nat. Rev. Drug. Discov.* **11**, 443–461 (2012).
3. Frye, R. A. Phylogenetic classification of prokaryotic and eukaryotic Sir2-like proteins. *Biochem. Biophys. Res. Commun.* **273**, 793–798 (2000).
4. Haigis, M. C. & Sinclair, D. A. Mammalian sirtuins: biological insights and disease relevance. *Annu. Rev. Pathol.* **5**, 253–295 (2010).
5. Verdin, E., Hirschey, M. D., Finley, L. W. & Haigis, M. C. Sirtuin regulation of mitochondria: energy production, apoptosis, and signaling. *Trends. Biochem. Sci.* **35**, 669–675 (2010).
6. Haigis, M. C. & Guarente, L. P. Mammalian sirtuins–emerging roles in physiology, aging, and calorie restriction. *Genes Dev.* **20**, 2913–2921 (2006).
7. Sebastian, C., Satterstrom, F. K., Haigis, M. C. & Mostoslavsky, R. From sirtuin biology to human diseases: an update. *J. Biol. Chem.* **287**, 42444–42452 (2012).
8. Banks, A. S. *et al.* SirT1 gain of function increases energy efficiency and prevents diabetes in mice. *Cell. Metab.* **8**, 333–341 (2008).
9. Kim, D. *et al.* SIRT1 deacetylase protects against neurodegeneration in models for Alzheimer's disease and amyotrophic lateral sclerosis. *EMBO. J.* **26**, 3169–3179 (2007).
10. Yoshizaki, T. *et al.* SIRT1 inhibits inflammatory pathways in macrophages and modulates insulin sensitivity. *Am. J. Physiol. Endocrinol. Metab.* **298**, E419–E428 (2009).
11. Yoshizaki, T. *et al.* SIRT1 exerts anti-inflammatory effects and improves insulin sensitivity in adipocytes. *Mol. Cell. Biol.* **29**, 1363–1374 (2009).
12. Milne, J. C. *et al.* Small molecule activators of SIRT1 as therapeutics for the treatment of type 2 diabetes. *Nature* **450**, 712–716 (2007).
13. Dai, H. *et al.* SIRT1 activation by small molecules: kinetic and biophysical evidence for direct interaction of enzyme and activator. *J. Biol. Chem.* **285**, 32695–32703 (2010).
14. Howitz, K. T. *et al.* Small molecule activators of sirtuins extend *Saccharomyces cerevisiae* lifespan. *Nature* **425**, 191–196 (2003).
15. Pacholec, M. *et al.* SRT1720, SRT2183, SRT1460, and resveratrol are not direct activators of SIRT1. *J. Biol. Chem.* **285**, 8340–8351 (2010).
16. Hubbard, B. P. *et al.* Evidence for a common mechanism of SIRT1 regulation by allosteric activators. *Science* **339**, 1216–1219 (2013).
17. Zhao, X. *et al.* The 2.5A crystal structure of the sirt1 catalytic domain bound to nicotinamide adenine dinucleotide (NAD(+)) and an indole (EX527 analogue) reveals a novel mechanism of histone deacetylase inhibition. *J. Med. Chem.* **56**, 963–969 (2013).
18. Davenport, A. M., Huber, F. M. & Hoelz, A. Structural and functional analysis of human SIRT1. *J. Mol. Biol.* **426**, 526–541 (2014).
19. Yuan, H. & Marmorstein, R. Structural basis for sirtuin activity and inhibition. *J. Biol. Chem.* **287**, 42428–42435 (2012).
20. Jin, L. *et al.* Crystal structures of human SIRT3 displaying substrate-induced conformational changes. *J. Biol. Chem.* **284**, 24394–24405 (2009).
21. Szczepankiewicz, B. G. *et al.* Synthesis of carba-NAD and the structures of its ternary complexes with SIRT3 and SIRT5. *J. Org. Chem.* **77**, 7319–7329 (2012).
22. Hamuro, Y. *et al.* Rapid analysis of protein structure and dynamics by hydrogen/deuterium exchange mass spectrometry. *J. Biomol. Tech.* **14**, 171–182 (2003).
23. Kang, H. *et al.* Peptide switch is essential for Sirt1 deacetylase activity. *Mol. Cell.* **44**, 203–213 (2011).
24. Pan, M., Yuan, H., Brent, M., Ding, E. C. & Marmorstein, R. SIRT1 contains N- and C-terminal regions that potentiate deacetylase activity. *J. Biol. Chem.* **287**, 2468–2476 (2012).
25. Robinson, C. R. & Sauer, R. T. Optimizing the stability of single-chain proteins by linker length and composition mutagenesis. *Proc. Natl. Acad. Sci. USA* **95**, 5929–5934 (1998).
26. Napper, A. D. *et al.* Discovery of indoles as potent and selective inhibitors of the deacetylase SIRT1. *J. Med. Chem.* **48**, 8045–8054 (2005).
27. Lakshminarasimhan, M. *et al.* Molecular architecture of the human protein deacetylase Sirt1 and its regulation by AROS and resveratrol. *Biosci. Rep.* **33**, 395–404 (2013).
28. Vu, C. B. *et al.* Discovery of imidazo[1,2-b]thiazole derivatives as novel SIRT1 activators. *J. Med. Chem.* **52**, 1275–1283 (2009).
29. Hsu, H. C. *et al.* (2013) Structural basis for allosteric stimulation of Sir2 activity by Sir4 binding. *Genes Dev.* **27**, 64–73 (2013).
30. Disch, J. S. *et al.* Discovery of thieno[3,2-d]pyrimidine-6-carboxamides as potent inhibitors of SIRT1, SIRT2, and SIRT3. *J. Med. Chem.* **56**, 3666–3679 (2013).
31. Sanders, B. D., Jackson, B. & Marmorstein, R. Structural basis for sirtuin function: what we know and what we don't. *Biochim. Biophys. Acta* **1804**, 1604–1616 (2010).
32. Smith, B. C., Hallows, W. C. & Denu, J. M. A continuous microplate assay for sirtuins and nicotinamide-producing enzymes. *Anal. Biochem.* **394**, 101–109 (2009).
33. Winter, G. xia2: An expert system for macromolecular crystallography data reduction. *J. Appl. Crystallogr.* **43**, 186–190 (2010).
34. McCoy, A. J. *et al.* Phaser crystallographic software. *J. Appl. Crystallogr.* **40**, 658–674 (2007).
35. Adams, P. D. *et al.* PHENIX: building new software for automated crystallographic structure determination. *Acta Crystallogr. D Biol. Crystallogr.* **58**, 1948–1954 (2002).
36. Emsley, P. & Cowtan, K. Coot: model-building tools for molecular graphics. *Acta Crystallogr. D Biol. Crystallogr.* **60**, 2126–2132 (2004).

Acknowledgements

We thank Meidy Lontoh, Sara Grab and Eli Schuman for compound plating and logistics. We are grateful for supervision of protein production and X-ray diffraction data collection by Derek Ren, Wentao Wei and Jianhua Cai at Viva Biotech. We thank Matthew Lochansky for HRMS analysis and Karen A. Evans, Minghui Wang and Yanqiu Qian for NMR analysis. The authors also thank Vipin Suri, Christine Loh, Nino Campobasso, Kevin Madauss, Marti Head, Andrew Maynard, William H. Miller, David A. Sinclair and Leonard P. Guarente for helpful discussion.

Author contributions

H.D.,D.Q.,and F.J. contributed to the structural biology experiments. H.D., A.W.C., T.V.R., T.C., B.P. and F.B. contributed to the enzymology experiments. H.D., J.E. and Y.H. contributed to the HDX-MS experiments. H.Z., Y.J., D.Q., B.W. and J.W. contributed to the protein expression, purification and characterization. C.A.B., J.S.D, R.C., B.S., C.O., P.Y.N., B.H.W., R.C., R.N., K.K. and M.W. contributed to the preparation and characterization of the final compounds or intermediates. H.D., T.V.R., S.M.S and B.S. designed the project. H.D., T.V.R., S.M.S, B.S., C.M., E.H., J.C.W., R.B.P., G.P.V. and J.L.E. supervised the project. H.D., T.V.R. J.C.W., R.B.P., G.P.V., and J.L.E. wrote the manuscript. All authors critically read and contributed to the manuscript.

Additional information

Accession codes. The atomic coordinates of the crystal structures of the mini-hSIRT1/1 complex, the mini-hSIRT1/2 complex, and the mini-hSIRT1/1/p53-7mer/carbaNAD complex have been deposited in the Protein Data Bank (accession codes 4ZZH, 4ZZI and4ZZJ).

Competing financial interests: H.D., A.W.C., T.V.R., T.C., H.Z., Y.J., S.M.S., B.P., B.S., C.A.B., J.S.D., R.C., B.S., C.O., P.Y.N., B.H.W., R.C., R.N., K.K., F.B., M.W., E.H., J.C.W., R.B.P., G.P.V. and J.L.E. are employees GlaxoSmithKline. Patent applications relating to the synthetic compounds have been filed.

13

Selenoether oxytocin analogues have analgesic properties in a mouse model of chronic abdominal pain

Aline Dantas de Araujo[1], Mehdi Mobli[1,2], Joel Castro[3,4], Andrea M. Harrington[3,4], Irina Vetter[1], Zoltan Dekan[1], Markus Muttenthaler[1,†], JingJing Wan[1], Richard J. Lewis[1], Glenn F. King[1], Stuart M. Brierley[3,4,5] & Paul F. Alewood[1]

Poor oral availability and susceptibility to reduction and protease degradation is a major hurdle in peptide drug development. However, drugable receptors in the gut present an attractive niche for peptide therapeutics. Here we demonstrate, in a mouse model of chronic abdominal pain, that oxytocin receptors are significantly upregulated in nociceptors innervating the colon. Correspondingly, we develop chemical strategies to engineer non-reducible and therefore more stable oxytocin analogues. Chemoselective selenide macrocyclization yields stabilized analogues equipotent to native oxytocin. Ultra-high-field nuclear magnetic resonance structural analysis of native oxytocin and the seleno-oxytocin derivatives reveals that oxytocin has a pre-organized structure in solution, in marked contrast to earlier X-ray crystallography studies. Finally, we show that these seleno-oxytocin analogues potently inhibit colonic nociceptors both *in vitro* and *in vivo* in mice with chronic visceral hypersensitivity. Our findings have potentially important implications for clinical use of oxytocin analogues and disulphide-rich peptides in general.

[1] Institute for Molecular Bioscience, The University of Queensland, St Lucia, Queensland 4072, Australia. [2] Centre for Advanced Imaging, The University of Queensland, St Lucia, Queensland 4072, Australia. [3] Nerve-Gut Research Laboratory, Discipline of Medicine, The University of Adelaide, Adelaide, South Australia 5000, Australia. [4] Department of Gastroenterology & Hepatology, Hanson Institute, Royal Adelaide Hospital, Adelaide, South Australia 5000, Australia. [5] Discipline of Physiology, Faculty of Health Sciences, The University of Adelaide, Adelaide, South Australia 5000, Australia. † Present address: Departments of Chemistry and Molecular Pharmacology, The Institute for Research in Biomedicine, C/Baldiri Reixac 10, 08028 Barcelona, Spain. Correspondence and requests for materials should be addressed to S.M.B. (email: stuart.brierley@adelaide.edu.au) or to P.F.A. (email: p.alewood@imb.uq.edu.au).

Since its discovery over a century ago, few bioactive peptides have proven to be more important and widely studied than the peptide hormone oxytocin (OT)[1]. OT was the first peptide hormone to be sequenced and synthesized, an achievement recognized with the award of the 1955 Nobel Prize in Chemistry to Vincent du Vigneaud[2]. OT has since become widely used in obstetrics to induce labour, prevent post-partum haemorrhage and stimulate lactation in nursing mothers[3]. In the central nervous system, OT functions as a neurotransmitter involved in complex social interactions, including maternal behaviour, partnership and social bonding[4]. Recent studies have shown that OT function (and that of the closely related hormone vasopressin) is impaired in brain disorders associated with social dysfunction such as autism, social anxiety, stress and schizophrenia, triggering an explosion of interest in the use of OT for treatment of mental conditions[5,6]. OT receptors have also attracted attention for their role in memory[7], breast cancer tumour growth[8] and visceral pain[9,10]. Nasal administration of OT reduces abdominal pain and discomfort in patients with chronic idiopathic constipation[9], whereas continuous intravenous OT significantly increases thresholds for visceral perception in patients with Irritable Bowel Syndrome (IBS)[10]. The mechanisms underlying these effects remain unclear and are important to determine as chronic abdominal pain represents a major clinical problem, with IBS alone affecting $\sim 11\%$ of the Western population[11].

With many clinical trials currently underway to investigate OT effects in a wide range of diseases[12] it is imperative to advance strategies that improve the metabolic stability and drug-like properties of this unique signaling hormone and neurotransmitter. In this study, we disclose several insights into OT. We describe the well-defined structure of OT in aqueous solution and present an efficient strategy for production of more stable analogues based on seleno-chemistry. Finally, we demonstrate that OT receptor expression and function is significantly upregulated in colonic neurons of mice with chronic visceral hypersensitivity (CVH) and show that stable OT analogues are potently analgesic in this animal model of chronic abdominal pain. Taken together, our results indicate that stable OT analogues have significant potential for the treatment of chronic abdominal pain associated with conditions such as IBS.

Results

OT analogues with an engineered selenoether bridge.
OT is a cyclic peptide comprising nine amino-acid residues with a single disulphide bridge between the first and sixth residues. The disulphide bond is critical for binding to the OT receptor; however, it renders the peptide susceptible to endogenous reductive degradation[3]. Although replacement of the labile bridge with a more redox-stable linkage is an attractive approach to improve the metabolic integrity of OT, it is non-trivial for OT, as its biological activity is sensitive to minute structural modifications within the cyclic framework. Even minor distortions such as increasing the 20-membered ring by one methylene group[13], substitution of Cys1 by penicillamine[14] or replacement of the disulphide bond by an amide[15], lanthionine[16] or dicarba[17] bond leads to a significant decrease in agonist activity. In contrast, OT bioactivity is retained when the OT S-S bond is replaced by chalcogen linkages such as cystathionine (CH$_2$-S, Ctt), diselenide (Se-Se), selenylsulphide (Se-S) and ditelluride (Te-Te) bonds, where the 20-membered ring framework is conserved[16]. Of particular interest for drug development is the close isomorphism between disulphides and non-reducible Ctt bonds[18,19]. Carbetocin, a Ctt analogue of desamino-OT, is an example of a long-acting disulphide bond mimetic that is approved as a drug[20].

Conventional intramolecular S-alkylation of cysteine used to build Ctt bridges in cyclic peptides is often problematic (Fig. 1a) and, with few exceptions[18,19,21,22], has not found broad application in the field of peptide chemistry. Here we describe a macrocyclization strategy that exploits the advantageous physicochemical properties of selenocysteine (Sec, U) instead of cysteine to accomplish effective crosslinking that can be applied not only to native OT but also to a wide range of other peptide sequences. In recent years, Sec has been incorporated into several bioactive peptides with innovative properties[23,24]. For example, substitution of S-S bonds by isosteric Se-Se bonds can improve peptide folding and stability[25–27]. We envisaged that replacement of a disulphide bond (S-S, bond length 2.03 Å)[28] by a non-reducible selenocystathionine (SeCtt) bond (Se-C, bond length 1.95–1.99 Å)[28] might enhance the metabolic stability of cyclic peptides with minimal structural perturbation. Furthermore, the low pK_a of the selenol in Sec[29] should allow selenide ring closure 1 to proceed efficiently under acidic to neutral conditions, largely preventing deterioration of labile electrophilic moieties at higher pH (Fig. 1b).

Synthesis of linear peptide precursors.
In order to investigate the scope of SeCtt cyclization in comparison with Ctt cyclization, a series of linear OT sequences featuring Sec, Cys and halogenated residues at the corresponding sites of the native Cys1–Cys6 disulphide bond were synthesized by solid-phase peptide

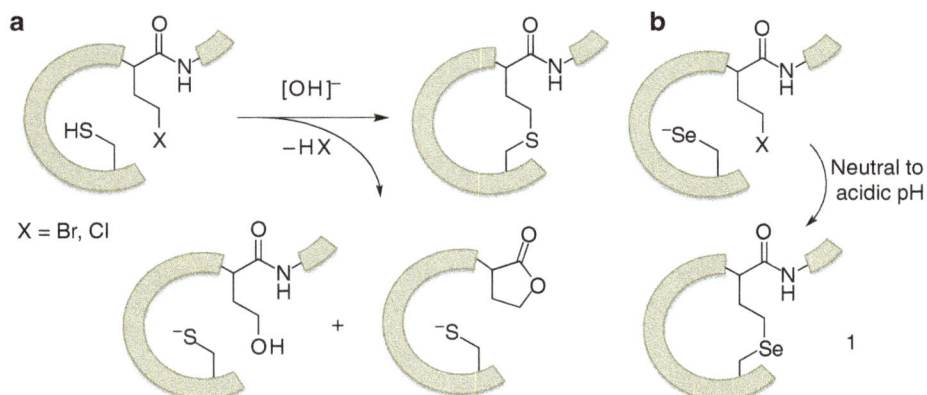

Figure 1 | Synthesis of Ctt and SeCtt cyclic peptides. (a) Synthesis of Ctt cyclic peptides by intramolecular S$_N$2-substitution of a γ-halo-homoalanine by cysteine[21,22] and possible degradation products of the linear precursor. Under the basic conditions required for monosulphide cyclization, the γ-halo-homoalanine residue can undergo intramolecular lactonization or be hydrolyzed to homoserine. **(b)** Intramolecular ring closure of a SeCtt cyclic peptide.

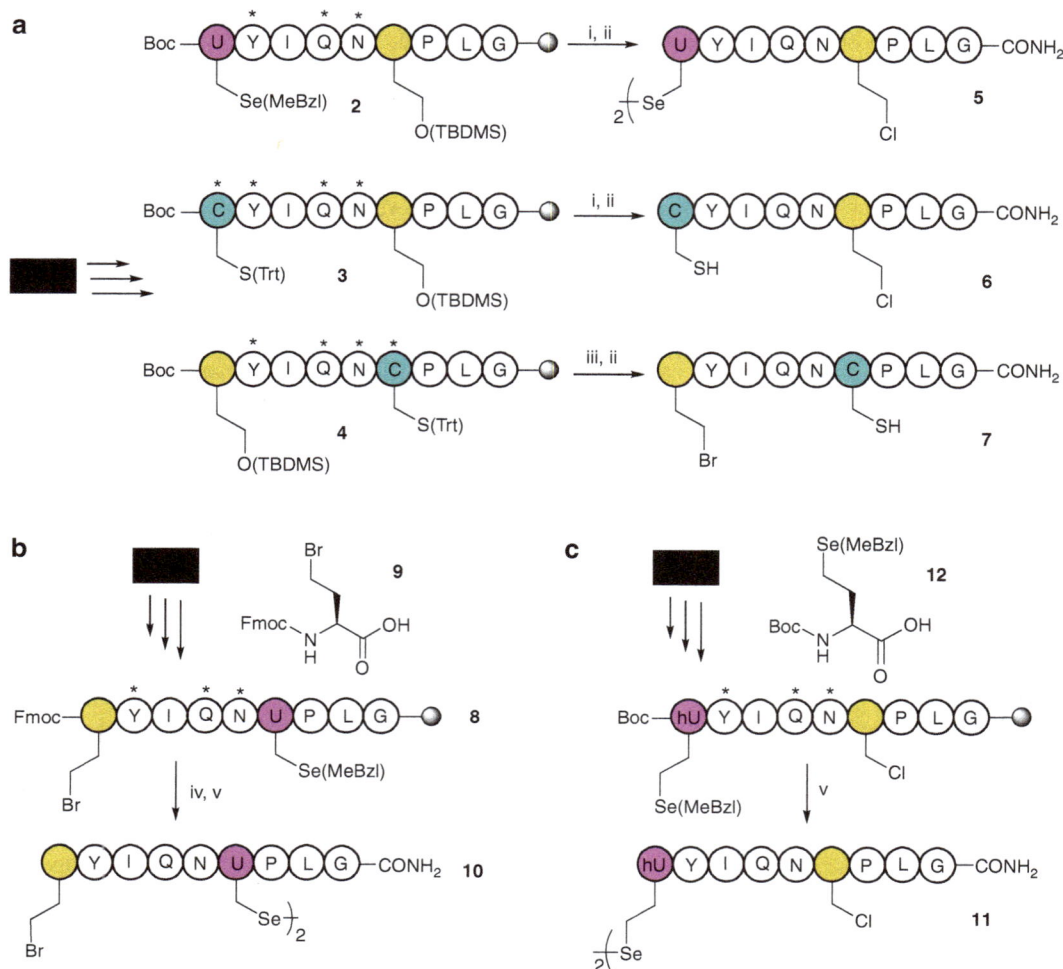

Figure 2 | Synthesis of the linear halogenated Sec- and Cys-containing OT precursors. (a) By Fmoc chemistry via chlorination or bromination on resin. (b) By Boc chemistry with coupling of a Fmoc-γBr-hAla residue. (c) By Boc chemistry via coupling of a β-chloro-alanine and SeHcy residues. Asterisks indicate that standard side-chain-protecting groups were used for the respective residues during SPPS. Reagents and conditions: (i) PPh₃/CCl₃CN, DMF, overnight; (ii) TFA:TIS:H₂O, 2 h; (iii) PPh₃Br₂, DCM, overnight; (iv) 20% piperidine in DMF, 1 min; (v) HF:p-cresol (9:1), 0 °C, 1h.

synthesis (SPPS) (Fig. 2). The linear precursors 2, 3 and 4 were assembled on a Rink amide resin using standard Fmoc chemistry (Fig. 2a)[30]. The crucial chlorination step, where the *tert*-butyl dimethylsilyl (TBDMS)-protected homoserine (Hse) is converted to γ-chloro-homoalanine (γCl-hAla)[18], was performed in a mixture of PPh₃ and CCl₃CN in dichloromethane (DCM) overnight. Surprisingly, chlorination treatment also removed the *p*-methylbenzyl (MeBzl) protecting group of the Sec residue in precursor 2, thus yielding diselenide 5 upon trifluoroacetic acid (TFA) cleavage. Likewise, the chlorinated intermediate 6 was prepared from Cys-peptide 3, while on-resin bromination of precursor 4 with PPh₃Br₂ transformed the TBDMS-protected Hse to a γ-bromo-homoalanine to give 7 in moderate yield. A similar bromination step was unsuccessful for peptides 2 and 3. Using Boc chemistry, the resin-bound 8 containing bromide and Sec moieties was prepared by coupling of Fmoc-γBr-hAla[21] 9 during peptide assembly as illustrated in Fig. 2b. Removal of the N-terminal Fmoc group using piperidine and subsequent cleavage from the resin by HF acidolysis afforded precursor 10 in modest yield. In a more efficient synthesis, the chlorinated Se-precursor 11 was prepared by Boc chemistry utilizing the β-chloro-alanine and selenohomocysteine (SeHcy, hU)-building blocks during peptide assembly (Fig. 2c).

Table 1 | Linear precursors to the cyclic OT analogues.

Linear precursor	Cyclic oxytocin		
	A	B	Name
10, 11	CH₂	Se	SeCtt 12
7	CH₂	S	Ctt 13
5	Se	CH₂	SeCtt 14
6	S	CH₂	Ctt 15
	Se		SeLan 16
	S	S	OT

OT, oxytocin.
See Fig. 3d for general cyclic OT structure.

Selenoether and thioether cyclizations. The key feature of the selenoether cyclization step is reduction of the diselenide peptide precursor by dithiothreitol (DTT) with concomitant intramolecular *Se*-alkylation of the generated selenolate (Fig. 3a)[31]. Cyclization of precursor peptides 5–7 and 10–11 was carried out with 100 μM precursor in sodium phosphate buffer at different pH using 40-fold excess DTT (Table 1). The ring-closing reaction was performed at room temperature (RT) and monitored via analytical reversed phase high-performance

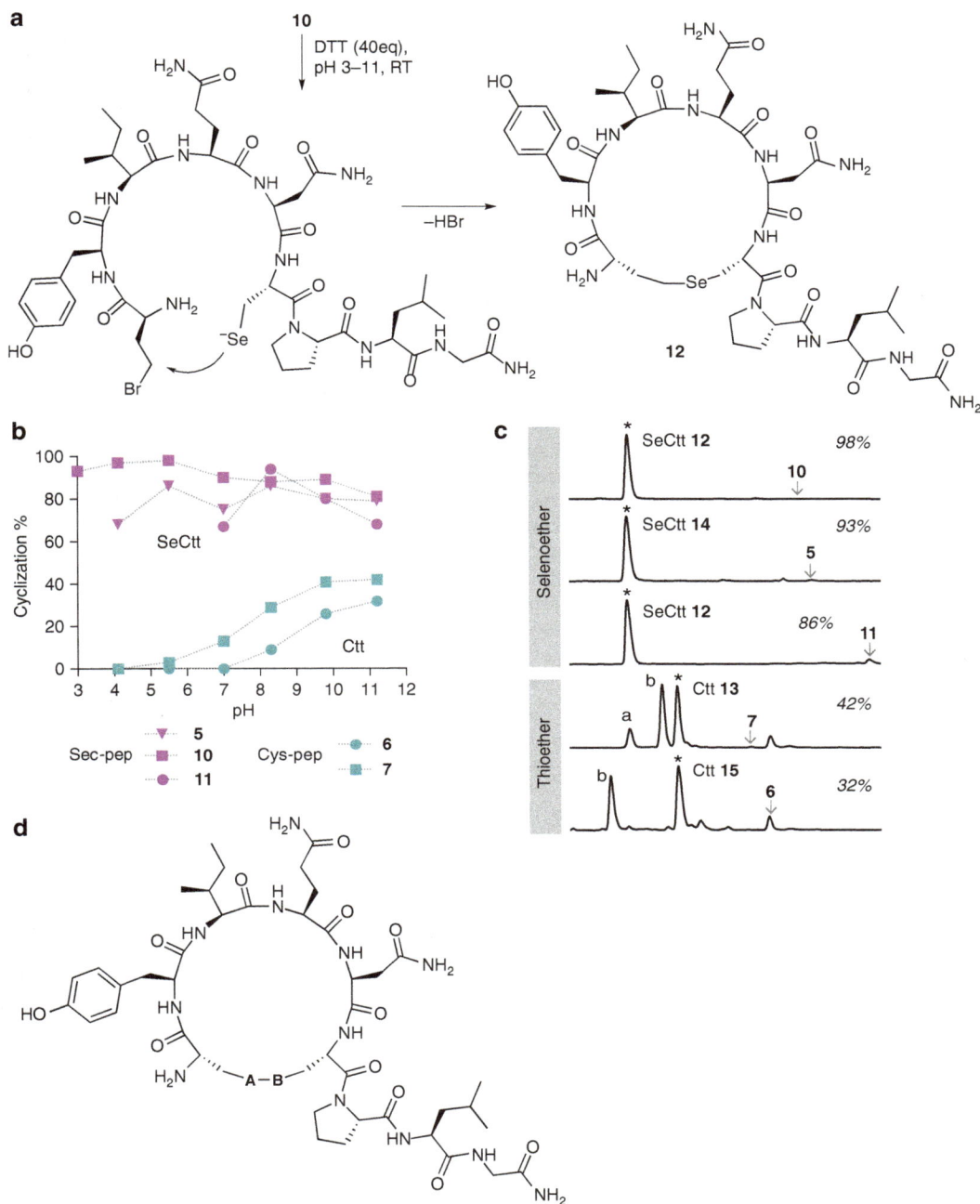

Figure 3 | Selenoether and thioether cyclizations. (**a**) Schematic representation of the cyclization of γ-bromo seleno-precursor **10** to selenoether **12**. (**b**) Conversion (%) of the precursors **10**, **5**, **11**, **6** and **7** into the respective cyclic products (Table 1) under DTT-reductive conditions at variable pH determined using HPLC. (**c**) HPLC analysis of the cyclization reaction under optimal conditions (Ctt **13** and **15**, pH 11; SeCtt **12**, pH 5.5 (from precursor **10**) and pH 8.3 (from precursor **11**); SeCtt **14**, pH 5.5). Asterisks mark the retention time for the cyclic products, while arrows indicate retention time of the respective linear precursors. The numbers in italics are the extent of conversion (%) of the linear precursor into the respective macrocycle. Major side products found during thioether cyclization (Fig. 1a) are indicated as peak 'a' (fragmentation by intramolecular lactonization) and 'b' (hydrolysis to homoserine). (**d**) General structure of the cyclic OT analogues. A, B: see Table 1.

liquid chromatography (RP-HPLC). Reduction of the γ-bromo-diselenide precursor **10** gave SeCtt **12** in excellent conversion (80–98% over a wide pH range) (Fig. 3a,b). At pH 5–11, **12** was formed within 2 h, whereas several hours were required for reactions at pH 3–4 (Supplementary Fig. 1). In contrast, the reaction time for thiolation using the analogous γ-bromo-thiol-precursor **7** took 2–4 times longer and macrocyclization was diminished (Fig. 3b). Under optimal conditions, γBr-hAla Cys-intermediate **7** was 42% converted to Ctt **13** (pH 11), while

γBr-hAla Sec-precursor **10** was quantitatively converted to SeCtt **12** (98%) at pH 5.5 (Fig. 3c). The formation of the selenoether or thioether ring was slower (8–72 h depending on pH) using γCl-hAla in comparison with the bromo-counterpart (Supplementary Fig. 1). The γCl-hAla Sec peptide **5** cyclized to SeCtt **14** in 68–86% transformation, while its cysteine-containing counterpart γCl-hAla Cys-peptide **6** cyclized to Ctt **15** poorly (< 32%) even at basic pH (Fig. 3b). SeCtt **12** was also produced from **11**; however, in this case, the intramolecular S_N2

substitution was only effective under basic conditions due to lower reactivity of the SeHcy synthon (Fig. 3b). Nevertheless, selenoether formation proceeded smoothly over 72 h at pH 8.3 with no detectable deterioration of the β-chloro-alanine moiety (Fig. 3c).

On the basis of the results obtained for synthesis of the linear precursors and their cyclization efficiency, we chose the chloro-peptides **11** and **5** for preparative synthesis of SeCtt OT analogues **12** and **14**, respectively. DTT-induced cyclization was performed directly on crude peptides after cleavage from resin. Selenoether crosslinking of **5** at pH 5.5 gave pure SeCtt **14** in 42% overall yield, whereas precursor **11** at pH 8.3 gave pure SeCtt **12** in 27% overall yield. All compounds were purified to >95% purity via RP-HPLC and characterized using mass spectrometry and nuclear magnetic resonance (NMR).

Thermal and plasma stability of the selenoether OT analogues. To evaluate their chemical stability, OT peptides were submitted to thermal stress at 55 °C, pH 7.2 (Fig. 4a). Native OT degraded significantly over 3 days at 55 °C, with a half-life of 2.2 days, as a result of disulphide bond disruption[32]. These side reactions were not observed with the SeCtt analogues and linkages remained mostly intact under these conditions (calculated half-lives for SeCtts **12** and **14** were 51.3 and 11.3 days, respectively). Metabolic stability studies yielded a half-life of 16 h for OT in human serum at physiological pH and 37 °C (Fig. 4b), whereas the half-lives for SeCtt **12** and **14** decay was 60 and 50 h, respectively. The three- to four fold increase in plasma stability is similar to that reported for Ctt **13** (ref. 16).

Functional activity of the selenoether OT analogues. The pharmacological activity of native OT, Ctt and SeCtt OT was assessed in a functional Ca^{2+} mobilization assay using the human neuroblastoma cell line SH-SY5Y that endogenously expresses OT receptors[33]. All SeCtt and Ctt OT analogues showed similar agonist activity to the parent hormone (Supplementary Table 1). In comparison, the selenoether derivative SeLan **16**, an OT surrogate with a selenolanthionine linker (Table 1) whose synthesis we recently reported[31], showed loss of bioactivity.

NMR structure analysis of OT and selenoether OT 14 and 16. Currently, there are two crystal structures available for OT unbound desamino-OT[34] and a complex of OT with its carrier protein neurophysin[35]. These OT structures are very different; the bound form reveals a helical fold for the OT ring, while the free form is more consistent with β-sheet structure (displaying Type II and III β-turns). The first NMR studies of OT conducted in the 1970s led the authors to propose a flexible structure for OT based solely on temperature coefficients and chemical shift information[36]. Later, NMR studies of OT were focused on its conformation when bound to neurophysin[37]. This latter study reported a lack of inter-residue dipolar connectivities in the absence of neurophysin, and subsequent studies have therefore assumed that OT is flexible and unstructured in solution[38]. This has led to the suggestion that binding to the OT receptor may occur through a receptor-induced fit[34]. Here we re-examined the solution structure of free OT using multidimensional heteronuclear NMR spectroscopy at ultra-high field (900 MHz).

The use of ultra-high magnetic field in combination with a cryogenically cooled probe enabled us to overcome the lack of cross peaks observed in nuclear Överhauser enhancement spectroscopy (NOESY) spectra acquired on less sensitive, lower-field instruments[38]. The frequencies of all ^1H atoms (except those absent due to fast exchange with solvent) were assigned using homonuclear total correlation spectroscopy and NOESY spectra, while all protonated heteroatoms were assigned using

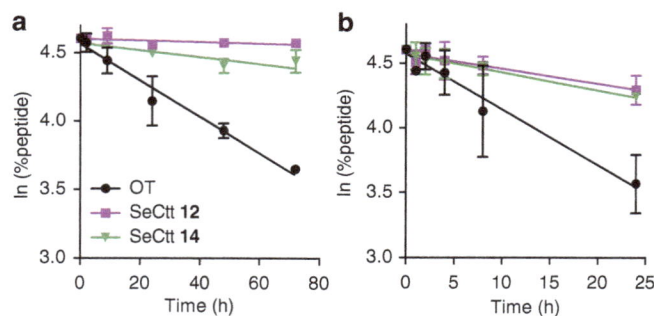

Figure 4 | Selenoether analogues are more stable than native OT. (**a**) Thermal stability of OT and SeCtt analogues **12** and **14** at pH 7 and 55 °C. (**b**) Stability of OT and analogues **12** and **14** in human plasma. Peptide levels were quantified using LC-MS ($n = 3$). All data are Mean ± SEM.

heteronuclear HSQC spectra. The selenoether bond was assigned using a ^1H-^{77}Se HMQC spectrum, where correlations from the Se atom could be observed to protons of neighbouring carbon atoms (Fig. 5a)[39]. Structures were calculated using the torsion angle dynamics program CYANA 3.0 (ref. 40) using torsion angle restraints derived from $^1H/^{13}C/^{15}N$ chemical shifts and distance restraints derived from ^1H-^1H NOEs. The results are summarized in Fig. 5 and Supplementary Tables 2,3.

All structures had excellent stereochemistry, although residue G9 is an outlier in the Ramachandran plot and poor side-chain rotamers were occasionally observed for residues Y2 and L8. In all structures, a hydrogen bond was identified between the backbone amide proton of residue X6 and the backbone carbonyl oxygen of Y2. An additional hydrogen bond was found between the backbone amide proton of N5 and the carbonyl oxygen of Y2. The backbone chemical shifts of residues 7–9 are consistent with random coil values and were predicted to be dynamic by Talos + [41], in agreement with previous studies (region coloured in red in Fig. 5b)[38]. The unfavourable NMR properties of sulphur make disulphide bonds largely 'invisible' in NMR studies[42]; in contrast, the SeCtt analogue provided structural constraints through ^{77}Se couplings to neighbouring methylenes while the additional methylene within the hydrophobic core **14** generated extra distance restraints.

Analgesic action of OT and selenoether analogues. In order to translate these findings to an intact physiological setting and to determine the mechanism of action of OT-induced analgesia in patients with abdominal pain associated with chronic idiopathic constipation[9] or IBS[10], we determined the level of OT receptor expression in colonic afferent dorsal root ganglion (DRG) neurons and tested the analgesic properties of native OT and the OT analogues SeCtt **12** and SeCtt **14** on sensory nociceptive afferents innervating the colon.

First, we examined expression of the OT receptor in colonic afferent neuronal cell bodies. As only 5% of DRG neurons innervate the colon, we used retrograde nerve tracing from the colon wall to specifically identify afferent neurons in the DRG supplying the colon[43–45]. Laser capture microdissection was then used to isolate the labelled neurons from dissociated DRG cultures, giving a pure colonic afferent neuron population. These studies were performed in healthy mice and in a mouse model of post-inflammatory CVH, which was induced with intra-colonic trinitrobenzene-sulphonic acid (TNBS), as described previously[46,47]. The TNBS-treated mice were allowed to recover for 28 days, at which stage inflammation had resolved and chronic colonic afferent mechanical hypersensitivity[46,47] and

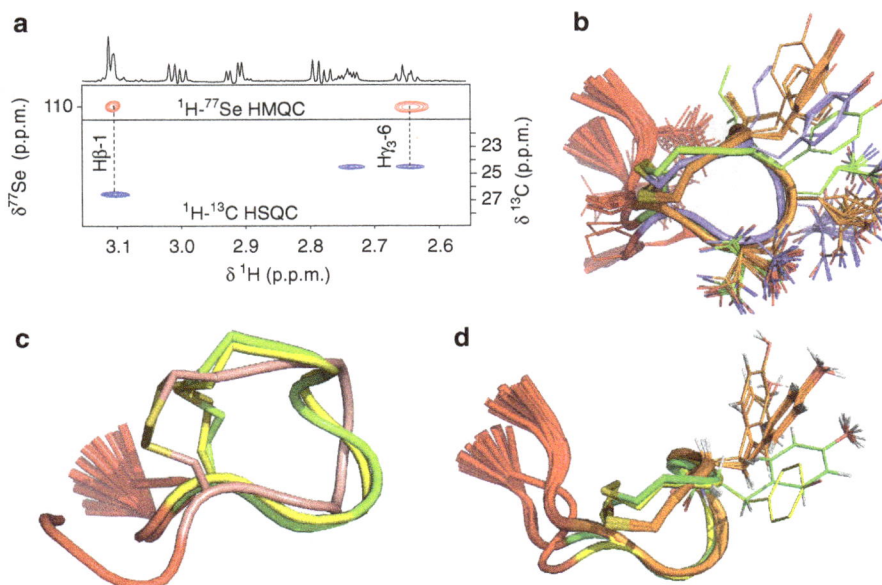

Figure 5 | Structural characterization. Structural characterization of OT and selenium analogues by NMR at 298 K and comparison to crystal structures. (**a**) Portions of ^1H-^{77}Se HMQC and ^1H-^{13}C HSQC spectra of the bioactive selenoether **14**. The ^1H-^{13}C HSQC spectrum shows correlations between the β carbons and their attached protons (at ^1H frequency of 900 MHz). The ^1H-^{77}Se HMQC spectrum shows correlations between the Se atom and protons two bonds away (at ^1H frequency of 500 MHz). A 900-MHz 1D ^1H NMR spectrum is shown above the 2D spectra. There are clear correlations between the Se atom and β protons on either side of the selenium bridge, confirming its position. (**b**) Ensemble of 10 NMR-derived solution structures for **14** (green), the inactive SeLan **16** (orange) and synthetic OT (blue). The flexible C-terminus is shown in red. (**c**) Overlay of the OT ring (residues 1–6) of **14** (green) and the crystal structure of 'free' (pink, PDB ID 1XY2) and bound OT (yellow, PDB ID 1NPO). (**d**) Overlay of the ring (residues 1–6) of active **14** (green), inactive **16** (orange) and bound OT (yellow) showing the difference in the position of the Se bridge.

hyperalgesia[48,49] were evident. We chose this model as it is being increasingly appreciated that gastrointestinal inflammation can precede IBS symptom development and that low-grade inflammation, mast cell infiltration, and immune dysfunction are evident in different subgroups of IBS patients[43,50–52]. Furthermore, chronic visceral mechanical hypersensitivity of colonic afferents is implicated in the development and maintenance of visceral pain in IBS[53–55]. As such these mice are termed CVH mice[46,47].

Quantitative RT–PCR analysis and gel electrophoresis showed that the OT receptor expression was below the level of detection in healthy thoracolumbar (TL; T10–L1) colonic DRG neurons (Fig. 6a,b). In contrast, OT receptor expression was significantly upregulated in colonic TL DRG neurons from CVH mice (Fig. 6a,b). We then determined the effects of native OT and the OT analogues on colonic afferent function[56]. We specifically targeted high-threshold nociceptive afferents in the splanchnic (thoracolumbar) pathway as we have shown that they normally respond to noxious levels of colonic distention/contraction[45,46]. These afferents are known to become hypersensitive[46,47] and hyper-excitable[57,58] in models of chronic visceral pain, which translates to increased signaling of noxious colorectal distention (CRD) within the thoracolumbar spinal cord[59] and enhanced behavioural responses to CRD[48,49]. We have also shown that specific functional deficits in these afferents translate to reduced sensory responses to noxious CRD in whole-animal studies[45]. Correspondingly, in the current study we show that with *in vitro* colonic afferent recordings[43–47,56] native OT, SeCtt **12** and SeCtt **14** had no effect on colonic nociceptor mechanosensitivity in healthy mice (Fig. 6c–e and Supplementary Fig. 2). However, in recordings from nociceptors from CVH mice we found that native OT, SeCtt **12** and SeCtt **14** all significantly and dose-dependently inhibited the mechanical hypersensitivity observed in CVH colonic nociceptors (Fig. 6f–h and Supplementary Fig. 2).

Overall, both SeCtt **12** and SeCtt **14** caused greater inhibition of colonic nociceptors than that induced by native OT (Fig. 6i–k and Supplementary Figs 2,3). Notably, we also found that the inhibitory effect of SeCtt **14** can be blocked by prior luminal administration of the OT receptor antagonist, atosiban (Supplementary Fig. 4).

Since native OT and OT analogues SeCtt **12** and SeCtt **14** inhibit colonic nociceptors *in vitro*, we hypothesized that this inhibition should correspondingly reduce signaling of noxious CRD within the spinal cord *in vivo*. We administered the OT analogue SeCtt **14** intra-colonically as this route of administration complements the conditions used in our *in vitro* studies. It also allowed us to ensure peripheral exposure to OT analogue SeCtt **14** for equal time durations, with minimal systemic actions. Furthermore, we recently used this route of administration to demonstrate the preclinical efficacy of a pharmacological treatment that reduces chronic abdominal pain and is poorly systemically absorbed and thus its effects are localized to the gastrointestinal tract[47]. We identified neurons in the dorsal horn (DH) of the thoracolumbar spinal cord activated by noxious CRD (Fig. 7a and Supplementary Fig. 5). In healthy mice, intra-colonic administration of SeCtt **14** had no effect on the number of DH neurons activated in the thoracolumbar spinal cord following noxious CRD (Fig. 7b–d and Supplementary Fig. 5), consistent with the lack of anti-nociceptive effect of native OT and OT analogues we showed *in vitro* (Fig. 6). In contrast, intra-colonic administration of SeCtt **14** in CVH mice resulted in a significant reduction in the number of DH neurons activated in the thoracolumbar spinal cord following noxious CRD (Fig. 7e–g and Supplementary Fig. 5). Overall, our data indicate that OT analogues reduce nociceptive signaling and reverse chronic visceral mechanical hypersensitivity both *in vitro* and *in vivo* but only during states of CVH and not in healthy mice.

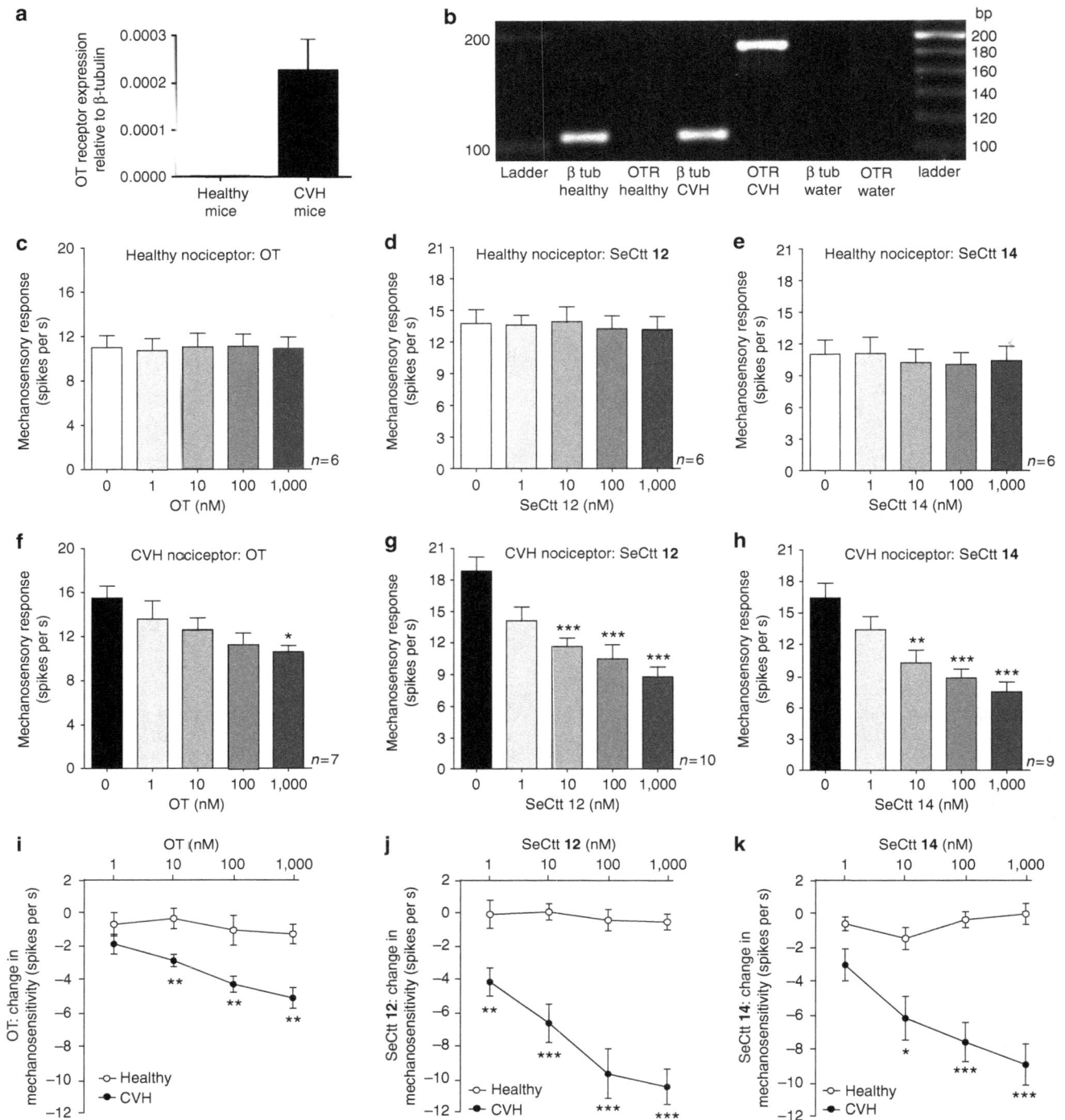

Figure 6 | OT receptor expression and function in colonic nociceptors during CVH. (**a**) Colonic DRG neurons from healthy mice lack OT receptor (OTR) expression (below the level of qRT–PCR detection), whereas expression of OT receptors is highly upregulated in colonic DRG neurons from CVH mice. (**b**) Gel electrophoresis confirming the lack of detectable OT receptor in healthy colonic DRG neurons, but expression in colonic DRG neurons from CVH mice. (**c–e**) *In vitro* luminal application of native OT (**c**), SeCtt **12** (**d**) and SeCtt **14** (**e**) had no effect at any dose on colonic nociceptor mechanosensitivity in healthy mice ($P > 0.05$). (**f**) In CVH mice, native OT inhibits nociceptor mechanosensitivity (*$P < 0.05$, $n = 7$). (**g,h**) In CVH mice, SeCtt **12** (**g**) and SeCtt **14** (**h**) caused a dose-dependent inhibition of colonic nociceptors, fully reversing the mechanical hypersensitivity of CVH mice (**$P < 0.01$, ***$P < 0.001$, one-way analysis of variance, Bonferroni *post hoc* test). (**i**) Native OT caused significantly greater nociceptor inhibition in CVH mice compared with healthy mice relative to baseline responses (**$P < 0.01$). (**j**) SeCtt **12** caused significantly greater nociceptor inhibition in CVH mice relative to healthy mice at all doses tested (**$P < 0.01$, ***$P < 0.001$). (**k**) SeCtt **14** caused significantly greater nociceptor inhibition in CVH mice relative to healthy mice at 10 nM (*$P < 0.05$, 100 nM (***$P < 0.001$) and 1,000 nM (***$P < 0.001$). All data are Mean ± SEM.

Discussion

In this study, we introduced a methodology for macrocyclization of peptides using non-reducible SeCtt crosslinkers that synthetically overpowers the limited Ctt cyclization strategy. The new procedure utilizes reductant DTT to release the highly reactive selenolate from the diselenide peptide precursor, allowing

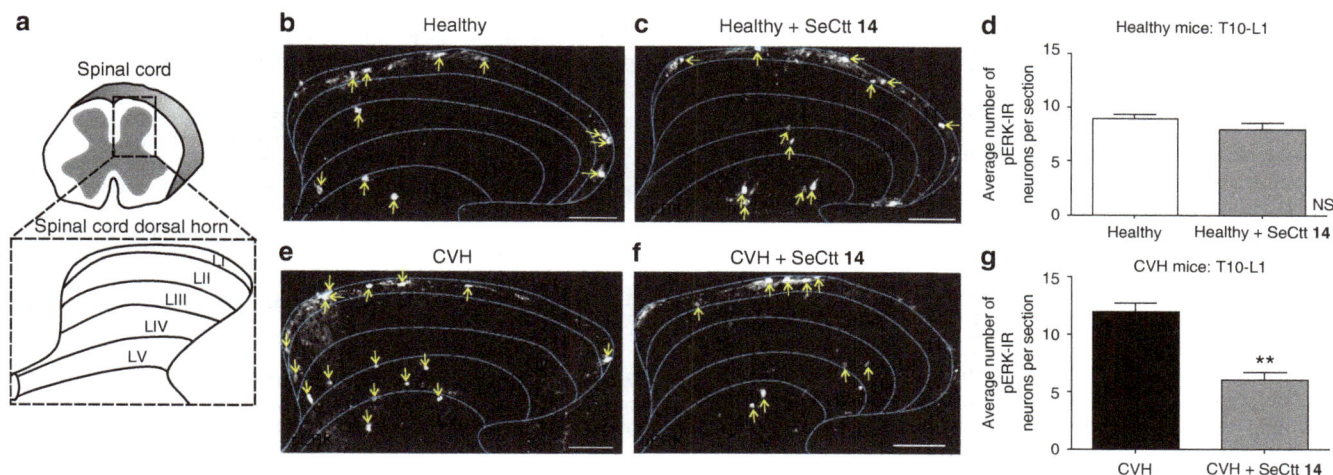

Figure 7 | In vivo studies. *In vivo* intra-colonic administration of SeCtt **14** reduces nociceptive signaling, but only during CVH. (**a**) Schematic representation of laminae I-V (LI-LV) in the dorsal horn of the thoracolumbar spinal cord. (**b**) In healthy mice, following noxious colorectal distension (CRD), pERK-immunoreactive neurons (pERK-IR; arrows) were predominantly located in laminae I and V of the thoracolumbar spinal cord (T10-L1) ($N = 6$). (**c,d**) Pretreatment with SeCtt **14** (1,000 nM) in healthy mice had no significant effect on the number of pERK-IR neurons in thoracolumbar dorsal horn following noxious CRD ($N = 4$). (**e**) In CVH mice, following noxious CRD (80 mm Hg), more pERK-IR neurons were activated at baseline than in healthy mice and they were predominantly located in the superficial DH laminae I-II and throughout laminae III-V. (**f,g**) In CVH mice, prior intra-colonic administration of SeCtt **14** (1,000 nM) significantly reduced the number of pERK-IR DH neurons in dorsal horn of the T10-L1 spinal cord (**$P < 0.01$, CVH: $N = 6$; CVH + SeCtt **14**: $N = 4$). Group data are combined from 10 sections per T10-T11, T11-T12 and T13-L1 thoracolumbar spinal cord. All scale bars are 100 µm. All data are Mean ± SEM.

efficient selenoether crosslinking to take place under mild conditions. The linear peptide precursor can be prepared using either Boc or Fmoc-SPPS with the halogenated moiety incorporated by a chlorination step or coupling of a halogenated building block. Selenide closure is chemoselective and can be applied to unprotected peptides in aqueous media at RT without a catalyst. This approach is particularly promising for the development of disulphide-containing peptide-drug candidates, with the surrogate SeCtt linkage showing substantial higher stability without disturbing the biological active structure of the OT peptide[32].

The structure of 'free' OT was determined for the first time by taking advantage of the unprecedented sensitivity of modern NMR spectrometers. Compared with previous studies of OT performed at 600 MHz using a conventional probe, we achieved a fourfold improvement in signal-to-noise by using a cryoprobe-equipped 900-MHz spectrometer (in addition to linear improvements in sensitivity at higher yields). In addition to being able to extract an unprecedented number of dipolar couplings, significant advances in predicting backbone dihedral angles of peptides and proteins based on backbone chemical shifts (^{15}N/^{13}C/^{1}H) allowed us to extract critical backbone ϕ and ψ angle restraints[41]. The new NMR data revealed that native OT and bioactive SeCtt **12** have similar well-defined structures in aqueous solution; the backbone of the OT rings (residues 1–6) are very similar, whereas the predicted dynamic region overlays poorly (red in Fig. 5). Surprisingly, the NMR structures overlay poorly with the crystal structure of the free form of dOT (PDB ID 1XY2) but are in good agreement with the crystal structure of OT bound to its carrier neurophysin. The heterogeneity found in the 'free' crystal form has been argued to be due to the inherent conformational flexibility of OT[34]. Furthermore, the large difference between the two crystal forms (0.9 Å) led to the suggestion that OT must undergo a conformational change upon binding its receptor[35]. However, the r.m.s.d. (root mean squared deviation) between the 'free' OT crystal structure and the NMR structure is ~1.0 Å, whereas the r.m.s.d. between the NMR structure of the active forms of OT and the complex structure is only 0.3–0.5 Å. This

difference is apparent when the backbones of the active OT rings are overlaid: the NMR and neurophysin-bound OT structures overlay well, while the free crystal form is more compressed, perhaps due to crystal packing forces (Fig. 5c). Thus, the new NMR data are not consistent with OT undergoing a major conformational change upon binding to neurophysin. Rather, the backbone conformation of OT in aqueous solution appears to be pre-optimized for receptor-binding. However, there are significant differences between the side-chain orientations in the neurophysin-bound OT structure and the NMR structure (0.8–1.1 Å), consistent with these flexible solvent-exposed side chains adopting a thermodynamically more favourable orientation upon binding. The inactive SeLan **16** OT analogue, which has a slightly shorter selenoether bridge in comparison to SeCtt **12**, has a similar overall fold to the other active OT rings, but with small perturbations in the positions of residues 1 and 2. The spatial displacement of the Y2-Cβ atom in SeLan **16** in comparison with the Cβ of bound OT (1NPO) is ~2 Å, while in SeCtt **14** the corresponding displacement is only 0.1 Å. Since the Y2 residue is critical for OT activity, these small structural changes might explain the loss of agonist activity in SeLan **16**.

It has generally been assumed that the reported analgesic properties of OT in clinical studies of patients with abdominal diseases[9,10] are due to a central effect of OT. However, there is a complete lack of evidence regarding the actual mechanism of action. The work described here reveals a very different scenario, whereby OT and OT analogues can act in the periphery on the endings of nociceptive afferents innervating the colon. In healthy mice, we were unable to detect expression of OT receptors in colonic DRG neurons. However, we found that OT receptor expression is massively upregulated in primary sensory DRG neurons innervating the colon from mice with CVH. Consistent with this high-level expression of OT receptors in CVH, *in vitro* luminal administration of native OT and the stable SeCtt OT analogues **12** and **14** were anti-nociceptive, as evidenced by their ability to reduce colonic nociceptor mechanosensitivity in a mouse model of chronic abdominal pain (Fig. 6g,h). This inhibitory effect was also blocked by the OT receptor antagonist atosiban, which was also applied to the lumen of the colon. This is an important finding as peripheral sensitization of nociceptors has been shown to occur in IBS patients[54,55]. This enhanced peripheral signaling facilitates aberrant processing within the spinal cord[59], which influences the manifestation of pain referred to other organs. Therefore, reducing peripheral signaling is an important component of symptom treatment. Our results represent the first definitive report of native OT, OT analogues and OT receptor actions specifically on peripheral sensory afferent endings in the colon. Critically, our *in vitro* data show that local luminal absorption of native OT and OT analogues in gut tissue significantly reduces colonic nociceptor function, without the need for systemic effects, but only under conditions of chronic abdominal pain. Correspondingly, we also show that intra-colonic luminal application of OT analogues *in vivo* significantly reduces signaling from colonic nociceptors into the spinal cord but again only under conditions of chronic abdominal pain. We found that mice intra-colonically administered with the OT analogue SeCtt **14** have a reduced capacity to detect and signal noxious CRD, as indicated by the reduction in activated DH neurons within the thoracolumbar spinal cord. In particular, fewer activated neurons were detected in the superficial lamina of the DH, which is the major termination zone for nociceptive afferents and consists of nociception-specific neurons responding to noxious inputs from afferent fibres[59]. Importantly, the OT analogue SeCtt **14** does not completely inhibit the capacity to signal noxious CRD into the spinal cord in CVH mice; however, it does reduce sensitivity to equivalent healthy levels. This is important, given the physiological importance of these afferents to detect and alert us to harmful events. Since we applied OT analogues to the lumen of the colon over a relatively short time period in both our *in vitro* and *in vivo* studies, their actions are predominantly localized in a topical manner to the gut wall. As such, we suggest that native OT and OT analogues act on the peripheral endings of nociceptors innervating the wall of the colon, thereby reducing the nociceptive signal at the first step of the pain pathway. This is an important finding, as targeting peptide therapeutics with poor oral bioavailability to the gastrointestinal tract has been demonstrated to be an effective approach for the clinical treatment of abdominal pain in IBS patients[47]. Such approaches maximize the anti-nociceptive effect of analgesic drugs to the site of action, the peripheral endings of nociceptors in the colon wall, while reducing the risk of systemic side effects. In this study, using the same approach, we identified anti-nociceptive actions of native OT and OT analogues that are of predictive clinical value for the treatment of chronic abdominal pain. Our findings are consistent with previous human studies where OT administration had no effect on pain thresholds in healthy subjects[60] but reduced chronic abdominal pain and discomfort in patients with IBS or chronic idiopathic constipation[9,10]. Importantly, the current study provides a mechanistic basis for these contrasting effects, whereby OT receptor expression and function are significantly increased on colonic nociceptors during states of chronic abdominal pain.

In conclusion, we improved OT stability by incorporating an isosteric non-reducible selenoether bond and revealed an unprecedented well-defined structure for free OT in solution that might guide future development of mimetics. We demonstrated that OT receptors are massively upregulated in mice with CVH and that the selenoether OT analogues, which are more resistant to redox degradation in the gut environment[61,62] than native OT, have analgesic activity in this model of chronic abdominal pain.

Methods

Peptide synthesis. Detailed procedures for the solid-phase assembly, cleavage and purification of the peptides are described in Supplementary Methods.

Synthesis of [UYIQN(γCl-hAla)PLG-*CONH$_2$*]$_2$ (5). The peptide sequence Boc-Sec(MeBzl)-Tyr(OtBu)-Ile-Gln(Trt)-Asn(Trt)-Hse(OTBDMS)-Pro-Leu-Gly **2** was assembled on a Rink Amide-MBHA resin following the general Fmoc-SPPS procedure (Supplementary Methods). Chlorination of the Hse residue was performed as follow: PPh$_3$ (10 equiv.) and Cl$_3$CCN (10 equiv.) were dissolved in DCM (1 ml per 0.1 g resin) at 0 °C. The cold solution was added to the resin and chlorination was carried out overnight at RT. Finally, the peptide was cleaved off the resin and purified using RP-HPLC or used directly for cyclization without further purification. HR-MS calculated for $[C_{88}H_{136}Cl_2N_{24}O_{24}Se_2 + 2H]^{2+}$: 1072.4006; found 1072.3978.

Synthesis of CYIQN(γCl-hAla)PLG-*CONH$_2$* (6). The peptide sequence Fmoc-Cys(Trt)-Tyr(BrZ)-Ile-Gln(Trt)-Asn(Trt)-Hse(OTBDMS)-Pro-Leu-Gly **3** was assembled on a Rink Amide-MBHA resin following the general Fmoc-SPPS procedure (Supplementary Methods). After full assembly of the peptide, the Fmoc group was removed by standard treatment with piperidine. Boc protection of the free *N*-terminal amine was carried out by treatment of the resin with Boc$_2$O (10 equiv.) and *N,N*-Diisopropylethylamine (DIPEA) (10 equiv.) in *N,N*-Dimethylformamide (DMF) for 10 min. The Boc group is preferred over the Fmoc group for protecting the *N*-terminal amino group in order to avoid any future exposure of the generated chloride moiety to base media. Chlorination was carried out by treating the resin with PPh$_3$ (10 equiv.) and Cl$_3$CCN (10 equiv.) in DCM overnight as described for compound **5**. Finally, the peptide was cleaved from the resin and purified using RP-HPLC. HR-MS calculated for $[C_{44}H_{69}ClN_{12}O_{12}S + H]^{+}$: 1025.4640; found 1025.4615.

Synthesis of (γBr-hAla)YIQNCPLG-*CONH$_2$* (7). The peptide sequence Fmoc-Hse(OTBDMS)-Tyr(OtBu)-Ile-Gln(Trt)-Asn(Trt)-Cys(Trt)-Pro-Leu-Gly was assembled on a Rink Amide-MBHA resin following the general Fmoc-SPPS procedure (Supplementary Methods). After removal of the Fmoc group of Hse1 by standard treatment with piperidine, Boc protection of the free *N*-terminal amine was carried out by treatment of the resin with Boc$_2$O (10 equiv.) and DIPEA (10 equiv.) in DMF for 10 min. Bromination of the Hse residue in **4** was performed by treating the resin with PPh$_3$Br$_2$ (10 equiv.) in DCM (1 ml per 0.1 g resin) at RT overnight. Finally, the peptide was cleaved from the resin and purified using RP-HPLC. HR-MS calculated for $[C_{44}H_{69}BrN_{12}O_{12}S + H]^{+}$: 1071.4115/1069.4135; found 1071.4106/1069.4112.

Synthesis of [(γBr-hAla)YIQNUPLG-*CONH$_2$*]$_2$ (10). The peptide sequence Tyr(BrZ)-Ile-Gln-Asn-Sec(MeBzl)-Pro-Leu-Gly was assembled on an MBHA resin using Boc-SPPS (Supplementary Methods). Upon removal of the Boc group of Tyr2, the resin was treated with 5% DIPEA in DMF for 2 min then washed with DMF. Fmoc-γ-bromo-homoalanine **9**[21] was coupled by combining the amino acid (5 equiv.) with HOAt (5 equiv.) and DIC (5 equiv.) in DMF:DCM (1:1). The resulting solution was added immediately to resin and the reaction mixture was shaken slowly for 2 h. The solvent was drained and the coupling procedure was repeated. After washing the resin with DMF, the *N*-terminal Fmoc group was removed by treatment with 20% piperidine in DMF for 1 min (2 ×). TFA cleavage of resin afforded crude peptide that was purified using RP-HPLC. HR-MS calculated for $[C_{88}H_{136}Br_2N_{24}O_{24}Se_2 + 2H]^{2+}$: 1116.3501/1117.3481; found 1116.3483/1117.3455.

Synthesis of [(hU)YIQN(βCl-Ala)PLG-*CONH$_2$*]$_2$ (11). The peptide sequence Boc-SeHcy(MeBzl)-Tyr(BrZ)-Ile-Gln-Asn-[βCl-Ala]-Pro-Leu-Gly was assembled on an MBHA resin using Boc-SPPS (Supplementary Methods). The β-chloro-alanine residue at position 6 was coupled in the following way: after removal of the Boc group in Pro3, the resin was treated twice with 5% DIPEA in DMF for 2 min and then washed with DMF. Boc-β-chloro-alanine (5 equiv.) was preactivated for 2 min with HOAt (5 equiv.) and DIC (5 equiv.) in DMF:DCM (1:1) and then coupled to the resin for 1 h. Upon complete assembly of the nonapeptide, HF cleavage of the resin afforded the crude peptide, which was either purified using RP-HPLC or used directly for cyclization without further purification. HR-MS calculated for $[C_{88}H_{136}Cl_2N_{24}O_{24}Se_2 + 2H]^{2+}$: 1072.4006; found 1072.3985.

Cyclization of the peptides under various pH conditions. Linear peptides (**5**, **6**, **7**, **10** or **11**) were dissolved in 0.1% TFA solution to a concentration of 1 mg ml^{-1}. The peptide solutions were then diluted 10-fold in a buffer solution containing DTT (40 equiv. for selenoether cyclization; 20 equiv. for thioether cyclization). The buffer solutions used were as follows: 0.1 M sodium phosphate buffer pH 3.0, 4.1, 5.5, 7.0, 8.3 or 9.8 or aqueous Na$_2$CO$_3$ (5 mg ml^{-1}, pH 11.2). Cyclizations were carried out at RT and monitored using RP-HPLC. Areas of peaks in analytical HPLC chromatograms were measured and used to quantify the ratio of starting material, cyclized product and side products and to determine the percentage conversion of linear precursors into cyclic products. Supplementary Figure 1 shows the reaction time for the seleno-peptides at different pH. It was important to check the level of DTT consumption throughout the cyclization step. Extra DTT (40 equiv.) was occasionally added to the reaction whenever total conversion of this reagent to its oxidized form was detected using RP-HPLC. The presence of DTT during thioether cyclization was not essential for reactions taking less than 6 h to complete; however, it was beneficial for those with longer reaction times.

Synthesis of selenoether OT SeCtt (12). Crude peptide **11** (20 mg, 0.00934 mmol) was dissolved in 0.1M sodium phosphate buffer pH 8.3 (200 ml) containing DTT (170 mg). Cyclization was allowed to take place over 3 days at RT, with occasional addition of DTT (170 mg) after the 1-day reaction. The solution was then diluted twofold with water and the final cyclized peptide was purified using RP-HPLC, affording 5.2 mg of SeCtt **12** in 27% overall yield (from first amino acid loading on resin). HR-MS calculated for $[C_{44}H_{68}N_{12}O_{12}Se + H]^+$: 1037.4318; found 1037.4295.

Synthesis of selenoether OT SeCtt (14). Crude peptide **5** (6.0 mg, 0.0028 mmol) was dissolved in 0.1 M sodium phosphate buffer pH 5.5 (40 ml) containing DTT (50 mg, 0.336 mmol). Cyclization was allowed to take place over 24 h at RT. The solution was then diluted twofold with water and the final cyclized peptide was purified using RP-HPLC, affording 2.45 mg of SeCtt **14** in 42% overall yield (from first amino acid loading on resin). HR-MS calculated for $[C_{44}H_{68}N_{12}O_{12}Se + H]^+$: 1037.4318; found 1037.4302.

Synthesis of thioether OT Ctt (13). Crude peptide **7** (7.8 mg, 0.0073 mmol) was dissolved in 0.1 M sodium phosphate buffer pH 9.8 (50 ml). Cyclization was allowed to take place over 4 h at RT. The solution was then diluted twofold with water and the final cyclized peptide **13** was purified using RP-HPLC, affording 1.0 mg of **13** (overall yield: 14% from first amino acid loading on resin). HR-MS calculated for $[C_{44}H_{68}N_{12}O_{12}S + H]^+$: 989.4873; found 989.4851.

Synthesis of thioether OT Ctt (15). Crude peptide **6** (4.1 mg, 0.0040 mmol) was dissolved in a solution of Na_2CO_3 (5 mg ml^{-1}, pH 11.2, 30 ml). DTT (12 mg, 0.078 mmol) was added and cyclization was allowed to take place over 3 days at RT. The solution was then diluted twofold with water and the final cyclized peptide was purified using RP-HPLC, affording 0.77 mg of **15** (overall yield: 19% from first amino acid loading on resin). HR-MS calculated for $[C_{44}H_{68}N_{12}O_{12}S + H]^+$: 989.4873; found 989.4869.

Thermal stability assay. OT and SeCtt **12** and **14** were dissolved in 50 mM sodium phosphate buffer pH 7.0 to a concentration of 20 µM. An aliquot (750 µl) of this solution was placed inside a glass vial, sealed and placed in an incubator at 55 °C. Samples (75 µl) were taken at $t = 0$, 2, 9, 24, 48 and 72 h, quenched with 5% TFA solution (20 µl) and analysed using RP-HPLC. The area of the peak corresponding to the starting peptide was measured and plotted as a percentage of the area at $t = 0$ (Fig. 4a). The data were plotted as ln (% of remaining peptide) versus time and the pseudo-first-order rate constant for degradation was used to calculate the half-life of the peptides (OT: 52 h, SeCtt **12**: 1,232 h, SeCtt **14**: 272 h).

Stability in human plasma. Human plasma (Sigma) was centrifuged at 13,000 r.p.m. for 15 min to separate lipids and then pre-warmed to 37 °C for 15 min before use. A 50 µl aliquot of peptide solution (~500 µM in water) was mixed with 300 µl plasma and incubated at 37 °C. Samples (50 µl) were taken at $t = 0$, 1, 2, 4, 8 and 24 h, quenched with 100 µl of 2% TFA/50% acetonitrile in water, cooled at 4 °C for 30 min and then centrifuged at 13,000 r.p.m. for 5 min. The supernatant was analysed via LC-MS using a Thermo Hypersil GOLD C18 2.1 × 100 mm column running at 0.3 ml min^{-1} with a gradient of 5–50% B over 30 min. Eluting peptides were detected using an API 150 mass spectrometer in positive ion mode within the mass range 400–1,800 Da. The area of the peak corresponding to the starting peptide was measured and plotted as a percentage of the area at $t = 0$ (Fig. 4b). The data were plotted as ln (% of remaining peptide) versus time, and the pseudo-first-order rate constant for degradation was used to calculate the half-life of the peptides (OT: 16 h, SeCtt **12**: 60 h, SeCtt **14**: 50 h).

Functional activity of the OT analogues. Intracellular Ca^{2+} mobilization in response to OT and its SeCtt and Ctt analogues was assessed in SH-SY5Y human neuroblastoma cells endogenously expressing OT receptors as previously described[63]. SH-SY5Y cells were routinely cultured in RPMI media supplemented with 15% fetal bovine serum and plated at a density of 50,000 cells per well on black-walled 384-well imaging plates 48 h prior to the assay. After removal of culture media, SH-SY5Y cells were loaded with Calcium 4 No-Wash dye (Molecular Devices, Sunnyvale, CA, USA) diluted in physiological salt solution (composition: NaCl 140 mM, glucose 11.5 mM, KCl 5.9 mM, $MgCl_2$ 1.4 mM, NaH_2PO_4 1.2 mM, $NaHCO_3$ 5 mM, $CaCl_2$ 1.8 mM, HEPES 10 mM) for 30 min at 37 °C. Ca^{2+} mobilization in response to the addition of OT and its selenocysteine analogues was measured using a FLIPR^{TETRA} plate reader (Molecular Devices; excitation/

emission: 470–495 nm/515–575 nm) for 300 s. Raw fluorescence values after addition of compounds were converted to ΔF/F values and the maximum increase in fluorescence after addition of compound plotted as a function of concentration using GraphPad Prism (version 5.03, San Diego, CA, USA). To establish concentration-response curves, a 4-parameter Hill equation with variable Hill coefficient was fitted to the data.

NMR spectroscopy. 1D ^1H NMR spectra and 2D ^1H–^1H total correlation spectroscopy (mixing time = 80 ms), 2D ^1H–^1H NOESY (mixing time = 350 ms) and ^1H–^{13}C HSQC NMR spectra were recorded using samples dissolved in 95% $H_2O/5\%$ D_2O on a Bruker AVANCE spectrometer equipped with a cryogenically cooled probe, operating at 298 K and a ^1H frequency of 900 MHz. All ^{77}Se experiments were performed at a ^1H frequency of 500 MHz on a Bruker AVANCE system equipped with a broadband probe. The chemical shifts of ^{77}Se sites were measured using ^1H–^{77}Se HMQC spectra; the optimal value of $^1J_{(77Se-1H)}$ was determined to be 25 Hz. These 2D experiments required, on average, 10 h of data acquistion time. Chemical shifts were referenced to Sec, as previously described[39]. All nonlabile ^1H as well as aliphatic ^{13}C and ^{77}Se chemical shifts were assigned (Supplementary Table 2).

Structure determination. NOESY spectra were assigned and structures were calculated automatically using the torsion angle dynamics program CYANA v3.0 (ref. 40). ^1H–^1H distance restraints from NOESY data were supplemented with φ and ψ dihedral-angle restraints derived from ^1H, ^{13}C and ^{15}N chemical shift data (where available) using the program TALOS + [41]. Three new templates were added to the CYANA default library in addition to a previously derived template for oxidized SEC[39]. The new templates were as follows: (1) a C-terminal amidation template; (2) a template based on selenomethionine where the S-C bond was substituted with Se-C bond properties and the Se atom was deprotonated (SME); (3) a template was generated based on the cysteine template where the S atom was removed (NSC). Thus, the OT analogues were created by fusing the NSC residue with either SEC or SME using distance restraints.

Colonic studies. For detailed descriptions of the methodology used, see the Supplementary Methods section. Experiments involving animals were approved by the Animal Ethics Committees of the Institute of Veterinary and Medical Science/ SA Pathology and The University of Adelaide.

CVH model. Intra-colonic TNBS (130 µl ml^{-1} in 30% ethanol, 0.1 ml bolus) was administered as described previously[46,47,59]. TNBS-treated mice were allowed to recover for 28 days, at which stage inflammation had resolved and chronic colonic afferent mechanical hypersensitivity was evident. These mice are termed CVH mice. For more information, see the Supplementary Methods.

***In vitro* colonic primary afferent recording preparation.** *In vitro* single-unit extracellular recordings of action potential discharge were made from colonic splanchnic colonic afferents. These recordings were made from C57BL/6 healthy or CVH mice using standard protocols[43–47,56]. Baseline mechanosensitivity was determined in response to application of a 2-g von Frey hair (vfh) probe to the afferent receptive field for 3 s. This process was repeated three to four times, separated each time by 10 s. Mechanosensitivity was then re-tested after the application of native OT (1, 10, 100 or 1,000 nM) or the OT analogues SeCtt **12** (1, 10, 100 or 1,000 nM) or SeCtt **14** (1, 10, 100 or 1,000 nM), respectively. In all cases, peptides were applied to the mucosal surface of the colon for a period of 5 min at each concentration via a small metal ring placed over the receptive field of interest. In some experiments, the OT receptor antagonist atosiban (10 µM) was pre-incubated on the colonic lumen for 10 min before the addition of a combination of atosiban (10 µM) and SeCtt **14** (100 nM). Data are presented as spikes per s and are expressed as mean ± s.e.m. *n* indicates the number of individual afferents.

Retrograde labelling to identify colonic neurons in DRG. Healthy and CVH mice of 16 weeks of age were anaesthetised with halothane and following midline laparotomy, three injections (10 µl total, 26 s gauge Hamilton syringe) of the fluorescent retrograde neuronal tracer cholera toxin subunit B conjugated to AlexaFluor-555 (CTB AF-555; Invitrogen, Carlsbad, CA, USA; 0.5% in 0.1 M phosphate buffer saline (PBS), pH 7.4) were made sub-serosally within the wall of the descending colon ~2 cm from the anus[44,45,59]. The viscera were carefully rinsed with sterile saline after each injection to ensure that dye was not incorporated into structures other than the colon wall, and the overlying muscle and skin were then sutured closed. Following surgery, but prior to regaining consciousness, mice were given an analgesic (5 mg kg^{-1} butorphanol subcutaneously; Intervet, Australia) and an antibacterial (10 mg kg^{-1} oxytetracycline; Pfizer, Groton, CT).

Dissociated DRG cell culture, laser capture microdissection. Mice were killed by CO_2 inhalation and DRGs from T10–L1 were surgically removed 4 days after injections of fluorescent dye into the colon (CTB-AF-555). DRGs were digested with $4\,mg\,ml^{-1}$ collagenase II (GIBCO, Invitrogen) and $4\,mg\,ml^{-1}$ dispase (GIBCO) for 30 min at 37 °C, followed by $4\,mg\,ml^{-1}$ collagenase II for 10 min at 37 °C[44,45]. Neurons were mechanically dissociated into a single-cell suspension via trituration through fire-polished Pasteur pipettes. Neurons were re-suspended in Hanks' buffered salt solution (GIBCO) and spot-plated on 50-mm Zeiss duplex dishes (Carl Zeiss, Oberkochen, Germany) and then maintained at 37 °C in 5% CO_2 for 2 h, allowing optimal cell adhesion[44,45]. Retrogradely labelled neurons were isolated using a PALM Microlaser Technologies microdissection system (Carl Zeiss) and catapulted directly into a lysis/stabilization buffer-containing carrier RNA ($4\,ng\,l^{-1}$) (Qiagen, Valencia, CA, USA). RNA was isolated from LCM cells using an RNeasy Micro-Kit (Qiagen) following the manufacturer's instructions.

Quantitative RT–PCR. Quantitative reverse transcription–polymerase chain reaction (qRT–PCR) was performed using a Chromo4 (MJ Research, Waltham, MA) real-time instrument attached to a PTC-200 Peltier thermal cycler (MJ Research) and Opticon Monitor software (MJ Research). Qiagen QuantiTect SYBR Green RT-PCR 1-step kits were used according to the manufacturer's specifications with the primers listed in the Supplementary Methods.

Colorectal distention and pERK immunohistochemistry. Mice received an enema of either saline or SeCt 14 (1,000 nM). Ten minutes later, under anaesthesia, a 4 cm CRD balloon catheter was inserted transanally into healthy or CVH mice. After regaining consciousness, CRD was performed (80 mm Hg for 10 s, then deflated for 5 s and repeated five times). Following killing via anaesthetic overdose, mice underwent fixation by transcardial perfusion, and the thoracolumbar (T10–L1) spinal cord was removed and cryoprotected. Frozen sections were cut and incubated with monoclonal rabbit anti-pERK with AlexaFluorR488 used for visualization.

References

1. Gimpl, G. & Fahrenholz, F. The oxytocin receptor system: structure, function, and regulation. *Physiol. Rev.* **81**, 629–683 (2001).
2. du Vigneaud, V., Ressler, C., Swan, J. M., Roberts, C. W. & Katsoyannis, P. G. The synthesis of oxytocin. *J. Am. Chem. Soc.* **76**, 3115–3121 (1954).
3. Jost, K., Lebl, M. & Brtnik, F. *CRC Handbook of Neurohypophyseal Hormone Analogs* (CRC Press, 1987).
4. Lee, H. J., Macbeth, A. H., Pagani, J. H. & Young, W. S. Oxytocin: the great facilitator of life. *Prog. Neurobiol.* **88**, 127–151 (2009).
5. Meyer-Lindenberg, A., Domes, G., Kirsch, P. & Heinrichs, M. Oxytocin and vasopressin in the human brain: social neuropeptides for translational medicine. *Nat. Rev.* **12**, 524–538 (2011).
6. Viero, C. et al. Oxytocin: crossing the bridge between basic science and pharmacotherapy. *CNS Neurosci. Ther.* **16**, e138–e156 (2010).
7. Kovacs, G. L. & Telegdy, G. Role of oxytocin in memory and amnesia. *Pharmacol. Ther.* **18**, 375–395 (1982).
8. Reversi, A., Cassoni, P. & Chini, B. Oxytocin receptor signaling in myoepithelial and cancer cells. *J. Mammary Gland Biol. Neoplasia* **10**, 221–229 (2005).
9. Ohlsson, B. et al. Effects of long-term treatment with oxytocin in chronic constipation; a double blind, placebo-controlled pilot trial. *Neurogastroenterol. Motil.* **17**, 697–704 (2005).
10. Louvel, D. et al. Oxytocin increases thresholds of colonic visceral perception in patients with irritable bowel syndrome. *Gut* **39**, 741–747 (1996).
11. Lovell, R. M. & Ford, A. C. Global prevalence of and risk factors for irritable bowel syndrome: a meta-analysis. *Clin. Gastroenterol. Hepatol.* **10**, 712–721 (2012).
12. Manning, M. et al. Oxytocin and vasopressin agonists and antagonists as research tools and potential therapeutics. *J. Neuroendocrinol.* **24**, 609–628 (2012).
13. Smith, C. W. & Ferger, M. F. Synthesis and some pharmacological properties of five analogs of oxytocin having L-homocysteine in position 6. *J. Med. Chem.* **19**, 250–254 (1976).
14. Meraldi, J. P., Hruby, V. J. & Brewster, A. I. R. Relative conformational rigidity in oxytocin and (1-penicillamine)-oxytocin: a proposal for the relationship of conformational flexibility to peptide hormone agonism and antagonism. *Proc. Natl Acad. Sci. USA* **74**, 1373–1377 (1977).
15. Smith, C. W., Walter, R., Moore, S., Makofske, R. C. & Meienhofer, J. Replacement of the disulfide bond in oxytocin by an amide group. Synthesis and some biological properties of (cyclo-(1-L-aspartic acid,6-L-alpha,beta-diaminopropionic acid))oxytocin. *J. Med. Chem.* **21**, 117–120 (1978).
16. Muttenthaler, M. et al. Modulating oxytocin activity and plasma stability by disulfide bond engineering. *J. Med. Chem.* **53**, 8585–8596 (2010).
17. Stymiest, J. L., Mitchell, B. F., Wong, S. & Vederas, J. C. Synthesis of biologically active dicarba analogues of the peptide hormone oxytocin using ring-closing metathesis. *Org. Lett.* **5**, 47–49 (2003).
18. Dekan, Z. et al. α-Conotoxin ImI incorporating stable cystathionine bridges maintains full potency and identical three-dimensional structure. *J. Am. Chem. Soc.* **133**, 15866–15869 (2011).
19. Knerr, P. J. et al. Synthesis and activity of thioether-containing analogues of the complement inhibitor compstatin. *ACS Chem. Biol.* **6**, 753–760 (2011).
20. Su, L. L., Chong, Y. S. & Samuel, M. Carbetocin for preventing postpartum haemorrhage. *Cochrane Database Syst. Rev.* **4**, CD005457 (2012).
21. Mayer, J. P., Heil, J. R., Zhang, J. & Munson, M. C. An alternative solid-phase approach to C1-oxytocin. *Tetrahedon Lett.* **36**, 7387–7390 (1995).
22. Yu, L., Lai, Y., Wade, J. V. & Coutts, S. M. A simple and efficient method for the synthesis of thioether cyclic peptides. *Tetrahedon Lett.* **39**, 6633–6636 (1998).
23. Metanis, N., Beld, J. & Hilvert, D. in The Chemistry of Selenocysteine (ed Rappoport, Z.) (Patai's Chemistry of Functional Groups) doi:10.1002/9780470682531.pat0582 (2011).
24. Craik, D. J. Protein folding: turbo-charged crosslinking. *Nat. Chem.* **4**, 600–602 (2012).
25. Steiner, A. M., Woycechowsky, K. J., Olivera, B. M. & Bulaj, G. Reagentless oxidative folding of disulfide-rich peptides catalyzed by an intramolecular diselenide. *Angew. Chem. Int. Ed.* **51**, 5580–5584 (2012).
26. de Araujo, A. D. et al. Total synthesis of the analgesic conotoxin MrVIB through selenocysteine-assisted folding. *Angew. Chem. Int. Ed.* **50**, 6527–6529 (2011).
27. Armishaw, C. J. et al. α-Selenoconotoxins, a new class of potent α_7 neuronal nicotinic receptor antagonists. *J. Biol. Chem.* **281**, 14136–14143 (2006).
28. Muttenthaler, M. & Alewood, P. F. Selenopeptide chemistry. *J. Pept. Sci.* **14**, 1223–1239 (2008).
29. Mobli, M., Morgenstern, D., King, G. F., Alewood, P. F. & Muttenthaler, M. Site-specific pK_a determination of selenocysteine residues in selenovasopressin by using ^{77}Se NMR spectroscopy. *Angew. Chem. Int. Ed.* **51**, 11952–11955 (2011).
30. Schnolzer, M., Alewood, P. F., Jones, A., Alewood, D. & Kent, S. B. In situ neutralization in Boc-chemistry solid phase peptide synthesis. Rapid, high yield assembly of difficult sequences. *Int. J. Pept. Protein Res.* **40**, 180–193 (1992).
31. de Araujo, A. D., Mobli, M., King, G. F. & Alewood, P. F. Cyclization of peptides via selenolanthionine bridges. *Angew. Chem. Int. Ed.* **51**, 10298–10302 (2012).
32. Hawe, A. et al. Towards heat-stable oxytocin formulations: analysis of degradation kinetics and identification of degradation products. *Pharm. Res.* **26**, 1679–1688 (2009).
33. Cassonie, P., Sapino, A., Stella, A., Fortunati, N. & Bussolati, G. Presence and significance of oxytocin receptors in human neuroblastomas and glial tumors. *Int. J. Cancer.* **77**, 695–700 (1998).
34. Woods, S. P. et al. Crystal structure analysis of deamino-oxytocin: conformational flexibility and receptor binding. *Science* **232**, 633–636 (1986).
35. Rose, J. P., Wu, C.-K., Hsiao, C.-D., Breslow, E. & Wang, B.-C. Crystal structure of the neurophysin-oxytocin complex. *Nat. Struct. Biol.* **3**, 163–169 (1996).
36. Brewster, A. I. & Hruby, V. J. 300-MHz nuclear magnetic resonance study of oxytocin aqueous solution: conformational implications. *Proc. Natl Acad. Sci. USA* **70**, 3806–3809 (1973).
37. Blumenstein, M. & Hruby, V. J. Interactions of oxytocin with bovine neurophysins I and II. Use of ^{13}C nuclear magnetic resonance and hormones specifically enriched with ^{13}C in the Glycinamide-9 and half-cystine-1 positions. *Biochemistry* **16**, 5169–5177 (1977).
38. Lippens, G. et al. Transfer nuclear overhauser effect study of the conformation of oxytocin bound to bovine neurophysin I. *Biochemistry* **32**, 9423–9434 (1993).
39. Mobli, M. et al. Direct visualization of disulfide bonds through diselenide proxies using ^{77}Se NMR. *Angew. Chem. Int. Ed.* **48**, 9312–9314 (2009).
40. Güntert, P. Automated NMR structure calculation with CYANA. *Methods Mol. Biol.* **278**, 353–378 (2004).
41. Shen, Y., Delaglio, F., Cornilescu, G. & Bax, A. TALOS + : a hybrid method for predicting protein backbone torsion angles from NMR chemical shifts. *J. Biomol. NMR* **44**, 213–223 (2009).
42. Mobli, M. & King, G. F. NMR methods for determining disulfide-bond connectivities. *Toxicon* **56**, 849–854 (2010).
43. Hughes, P. A. et al. Sensory neuro-immune interactions differ between IBS subtypes. *Gut* **62**, 1456–1465 (2013).
44. Harrington, A. M. et al. A novel role for TRPM8 in visceral afferent function. *Pain* **152**, 1459–1468 (2011).
45. Brierley, S. M. et al. Selective role for TRPV4 ion channels in visceral sensory pathways. *Gastroenterology* **135**, 2059–2069 (2008).
46. Hughes, P. A. et al. Post-inflammatory colonic afferent sensitization: different subtypes, different pathways, and different time-courses. *Gut* **58**, 1333–1341 (2009).
47. Castro, J. et al. Linaclotide inhibits colonic nociceptors and relieves abdominal pain via guanylate cyclase-C and extracellular cyclic GMP. *Gastroenterology* **145**, 1334–1346, e11 (2013).

48. Adam, B. *et al.* Severity of mucosal inflammation as a predictor for alterations of visceral sensory function in a rat model. *Pain* **123**, 179–186 (2006).

49. Gschossmann, J. M. *et al.* Long-term effects of transient chemically induced colitis on the visceromotor response to mechanical colorectal distension. *Digest. Dis. Sci.* **49**, 96–101 (2004).

50. Barbara, G. *et al.* Activated mast cells in proximity to colonic nerves correlate with abdominal pain in irritable bowel syndrome. *Gastroenterology* **126**, 693–702 (2004).

51. Liebregts, T. *et al.* Immune activation in patients with irritable bowel syndrome. *Gastroenterology* **132**, 913–920 (2007).

52. Ohman, L. & Simren, M. Pathogenesis of IBS: role of inflammation, immunity and neuroimmune interactions. *Nat. Rev. Gastroenterol. Hepatol.* **7**, 163–173 (2010).

53. Azpiroz, F. *et al.* Mechanisms of hypersensitivity in IBS and functional disorders. *Neurogastroent. Motil.* **19**, 62–88 (2007).

54. Lembo, T. *et al.* Evidence for the hypersensitivity of lumbar splanchnic afferents in irritable bowel syndrome. *Gastroenterology* **107**, 1686–1696 (1994).

55. Price, D. D., Zhou, Q., Moshiree, B., Robinson, M. E. & Verne, G. N. Peripheral and central contributions to hyperalgesia in irritable bowel syndrome. *J. Pain* **7**, 529–535 (2006).

56. Brierley, S. M., Jones, III R. C. W., Gebhart, G. F. & Blackshaw, L. A. Splanchnic and pelvic mechanosensory afferents signal different qualities of colonic stimuli in mice. *Gastroenterology* **127**, 166–178 (2004).

57. Ibeakanma, C. *et al. Citrobacter rodentium* colitis evokes post-infectious hyperexcitability of mouse nociceptive colonic dorsal root ganglion neurons. *J. Physiol.* **587**, 3505–3521 (2009).

58. Ibeakanma, C. *et al.* Brain-gut interactions increase peripheral nociceptive signaling in mice with postinfectious irritable bowel syndrome. *Gastroenterology* **141**, 2098–2108 (2011).

59. Harrington, A. M. *et al.* Sprouting of colonic afferent central terminals and increased spinal mitogen-activated protein kinase expression in a mouse model of chronic visceral hypersensitivity. *J. Comp. Neurol.* **520**, 2241–2255 (2012).

60. Ohlsson, B., Ringstrom, G., Abrahamsson, H., Simren, M. & Bjornsson, E. S. Oxytocin stimulates colonic motor activity in healthy women. *Neurogastroent. Motil.* **16**, 233–240 (2004).

61. Circu, M. L. & Aw, T. Y. Redox biology of the intestine. *Free Radic. Res.* **45**, 1245–1266 (2011).

62. Fjellestad-Paulsen, A., Sijderberg-Ahlm, C. & Lundin, S. Metabolism of vasopressin, oxytocin, and their analogs in the human gastrointestinal tract. *Peptides* **6**, 1141–1147 (1995).

63. Vetter, I. & Lewis, R. J. Characterization of endogenous calcium responses in neuronal cell lines. *Biochem. Pharmacol.* **79**, 908–920 (2010).

Acknowledgements

This work was funded in part by the National Health and Medical Research Council of Australia (NHMRC) Project Grant no. 1063803 to P.F.A. and S.M.B. A.M.H received funding via the Australian Research Council Discovery Early Career Research Award. S.M.B received funding via an NHMRC R.D Wright Biomedical Research Fellowship.

Author contributions

A.D.A. and M.Mo. contributed equally to the work. A.D.A. designed and performed the synthesis of the oxytocin analogues. M.Mobli designed and performed the NMR structure analysis. S.M.B., J.C., A.M.H. and M. Muttenthaler discovered OT analgesic activity and performed the colonic assays and expression studies. I.V. performed the functional Ca mobilization assays. Z.D. performed the plasma stability assay. J.W. synthesized OT. P.F.A., S.M.B, R.J.L. and G.F.K directed the project. A.D.A., S.M.B, M. Mobli and P.F.A wrote the paper. All authors contributed to the discussion and interpretation of the results.

Additional information

Competing financial interests: The authors declare no competing financial interests.

14

Assembly of a π–π stack of ligands in the binding site of an acetylcholine-binding protein

Mariano Stornaiuolo[1], Gerdien E. De Kloe[2], Prakash Rucktooa[1], Alexander Fish[1], René van Elk[3], Ewald S. Edink[2], Dariel Bertrand[4], August B. Smit[3], Iwan J. P. de Esch[2] & Titia K. Sixma[1]

Acetylcholine-binding protein is a water-soluble homologue of the extracellular ligand-binding domain of cys-loop receptors. It is used as a structurally accessible prototype for studying ligand binding to these pharmaceutically important pentameric ion channels, in particular to nicotinic acetylcholine receptors, due to conserved binding site residues present at the interface between two subunits. Here we report that an aromatic conjugated small molecule binds acetylcholine-binding protein in an ordered π–π stack of three identical molecules per binding site, two parallel and one antiparallel. Acetylcholine-binding protein stabilizes the assembly of the stack by aromatic contacts. Thanks to the plasticity of its ligand-binding site, acetylcholine-binding protein can accommodate the formation of aromatic stacks of different size by simple loop repositioning and minimal adjustment of the interactions. This type of supramolecular binding provides a novel paradigm in drug design.

[1] Division of Biochemistry and Center for Biomedical Genetics, Netherlands Cancer Institute, Plesmanlaan 121, 1066 CX Amsterdam, The Netherlands. [2] Division of Medicinal Chemistry, Faculty of Sciences, Amsterdam Institute for Molecules, Medicines and Systems, VU University Amsterdam, De Boelelaan 1083, 1081 HV Amsterdam, The Netherlands. [3] Department of Molecular and Cellular Neurobiology, Center for Neurogenomics and Cognitive Research, VU University, 1081 HV Amsterdam The Netherlands. [4] HiQScreenSàrl, 6, rue de Compois, 1222 Vésenaz, Geneva, Switzerland. Correspondence and requests for materials should be addressed to T.K.S. (email: t.sixma@nki.nl).

Screening compound libraries for biologically active molecules results in hit structures considered to be interesting starting points for drug design. Although it is often assumed that a single small drug molecule interacts with one protein-binding site, compounds binding to target proteins with higher stoichiometry can be found during library screening[1]. Here, we show an unexpected ligand interaction where three identical molecules interact within a single binding site. The binding of preorganized and/or in situ-organizing small binder molecules was shown to happen on the surface of proteins but examples of supramolecular assembly happening at the canonical-binding site of a target are still rare[2,3]. Recently two molecules of the IRE1 inhibitor quercetin were found binding at the dimer interface of the target and proved to induce its dimerization[4] (PDB: 3LJ0). An example of ligand supramolecular assembly was described also for a flavine-binding enzyme in complex with the cofactors FMN and NADH at the surface of the protein[5] (PDB: 2VZH, 2VZJ).

Cys-loop receptors are important ligand-gated ion channels in the central and peripheral nervous systems[6–10]. Members include the nicotinic acetylcholine receptors (nAChR), GABA$_A$ receptors, 5HT$_3$ serotonin and glycine receptors, and all

Table 1 | Chemical formula, numbering and IUPAC name of the fragments.

	2	1-Amino-3-(2-pyridyl)isoquinoline
	3	1-Amino-3-(3-pyridyl)isoquinoline
	4	6-Amino-2,2′-bipyridine
	5	4-(4-Methylpiperazin-1-yl)-6-phenylpyrimidin-2-amine
	6	2-(1-Methylimidazol-2-yl)-4,6-dipyridine

IUPAC, International Union of Pure and Applied Chemistry.

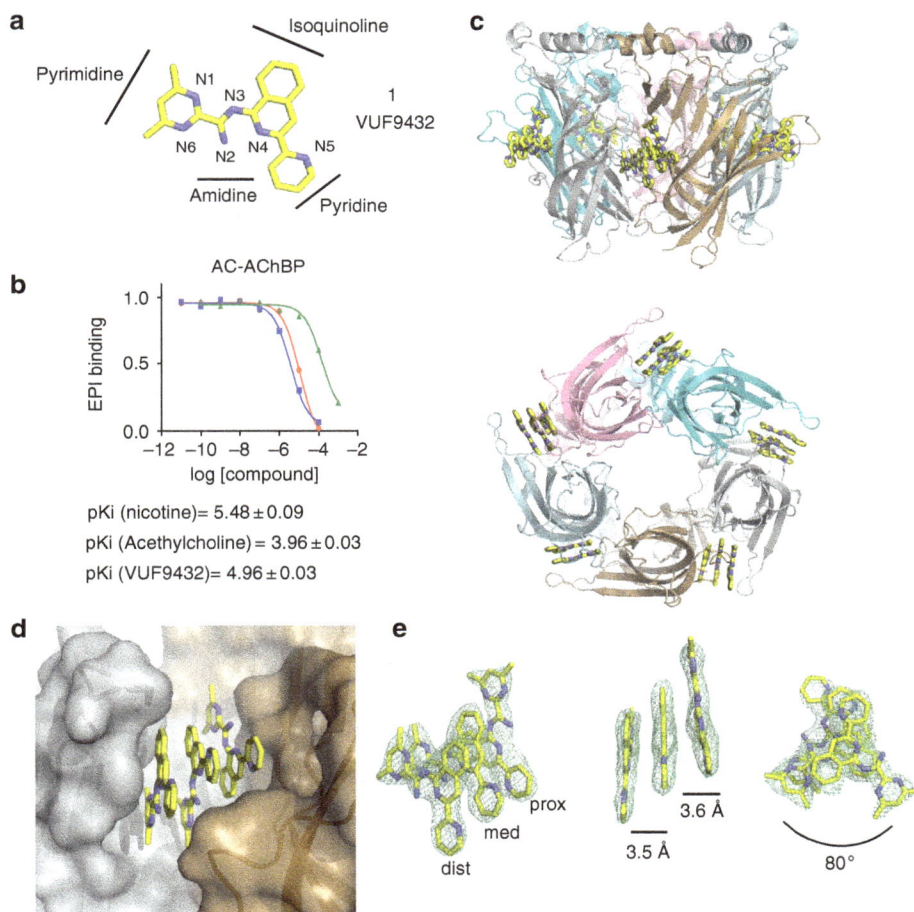

Figure 1 | VUF9432 binds as a triple stack to Ac-AChBP. (**a**) Chemical structure of VUF9432 (carbon atoms in yellow, nitrogen atoms in blue). (**b**) Displacement of radio-labelled epibatidine (EPI) by VUF9432 (red curves), nicotine (blue curves) and acetylcholine (green curves) on Ac-AChBP (purified proteins). Data are the mean ± s.e.m. of three experiments and are reported below the panel. (**c**) Side and bottom side view of Ac-AChBP-VUF9432 complex structure, showing VUF9432 molecules (yellow sticks) in the five binding sites. (**d**) Protomer–protomer interfaces (surface representation) of Ac-AChBP-VUF9432 complex. Principal side is depicted in silver and complementary side in sand colours. Ligand-binding site are shown in transparency. (**e**) Electron density map displaying VUF9432 molecules in the ligand-binding site formed by subunit A and B (experimental density contoured at 1 σ), different orientation of the stacking molecules are shown together with the nomenclature used to distinguish the three molecules in the text. Intermolecular distances and angles are depicted as lines between the planes. dist, distal; med, medial; prox, proximal.

important pharmacological targets for various diseases and conditions[10]. nAChRs are targets for the endogenous neurotransmitter acetylcholine and for a series of compounds aimed at the treatment of cognitive decline in Alzheimer's disease, certain forms of epilepsy[11] or nicotine addiction[12].

In the homo- or heteropentameric ion channels of the cys-loop receptor family, an extracellular ligand-binding site, is located at the interface between a 'principal' and a 'complementary' subunit, each of which contributes three loops (A–C and D–F, respectively) to the binding[6–8,13]. Agonist binding triggers conformational changes in cys-loop receptors and leads to opening of the channel and a flux of ions through the channel pore[14]. Ligand-binding sites in cys-loop receptors are highly plastic, allowing binding of various molecules ranging from small neurotransmitters all the way to large peptide neurotoxins, such as conotoxins and snake toxin[6–10]. Flexibility for different-sized ligands is generated by the positioning of loop C that contributes two conserved tyrosines and a vicinal disulphide bridge to the ligand-binding site.

Most high-resolution structural information on cys-loop receptor–ligand interactions is available from a molluscan acetylcholine-binding protein (AChBP)[15–18]. AChBP structurally resembles the ligand-binding domains of cys-loop receptors, but lacks a transmembrane domain[16]. Their ligand-binding site resembles the α7 subtype of the nAChRs most (20–24% sequence identity) and their high-resolution crystal structures[16–23] reveal a structural fold closely related to cys-loop receptors as well as to their bacterial homologs[24–29].

Here we show that AChBP binds an ordered aromatic π–π stack of three identical ligands. The high-resolution X-ray crystal structure of this molecule in complex with *Aplysia californica* (Ac)-AChBP reveals a new example of protein–ligand interaction controlled by supramolecular ligand assembly. The nature of the binding mode, the analysis of protein residues contributing to the stabilization of the stack and the kinetics of the binding events are described. Finally, we identify acridine orange (AO) as a ligand with similar binding that could potentially be used as competitive inhibitor for α7 nAChR.

Results

Identification of VUF9432. A fragment[30,31] screening assay using online fluorescence enhancement led to the identification of fragments 2–6 (Table 1) as hits for AChBP (refs 32,33). In a subsequent analogue screening, VUF9432 (1), (IUPAC name: 4,6-dimethyl-N-(3-(pyridin-2-yl)isoquinoline-1-yl)-pyrimidine-2-carboximidamide) (Fig. 1a) was shown to have micromolar affinity for AChBP. VUF9432 was originally synthesized as a copper-dependent antimycoplasmal agent active against *Mycoplasma gallisepticum* proliferation and later identified in a screen as ligand for adenosine A₃ receptors[34].

Binding affinities of VUF9432 for Ac-AChBP and α7 nAChR were measured in a radioligand displacement assay with [³H] epibatidine and [³H] methyllycaconitine (MLA) as displaceable ligands for AChBPs (Fig. 1b) and α7 nAChR (Supplementary Fig. S1), respectively. VUF9432 behaves as competitive binder for AChBP, showing a pKi value of 4.96 ± 0.03 for Ac-AChBP. The compound also displays some binding to α7 nAChR (pKi around five) but the radioligand is not fully displaced at the highest concentration tested, possibly due to low solubility of the compound under the assay conditions.

In contrast to typical nAChR targeting molecules, VUF9432 lacks the canonical cation center involved in cation-π interactions with aromatic residues in the binding site[13,14]. The binding mode, interaction of VUF9432 to Ac-AChBP, was investigated by cocrystallization trials and X-ray analysis.

Table 2 | Data collection and refinement statistics.

	AChBP-VUF9432
Data collection	PX1 (SLS)
Space group	P21
Cell dimensions	
a, b, c (Å)	80.73, 78.33, 106.53
α, β, γ (°)	90.00, 102.67, 90.00
Resolution (Å)	43.30–2.4 (2.53–2.4)*
Rmerge	12.9 (76.1)
I/σI	5.9 (1.8)
Completeness (%)	93.0 (92.6)
Redundancy	2.4
Refinement	
Resolution (Å)	41.26–2.4 (2.53–2.4)
No. of reflections	44,879
Rwork/Rfree	0.21/0.25
No. of atoms	
Protein	8,188
Ligand/ion	384
Water	129
B-factors	
Protein	36.80
Ligand/ion	63.48
Water	27.41
R.m.s deviations	
Bond lengths (Å)	0.009
Bond angles (°)	1.315

*Highest resolution shell is shown in parenthesis

VUF9432 binds AChBP in a triple stacked configuration. The 2.4-Å crystal structure of the complex between Ac-AChBP and VUF9432 revealed the unexpected presence of three VUF9432 molecules in four out of the five ligand-binding sites in the pentamer (the fifth site is discussed separately below) (Fig. 1c,d). Careful refinement of the protein and the asymmetric shape of the VUF9432 molecule allowed the unambiguous fitting into the electron densities (Fig. 1e and Supplementary Fig. S2), resulting in a refined structure with R = 21%/Rfree = 25% and excellent stereochemistry (Table 2).

Within each ligand-binding site, the three conjugated molecules of VUF9432 stack on each other (Fig. 1e) in a flat planar configuration. The three molecules are organized in a columnar stack, with an off-centred parallel displaced geometry. The distal molecule of VUF9432, closest to the C-loop and the medial one (Fig. 1e) are identically oriented with the pyrimidine rings pointing towards the inner part of the ligand-binding site, whereas the proximal molecule is twofold rotated relative to the other VUF9432 molecules. The distance between the medial molecule and the proximal and distal ones are 3.5 and 3.6 Å, respectively, consistent with previously measured π–π stacking distances between aromatic molecules[35]. The angle between the planes is at most 3.8 ± 0.8° and 6.2 ± 2.1°, due to slight tilting of the medial and proximal molecules towards the distal one, respectively, confirming the almost perfectly parallel displaced orientation (Fig. 1e). The proximal and distal copies of the molecule occupy slightly variable tilt angles within these planes, and hence have somewhat higher average B factors (58.4 ± 10.23, 60.28 ± 10.16 and 74.45 ± 11.8 Å² for the medial, proximal and distal copy of VUF9432, respectively). Nevertheless it is clear that all three sites are fully occupied and the excellent quality of the electron density of the C-loop indicates full occupancy of these ligands.

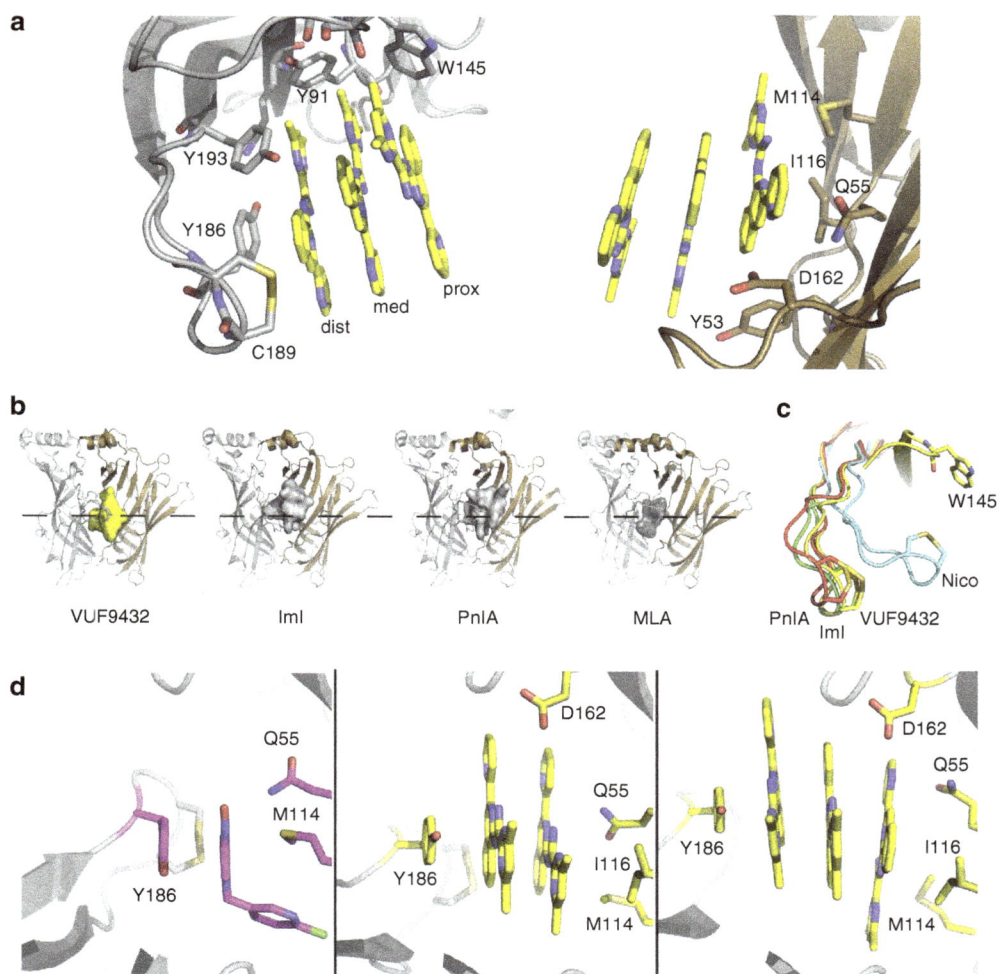

Figure 2 | Details of VUF9432 binding to Ac-AChBP. (**a**) Ball-and-stick representation showing Ac-AChBP residues on principal and complementary subunits interacting with VUF9432 (colours as in Fig. 1). The triple stack is held up like a row of books by Y186, Q55 and M114. Edge interactions with aromatic residues, D162 and the vicinal disulphide are indicated. (**b**) Protomer–protomer interfaces of VUF9432-Ac-AChBP structure illustrating how VUF9432 (surface, yellow) is occupying a lower part of the ligand-binding site if compared with the toxin IMI (surface, grey), PnIA (surface, grey) and MLA (surface, grey). (**c**) Comparison of C-loop opening in AChBP- nicotine (cyan), AChBP-PnIA (red), AChBP-IMI (green) and AChBP-VUF9432 (yellow) complex. Position assumed by the C-loop after VUF9432 binding resembles that in conotoxins. (**d**) Comparison of binding modes of Imidacloprid (magenta) and VUF9432 (yellow) to AChBP showing the two ligands establishing similar interactions with the ligand-binding site. Repositioning of the C-loop provides the space for either one, two or three flat aromatic moieties.

The stack of aromatic VUF9432 molecules is held in place like a pile of books, at one end by the stacking of well-conserved principal face residue Y186 (Fig. 2a), which has an off-centred displaced parallel π–π interaction with the distal molecule, tilted at $12.3 \pm 2.4°$. At the other end the stack is positioned through van der Waals interactions with complementary side residues Q55 and M114. The side chain of I116 is positioned towards the stack, but does not interact with the proximal molecule.

Aromatic groups on the principal (Y91, W145, Y193) and complementary faces (Y53) stabilize the sides of the stack of ligands via edge-to-face interactions, establishing T-shaped aromatic contacts with the molecules (Fig. 2a). Finally, the F-loop D162 and the vicinal disulphide in the C-loop also interact with the sides of the stacked VUF9432 molecules.

Taken together, the three stacked molecules of VUF9432 occupy a large volume and bury a substantial surface area in AChBP ($959.9 \pm 4.8 Å^2$) comparable with the area buried by conotoxins IMI[20] (PDB:2C9T) and PnIA[19] (PDB:2BR8) ($1164 Å^2$ and $1468 Å^2$, respectively). However, the position of VUF9432 in

the binding site is different, as can be seen in Fig. 2b. The space occupied by the conotoxins is above the midline of the pentamer, away from the transmembrane domain in the cys-loop receptors, whereas the VUF9432 molecules are placed lower, close to the membrane, not far from the binding site for MLA (ref. 36). However, MLA (PDB:2BYR) is in a different site closer to the five-fold axis than VUF9432, which uses a lower, more external cavity (Fig. 2b). It does not address the so-called 'lobeline pocket' and Y91 is in the g-conformation, interacting with S144[37]. The combination of this novel position and slightly smaller buried surface area result in a C-loop position that is similar to that for the conotoxins, in its most open state (Supplementary Fig. S3).

In one of the five ligand-binding sites only two molecules of VUF9432 are bound, positioned in parallel manner, similarly to the medial and the distal copy in the other ligand-binding sites (Fig. 3a,b). This state is most likely stabilized by crystal contacts (Fig. 3f). Although the double stack is tilted 15° relative to the triple stack in the other binding sites (Fig. 3c), the direct contacts are retained. Thus, the stack is upheld by Y186 at one end and

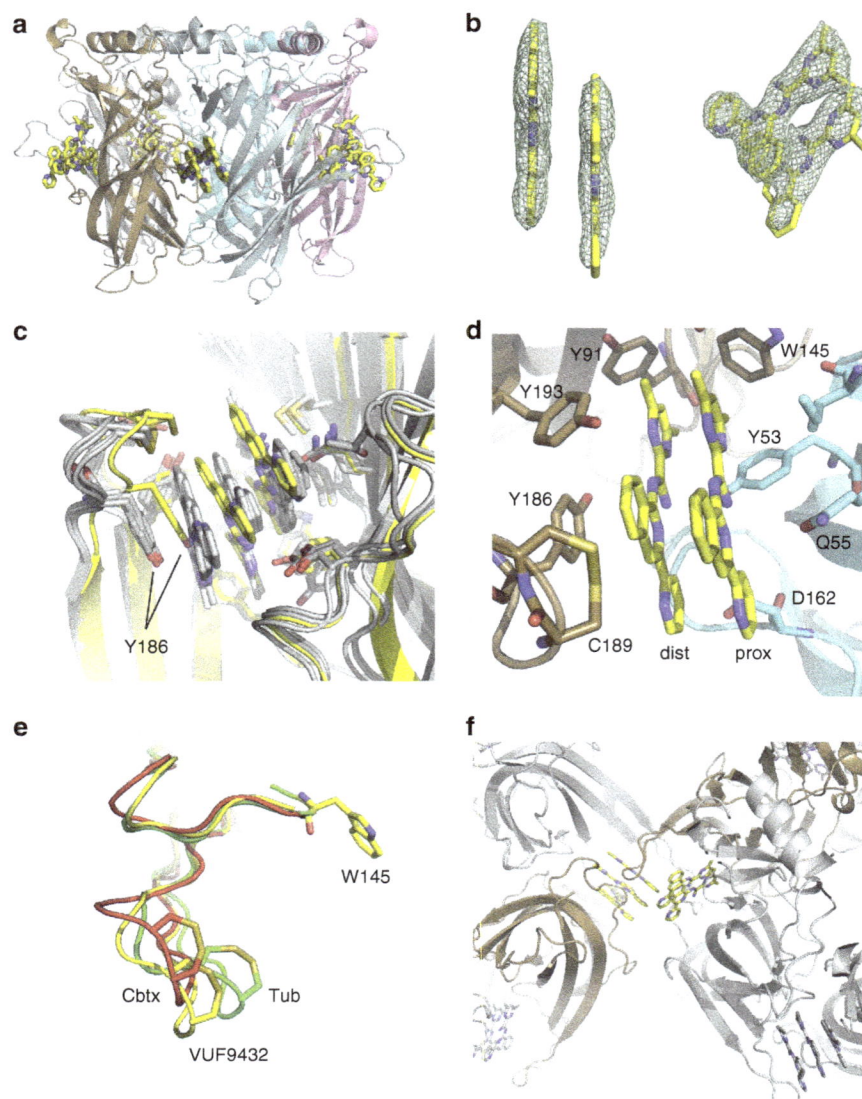

Figure 3 | AChBP can accommodate a double stack of VUF9432. (**a**) Side view of Ac-AChBP-VUF9432 complex structure, showing two VUF9432 molecules (yellow sticks) in the binding site formed by subunit B (sand) and C (cyan). (**b**) Electron density map displaying VUF9432 molecules in the ligand-binding site formed by subunit B and C (experimental density contoured at 1 σ). (**c**) Superposition of the four ligand binds site binding triple stacks of VUF9432 (grey cartoon and sticks) and the one binding the double stack of molecule (yellow cartoon and sticks), showing the movement of the Y186 to accommodate the third molecule of the stack. (**d**) Ball-and-stick representation showing AChBP residues on principal and complementary subunits interacting with the double stack of VUF9432 (colours as in **a**). (**e**) Comparison of C-loop opening in AChBP-tubocurarine (Tub, green), AChBP-α-cobratoxin (Cbtx, red), AChBP-VUF9432 (the shown C-loop is the one of the ligand-binding site containing two copies of the stack, yellow) complex. Position assumed by the C-loop after VUF9432 binding resembles that in cobratoxin. (**f**) Interaction of an AChBP-VUF9432 molecule with the symmetry-related molecule that form intermolecular contacts. The open C-loop of subunit B contacts the F-loop of a symmetry-related molecules. The bound VUF9432 molecules are shown in ball and sticks.

M114 and Q55 at the other end with similar side interactions (Fig. 3d). The major difference for this binding site is caused by the loop C position, which in this case is in an intermediate open state, similar to that found for ligands such as tubocurarine[38] (PDB:2XYT) and α-cobratoxin[39] (PDB:1YI5) (Fig. 3e).

Interestingly, these contacts resemble those described for the pentameric ring of imidacloprid[40,41]. In that case, the flat aromatic imidazolinic part of the molecule is held in place by face to face stacking with Y186 and upheld by van der Waals contacts with M114. A H-bond connects the Q55 to an oxygen of the nitro group of imidacloprid (Fig. 2d), now held in place by a maximally closed C-loop.

Here, we show that the binding site of AChBP provides space for either one, as in imidacloprid, two or three flat aromatic moieties as seen here for VUF9432, all with similar contacts. This remarkable plasticity is organized primarily by repositioning of the C-loop (Fig. 2d).

Ligand stacking promoted by aromaticity and planarity. To exclude that the unusual configuration of these ligands is a crystallographic artifact, we analysed the binding in several ways. First we confirmed the VUF9432 binding to the ligand-binding site, by mutating interacting amino acids. Mutation of either

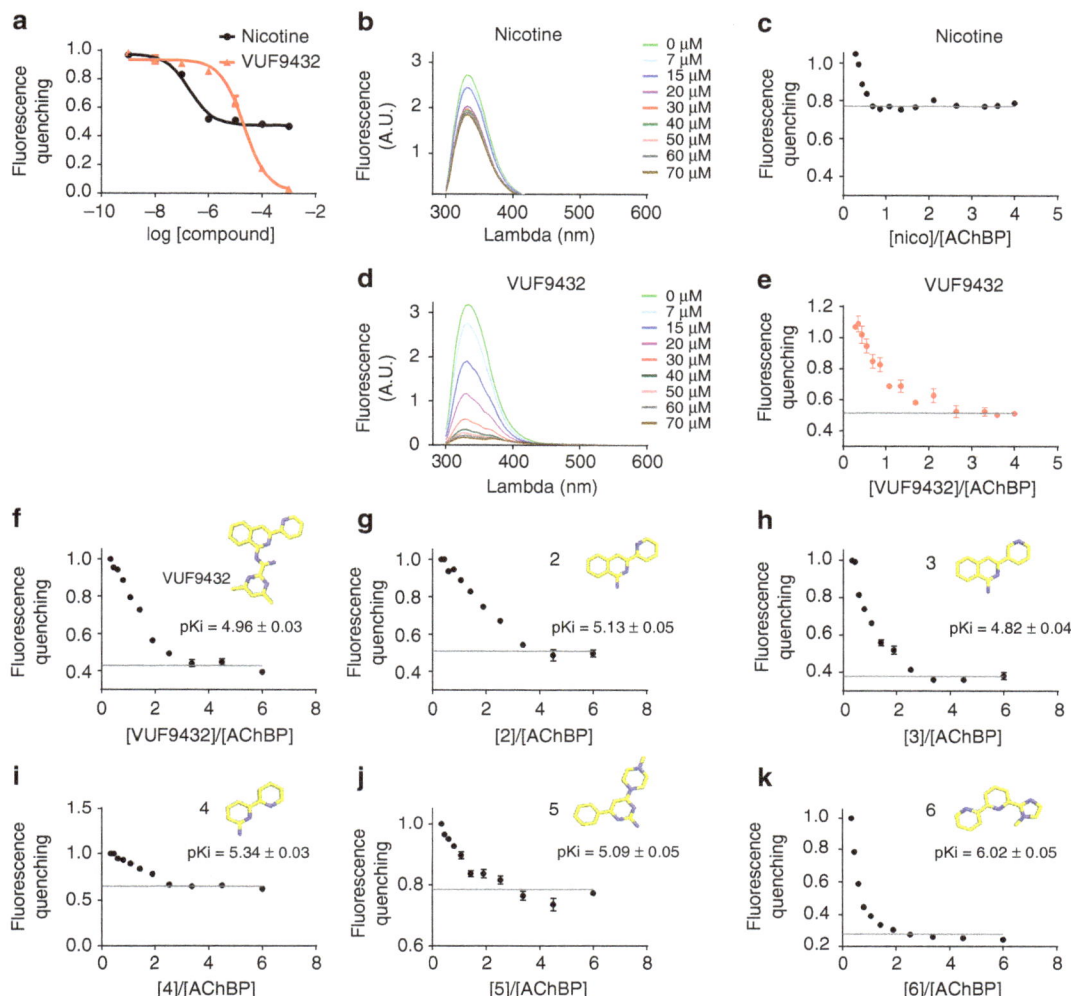

Figure 4 | Aromaticity and planarity determine multiple ligand binding to AChBP. (**a**) Comparison of affinity of Ac-AChBP for VUF9432 (red curve) and nicotine (black curve) measured with tryptophan fluorescence quenching. Titration of binding sites for nicotine (**b,c**) and VUF9432 (**d,e**) on Ac-AChBP by fluorescence quenching. Ac-AChBP at 20 μM binding sites was titrated with incremental quantities of ligand. Fluorescence excitation was at 280 nm. Full emission spectra were recorded and maxima were measured over the range 335–345 nm (**b,d**) and plotted versus the nicotine/AChBP (**c**, black dots) or VUF9432/AChBP (**e**, red dots) stoichiometric ratio. A straight line was fit through the plateau points (grey line) as described in the methods section. (**f–k**) Titration of binding sites for the VUF9432 and analogues on Ac-AChBP by fluorescence quenching. Affinity for AChBP (mean ± s.e.m. measured with radiodisplacement assay) and structure of the ligands (colours as in figure 1) are indicated. AChBP at 20 μM was titrated with incremental quantities of ligands as described above (fluorescence maxima plotted as in **c**).

Y186 or Y193 to alanine resulted in the loss of affinity for VUF9432 (Supplementary Fig. S4), confirming, also in solution, the binding to the canonical pocket.

We then tested the stoichiometry of VUF9432 binding to Ac-AChBP in solution, using equilibrium titration. Binding was analysed by the change in the fluorescence emission of W145 of AChBP, which correlates with the binding of agonists or antagonists[42]. Titration of nicotine binding at high protein concentrations showed that the fluorescence quenching reaches a plateau at the stoichiometric ratio ligand/AChBP close to one nicotine molecule bound per protomer (Fig. 4b,c). In contrast the titration profile of VUF9432 binding does not saturate until a stoichiometry of three ligands per protomer is reached (Fig. 4d,e), confirming the crystallographic data.

We wondered what properties of VUF9432 are necessary for the supramolecular binding. Conformational analysis in the gas phase (Supplementary Fig. S5a) shows that VUF9432 can adopt a series of relatively planar conformations, with minimal rotational freedom of the pyridine ring and of the amidine bond. In the

structure a conformation is selected where the pyridine, isoquinoline and pyrimidine rings are coplanar stabilized by a hydrogen bond between the amidine N2 and the isoquinolinic N4.

We then analysed the original fragment hits for their ligand-binding stoichiometries using fluorescence quenching. Affinity of these fragments for Ac-AChBP was relatively weak (Supplementary Fig. 6, numbers presented as mean pKi in Fig. 4f–k), which meant that we could only use a relative small excess of Ac-AChBP in these experiments. Nevertheless, we could clearly observe that several fragments retain the ability to bind in a three-to-one ratio.

Derivatives, VUF6141 (**2**) and VUF5954 (**3**) (Fig. 4g,h), that lack the pyrimidine ring show similar affinity to Ac-AChBP compared with VUF9432, in line with the lack of interaction with Ac-AChBP for this moiety. In computational analysis, both compounds are able to adopt a planar configuration (Supplementary Fig. S5b,c), especially compound **2**, where the planar configuration is the most stable, thanks to the N in position 6 of the pyridine, that prevents clashing between the hydrogen

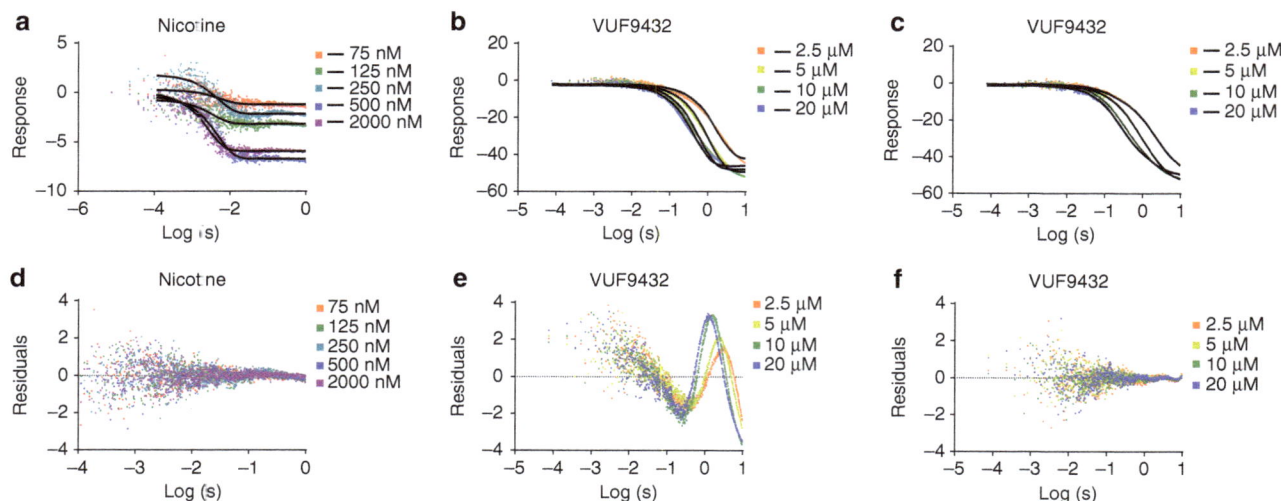

Figure 5 | Binding of VUF9432 is a multistep process. Kinetic studies of ligand association with AChBP. Stopped-flow traces of tryptophan fluorescence quenching on Ac-AChBP binding to nicotine (**a**) and VUF9432 (**b,c**). Upper panels show typical traces of observed fluorescence during and after stop page of flow at the indicated ligand concentrations. Panel **d** reports the residuals of the fitting for one-step nicotine binding to AChBP. Panels **e** and **f** report the residuals of the fitting for one (**e**) or two steps binding (**f**) of VUF9432 to AChBP, respectively.

atoms of the isoquinolinic and the pyridine rings (Supplementary Fig. S5b,c). Equilibrium fluorescence titration clearly indicates that Ac-AChBP can bind multiple copies of ligand **2** and **3** per binding site (Fig. 4g,h).

Interestingly, supramolecular binding was also seen for the bi-pyrimidinic compound VUF11370 (**4**) (Fig. 4i) showing that different aromatic planar molecules can self-assemble in Ac-AChBP. As seen for **2**, compound **4** prefers the planar conformation (Supplementary Fig. S5d). In compound VUF10460 (**5**), a piperazine moiety is present. As seen for nicotine (Fig. 4c) and many other canonical AChBP ligands[42], this compound induces less fluorescence quenching after binding to AChBP. Equilibrium fluorescence titration indicates the stoichiometry is changed to 1:1, although the affinity for the receptor was maintained (Fig. 4j). This molecule is not fully aromatic resulting in non-planarity of the piperazine moiety (Supplementary Fig. S5e), which most likely prevents the stacking observed in compounds **1–4**. Moreover, the compound is slightly basic, which could allow a cation-π interaction and an alternative binding mode.

The presence of an imidazolinic moiety like in compound VUF14476 (**6**) could result in a loss of the binding of multiple copies (Fig. 4k). In compound **6**, the methyl group attached to the imidazole ring is located at the centre of the molecule (Supplementary Fig. S5f), possibly preventing the formation of stacked molecules. Although there are two methyl groups present on the pyrimidine ring of VUF9432, these are at the edge of the molecule. The slight displacement of the molecules in the stacks may just be enough to ensure the absence of clashes between the hydrogen atoms of the methyl present on the distal and the medial molecules, when located at the edge of the molecule. Even assembling in a similar displaced configuration, the clashes between the hydrogen atoms of the methyl group of **6** could probably not be avoided, explaining the one to one stoichiometry to AChBP.

Binding of VUF9432 molecules occurs in steps. An interesting question is whether the three molecules bind as a 'package' or whether they bind sequentially. For this we first analysed the shape of the binding curves of the three molecules in VUF9432 and derivatives **2–4** (Fig. 4a,g–i), some of which may be non-linear.

This non-linearity could reflect differences in affinities for the three VUF9432 sites, resulting in differently shaped binding curves. Alternatively, the effect of binding of the three individual molecules could have differential effects on the tryptophan quenching. One could even imagine that a stack of more than one ligand will receive increased levels of resonance energy transferred from remote aromatic residues, otherwise unaffected by the binding of a single molecule. It will not be trivial to uncouple these possibilities, but it seems likely that the binding event is not a single-step transition of a single package of three ligands into the binding site.

To analyse the binding process in more detail, we used stopped-flow kinetic studies to monitor this assembly process (Fig. 5). Titration of nicotine shows simple association to Ac-AChBP (Fig. 5a)[42] that can be fitted with a one-step binding model (Fig. 5d). In contrast, the binding profile of VUF9432 cannot be fitted with a simple model (Fig. 5b,c). In practice a two-step fitting of the binding is sufficient to achieve acceptable residuals (Fig. 5e,f), confirming a more complex binding process. In contrast to the proposed binding of bungarotoxin[42], where the second step is concentration independent and most likely due to a conformational adjustment, for VUF9432 the second step varies with concentration, indicating the stepwise binding of the ligands.

Multiple binding of a fluorescent aromatic molecule to AChBP. We wondered whether different molecules could bind in this manner and searched for planar aromatic molecules. AO[43–45] is a fluorescent planar aromatic molecule with increased solubility compared with VUF9432. We found that AO (Fig. 6a) binds the ligand-binding site of AChBP with micromolar affinity (pKi = 5.8, Fig. 6b). An analogue of AO, *N*-methylacridinium, was shown to bind in the active site of the enzyme acetylcholinesterase, which also displays affinity for acetylcholine[46]. When AO binding to Ac-AChBP was tested using tryptophan fluorescence quenching at high concentration, we observed that as for VUF9432 the binding has a stoichiometric ratio higher than one (Fig. 6c). In agreement with this, titration of Ac-AChBP into an AO solution, Ac-AChBP quenched AO fluorescence at a stoichiometric ratio of 0.3 (Fig. 6d, black dots). This quenching of AO by Ac-AChBP is inhibited in the presence of an excess of nicotine, confirming that AO is

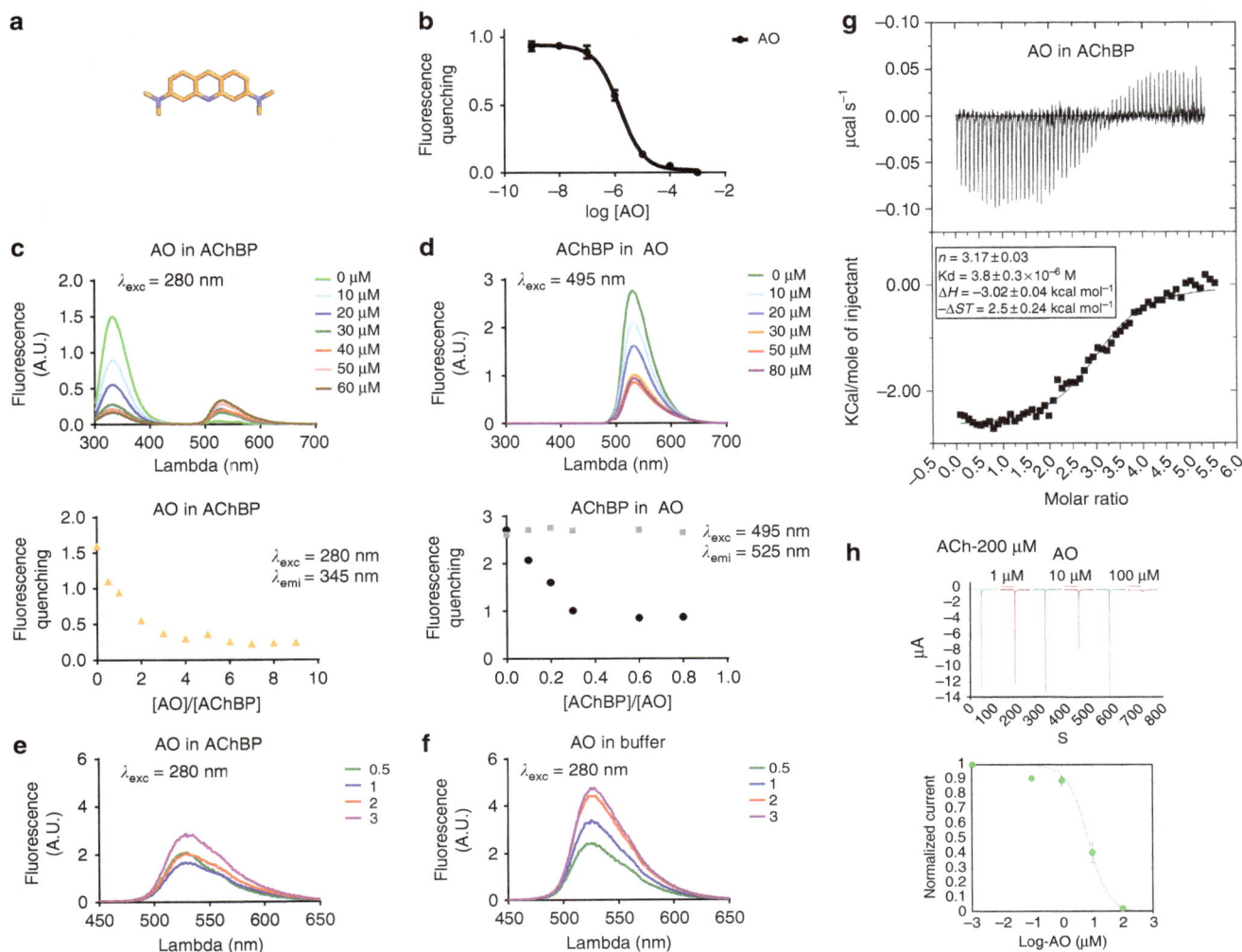

Figure 6 | AO orange mimics the triple stacking ligand. (**a**) Chemical structure of AO (carbon in orange, nitrogen in blue) (**b**) Affinity of Ac-AChBP for AO measured with fluorescence quenching (as described in Figure4). (**c**) Titration of binding sites for AO on Ac-AChBP by tryptophan fluorescence quenching. Ac-AChBP at 20 μM was titrated with incremental quantities of AO. Fluorescence excitation was at 280 nm and full emission spectra were collected between 300 and 700 nm, and emission maxima were measured over the range 335–345 nm and plotted versus the AO/AChBP stoichiometric ratio. (**d**) Titration of binding sites for AO on Ac-AChBP by AO fluorescence quenching. AO at 100 μM was titrated with incremental quantities of AChBP in presence (grey dots) or in absence of 1mM nicotine (black dots). Fluorescence excitation was at 495nm and full emission spectra were collected between 300 and 700 nm: emission maxima were measured over the range 525–535 nm and plotted versus the AO-AChBP stoichiometric ratio. Comparison of the fluoresce emission of free AO (**f**) or AChBP-AO complex (**e**) at stoichiometric ratio AO-AChBP of 0.5 (green curve), 1 (blue curve), 2 (red curve) and 3 (purple curve). (**g**) Calorimetric data of AO binding to AChBP. Top panel shows the raw heat measured over a series of AO injections (500 μM). Each heat signal is integrated and shown as data point in the bottom panel. Data points were fitted to a model describing a single set of binding sites and best-fit parameters for AO binding were calculated using least-squares fitting. (**h**) Acridine orange inhibits half of ACh-evoked currents at α7 nAChR receptors expressed in oocytes at concentrations around 10 μM and gives almost full inhibition of the current at 100 μM.

binding competitively to the binding pocket of Ac-AChBP (Fig. 6d, grey dots).

The formation of the AO stack in Ac-AChBP should determine differences in the emission spectra of the molecules as seen for aromatic π–π stacking in organic aromatic cages[47]. The fluorescence spectra of AO in complex with Ac-AChBP and those free in solution were compared. Emission at 525nm (π–π* transition)[43] of the complexed acridine moiety is quenched in the presence of Ac-AChBP due to the interaction of AO with the aromatic environment. During the titration the intensity at 525 nm increases without further shifts (Fig. 6f), as expected[47].

AO is highly soluble allowing us to use isothermal titration calorimetry (ITC) to follow its binding to AChBP. Our data indicate that AO binds to Ac-AChBP with a stoichiometric ratio of 3–4, with a Kd of 1.86 μM and that the sequential binding is enthalpically favoured (Fig. 6g). Fitting of the experimental data to a model indicates the existence of three events of AO binding per ligand-binding domain of Ac-AChBP. This confirms that other planar molecules can bind to the Ac-AChBP ligand-binding site in a similar manner to VUF9432. Interestingly, when AO was tested in electrophysiology experiments on α7 nAChR-expressing oocytes, it behaved as competitive inhibitor with an IC50 of 7.3 μM, showing an affinity similar to the one measured for Ac-AChBP (Fig. 6h). Thus, ligands with the potential of supramolecular binding can be relevant for drug design on nAChRs.

Discussion

To our knowledge Ac-AChBP is the first example of a target protein binding a triple π–π stack of ligand molecules. In this paper, we prove that Ac-AChBP binds VUF9432 (Figs 1–5), fragments **2**, **3**, **4**, and AO with stoichiometry higher than one (Figs 4 and 6). All these compounds address the canonical-binding site of Ac-AChBP and behave as competitive binders (Figs 1, 4 and 6). Aromaticity and planarity of the molecule positively influence the super-stoichiometry (Fig. 4 and Supplementary Fig. S5).

VUF9432 is not very soluble and binds only weakly to α7 nAChR. When tested in electrophysiology experiments, we did not observe any effect of VUF9432 on α7 nAChR expressed in oocytes, probably due to the low solubility (data not shown). However, we identified AO as a molecule that binds AChBP with similar binding properties and stoichiometry. Interestingly, this highly soluble ligand has robust inhibitory properties on nAChR in oocytes, showing the potential for exploitation of these types of ligand binding.

The crystal structure of VUF9432 in Ac-AChBP allows analysis of the supramolecular binding mode. The three molecules of VUF9432 stack in a parallel displaced orientation. The latter was reported to be one of the lowest energetic conformations that such a stack can acquire[35]. In addition several edge-to-face interactions are observed, contributing to the binding properties.

The non-linearity of the binding curves of VUF9432, compound **2**–**4** and AO, the stopped-flow analysis of VUF9432 binding to Ac-AChBP and the ITC measurement of AO binding to Ac-AChBP suggest that likely the stacking of the molecules is happening *in situ* and not as preassembled stack (Figs 4–6). However, we cannot exclude other scenarios. Stopped-flow fluorescence measurement of the binding of α-bungarotoxin to Ac-AChBP was shown to not be a one-step event[43]. This result was interpreted, suggesting multiple binding modes of the toxin to the binding site of Ac-AChBP. As postulated for the toxin also a stack of VUF9432 could just bind preassembled and have multiple binding modes.

Conformational search performed in gas phase would suggests that this unusual stacking is not present for VUF9432 in solution and that the assembly *in situ* at the protein-binding site would be energetically more favoured. In particular, the dipole on VUF9432 would disfavour the parallel stacking that is observed for the distal and medial copies of the compound (Figs 1–3). Hence, it is clear that interactions with Ac-AChBP could contribute to stabilize these configurations and that each VUF9432 molecule orients in the ligand-binding site according to the electrostatic environment of the protein rather than their individual local dipole moment.

Entropic factors hamper the intentional creation of parallel π–π stacks of molecules. 'Tweezer' molecules have been used to stabilize columns of aromatic molecules[48]. Also, reconstitution of a discrete columnar stack of aromatic molecules has been achieved using box-shaped coordination cage[47]. Here, we show that a protein can enable the formation of a π–π stack of molecules. The stacking is stabilized by the contribution of the aromatic side chains of the ligand-binding site. Although π–π interactions are thought to be weak[35], they have been recognized to have an important role in the folding and in the thermal stability of proteins and the binding to ligands.

The binding site in Ac-AChBP is closely related to that of other cys-loop receptors, where specificity for different ligands is provided by amino-acid changes in the loops A–C and D–F. The remarkable plasticity of the ligand-binding site, allowing the binding of differently sized ligands in cys-loop receptors, is tuned by the positioning of the C-loop and has a pivotal role in dictating the dimension of the stack. Recently, Ac-AChBP was found to be capable of accommodating two molecules of acetylcholine it its binding sites, although relative occupancies are very different between the two molecules[49] (PDB: 2XZ5). Here, we show that the binding site offers a variety of binding possibilities, by simple repositioning of the C-loop (Figs 2 and 3) to accommodate either one, two or three ligand molecules (Fig. 2), with relatively little adjustment in the interactions.

The binding site AChBP was recently shown to accommodate *in situ* Huisgen cycloaddition 'click' reactions[50]. Thus, these binding sites can serve as a reaction vessel for chemical reactions. In combination with the ability to promote supramolecular self-assembly, this binding site provides a unique environment for novel chemistry, which can be further tuned by amino-acid variations of loops A–F, varying the properties of the binding pocket.

Multiple binding in a specific manner within a ligand-binding site provides a novel paradigm for ligand binding. Aggregation of molecules and the presence of multiple independent binding sites have been discussed in the area of drug design previously[51]. However, the interdependent binding required to make a ligand stack is different. It provides specific opportunities as well as novel challenges. Clearly, it will become important to take the stacking possibility into account when analysing ligand binding. Stoichiometry analysis will be important, in particular when considering binding profiles that could potentially provide this type of stacking. Meanwhile, one can see this as a novel opportunity, providing previously unexplored avenues for drug design. Not necessarily trivial, as large flat molecules have obvious disadvantages in design strategies compared with three-dimensional fragments[51], but definitely a new and unexplored opportunity, where a ligand induces different opening of a ligand-binding site while establishing the same interactions with the target protein. In addition, the growing literature on 'tweezer' molecules[48] and on biocatalytic induction of supramolecular order[52] may well prove helpful in exploring the possibilities of purposely designing stacks of ligands in proteins.

Methods

Proteins. Untagged wild-type (wt) and mutants Ac-AChBPs were purified from Sf21 insect cells as previously described[19]. The complementary DNAs for the Ac-AChBP mutants, Ac-AChBP Y186A and Ac-AChBP Y193A, were generated using Quik Change Mutagenesis following the manufacturer's protocols. Mutant proteins were expressed from baculovirus in Sf21 cells. SHS5Y neuroblastoma cell membranes were used as source of α7 nAChR in radiodisplacement assays[15].

Conformational search. A stochastic conformational search was performed using MOE (version 2011.10, Chemical Computing Group Montreal, Canada), using default settings.

Crystallization. The VUF9432-Ac-AChBP complex was formed by mixing the protein at 3.5 mg ml^{-1} with 1 mM VUF9432 and incubating on ice for 1 h. Cocrystals were grown using the vapour diffusion method in a solution consisting of 0.2 M Li$_2$SO$_4$ and 0.8 M ammonium sulphate in MMT buffer (pH 8.0) at 19 °C. Crystals were cryoprotected in mother liquor supplemented with 20% glycerol and flash-frozen in liquid nitrogen.

Structure solution and refinement. Data were collected on beamline PX1 at the SLS (Switzerland), and processed using iMOSFLM/SCALA software[55]. The VUF9432-Ac-AChBP cocrystal was in space group P2$_1$ and diffracted to a resolution of 2.4 Å. The structure was solved by molecular replacement using PHASER[53] and the Ac-ACHBP-HEPES structure (2BR7) (ref. 19) as model. Iterative structure refinement was performed using REFMAC[54] from the CCP4 suite[56] or BUSTER[57]. Non-crystallographic symmetry restraints (NCSR) were maintained during refinement, using local NCS restraints as implemented in REFMAC or local structure similarity restraints in BUSTER. One TLS group per chain was used in refinement, and both the X-ray weight and B-factor restraint weight were optimized using a local version of the PDB_REDO script[58]. Ligands and water molecules were built in the final stages of refinement. Validation, performed using molprobity[59] and PDB_REDO, identified 0% of Ramachandran outliers and 2% of poor rotamers (overall score: 99th percentile). Distances, angles and buried surface areas were measured in Pymol (DeLano Scientific, LLC). Values and errors in text refer to the average over the four ligand-binding sites with three ligands bound. C-loop opening was calculated measuring the distance between Nε of W145 and Sγ of Cys 189. Tilting angles of aromatic planes was obtained by calculating the angle between the normal to the planes and averaged over four ligand-binding sites.

Ligand radiodisplacement assays. Competition binding assays were performed with Ac-AChBP (wt or mutants) in buffer (PBS, 20 mM Tris, pH 7.4/0.05% Tween) in a final assay volume of 100 μl in Optiplates (PerkinElmer Life Science, Inc., USA). Ligands were added at 10^{-3}–10^{-11} M. Radioligand, [^{3}H] epibatidine (PerkinElmer, specific activity $\sim$56 Ci mmol^{-1}), was added at 2.25 nM. The amount of protein was chosen such that we obtained a counting window in the displacement curve of <5% of the total amount of radioligand, generally 2–20 ng. Copper His-Tag PVT SPA beads (PerkinElmer) were added at 2 mg ml^{-1} final concentration. Plates were incubated at room temperature under continuous shaking, protected from light, for 1.5 h. SPA beads were allowed to settle for 3 h in the absence of light before counting. The label-bead complex was counted in a Wallac Trilux 1450 Microbeta (PerkinElmer).

Binding assays with α-bungarotoxin-[^{125}I] (IBTX) were performed as above at 1.8 nM IBTX.

Binding assays with the human α7 receptor were performed as above, but without the SPA beads, as a filtration assay. Human neuroblastoma cells (SH-SY5Y) expressing human α7 nAChRs (from Christian Fuhrer, Department of Neurochemistry, Brain Research Institute, Zurich) were cultured. The cells were washed three times, and pelleted aliquots were stored frozen at −80 °C. Before use the cells were resuspended in ice-cold buffer and sonicated. [^{3}H]MLA (American Radiolabeled Chemicals, Inc., specific activity $\sim$100 Ci mmol^{-1}) was used at a final concentration of 2 nM. Bound radioligand was collected on 0.3% poly-ethyleneimine-pretreated Unifilter-96 GF/C filters (PerkinElmer). Plates were washed with ice-cold 50 mM Tris buffer at pH 7.4. After drying the filters, scin-tillation fluid (MicroScint, PerkinElmer) was added and the radioactivity was counted as above.

All radioligand binding data were evaluated by a non-linear, least-squares curve fitting procedure using GraphPad Prism (version 5, GraphPad Software, Inc., San Diego, CA). All data are represented as mean ± s.e.m. from at least three inde-pendent experiments.

Trp and AO fluorescence quenching. Ac-AChBP, 1 μM in binding site, was equilibrated with dilution of the ligands 1 h before fluorescence measurement. Equilibrium fluorescence was monitored using a PheraStar fluorescence plate reader in the 96-well plates. Ac-AChBP was excited at 280 nm, and emission intensity was monitored at 340 nm with an emission slit of 8 nm. AO was excited at 495 nm and emission monitored at 525 nm with an emission slit of 10 nm. Data were normalized, and pKi values were calculated by fitting to a sigmoidal dose–response curve with GraphPad.

To determine ligand stoichiometries, Ac-AChBP (20 μM in binding site) was titrated with increasing concentration of ligand until <8% quenching was apparent. A straight line was fit through the average of the plateau points. For AO titration by Ac-AChBP, AO (100 μM) was titrated with increasing con-centration of protein. When indicated 1 mM nicotine was added to the assay to compete with AO. Full fluorescence spectra were recorded with a QuantaMaster 3 Fluorometer.

Isothermal calorimetry. ITC experiments were performed on a VP-ITC microcalorimeter (Microcal) at 25°as described[17]. Ac-AChBP used in these experiments was dialysed in PBS, and the AO was solubilized in the same buffer. For a typical experiment, the ligand at a concentration of 0.5 mM was titrated into 20 μM Ac-AChBP. Titration of ligand in buffer alone was performed to determine the change in enthalpy caused by the dilution of the ligand and subtracted as background from the actual ligand-binding experiment. Corrected data were analysed using software supplied by the manufacturer and fitted using a non-linear least-squares method to a model describing one set of binding sites.

Stopped-flow kinetics. Stopped-flow measurement were obtained using a TgK Scientific stopped-flow system (model SF-61DX2). Ac-AChBP was excited at 280 nm, and emission was recorded with a band filters WG320 and VG11. Changes in fluorescence emission intensity were fit to a first- (nicotine) or a second- (VUF9432) order equation.

Electrophysiology. To probe effects of VUF9432 and AO at the α7 nAChR receptors, experiments were conducted at Xenopus oocytes expressing the homo-meric human α7 nAChRs. Expression was obtained by intranuclear injection of 10 nl of a solution containing the cDNA encoding for the human α7 subunit at a concentration of 0.2 μg ml^{-1} using an automated injector (roboinject, Multi-channelsystems, Germany). Oocyte preparation and injection was done using the standard procedures as previously described[60]. Three or more day later, electro-physiological properties of the cells were assessed using an automated electrophysiological setup (HiClamp, Multichannelsystems, Germany). Recordings

electrodes were filled with 3 M KCl and oocytes superfused with OR2 medium containing in mM: NaCl 82.5, KCl 2.5, HEPES 5, CaCl$_2$.2H$_2$O 1.8, MgCl$_2$.6H$_2$O 1, pH 7.4. Cells were held at − 80 mV, and α7 expression was tested responses by a brief exposure to 1 mM acetylcholine. Cells displaying robust currents were subsequently tested for their sensitivity to the compound.

References

1. Murray, C. W. & Rees, D. C. The rise of fragment-based drug discovery. *Nat. Chem.* **1**, 187–192 (2009).
2. Shokat, K. M. A drug-drug interaction crystallizes a new entry point into the UPR. *Mol. Cell* **38**, 161–163 (2010).
3. Potter, A. J. et al. Structure-guided design of alpha-amino acid-derived Pin1 inhibitors. *Bioorg. Med. Chem. Lett.* **20**, 586–590 (2010).
4. Wiseman, R. L. et al. Flavonol activation defines an unanticipated ligand-binding site in the kinase-RNase domain of IRE1. *Mol. Cell.* **38**, 291–304 (2010).
5. Nissen, M. S. et al. Crystal structures of NADH:FMN oxidoreductase (EmoB) at different stages of catalysis. *J. Biol. Chem.* **283**, 28710–28720 (2008).
6. Sine, S. M. & Engel, A. G. Recent advances in Cys-loop receptor structure and function. *Nature* **440**, 448–455 (2006).
7. Taly, A., Corringer, P. J., Guedin, D., Lestage, P. & Changeux, J. P. Nicotinic receptors: allosteric transitions and therapeutic targets in the nervous system. *Nat. Rev. Drug Discov.* **8**, 733–750 (2009).
8. Karlin, A. Emerging structure of the nicotinic acetylcholine receptors. *Nat. Rev. Neurosci.* **3**, 102–114 (2002).
9. Changeux, J. P. & Taly, A. Nicotinic receptors, allosteric proteins and medicine. *Trends Mol. Med.* **14**, 93–102 (2008).
10. Thompson, A. J., Lester, H. A. & Lummis, S. C. The structural basis of function in Cys-loop receptors. *Q Rev. Biophys.* **43**, 449–499 (2010).
11. Arneric, S. P., Holladay, M. & Williams, M. Neuronal nicotinic receptors: a perspective on two decades of drug discovery research. *Biochem. Pharmacol.* **74**, 1092–1101 (2007).
12. Dwoskin, L. P. et al. Nicotinic receptor-based therapeutics and candidates for smoking cessation. *Biochem. Pharmacol.* **78**, 732–743 (2009).
13. Sine, S. M. The nicotinic receptor ligand binding domain. *J. Neurobiol.* **53**, 431–446 (2002).
14. Xiu, X., Puskar, N. L., Shanata, J. A., Lester, H. A. & Dougherty, D. A. Nicotine binding to brain receptors requires a strong cation-pi interaction. *Nature* **458**, 534–537 (2009).
15. Smit, A. B. et al. A glia-derived acetylcholine-binding protein that modulates synaptic transmission. *Nature* **411**, 261–268 (2001).
16. Brejc, K. et al. Crystal structure of an ACh-binding protein reveals the ligand-binding domain of nicotinic receptors. *Nature* **411**, 269–276 (2001).
17. Celie, P. H. et al. Crystal structure of acetylcholine-binding protein from *Bulinus truncatus* reveals the conserved structural scaffold and sites of variation in nicotinic acetylcholine receptors. *J. Biol. Chem.* **280**, 26457–26466 (2005).
18. Hansen, S. B. et al. Structural characterization of agonist and antagonist-bound acetylcholine-binding protein from *Aplysia californica*. *J. Mol. Neurosci.* **30**, 101–102 (2006).
19. Celie, P. H. et al. Crystal structure of nicotinic acetylcholine receptor homolog AChBP in complex with an alpha-conotoxin PnIA variant. *Nat. Struct. Mol. Biol.* **12**, 582–588 (2005).
20. Ulens, C. et al. Structural determinants of selective alpha-conotoxin binding to a nicotinic acetylcholine receptor homolog AChBP. *Proc. Natl Acad. Sci. USA* **103**, 3615–3620 (2006).
21. Rucktooa, P., Smit, A. B. & Sixma, T. K. Insight in nAChR subtype selectivity from AChBP crystal structures. *Biochem. Pharmacol.* **78**, 777–787 (2009).
22. Celie, P. H. et al. Nicotine and carbamylcholine binding to nicotinic acetylcholine receptors as studied in AChBP crystal structures. *Neuron* **41**, 907–914 (2004).
23. Billen, B. et al. Molecular actions of smoking cessation drugs at alpha4beta2 nicotinic receptors defined in crystal structures of a homologous binding protein. *Proc. Natl Acad. Sci. USA* **109**, 9173–9178 (2012).
24. Unwin, N. Refined structure of the nicotinic acetylcholine receptor at 4A resolution. *J. Mol. Biol.* **346**, 967–989 (2005).
25. Dellisanti, C. D., Yao, Y., Stroud, J. C., Wang, Z. Z. & Chen, L. Crystal structure of the extracellular domain of nAChR alpha1 bound to alpha-bungarotoxin at 1.94 A resolution. *Nat. Neurosci.* **10**, 953–962 (2007).
26. Hilf, R. J. & Dutzler, R. X-ray structure of a prokaryotic pentameric ligand-gated ion channel. *Nature* **452**, 375–379 (2008).
27. Bocquet, N. et al. X-ray structure of a pentameric ligand-gated ion channel in an apparently open conformation. *Nature* **457**, 111–114 (2009).
28. Li, S. X. et al. Ligand-binding domain of an alpha7-nicotinic receptor chimera and its complex with agonist. *Nat. Neurosci.* **14**, 1253–1259 (2011).
29. Hibbs, R. E. & Gouaux, E. Principles of activation and permeation in an anion-selective Cys-loop receptor. *Nature* **474**, 54–60 (2011).
30. de Kloe, G. E., Bailey, D., Leurs, R. & de Esch, I. J. Transforming fragments into candidates: small becomes big in medicinal chemistry. *Drug Discov. Today* **14**, 630–646 (2009).

31. Boyd, S. & de Kloe, G. E. Fragment library design: efficiently hunting drugs in chemical space. *Drug Discov. Today Technol.* **7**, e173–e180 (2010).

32. Kool, J. *et al.* High-resolution bioactivity profiling of mixtures toward the acetylcholine binding protein using a nanofractionation spotter technology. *J. Biomol. Screen* **16**, 917–924 (2011).

33. de Kloe, G. E. *et al.* Online parallel fragment screening and rapid hit exploration for nicotinic acetylcholine receptors. *Med. Chem. Commun.* **2**, 590–595 (2011).

34. van Muijlwijk-Koezen, J. E., Timmerman, H., Link, R., van der Goot, H. & AP, I. J. A novel class of adenosine A3 receptor ligands. 1.3-(2-Pyridinyl) isoquinoline derivatives. *J Med. Chem.* **41**, 3987–3993 (1998).

35. Meyer, E. A., Castellano, R. K. & Diederich, F. Interactions with aromatic rings in chemical and biological recognition. *Angew. Chem. Int. Ed.* **42**, 1210–1250 (2003).

36. Hansen, S. B. *et al.* Structures of Aplysia AChBP complexes with nicotinic agonists and antagonists reveal distinctive binding interfaces and conformations. *EMBO J.* **24**, 3635–3646 (2005).

37. Edink, E. *et al.* Fragment growing induces conformational changes in acetylcholine-binding protein: a structural and thermodynamic analysis. *J. Am. Chem. Soc.* **133**, 5363–5371 (2012).

38. Brams, M. *et al.* A structural and mutagenic blueprint for molecular recognition of strychnine and d-tubocurarine by different cys-loop receptors. *PLoS Biol.* **9**, e1001034 (2011).

39. Bourne, Y., Talley, T. T., Hansen, S. B., Taylor, P. & Marchot, P. Crystal structure of a Cbtx-AChBP complex reveals essential interactions between snake alpha-neurotoxins and nicotinic receptors. *EMBO J.* **24**, 1512–1522 (2005).

40. Ihara, M. *et al.* Crystal structures of *Lymnaea stagnalis* AChBP in complex with neonicotinoid insecticides imidacloprid and clothianidin. *Invert. Neurosci.* **8**, 71–81 (2008).

41. Talley, T. T. *et al.* Atomic interactions of neonicotinoid agonists with AChBP: molecular recognition of the distinctive electronegative pharmacophore. *Proc. Natl Acad. Sci. USA* **105**, 7606–7611 (2008).

42. Hansen, S. B. *et al.* Tryptophan fluorescence reveals conformational changes in the acetylcholine binding protein. *J. Biol. Chem.* **277**, 41299–41302 (2002).

43. Feng, X. Z., Lin, Z., Yang, L. J., Wang, C. & Bai, C. L. Investigation of the interaction between acridine orange and bovine serum albumin. *Talanta* **47**, 1223–1229 (1998).

44. Wang, H., Zhang, W., Dong, X. & Yang, Y. Thermo-reversibility of the fluorescence enhancement of acridine orange induced by supramolecular self-assembly. *Talanta* **77**, 1864–1868 (2009).

45. Jimenez-Millan, E., Giner-Casares, J. J., Munoz, E., Martin-Romero, M. T. & Camacho, L. Self-assembly of acridine orange into H-aggregates at the air/water interface: tuning of orientation of headgroup. *Langmuir* **27**, 14888–14899 (2011).

46. Mooser, G. & Sigmand, D.S. Ligand binding properties of acetylcholinesterase determined with fluorescent probes. *Biochemistry* **13**, 2299–2307 (1974).

47. Yamauchi, Y., Yoshizawa, M., Akita, M. & Fujita, M. Molecular recognition and self-assembly special feature: discrete stack of an odd number of polarized aromatic compounds revealing the importance of net vs. local dipoles. *Proc. Natl Acad. Sci. USA* **106**, 10435–10437 (2009).

48. Leblond, J. & Petitjean, A. Molecular tweezers: concepts and applications. *Chemphyschem* **12**, 1043–1051 (2011).

49. Brams, M. *et al.* Crystal structures of a cysteine-modified mutant in loop D of acetylcholine-binding protein. *J. Biol. Chem.* **286**, 4420–4428 (2011).

50. Grimster, N. P. *et al.* Generation of candidate ligands for nicotinic acetylcholine receptors via in situ click chemistry with a soluble acetylcholine binding protein template. *J. Am. Chem. Soc.* **134**, 6732–6740 (2012).

51. Hung, A. W. *et al.* Route to three-dimensional fragments using diversity-oriented synthesis. *Proc. Natl. Acad. Sci. USA* **108**, 6799–6804 (2011).

52. Hirst, A. R. *et al.* Biocatalytic induction of supramolecular order. *Nat. Chem.* **2**, 1089–1094 (2010).

53. McCoy, A. J. *et al.* Phaser crystallographic software. *J. Appl. Crystallogr.* **40**, 658–674 (2007).

54. Murshudov, G. N., Vagin, A. A. & Dodson, E. J. Refinement of macromolecular structures by the maximum-likelihood method. *Acta Crystallogr. D Biol. Crystallogr.* **53**, 240–255 (1997).

55. Evans, P. Scaling and assessment of data quality. *Acta crystallographica. Sec. D Biol. Crystallogr.* **62**, 72–82 (2006).

56. Winn, M. D. *et al.* Overview of the CCP4 suite and current developments. *Acta crystallographica. Sec. D Biol. Crystallogr.* **67**, 235–242 (2011).

57. Global Phasing Ltd.. *BUSTER v. 2.8.0.* (Global Phasing Ltd., 2011).

58. Joosten, R. P., Joosten, K., Cohen, S. X., Vriend, G. & Perrakis, A. Automatic rebuilding and optimization of crystallographic structures in the Protein Data Bank. *Bioinformatics* **27**, 3392–3398 (2011).

59. Chen, V. B. *et al.* MolProbity: all-atom structure validation for macromolecular crystallography. *Acta Crystallogr. Sec. D Biol. Crystallogr.* **66**, 12–21 (2010).

60. Hogg, R. C., Bandelier, F., Benoit, A., Dosch, R. & Bertrand, D. An automated system for intracellular and intranuclear injection. *J. Neurosci. Methods* **169**, 65–75 (2008).

Acknowledgements

We thank J. W. Borst and T. Visser for critically reading the manuscript. We thank the staff from SLS PXI and ESRF for assistance during data collection and R. Joosten and A. Perrakis for useful discussions during the refinement and data validation steps. We thank T. Schaer and E. Neveu for their help in the electrophysiological experiments. We thank A. Perrakis, P. Taylor, P. Celie, A. Amore., H. Ovaa, J. Hausmann, J. E. van Muijlwijk-Koeze and C. Verlinde for fruitful discussions. This work was supported by the European Union Seventh Framework Programme under Grant agreement HEALTH-F2-2007-202088 (Neurocypres project) (to T.K.S., A.B.S. and I.J.P.E.) and by TIPharma Grant D2-103 (to T.K.S., A.B.S. and I.J.P.E.).

Author contributions

The experimental work was performed by M.S., with contribution from P.R. for the structure refinement and from A.F. for the biophysical experiments. G.E.K. and E.S.E. performed the chemical analysis of the compounds by NMR and high-resolution mass spectral analysis, and they also performed their conformational analysis. R.v.E. performed the affinity measurement of the ligands for AChBP and the nAChR receptors. D.B. performed the electrophysiology measurement. M.S., T.K.S. and P.R. planned the work and analysed the results. The paper was written by T.K.S and M.S. with assistance from the other authors.

Additional information

Accession codes: Atomic coordinates and structure factors for the reported crystal structure have been deposited in the Protein Data Bank with accession code 4bfq.

15

Triggering HIV polyprotein processing by light using rapid photodegradation of a tight-binding protease inhibitor

Jiří Schimer[1,2], Marcela Pávová[1], Maria Anders[3], Petr Pachl[1], Pavel Šácha[1,2], Petr Cígler[1], Jan Weber[1], Pavel Majer[1], Pavlína Řezáčová[1], Hans-Georg Kräusslich[3,4], Barbara Müller[3,4] & Jan Konvalinka[1,2]

HIV protease (PR) is required for proteolytic maturation in the late phase of HIV replication and represents a prime therapeutic target. The regulation and kinetics of viral polyprotein processing and maturation are currently not understood in detail. Here we design, synthesize, validate and apply a potent, photodegradable HIV PR inhibitor to achieve synchronized induction of proteolysis. The compound exhibits subnanomolar inhibition in vitro. Its photo-labile moiety is released on light irradiation, reducing the inhibitory potential by 4 orders of magnitude. We determine the structure of the PR-inhibitor complex, analyze its photolytic products, and show that the enzymatic activity of inhibited PR can be fully restored on inhibitor photolysis. We also demonstrate that proteolysis of immature HIV particles produced in the presence of the inhibitor can be rapidly triggered by light enabling thus to analyze the timing, regulation and spatial requirements of viral processing in real time.

[1] Institute of Organic Chemistry and Biochemistry, Academy of Sciences of the Czech Republic, Gilead Sciences and IOCB Research Center, Flemingovo n.2, 166 10, Prague 6, Czech Republic. [2] Department of Biochemistry, Faculty of Science, Charles University in Prague, Hlavova 8, 128 43, Prague 2, Czech Republic. [3] Department of Infectious Diseases, Virology, University Hospital Heidelberg, Im Neuenheimer Feld 324, 69120 Heidelberg, Germany. [4] Molecular Medicine Partnership Unit, Heidelberg, Germany. Correspondence and requests for materials should be addressed to J.K. (email: konval@uochb.cas.cz) or to B.M. (email: Barbara_Mueller@med.uni-heidelberg.de).

HIV-1 protease (HIV-1 PR) is among the best-studied enzymes in biochemistry. This 99 amino acid long homodimeric aspartic PR plays a pivotal role in the viral replication cycle[1]. PR is synthesized as part of the viral Gag-Pol polyprotein. Approximately 125 molecules of Gag-Pol co-assemble at the plasma membrane with $\sim$2,500 molecules of the main structural polyprotein Gag to create an immature virion. In the assembled immature particle, the PR domain of Gag-Pol cleaves Gag and Gag-Pol at nine distinct sites to create the mature, functional subunits. Proteolytic processing results in a dramatic rearrangement of the particle core termed maturation, which is a prerequisite for HIV-1 infectivity. Consequently, inhibitors of HIV-1 PR are powerful virostatics. Due to major efforts from both academia and industry 10 specific HIV-1 PR inhibitors are currently available for antiretroviral therapy (for review, see ref. 2).

While the structure and the enzymatic properties of HIV-1 PR *in vitro* are well characterized, key questions concerning proteolytic maturation remain unanswered. Virological studies from many groups indicate that the maturation process needs to be tightly controlled. Not only inhibition, but also premature activation of PR is detrimental for virus replication[3], and blocking or even partially inhibiting processing at one of the cleavage sites strongly reduces HIV-1 infectivity[4]. According to current understanding, Gag proteolysis occurs when the polyprotein has already assembled into a tight hexameric lattice, but it is unclear what prevents premature proteolysis and how PR is activated once the immature virion has been assembled[5]. Furthermore, the sequence, timing, and topology of cleavage events during particle maturation remain largely unclear. The key obstacle in dissecting this complex process is the asynchronous formation of mature HIV-1 particles in tissue culture, since any virus population harvested from culture media constitutes an ensemble of particles in different stages of polyprotein processing and maturation. Overcoming this fundamental obstacle requires an experimental tool for triggering HIV-1 PR activity at a defined moment, thus inducing and synchronizing the viral maturation process.

Several approaches can in principle be used to achieve synchronization. Temperature-sensitive PR mutants have been developed to analyze individual steps of the replication cycle of picorna and other viruses[6]. However, attempts to prepare temperature-dependent mutants of HIV-1 PR have met with limited success. Although several HIV-1 PR mutants with temperature-dependent differences in proteolytic activity have been reported, none of these allowed switching from a non-active to an active enzymatic state, which would be required to trigger HIV-1 maturation[7,8].

Alternatively, one may induce proteolysis by wash-out of a specific PR inhibitor from immature particles produced in the presence of the inhibitor. We have recently explored this strategy by systematic testing of a panel of available and experimental PR inhibitors and found that PR activation can indeed be accomplished by inhibitor wash-out, provided that inhibitors with a high off-rate are used[9]. With a half-time of 4–5 h, the kinetics of proteolysis were slow, however, and morphologically mature virus particles and virus infectivity were not recovered[9]. Accordingly, inhibitor wash-out does not appear to trigger functional maturation and more efficient and faster induction of proteolysis inside the immature virion may be needed.

A possible way to overcome this limitation is the use of caged compounds that are released on irradiation with light of a specific wavelength. The release of effector molecules by light-induced cleavage of inactive precursors is well-established in chemical biology. Following pioneering studies describing photocaged cAMP and ATP[10,11], photocaged small molecules acting as secondary messengers, for example, calcium[12] and nitric oxide[13],

as well as caged hormones[14,15], neurotransmitters[16,17], nucleic acids[18,19] and diacylglycerols[20] were developed. Whole proteins have also been caged to analyze signalling and other regulatory events in the cell (for example, refs 21,22; for recent reviews covering caged small molecules, see refs 23–25).

To trigger the activity of an enzyme in the absence of a specific small molecule activator would require a caged version of the enzyme of interest. However, caging of a large biomolecule presents a major technical challenge. Furthermore, the caged protein must be delivered into the cell (for example, by microinjection), and would compete with the endogenously expressed protein[26]. In the specific case of HIV-1 PR, the enzyme is part of a polyprotein which needs to be incorporated into the nascent virus particle, rendering this strategy not feasible.

An alternative to protein caging is the use of a photolabile enzyme inhibitor that could be inactivated by light, to trigger enzyme activity. An effective photodegradable enzyme inhibitor is characterized by a substantial decrease in inhibitory activity on photolysis, and a few examples for this strategy have been published. Li *et al.*[26] connected two peptidic inhibitors of two distinct domains of Src kinase via a photodegradable linker. Separation of the bivalent inhibitor into two compounds, each binding the target with lower affinity, reduced inhibitory potency by $\sim$50-fold. Porter *et al.*[27] developed a mechanism-based approach to analyze activation of a serine PR. Photolysis of a covalent adduct in the active site of the PR led to PR activation.

The wealth of structure-activity data accumulated on purified HIV-1 PR and its inhibitors renders HIV-1 polyprotein processing and maturation an excellent target for the development of a specific photoinactivatable inhibitor. We thus set out to develop a method to activate HIV-1 maturation by photodegradation of a specific and potent PR inhibitor. Here we describe the design, synthesis, validation and application of a subnanomolar HIV-1 PR inhibitor that is cleaved on irradiation by 405-nm light. After irradiation, the inhibitor's potency decreases by 4 orders of magnitude, leading to nearly full restoration of enzyme activity and to rapid induction of polyprotein processing in assembled HIV-1 particles in tissue culture.

Results

Kinetic analysis of inhibitor and its photodegradation product. The design of a photoinactivable inhibitor of HIV-1 PR (**1**) was based on the structure of the PR inhibitor ritonavir (RTV; Fig. 1a)[28]. Compound **1** contains a photolabile 7-diethylamino-4-(hydroxymethyl)coumarin group connected via a carbamate linker to a RTV fragment (Fig. 1b), and is a tight-binding inhibitor of HIV-1 PR, displaying subnanomolar inhibition potency ($K_i = 170 \pm 20$ pM, for detailed synthesis see Supplementary Fig. 1). The degradation fragment **2** displayed only weak inhibitory activity, with a K_i value of 3.2 ± 0.3 μM (Fig. 1b). The other product of photolysis, the coumarin group, did not show any inhibitory activity at a concentration of 10 μM. The identities of the photodegradation fragments of compound **1** were confirmed by independent measurement using analytical high-performance liquid chromatography (HPLC; Supplementary Fig. 2).

Determination of binding mode into HIV-1 PR. To investigate the binding modes of compounds **1** and **2**, we co-crystallized both with HIV-1 PR and determined the corresponding structures at resolutions of 1.6 Å and 1.4 Å, respectively. Both crystals were of identical space group ($P6_1$), and contained one PR dimer in the asymmetric unit. The structures were refined with two inhibitor molecules bound in alternative orientations related by 180° rotation with 50% relative occupancy. The quality of the electron density map for residues 35–60 for 35–45 for HIV-1 PR-**1** and HIV-1 PR-**2** complex, respectively, was limited, suggesting that these regions of flaps are partially disordered. The electron density for the remaining part of the protein as well as compounds bound to the active site were of good quality enabling unambiguous modelling (Supplementary Fig. 3).

The crystal structures revealed that compounds **1** and **2** both occupy enzyme subsites S2, S1, S1′ and S2′. In addition, compound **1** interacted with the S3 enzyme subsite through the coumarin moiety. The extent of interactions with S3 residues was rather limited, however, and the coumarin moiety protruded from the enzyme active site cavity (Fig. 2a). The suboptimal interaction in the S3 pocket, compared with the interaction of the P3 moiety of RTV, is likely to contribute to the 10-fold difference in K_i values for RTV and compound **1**. Binding of the P2′, P1′ and P2 substituents of compound **1** was similar to that of RTV (Fig. 2b), whereas differences were observed for interactions in the S1 and S2 pockets. In the HIV-1 PR-compound **1** complex, the carbamate between the coumarin moiety and the inhibitor formed a hydrogen bond with the Asp29A side chain, similar to the interaction of the corresponding group of RTV.

Interestingly, the positions and conformations of moieties common to compound **1** and **2** as well as their interactions within the S2 to S2′ subsites were quite different (Fig. 2c). The largest difference was observed in the P1 and P2′ moieties, where the extent of interactions was much lower for compound **2** compared with compound **1**. This might provide a structural explanation for the observation that compound **2** displayed a low inhibitory activity against HIV-1 PR, considering that it occupies the S2 to S2′ enzyme binding subsites. In addition, compound **2** differs from compound **1** in that it has a free terminal amine group, which is charged at lower pH and likely repulsed from the enzyme cavity. In support of this hypothesis, acetylation of the free amine of compound **2** led to a major increase in inhibitory activity.

Reactivation of HIV-1 PR by photolysis of compound 1. To evaluate the efficacy of photodegradation, we analyzed the restoration of HIV-1 PR activity that had been inhibited by compound **1** (Fig. 3a) on irradiation at 405 nm. For irradiation, two lasers with outputs of 130 mW and 170 mW, respectively, were used in parallel. First, we tested a standard cuvette set up, in which 8 nM purified recombinant HIV-1 PR (final concentration of compound **1**: 10 or 100 nM; Fig. 3b) in 1 ml cleavage buffer was irradiated. At the lower concentration, irradiation led to a significant restoration of enzyme activity (65% compared with the uninhibited enzyme reaction). At the higher concentration of compound **1**, however, PR reactivation was limited even after prolonged irradiation (only 35% activity after 5 min of

irradiation). We reason that the product of photodegradation (compound **2**) interferes with degradation of compound **1** in this set up, because the absorption spectrum of compound **2** is almost identical to that of compound **1**. Therefore, we investigated a number of alternative irradiation set ups, and obtained optimal results when the inhibitor solution was irradiated while being pumped through a thin glass capillary at which the two lasers were focused (Fig. 3c). This set up ensured homogeneous irradiation throughout the sample and prevented absorption of light by the released coumarin product. At a flow rate of 15 μl min^{-1}, up to 75% of original PR activity was recovered, despite an inhibitor concentration 4 orders of magnitude above its K_i value ($K_i = 170$ pM, inhibitor concentration 100 nM). Considering that compound **1** is a tight-binding inhibitor (see Fig. 3a) and 75% of the PR activity was restored, we estimate that up to 98% of compound **1** was degraded.

Reactivation of HIV-1 PR inside immature virions. Based on these results, we analyzed whether photodegradation of compound **1** can be used to trigger HIV-1 PR activity inside intact immature HIV-1 particles produced in tissue culture in the presence of the inhibitor. PR-mediated cleavage of the Gag polyprotein yields the mature structural proteins and two small spacer peptides (Fig. 4a), and different rates of cleavage at individual sites result in the generation of characteristic processing intermediates[29]. First, we assessed the inhibitory potency of compound **1** on HIV-1 Gag polyprotein processing in virus producing cells. For this, particles were purified from the supernatant of HEK293T cells transfected with an HIV-1 proviral plasmid and incubated in the presence of various concentrations of compound **1**. Gag processing was efficiently inhibited with ∼50% reduction in Gag cleavage at ∼500 nM compound **1** (Fig. 4b). Previous studies had indicated that infectivity is severely impaired at concentrations where polyprotein processing is only inhibited to a minor extent[30,31]. Accordingly, compound **1** inhibited HIV-1 replication in the MT-4T-cell line with an EC$_{50}$ of 8.1 nM, although almost no effect on Gag processing could be seen at this concentration (Supplementary Fig. 5). Compound **1** was soluble and noncytotoxic at a concentration of 2 μM in 0.5% DMSO (CC$_{50}$ = 7.3 μM for MT4, CC$_{50}$ > 50 μM for HEK293T cells; for more detailed information see Supplementary Chapter 5).

Having established conditions for the inhibition of HIV-1 polyprotein processing by compound **1**, we proceeded to prepare immature particles for *in situ* activation of PR. For this, virus particles were produced in transfected HEK293T cells grown in the presence of 2 μM inhibitor. The experimental set up is schematically illustrated in Fig. 5a. Particles collected from inhibitor-treated cells were either subjected to inhibitor wash-out

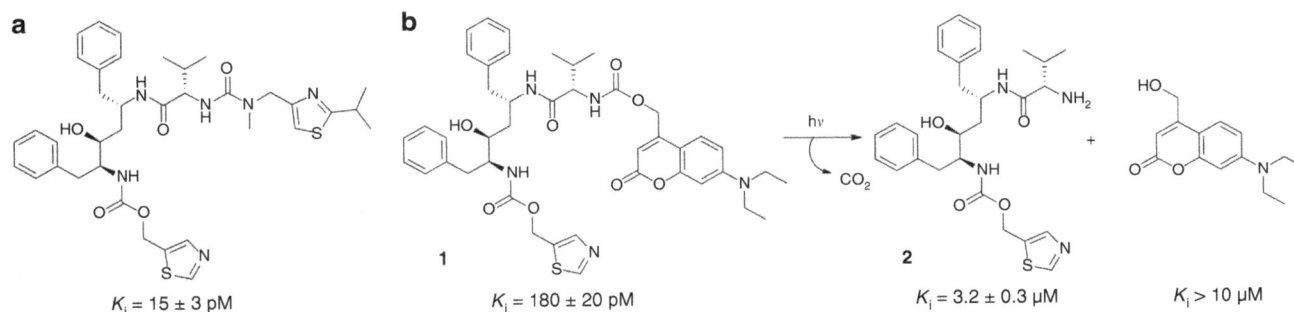

$K_i = 15 \pm 3$ pM $K_i = 180 \pm 20$ pM $K_i = 3.2 \pm 0.3$ μM $K_i > 10$ μM

Figure 1 | A photolabile inhibitor of HIV-1 PR and its degradation triggered by light. (**a**) HIV-1 protease inhibitor Ritonavir; (**b**) Photodegradable inhibitor of HIV-1 PR (compound **1**) and products resulting from photolysis (compound **2** and coumarin derivative). Inhibition constants determined as in Fig. 3a are shown for each compound.

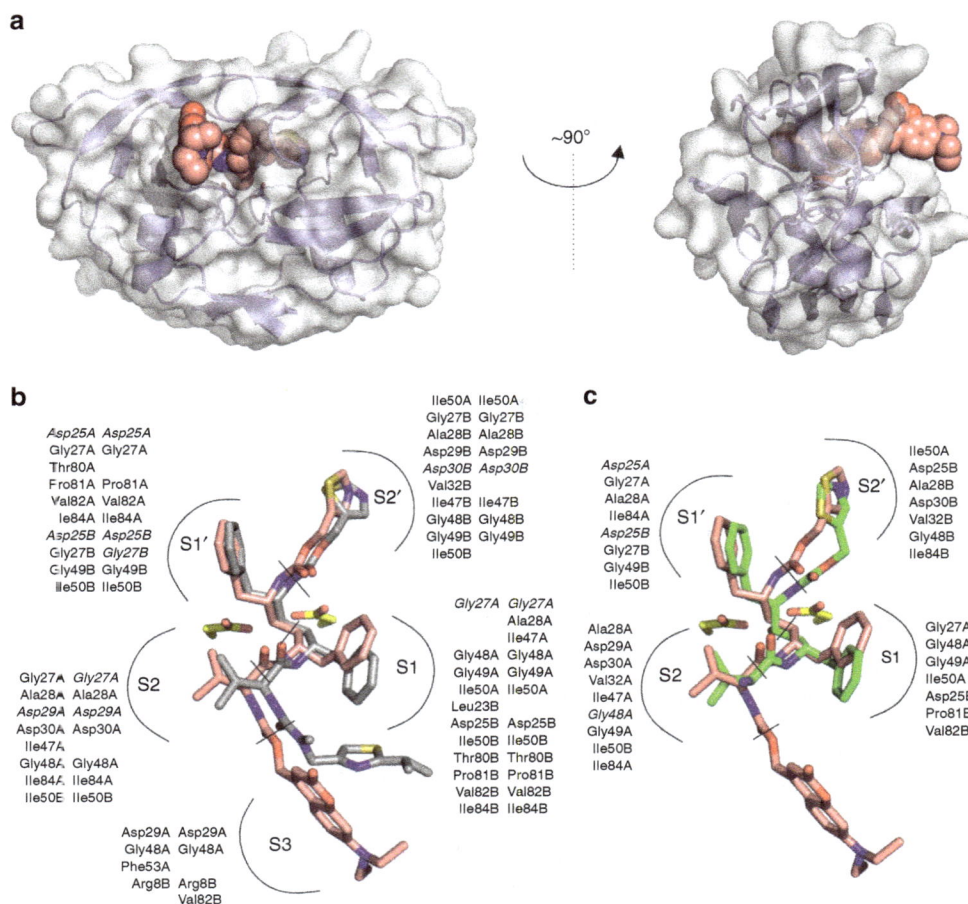

Figure 2 | Comparison of binding mode of compounds 1 and 2 to HIV-1 PR. (**a**) Two views of the HIV-1 PR-**1** complex (PDB code 4U7Q). The protein is shown in cartoon representation with a transparent surface, while the inhibitor atoms are represented by spheres. The coumarin moiety protrudes from the enzyme active site cavity. (**b**) Superposition of **1** (pink carbon atoms) and RTV (ritonavir; grey carbon atoms) bound in the HIV-1 PR active site. (**c**) Superposition of **1** with **2** (in green, PDB code 4U7V) bound to HIV-1 PR (PDB code 1HXW (ref. 28)). (**b,c**) Residues interacting with **1**, **2** and RTV are indicated in the corresponding colours for individual enzyme subsites. Residues forming polar interactions are highlighted in bold italics. To identify non-polar interactions, the cut-off for distance between any atom of residue and any atom of inhibitor was 4 Å. For polar interaction, the cut-off for distance between hydrogen bond donor and acceptor was 3.5 Å. Active site aspartates are shown in stick representation.

by two subsequent ultracentrifugation steps (Fig. 5b), or only filtered to remove cell debris (Fig. 5c). In both cases, samples were then either irradiated (405 nm) in a glass capillary (Fig. 5b,c, bottom panels) or passed through the capillary in the absence of irradiation (Fig. 5b,c, top panels).

Wash-out of compound **1** in the absence of irradiation resulted in slow PR activation and Gag processing (Fig. 5b, top), with kinetics closely resembling those observed in our previous study (Fig. 5d)[9]. In contrast, mature CA was produced much more rapidly in the irradiated sample (Fig. 5b, bottom), yielding ∼30% mature CA within 15 min (Fig. 5d). Gag processing remained incomplete, however, with ∼50% unprocessed or partially processed products remaining at 6 h of incubation. Direct irradiation of particle-containing culture medium without prior ultracentrifugation allowed us to process samples much more rapidly, thereby protecting sample integrity and PR activity. In this set up, no induction of proteolysis was observed in the absence of irradiation even after prolonged incubation (Fig. 5c, top). In contrast, irradiation of culture medium without any inhibitor removal resulted in rapid PR activation and virtually complete Gag processing (Fig. 5c, bottom). The irradiated sample exhibited a level of Gag processing comparable to that observed for an uninhibited control virus after ∼2 h of incubation, yielding an apparent half-time of ∼20 min for Gag processing (Fig. 5e).

Discussion

This report demonstrates that a photodestructible inhibitor can be used to trigger HIV-1 PR activation and polyprotein processing *in situ* inside the assembled immature virus. This was accomplished by design, synthesis and validation of a photolabile tight-binding inhibitor of HIV-1 PR ($K_i = 170 \pm 20$ pM) that demonstrates a 4-order-of-magnitude loss of potency on irradiation with a 405 nm laser. The inhibitor thus served as a photocage for HIV-1 PR activity and allowed initiating HIV-1 polyprotein processing within the assembled virion in a controlled manner. Analysis of Gag processing kinetics under these conditions revealed that the mature CA subunit was released with a half-time of ∼20–30 min, which is substantially faster than the half-time of 4–5 h observed using an optimized inhibitor wash-out strategy[9]. The direct comparison between wash-out and photodestruction of the newly described inhibitor (Fig. 5) clearly showed that much more rapid activation is accomplished by photodestruction. Furthermore, processing rates were not enhanced by including a wash-out step prior to irradiation, demonstrating the effectiveness of photodestruction.

At first glance, the half-time of 20–30 min measured in the experiments shown in Fig. 5 appears rather slow. It needs to be considered, however, that the experiments with immature virus do not directly measure the kinetics of PR activation by

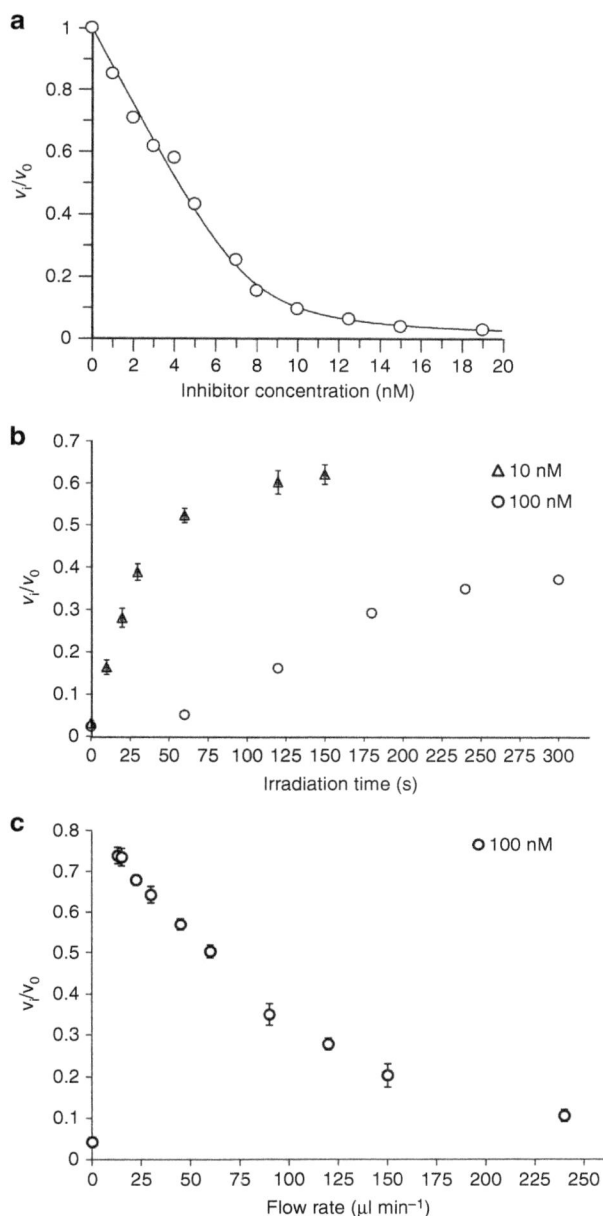

Figure 3 | Kinetic analysis of HIV-1 PR reactivation by inhibitor photodegradation. (**a**) A non-linear fit of Morrison equation of inhibition of HIV-1 PR by compound **1**. The activity of purified recombinant HIV-1 PR was determined *in vitro* as described in the experimental section in the presence of the indicated inhibitor concentrations. Two independent experiments yielded very similar results; (**b,c**) Reactivation of purified recombinant HIV-1 PR in buffer (100 mM sodium acetate, 300 mM NaCl, 4 mM EDTA, pH 4.7) by photodegradation of **1** using either the cuvette set up (**b**) or the capillary set up (**c**): (**b**) Purified recombinant HIV-1 PR (8 nM) incubated with compound **1** at the indicated concentrations was irradiated with two 405 nm lasers (combined output of 300 mW) for various time intervals. The PR activity was then measured using a chromogenic substrate. The plot shows relative PR activity as a function of time. (**c**) Purified recombinant HIV-1 PR (160 nM) incubated with 2 µM compound **1** was pumped at different flow rates through a thin glass capillary onto which two 405 nm lasers (combined output of 300 mW) were focused (for set up see Supplementary Fig. 4). Relative PR activity was determined as in **b** after 20-fold dilution into cleavage buffer using the same chromogenic substrate (for details, see Experimental section) and plotted against the flow rate of the sample through the capillary. Flow rate 0 represents a non-irradiated sample. The graph shows mean values and s.d. from three independent experiments.

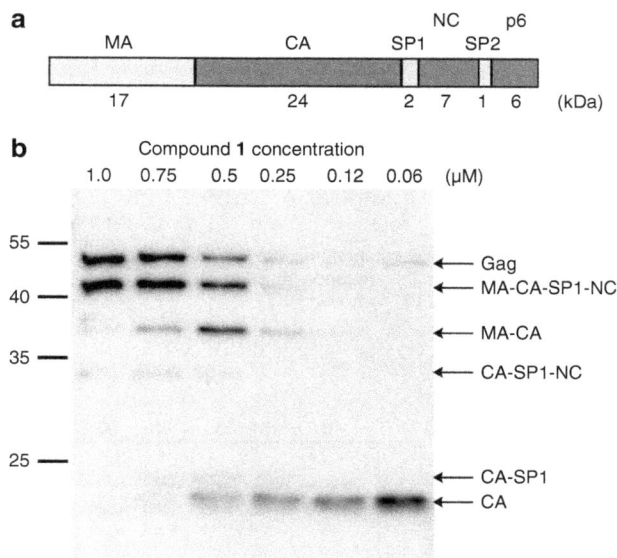

Figure 4 | Inhibition of HIV-1 Gag processing by compound 1.
(**a**) Schematic representation of the 55 kDa HIV-1 Gag polyprotein and its cleavage products. (**b**) Inhibition of HIV-1 Gag processing by compound **1**. HIV-1 particles were produced in HEK293T cells in the presence of the indicated inhibitor concentrations. The experiment was performed in duplicate and a representative result is shown. Molecular mass standards are shown on the left; Gag and its respective cleavage products are identified on the right. CA, capsid; MA, matrix; NC, nucleocapsid; p6, p6 protein; SP1, spacer peptide 1; SP2, spacer peptide 2.

photodestruction, as the biochemical experiments shown in Fig. 3, but rather reflect the production of mature CA by processing of the Gag polyprotein assembled in a tight hexagonal lattice. Although HIV-1 proteolytic maturation presumably involves only the viral PR and its substrates Gag and Gag-Pol in the relatively defined environment of the virus particle, the reaction entails at least 66 distinct substrates, intermediates or products, and numerous competing intermolecular interactions occurring simultaneously[32]. Arrangement of the substrate in a multimeric lattice presents further constraints that likely reduce processing rates. The time course of this complex reaction in the virus is currently unknown, and our current study provides an upper time limit for HIV-1 polyprotein processing. Estimates for the period required for polyprotein processing in retroviruses in the literature are based almost exclusively on indirect and very limited evidence and range from a few minutes up to several hours[33] for completion of proteolytic maturation. Modelling based on simplified assumptions from *in vitro* data yielded an estimate of 30 min for completion of HIV proteolysis[32], which would be in good agreement with our results. We want to emphasize, however, that our results provide an upper limit for the half-time of Gag proteolysis, assuming instantaneous and complete photodestruction and concomitant PR activation inside the immature particle. Conceivably, authentic polyprotein processing may be even faster, while the slower rates of Gag proteolysis reported in a previous study[33] are clearly inconsistent with our results.

The possibility to trigger HIV-1 PR activity by light in precisely defined time and space enabled us to induce HIV-1 polyprotein processing inside the native immature virion, and to analyze the timing, regulation, spatial requirements and kinetics of Gag proteolysis in real time. This system now provides the opportunity for a targeted analysis of HIV-1 maturation, which should eventually lead to an understanding of the dynamics of

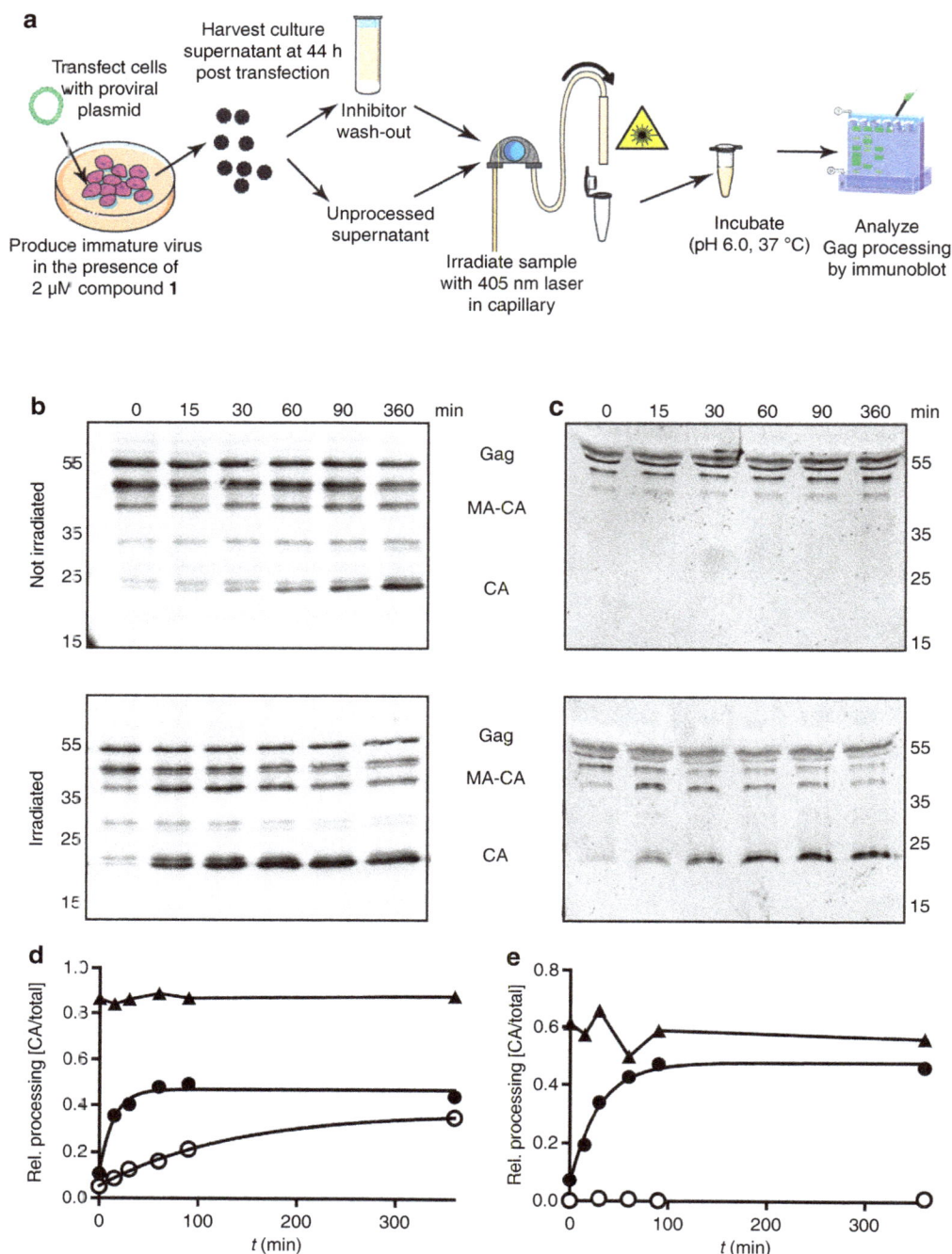

Figure 5 | Photoinduced Gag processing in the context of the assembled virion. (**a**) Schematic illustration of the irradiation experiment to trigger HIV-1 maturation using photoinactivation of compound **1**. HEK293T cells were transfected with a proviral HIV-1 plasmid and particles were produced in the presence of 2 μM compound **1** At 44 h post transfection, tissue culture supernatant was harvested and either subjected to ultracentrifugation (**b,d**) or used directly (**c,e**). In both cases, samples were then pumped through the capillary set up shown in Supplementary Fig. 4 either with or without ultraviolet irradiation. Subsequently, samples were incubated for various lengths of time. (**b,c**) Immunoblot analysis of Gag processing products. Samples were separated by SDS–PAGE, and products of Gag processing were detected by quantitative immunoblot (LiCor) using antiserum raised against recombinant HIV-1 CA. The figures show samples incubated for the indicated times without prior irradiation or following irradiation, respectively. Positions of Gag-derived proteins are indicated. (**d,e**) Quantitative analysis of the experiments shown in **b** or **c**, respectively. Anti-CA reactive bands from the immunoblots shown and from corresponding blots from irradiated mature control virus produced in the absence of inhibitor (not shown here) were quantified using Image Studio Light. The graphs show the proportion of mature CA relative to the sum of all anti-CA reactive bands in the respective lane. Filled triangles, irradiated control virus; open circles, inhibitor-treated virus, not irradiated; filled circles, inhibitor-treated virus, irradiated. Curves through data from inhibitor-treated samples represent fits to a single exponential equation. The results are representative of several independent experiments with a slight variation in the half-time of Gag polyprotein processing between 20 and 30 min. CA, capsid; MA, matrix.

this crucial step in the HIV-1 life cycle. We suggest that a similar approach, that is, design of specific photolabile inhibitors that can be photolysed to inactive products, thus triggering enzymatic activity, can be used for photocaging of other regulatory PRs to analyze their roles *in situ*.

Methods

Chemical synthesis. The synthesis of all intermediates and their full chemical analyses are described in the Supplementary Information. All compounds tested in biochemical assays were of at least 99% purity. All peaks in NMR spectra for all compounds were assigned using standard 2D NMR techniques (COSY, HMBC, HSQC).

Compound **1**: Compound **2** (20 mg, 31.3 μmol, 1.0 equiv.) was dissolved in 0.5 ml tetrahydrofurane along with 16 μl + N,N-Diisopropylethylamine (93.9 μmol, 3.0 equiv.). (7-(Diethylamino)-2-oxo-2H-chromen-4-yl)methyl(2,5-dioxopyrrolidin-1-yl) carbonate (13.5 mg, 34.4 μmol, 1.1 equiv. (for preparation, see Supplementary Information) was added in one portion, and the reaction was stirred overnight. The crude product obtained after removal of all volatiles was purified on preparative scale HPLC (gradient 50–100% acetonitrile in 30 min. $R_t = 16$ min). Yellow powder was obtained on lyophilization (10 mg, isolated yield = 35%). Analytical HPLC (gradient 2–100% in 30 min, flow rate 1 ml min^{-1}; $R_t = 25.5$ min). ^{1}H NMR (500 MHz, DMSO-d6):δ 9.05 (d, $J = 0.8$, 1H, N-CH-S), 7.86 (q, $J = 0.8$, 1H, S-C-CH-N), 7.79 (d, $J = 8.7$, 1H, CH-NH-Val), 7.45 (d, $J = 9.7$, 1H, Val-NH-COO), 7.45 (d, $J = 9.1$, 1H, C-CH-CH-C-N-Et$_2$), 7.23-7.07 (m, 10H, 2 × Ph), 6.91 (d, $J = 9.4$, 1H, NH-CH-CH-OH), 6.68 (dd, $J = 9.1$, 2.5, 1H, C-CH-CH-C-N-Et$_2$), 6.55 (d, $J = 2.5$, 1H, C-CH-C-N-Et$_2$), 6.08 (t, $J = 1.3$, 1H, O-C(O)-CH-C), 5.25 and 5.25 (2 × dd, $J = 16.1$, 1.3, 2 × 1H, O-CH$_2$-coumarin), 5.11 and 5.16 (2 × d, $J = 13.0$, 2 × 1H, O-CH$_2$-thiazole), 4.15 (bm, 1H, CH-NH-Val), 3.80 (bm, 1H, NH-CH-CH-OH), 3.78 (dd, $J = 9.2$, 7.3, 1H, NH-C(O)-CH(iPr)-NH), 3.59 (td, $J = 6.7$, 2.1, 1H, NH-CH-CH-OH), 3.42 (q, $J = 7.0$, 4H, CH$_2$-CH$_3$), 2.69 (bdd, $J = 13.5$, 4.9, 1H, CH$_2$-CH-NH-Val), 2.67 (bd, $J = 7.6$, 2H, CH$_2$-CH-NH-C(O)o-thiazole), 2.59 (bdd, $J = 13.5$, 8.0, 1H, CH$_2$-CH-NH-Val), 1.85 (dsept, $J = 7.3$, 6.8, 1H, -CH(CH$_3$)$_2$), 1.45 (m, 2H, OH-CH$_2$-CH$_2$-CH-NH), 1.11 (t, $J = 7.0$, 6H, CH$_2$-CH$_3$), 0.76 and 0.79 (2 × d, $J = 6.8$, 6H, -CH(CH$_3$)$_2$). ^{13}C NMR (125.7 MHz, DMSO-d6):δ 161.01 (NH-(O)CVal-NH), 155.92 (O-C-CH-C-N-Et$_2$), 155.79 (thizaole-O-C-N), 155.74 (N-CH-S), 155.53 (Val-NH-C(O)-O), 152.07 (Val-NH-C(O)-O -CH$_2$-C), 150.58 (C-N-Et$_2$), 143.21 (S-C-CH-N), 139.640 (i-Ph-CH$_2$-CH-NH-thiazol), 138.86 (i-Ph-CH$_2$-CH-NH-Val), 134.29 (S-C-CH-N), 129.19 and 129.52 (2 × o-Ph), 128.18 and 128.03 (2 × m-Ph), 126.00 and 125.94 (2 × p-Ph), 125.50 (C-CH-C-N-Et$_2$), 108.91 (C-CH-CH-C-N-Et$_2$), 105.43 (C-CH-CH-C-N-Et$_2$), 104.63 (O-CH-C(O)-C), 97.05 (C-CH-C-N-Et$_2$), 69.15 (HO-CH), 61.16 (O-CH$_2$-coumarin), 60.57 (NH-C(O)-CH(iPr)-NH), 57.37 (C(O)O-CH$_2$-thiazole), 55.73 (NH-CH-CH-OH), 47.30 (OH-CH-CH$_2$-CH-NH), 44.20 (CH$_2$-CH$_3$), 39.53 (Val-NH-CH-CH$_2$-Ph), 38.29 (OH-CH-CH$_2$-CH-NH), 37.34 (CH$_2$-CH-NH-C(O)o-thiazole), 30.55 (CH(CH$_3$)$_2$), 19.43 and 18.33 (2 × CH$_3$), 12.50 (CH$_2$-CH$_3$). HRMS (m/z; ESI +): calculated for C$_{43}$H$_{51}$O$_8$N$_5$S [MNa]$^+$ 820.33506; found 820.33470.

Purification of HIV PR. The recombinant PR was overexpressed in *Escherichia coli* BL21(DE3) RIL (Novagen). Protein expression and isolation of inclusion bodies were carried out as previously described[34]. Inclusion bodies were solubilized in 67% (v/v) acetic acid and refolded by dilution into a 25-fold excess of water, followed by overnight dialysis at 4 °C against water and then against 50 mM MES (pH 5.8), 10% (v/v) glycerol, 1 mM EDTA and 0.05% (v/v) 2-mercaptoethanol. The PR was purified by cation exchange chromatography using MonoSFPLC (Pharmacia). The enzyme was stored at 70 °C until further use[34].

Inhibition of HIV-1 PR. K_i values were determined by spectrophotometric assay using purified recombinant HIV-1 PR and the chromogenic substrate KARVN-leNphEaNle-NH$_2$. Data were analyzed using the Morrison equation[35].

Crystallization experiments. The HIV PR-compound **1** complex was prepared by mixing the enzyme with an equimolar amount of **1** dissolved in DMSO. The protein was pre-concentrated to 4 mg ml^{-1} by ultrafiltration using Microcon-10 filters (Millipore, Billerica, MA, USA). The complex was then centrifuged for 25 min at 16,000 g to reduce the number of crystallization nuclei. Crystals were then grown by the hanging drop vapour diffusion technique at 19 °C. The crystallization drops contained 2 μl protein-inhibitor complex and 1 μl reservoir solution (0.2 M lithium sulfate, 0.1 M phosphate/citrate pH 4.2 and 20% (w/v) PEG 1000; JSCG + condition 6). The HIV PR-compound **2** complex was prepared by incubation HIV PR with fourfold molar excess of **2** for 30 min and it was then concentrated to a protein concentration of 4 mg ml^{-1} by the above described procedure. Crystals were grown as described above. The reservoir solution was 0.2 M magnesium chloride, 0.1 M Tris pH 8.5 and 20% (w/v) PEG 8000. For diffraction measurements, crystals were soaked in reservoir solution supplemented with 25% (v/v) glycerol and cooled in liquid nitrogen. The diffraction data collection and structure refinement are described in Supplementary Information in chapter 3.3.

Photolysis of the inhibitor. Irradiation was performed in two distinct set ups.

Cuvette set up. A 1 ml reaction mixture (8 nM purified recombinant HIV-1 PR in cleavage buffer—100 mM sodium acetate, 0.3 M NaCl, 4 mM EDTA, pH 4.7, various concentrations of inhibitor) at 4 °C was irradiated with two defocused 405 nm lasers (130 and 170 mW) in a quartz cuvette for various periods of time. The cuvette was then equilibrated to 37 °C, and the enzymatic reaction was started by adding 4 μl of 3.8 μM chromogenic substrate (KARVNleNphEaNle-NH$_2$)[27]. The enzyme activity (and thus the efficacy of photodegradation) was followed by the decrease in absorbance at 305 nm.

Capillary set up. Two 405 nm focusable lasers (130 and 170 mW, checked for both intensity and wavelength before use) were used for irradiation in a capillary set up. The solution (either purified HIV-1 PR or a suspension of immature virions) was linearly pumped through a 250 μm glass capillary (Hirschmann ring caps) at which both laser beams were focused (for an illustrative photo, see Supplementary Fig. 4). To 47.5 μl of cleavage buffer (100 mM sodium acetate, 0.3 M NaCl, 4 mM EDTA, pH 4.7) on ice, 2 μl of 4 μM HIV-1 PR and 0.5 μl of 200 μM compound **1** were added. The solution was irradiated at different flow rates, diluted in a 1 ml cuvette with 950 μl of cleavage buffer (100 mM sodium acetate, 0.3 M NaCl, 4 mM EDTA, pH 4.7, 37 °C) and the enzymatic reaction was started by adding 4 μl of 3.8 μM chromogenic substrate.

Analysis of photodegradation products. The photodegradation of the inhibitor was analyzed with an analytical Jasco PU-1580 HPLC (flow rate 1 ml min^{-1}, invariable gradient 2–100% ACN in 30 min, Watrex C18 Analytical Column, 5 μm, 250 × 5 mm), and the retention times were compared with those of synthetic standards (the degradation product was also an intermediate during synthesis of compound **1**).

Plasmids and cell cultures. Proviral plasmid pNL4-3 (obtained through the NIH AIDS Reagent Program from Dr Malcolm Martin) has been described before[36]. Plasmid pCHIV, which encodes all HIV-1 NL4-3 proteins except Nef, but lacks both long terminal repeat regions required for infectivity, has also been described[37]. HEK293T cells were kept in high-glucose Dulbecco's modified Eagle's medium (DMEM, Life Technologies) supplemented with penicillin/streptomycin and 10% foetal calf serum at 37 °C, 5% CO$_2$. For the analysis of inhibitor activity on viral particle processing, HEK293T cells were transfected with pNL4-3 using calcium phosphate, and inhibitor was added at the indicated concentrations. At 48 h post transfection, supernatants were harvested, cleared by filtration through a 0.45-μm filter and concentrated by ultracentrifugation through a 20% (w/w) sucrose cushion.

Photoactivation of HIV-1 PR *in situ*. HEK293T cells were seeded in six-well plates in high-glucose, phenol red-free DMEM supplemented with penicillin/streptomycin and 10% foetal calf serum. On the following day, cells were transfected with plasmid pCHIV[37] using polyethylenimine according to standard procedures. A final concentration of 2 μM compound **1** or DMSO (vehicle) was added to the tissue culture medium at the time of transfection. At 44 h post transfection, tissue culture supernatants were harvested, adjusted to pH 6.0 using PR buffer (50 mM MES, pH 6.0, 150 mM NaCl, 2 mM DTT, 1 mM EDTA). Alternatively, supernatants were harvested, filtered, inhibitor was removed by two successive ultracentrifugation steps through a 20% sucrose cushion and the particle pellet was resuspended in PR buffer. In both cases, samples were then split into two aliquots, one of which was subjected to ultraviolet irradiation using the capillary set up described above, whereas the control aliquot was pumped through the capillary set up without ultraviolet irradiation. Subsequently, samples were incubated at 37 °C, and 20 μl aliquots were taken before incubation ($t = 0$) and at $t = 15$, 30, 60, 90 and 360 min. At these time points, the processing reaction was stopped by addition of SDS sample buffer and heat treatment (5 min, 90 °C).

Analysis of HIV polyprotein processing by immunoblot. Samples were separated by SDS–PAGE (17.5%; acrylamide:bisacrylamide 200:1), and proteins were transferred to a nitrocellulose membrane by semi-dry blotting. HIV-1 Gag-derived proteins were detected using rabbit polyclonal antiserum raised against HIV-1 CA, followed by fluorescently labelled goat-anti rabbit secondary antibody (LiCor). Quantification of anti-CA reactive bands was performed using an infrared imaging system (LiCor Odyssey) and Image Studio Lite software. Data were analyzed with GraphPad prism.

References

1. Krausslich, H. G. *et al.* Activity of purified biosynthetic proteinase of human immunodeficiency virus on natural substrates and synthetic peptides. *Proc. Natl Acad. Sci. USA* **86**, 807–811 (1989).

2. Pokorna, J., Machala, L., Rezacova, P. & Konvalinka, J. Current and novel inhibitors of HIV protease. *Viruses* **1**, 1209–1239 (2009).

3. Krausslich, H. G. Human immunodeficiency virus proteinase dimer as component of the viral polyprotein prevents particle assembly and viral infectivity. *Proc. Natl Acad. Sci. USA* **88**, 3213–3217 (1991).

4. Wiegers, K. et al. Sequential steps in human immunodeficiency virus particle maturation revealed by alterations of individual Gag polyprotein cleavage sites. J. Virol. **72**, 2846–2854 (1998).

5. Debouck, C. et al. Human immunodeficiency virus protease expressed in Escherichia coli exhibits autoprocessing and specific maturation of the gag precursor. Proc. Natl Acad. Sci. USA **84**, 8903–8906 (1987).

6. Krausslich, H. G., Nicklin, M. J., Lee, C. K. & Wimmer, E. Polyprotein processing in picornavirus replication. Biochimie **70**, 119–130 (1988).

7. Manchester, M., Everitt, L., Loeb, D. D., Hutchison, 3rd C. A. & Swanstrom, R. Identification of temperature-sensitive mutants of the human immunodeficiency virus type 1 protease through saturation mutagenesis. Amino acid side chain requirements for temperature sensitivity. J. Biol. Chem. **269**, 7689–7695 (1994).

8. Konvalinka, J. Structural and molecular biology of protease function and inhibition. J. Cell Biochem. **56**, 117–177 (1994).

9. Mattei, S. et al. Induced maturation of human immunodeficiency virus. J. Virol. **88**, 13722–13731 (2014).

10. Engels, J. & Schlaeger, E. J. Synthesis, structure, and reactivity of adenosine cyclic 3′,5′-phosphate benzyl triesters. J. Med. Chem. **20**, 907–911 (1977).

11. Kaplan, J. H., Forbush, 3rd B. & Hoffman, J. F. Rapid photolytic release of adenosine 5′-triphosphate from a protected analogue: utilization by the Na:K pump of human red blood cell ghosts. Biochemistry **17**, 1929–1935 (1978).

12. Ellis-Davies, G. C. Neurobiology with caged calcium. Chem. Rev. **108**, 1603–1613 (2008).

13. Makings, L. R. & Tsien, R. Y. Caged nitric oxide. Stable organic molecules from which nitric oxide can be photoreleased. J. Biol. Chem. **269**, 6282–6285 (1994).

14. Cruz, F. G., Koh, J. T. & Link, K. H. Light-activated gene expression. J. Am. Chem. Soc. **122**, 8777–8778 (2000).

15. Lin, W., Albanese, C., Pestell, R. G. & Lawrence, D. S. Spatially discrete, light-driven protein expression. Chem. Biol. **9**, 1347–1353 (2002).

16. Breitinger, H. G., Wieboldt, R., Ramesh, D., Carpenter, B. K. & Hess, G. P. Synthesis and characterization of photolabile derivatives of serotonin for chemical kinetic investigations of the serotonin 5-HT(3) receptor. Biochemistry **39**, 5500–5508 (2000).

17. Callaway, E. M. & Yuste, R. Stimulating neurons with light. Curr. Opin. Neurobiol. **12**, 587–592 (2002).

18. Mikat, V. & Heckel, A. Light-dependent RNA interference with nucleobase-caged siRNAs. RNA **13**, 2341–2347 (2007).

19. Shah, S., Jain, P. K., Kala, A., Karunakaran, D. & Friedman, S. H. Light-activated RNA interference using double-stranded siRNA precursors modified using a remarkable regiospecificity of diazo-based photolabile groups. Nucleic Acids Res. **37**, 4508–4517 (2009).

20. Nadler, A. et al. The fatty acid composition of diacylglycerols determines local signaling patterns. Angew. Chem. Int. Ed. **52**, 6330–6334 (2013).

21. Hiraoka, T. & Hamachi, I. Caged RNase: photoactivation of the enzyme from perfect off-state by site-specific incorporation of 2-nitrobenzyl moiety. Bioorg. Med. Chem. Lett. **13**, 13–15 (2003).

22. Chang, C. Y., Fernandez, T., Panchal, R. & Bayley, H. Caged catalytic subunit of cAMP-dependent protein kinase. J. Am. Chem. Soc. **120**, 7661–7662 (1998).

23. Riggsbee, C. W. & Deiters, A. Recent advances in the photochemical control of protein function. Trends Biotechnol. **28**, 468–475 (2010).

24. Brieke, C., Rohrbach, F., Gottschalk, A., Mayer, G. & Heckel, A. Light-controlled tools. Angew. Chem. Int. Ed. **51**, 8446–8476 (2012).

25. Lee, H. M., Larson, D. R. & Lawrence, D. S. Illuminating the chemistry of life: design, synthesis, and applications of "caged" and related photoresponsive compounds. ACS Chem. Biol. **4**, 409–427 (2009).

26. Li, H., Hah, J. M. & Lawrence, D. S. Light-mediated liberation of enzymatic activity: "small molecule" caged protein equivalents. J. Am. Chem. Soc. **130**, 10474–10475 (2008).

27. Porter, N. A., Bush, K. A. & Kinter, K. S. Photo-reversible binding of thrombin to avidin by means of a photolabile inhibitor. J. Photochem. Photobiol. B **38**, 61–69 (1997).

28. Kempf, D. J. et al. ABT-538 is a potent inhibitor of human immunodeficiency virus protease and has high oral bioavailability in humans. Proc. Natl Acad. Sci. USA **92**, 2484–2488 (1995).

29. Sundquist, W. I. & Krausslich, H. G. HIV-1 assembly, budding, and maturation. Cold Spring Harb. Symp. Quant. Biol. **2**, a006924 (2012).

30. Muller, B. et al. HIV-1 Gag processing intermediates trans-dominantly interfere with HIV-1 infectivity. J. Biol. Chem. **284**, 29692–29703 (2009).

31. Kaplan, A. H. et al. Partial inhibition of the human immunodeficiency virus type 1 protease results in aberrant virus assembly and the formation of noninfectious particles. J. Virol. **67**, 4050–4055 (1993).

32. Konnyu, B. et al. Gag-Pol processing during HIV-1 virion maturation: a systems biology approach. PLoS Comput. Biol. **9**, e1003103 (2013).

33. Dale, B. M. et al. Cell-to-cell transfer of HIV-1 via virological synapses leads to endosomal virion maturation that activates viral membrane fusion. Cell Host Microbe **10**, 551–562 (2011).

34. Saskova, K. G. et al. Enzymatic and structural analysis of the I47A mutation contributing to the reduced susceptibility to HIV protease inhibitor lopinavir. Protein Sci. **17**, 1555–1564 (2008).

35. Richards, A. D. et al. Sensitive, soluble chromogenic substrates for HIV-1 proteinase. J. Biol. Chem. **265**, 7733–7736 (1990).

36. Adachi, A. et al. Production of acquired immunodeficiency syndrome-associated retrovirus in human and nonhuman cells transfected with an infectious molecular clone. J. Virol. **59**, 284–291 (1986).

37. Lampe, M. et al. Double-labelled HIV-1 particles for study of virus-cell interaction. Virology **360**, 92–104 (2007).

Acknowledgements

We would like to thank Hana Prouzová for expert technical help, Hillary Hoffman for language editing, and Petr Klán for insightful advice in field of caged compounds. We also acknowledge the Grant Agency of the Czech Republic, Grant No. P208-12-G016 (Center of Excellence), BIOCEV; Grant number: CZ.1.05/1.1.00/02.0109 and Inter-BioMed Project LO1302 from the Ministry of Education of the Czech Republic for financial support. This work was funded in part by grants from the Deutsche Forschungsgemeinschaft to B.M. (MU885/5-1) and H.-G.K. (DFG grant number KR906/7-1). H.-G.K. and B.M. are investigators of the CellNetworks Cluster of Excellence (EXC81).

Author contributions

J.S. designed the compounds; J.S. with P.M. and P.C. synthesized the compounds; J.S. evaluated the compounds in vitro; J.W., M.P., M.A. and B.M. analyzed the antiviral activity and inhibition of polyprotein processing; J.S. and P.Š. designed the irradiation apparatus; J.S., P.P. and P.Ř. crystallized the PR complexes and solved the structures; M.A., J.S., B.M. and H.-G.K. analyzed the polyprotein processing by photoactivation; J.K. conceived and lead the project; J.S., J.K., H.-G.K. and B.M. analyzed the data, J.S., H.-G.K., P.Ř., B.M. and J.K. wrote the manuscript.

Additional information

Accesion codes: Atomic coordinates and experimental structure factors have been deposited in the Protein Data Bank under codes 4U7Q and 4U7V for complexes with compounds 1 and 2, respectively.

16

Identification and optimization of small-molecule agonists of the human relaxin hormone receptor RXFP1

Jingbo Xiao[1,*], Zaohua Huang[2,*], Catherine Z. Chen[1], Irina U. Agoulnik[3], Noel Southall[1], Xin Hu[1], Raisa E. Jones[1], Marc Ferrer[1], Wei Zheng[1], Alexander I. Agoulnik[2] & Juan J. Marugan[1]

The anti-fibrotic, vasodilatory and pro-angiogenic therapeutic properties of recombinant relaxin peptide hormone have been investigated in several diseases, and recent clinical trial data has shown benefit in treating acute heart failure. However, the remodelling capacity of these peptide hormones is difficult to study in chronic settings because of their short half-life and the need for intravenous administration. Here we present the first small-molecule series of human relaxin/insulin-like family peptide receptor 1 agonists. These molecules display similar efficacy as the natural hormone in several functional assays. Mutagenesis studies indicate that the small molecules activate relaxin receptor through an allosteric site. These compounds have excellent physical and *in vivo* pharmacokinetic properties to support further investigation of relaxin biology and animal efficacy studies of the therapeutic benefits of relaxin/insulin-like family peptide receptor 1 activation.

[1] NIH Chemical Genomics Center, Discovery Innovation, National Center for Advancing Translational Sciences, National Institutes of Health, 9800 Medical Center Drive, Rockville, Maryland 20850, USA. [2] Department of Human and Molecular Genetics, Herbert Wertheim College of Medicine, Florida International University, 11200 SW 8th Street, Miami, Florida 33199, USA. [3] Department of Cellular Biology and Pharmacology, Herbert Wertheim College of Medicine, Florida International University, 11200 SW 8th Street, Miami, Florida 33199, USA. * These authors contributed equally to this work. Correspondence and requests for materials should be addressed to J.J.M. (email: maruganj@mail.nih.gov).

Despite great advances in medical science, 1 of every 2.9 deaths in the United States is due to cardiovascular disease[1]. Each year about 795,000 people experience a new or recurrent stroke, and one in nine death certificates in the United States mention heart failure. In addition, 33.5% of US adults over 20 years of age have hypertension[1]. These statistics clearly illustrate both the grave need for more effective treatments and the limitations of current therapies to address cardiovascular disease in general and acute heart failure in particular.

The peptide hormone relaxin was discovered in 1926 as a hormone of pregnancy[2], due to its relaxation effects on pubic ligaments (hence the name) and softening the cervix to facilitate parturition[3]. It has been shown that concentration of relaxin in blood rises during the first trimester of pregnancy, promoting cardiovascular and renal adjustments to meet the increased nutritional demands of the growing fetus, and the elevated requirements for renal clearance of metabolic wastes[4]. Relaxin induces a 20% increase in cardiac output, 30% decrease in systemic vascular resistance, 30% increase in global arterial compliance and 45% increase in renal blood flow during pregnancy[5]. Numerous clinical and nonclinical studies using this hormone have now recapitulated these cardiovascular effects in both males and females, demonstrating its potential pharmacological utility in modulating cardiovascular and renal function.

The clinically observed physiological effects of relaxin are mediated though its interaction with the G-protein-coupled receptor, relaxin/insulin-like family peptide receptor 1 (RXFP1), leading to the modulation of several signal transduction pathways[6]. Activation of RXFP1 by relaxin induces: (1) upregulation of the endothelin system that leads to vasodilation; (2) extracellular matrix remodelling through regulation of collagen deposition, matrix metalloproteinase and tissue inhibitor of metalloproteinase expression, and overall tissue homoeostasis; (3) a moderation of inflammation by reducing levels of inflammatory cytokines, such as tumour necrosis factor-alpha and transforming growth factor beta; and (4) angiogenesis by activating transcription of vascular endothelial growth factor (VEGF)[6–8]. The understanding of the biological effects of RXFP1 activation by relaxin has led to the evaluation of relaxin as a pharmacological agent for the treatment of patients with acute heart failure[9,10], preeclampsia[11] and hypertensive diseases[12,13]. Given its anti-inflammatory and extracellular matrix remodelling function, several clinical trials have also evaluated the potential of relaxin as treatment for scleroderma, cervical ripening, fibromyalgia and orthodontics[8].

A similar anti-inflammatory and remodelling need also exists for cardiac rehabilitation. None of the current methodologies, such as surgery, medical devices or approved medications (angiotensin-converting enzyme inhibitors, angiotensin II receptor blockers, digoxin, beta blockers and aldosterone antagonists), are able to prevent the development of heart tissue scar after acute heart failure, or repair heart tissue after damage is incurred. The anti-fibrotic and remodelling properties of relaxin[9,14], together with its capacity to normalize blood pressure, increase blood and renal flow[15], seem to be ideal for the treatment of patients with cardiovascular diseases. Clinical trial data support this theory[9,16]. Relaxin relieves systemic and renal vasoconstriction and increases vascular compliance, including normalization of high blood pressure, reduction of pulmonary capillary wedge pressure, increase of cardiac output, increase renal blood flow, natriuresis and decongestion[17]. Recent data from the RELAX-AHF phase III clinical trial showed that the early administration of serelaxin, a recombinant analogue of the natural hormone, reduced overall mortality at 6 months and promoted a more rapid relief of congestion with fewer signs of organ damage during the initial days after admission[9,10]. In addition, animal pharmacology data indicate that relaxin hormone has anti-inflammatory and cardiac protection effects, including reduction of myocardial ischaemia and reperfusion injury, increase of wound healing, reduction of ventricular fibrosis[14] and increase of endothelial progenitor cell mobilization[18].

Recombinant relaxin hormone has produced promising responses in clinical trials for the treatment of heart failure and is close to commercialization[9]. However, the peptide is difficult to administer as a chronic therapy. The half-life of this peptide hormone is < 10 min and it has to be administrated intravenously[13]. The development of small-molecule agonists of RXFP1 as an alternative to recombinant hormone would have numerous benefits and will enable the investigation of additional therapeutic applications that may require chronic administration. In this article, we report the first series of small-molecule agonists of RXFP1. These small molecules are potent, highly selective, orally bioavailable and easy to synthesize.

Results

Identification of hits as small-molecule agonists of RXFP1.
More than 350,000 compounds of the Molecular Libraries Probe Center Network library[19] were tested in a quantitative high-throughput screening[20] campaign searching for small-molecule agonists of RXFP1, by measuring the ability of compounds to elevate cyclic adenosine monophosphate (cAMP) levels in a HEK293 cell line stably transfected with human $RXFP1$[21]. Maximal cAMP signal was established by treatment with porcine relaxin (1.66 nM) or the adenylyl cyclase activator forskolin (57 µM). Confirmed active compounds were further interrogated using the naive parental HEK293 cell line and cells transfected with the related receptors insulin-like 3 peptide receptor, $RXFP2$, or arginine vasopressin receptor 1B, $AVPR1B$, using the same cAMP detection kit as screens for selectivity and to eliminate compounds which non-specifically increase the cAMP signal through an RXFP1-independent mechanism. Two molecules **1** and **2** with modest activity in the primary screen were validated using these counter-screen assays[21] and then resynthesized in-house. Both confirmed hits displayed similarities in their chemical scaffold containing a 2-acetamido-N-phenylbenzamide core in their structures (Fig. 1, in blue).

Hit-to-lead medicinal chemistry optimization.
The initial screening was followed up by an extensive structure activity relationship campaign to improve the potency, efficacy and physical properties of the compounds (Fig. 2; Supplementary Table S1). Compound activity is reported through two measurements: EC_{50} (concentration necessary to reach 50% of the maximum cAMP signal produced by the molecule) and maximum response (efficacy, corresponding with the level of cAMP elevation normalized to relaxin control). Both EC_{50} and maximum response were evaluated and optimized through these efforts. Our studies on the aniline ring indicated the importance

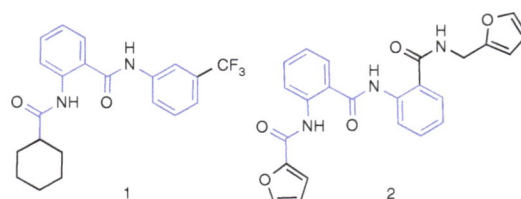

Figure 1 | Chemical structures of hit molecules 1 and 2 identified in a RXFP1 cAMP primary screening assay. Both molecules share a common chemical scaffold containing a core substructure of 2-acetamido-N-phenylbenzamide (in blue).

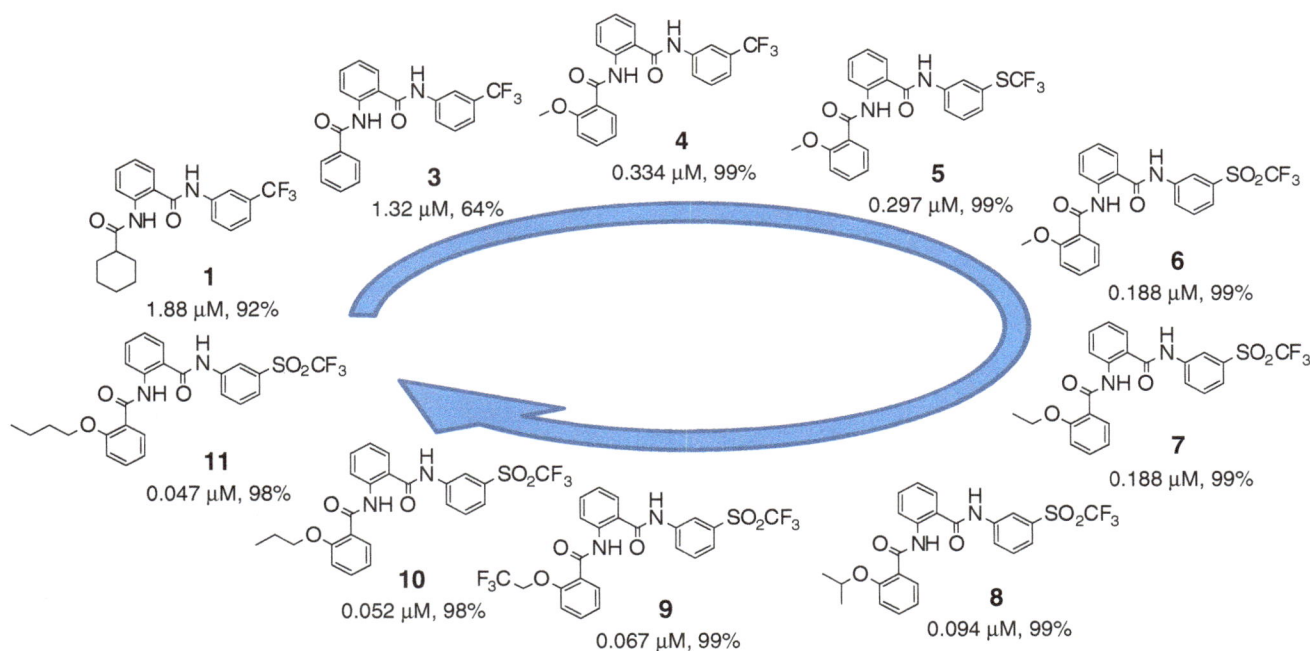

Figure 2 | Structure activity relationship optimization campaign. Ten representative compounds, **1** and **3–11**, highlight the key steps in the hit-to-lead evolution. The EC_{50} and relative activity for each compound are shown using the RXFP1 primary screening assay. 100% relative activity was normalized to 57.7 μM forskolin stimulation, and 0% relative activity was normalized to compound vehicle control (0.58% DMSO). Complete concentration-response data are also provided (Supplementary Fig. S1).

Table 1 | Profiles of potent analogues 5–11 with EC_{50} <300 nM in the RXFP1-transfected HEK293 cAMP assay.

ID	HEK-RXFP1 EC_{50} (μM)	THP1 EC_{50} (μM)	HEK-RXFP2 EC_{50} (μM)	HEK-V1b EC_{50} (μM)	ATP toxicity EC_{50} (μM)	PBS solubility (μM)	MLM stability ($T_{1/2}$ in min)
5	0.297	0.523	3.34	Inactive	3.7	2.9	N/A
6	0.188	0.358	Inactive	Inactive	29.7	6.3	N/A
7	0.188	0.362	7.47	Inactive	18.8	<1.1	1732
8	0.094	0.200	Inactive	Inactive	9.4	7.0	122
9	0.067	0.107	Inactive	Inactive	29.7	3.3	100
10	0.052	0.105	Inactive	Inactive	9.4	17.0	133
11	0.047	0.124	Inactive	Inactive	59.3	5.3	178

Abbreviation: MLM, mouse liver microsome.
EC_{50} of compounds are given in micromolar units for the HEK293 cells stably transfected with *RXFP1* (HEK-RXFP1), THP1 cells that endogenously express RXFP1, HEK293 cells stably transfected with *RXFP2* (HEK-RXFP2), as well as the vasopressin receptor (HEK-V1b) and cytotoxicity at 72 h using the HEK293 cells stably transfected with *RXFP1* (HEK-RXFP1). Replicate compound concentration-response data is also provided (Supplementary Fig. S1). The series has good selectivity against RXFP2 and AVPR1B receptors stably transfected into HEK293 cells. PBS solubility analysis was performed by Analiza Inc. and based upon quantitative nitrogen detection as described (www.analiza.com). MLM stability analyses were performed by Pharmaron and are based upon duplicate incubations of test reagent in pooled male MLMs (www.pharmaron.com). Analysis in the absence and presence of glutamate synthase (NADPH) was performed to assess NADPH-free degradation. Half-lifes ($T_{1/2}$) were calcuated only in NADPH (+) degradation (Supplementary Table S2).

of a hydrophobic functional group having the proper field effect[22] at the *meta*-position of this aromatic ring, with a trifluoromethylsulfonyl group providing the best activity. *Meta*-substituents with incremental field-effect values at this position (SO_2CF_3, F = 0.73; SCF_3, F = 0.35; and CF_3, F = 0.38)[22] provide increasingly potent activity. We also investigated the impact of modifying the cyclohexane ring moiety and found that aromatic replacements, especially those with an alkoxy aliphatic chain in *ortho*-position, increased compound potency. Finally, most substituents and replacement modifications of the middle phenyl ring core and amide functional groups produced analogues with the same or lower activity than the corresponding parent compound.

Profiling of representative lead compounds. Table 1 displays the profile of compounds **5–11** with an EC_{50} <300 nM in the *RXFP1*-transfected cAMP assay, and also includes their activities

in a human monocytic leukaemia cell line (THP1), which endogenously expresses the RXFP1 receptor, their selectivity against HEK293 cells transfected with the receptors *RXFP2* and *AVPR1B*, adenosine triphosphate (ATP) cytotoxicity, aqueous PBS solubility and mouse liver microsomal stability (Supplementary Table S2). As expected, because of the lipophilic character of our molecules, these compounds have poor water solubility, although our most potent compounds (**8–11**, EC_{50} <100 nM) display a solubility of 3.3–17.0 μM, which is 49–327 times higher than their corresponding EC_{50} for RXFP1 in HEK293 cells.

Lead compounds increase *VEGF* expression in THP1 cells. Beyond inducing elevated intracellular cAMP levels, we also evaluated the ability of the most potent compounds **5–11** to activate the transcription of the known relaxin target gene, *VEGF*, in THP1 cells[23,24]. The addition of 10 ng ml^{-1} (1.66 nM) of relaxin hormone induces a significant increase (2.4 fold) in the

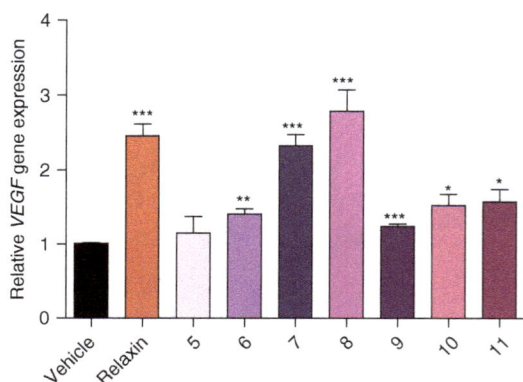

Figure 3 | Activation of *VEGF* gene expression in THP1 cells. THP1 cells were treated with compound vehicle control (0.58% DMSO), relaxin (10 ng ml^{-1}; 1.66 nM) or seven representative compounds **5–11** at 250 nM for 2 h. The level of *VEGF* gene expression was measured by quantitative real-time PCR and normalized to *GAPDH* expression and vehicle control as 1 ($n = 4$ for each). All analogues other than compound **5** show significant (*$P < 0.05$; **$P < 0.01$; and ***$P < 0.001$) upregulation of *VEGF* gene expression between treatment groups and vehicle control. Scale bars, mean values ± s.e.m.; statistical analysis was performed using two-tailed, Student's *t*-test.

relative expression of *VEGF* mRNA as measured by quantitative real-time PCR. Similar effects were obtained in cells stimulated with compound (Fig. 3).

Lead compound 8 increases cell impedance in HEK293 cells. Cellular impedance was measured using xCELLigence Analyzer (Roche Diagnostics, Indianapolis, IN), which allows for continuous time-resolved measurement of cellular index without additional labelling[25]. Cells were treated with compound for 30 min. Given this short incubation time, changes in cell number were unlikely to contribute to the overall effect. The results indicate that compound 8 treatment generated a dose-dependent response similar to that of relaxin hormone (Fig. 4a,b). Neither treatment affected cell impedance in the corresponding parental HEK293 cells (Fig. 4c), indicating that changes in cell impedance were mediated through RXFP1.

Three-dimensional conformation and stability of the lead compound 8. The minimum energy conformation of compound **8** was determined in solid state by X-ray crystallography (Fig. 5; Supplementary Table S3) and in solution by variable temperature NMR and Nuclear Overhauser Effect (NOE) spectroscopy studies (Supplementary Fig. S2). The two intramolecular hydrogen-binding interactions found in compound **8** rigidify its three-dimensional conformation, possibly contributing to its remarkable stability. Moreover, stability studies using mouse and human plasma demonstrated that compound **8** has excellent plasma stability *in vitro* (Supplementary Table S4), with no significant decrease after 2 h of exposure.

***In vivo* pharmacokinetic of the lead compound 8 in mice.** We measured the plasma and heart concentration of compound **8** in C57BL/6 mice after a single intraperitoneal administration at a dose of 30 mg kg^{-1} (Fig. 6; Supplementary Table S5). Compound **8** has a long half-life in both plasma ($T_{1/2} = 8.56$ h) and heart ($T_{1/2} = 7.48$ h). In addition, exposure in heart was generally three to four times higher than plasma levels. Furthermore, no abnormal clinical behaviours or acute toxicity were observed in animals throughout the study.

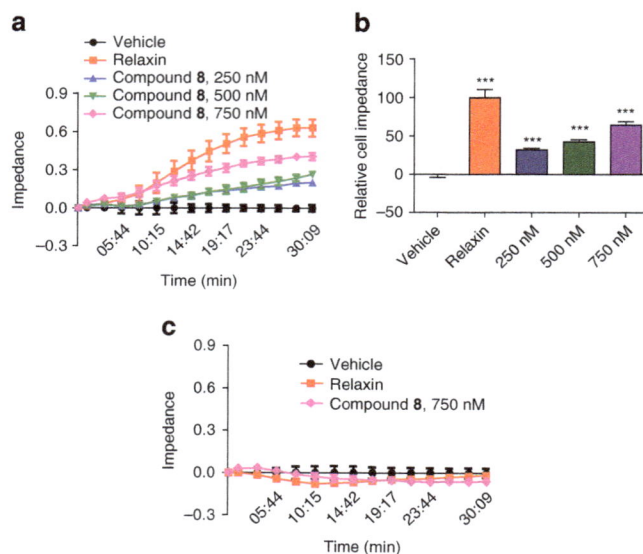

Figure 4 | Compound 8 exhibits concentration-dependent increase of cellular impedance in *RXFP1*-transfected HEK293 cells. (**a**) Effect of relaxin (10 ng ml^{-1}; 1.66 nM), compared with compound **8** at 250 nM, 500 nM and 750 nM on cell impedance in HEK293 cells stably transfected with *RXFP1* ($n = 4$ for each). The values at each point were normalized to the values of vehicle treatment. The subset of data points was used for the graph drawing. All points represent the mean values ± s.e.m. (**b**) Relative cell impedance normalized to the relaxin treatment group (100) at 30 min after addition of relaxin or compound **8**. Columns represent the mean values ± s.e.m. Differences, evaluated by two-tailed, Student's *t*-test, between treatment groups and vehicle control are significant (***$P < 0.001$). (**c**) Relaxin (10 ng ml^{-1}; 1.66 nM) and compound **8** at 750 nM did not affect cell impedance in parental HEK293 cells.

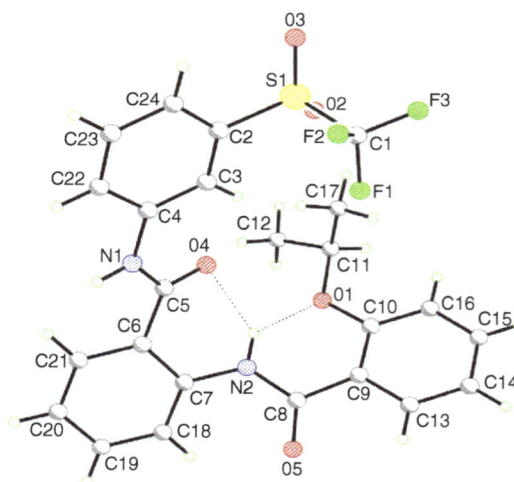

Figure 5 | Three-dimensional conformation of compound 8 determined by X-ray diffraction crystallography. Two intramolecular hydrogen-binding interactions (dash lines) are identified with a bond length of 2.03 and 2.12 Å, respectively. Full parameters are also provided (Supplementary Table S3).

RXFP1 region responsible for activation by compound 8. The majority of preclinical studies with relaxin peptide have been performed on mouse and rat models. Therefore, we analysed the performance of our series of agonists on HEK293 cells transfected with mouse *RXFP1* (89% identity to human sequence) and found that the compounds are significantly better agonists for the human RXFP1 than for the mouse clone (Fig. 7). We took

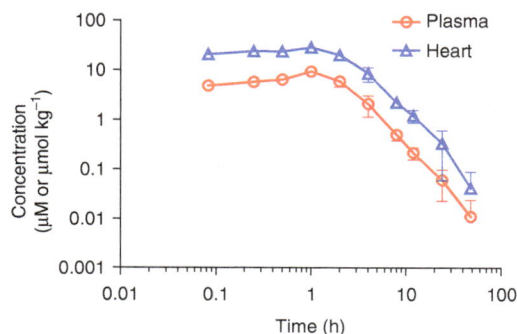

Figure 6 | In vivo PK profile of compound 8. Mean plasma and heart concentration-time profiles of compound **8** ± s.e.m. after a single intraperitoneal (IP) dose of 30 mg kg^{-1} in male C57BL/6 mice ($n = 3$). No abnormal clinical observation was found during the in-life phase. The IP dosing formulation solution was prepared in 10% NMP + 10% Solutol HS15 + 10% PEG400 + 70% saline. Full PK data and parameters are also provided (Supplementary Table S5).

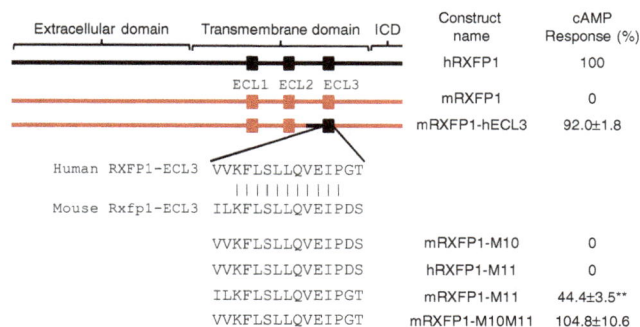

Figure 7 | Identification of RXFP1 region responsible for activation by compound 8. Human RXFP1 (hRXFP1 denoted for clarity in black) is fully activated (100%) after treatment with relaxin (15 nM) or compound **8** (66 μM). Mouse RXFP1 (mRXFP1 denoted in red) does not respond to compound **8** (marked as 0%) at 66 μM. RXFP1 contains extracellular, transmembrane and intracellular domains (ICDs). Using chimeric mouse-human receptors, the region responsible for RXFP1 activation by compound **8** was mapped to the part containing ECL3 of the transmembrane domain. Alignment of hRXFP1 and mRXFP1 shows two pairs of divergent amino acids within ECL3. The N-terminal IL to VV substitution in the mouse construct (mRXFP1-M10) did not rescue mouse receptor response, whereas C-terminal GT to DS substitution in human RXFP1 (hRXFP1-M11) abolished its compound **8**-dependent activation. The mouse construct with (mRXFP1-M11) mutant was partially active and the mouse receptor with humanized ECL3 (mRXFP1-M10M11) was fully active after stimulation with compound **8**. The cAMP response to compound **8** (66 μM) in cells transfected with a specific construct was normalized to the response of the same cells to relaxin (15 nM). The results represent the average of three independent experiments ± s.e.m. repeated in quadruplicates. **$P < 0.01$ versus mRXFP1 by Student's t-test.

advantage of this difference in species activity to map out the regions of the human receptor that determine such specificity. We tested a number of chimeric mouse/human RXFP1 constructs and found that the human receptor region of transmembrane helix 5 to extracellular loop 3 (ECL3) is required for the activation by compound **8**. Importantly, all receptor constructs responded to relaxin. Further site-specific mutagenesis studies demonstrated that the substitution of mouse ECL3 sequence with the human ECL3 resulted in full activation of the mouse receptor

after treatment with compound **8**. Conversely, applying mouse $_{659}GT_{660}/_{659}DS_{660}$ mutations to ECL3 of human receptor completely abolished compound **8**-induced cAMP activation, whereas a mouse construct with the $_{659}DS_{660}/_{659}GT_{660}$ equivalent mutation recovered partial activity (Fig. 7).

Discussion

We have identified the first novel series of small-molecule agonists of RXFP1 through a screening of > 350,000 compound libraries in quantitative high-throughput screening format with > 100-fold selectivity over RXFP2 receptor (Fig. 1). Through extensive medicinal chemistry efforts, a pool of lead compounds with improved potency and selectivity were discovered (Fig. 2). Analogue **3** was obtained by replacement of the cyclohexyl group in hit compound **1** with a phenyl ring. Analogue **4** was obtained from **3** by introduction of an *ortho*-methoxy group within this benzoic substituent. *Meta*-substituents with increased field-defect values on the aniline ring yield compounds **4–6**. Lastly, compounds **7–11** were produced from analogue **6** through the introduction of longer aliphatic chains within the *ortho*-alkoxy substituent of the benzoic ring. Optimized compounds show a remarkable increase in activity from the high micromolar EC$_{50}$ of the initial hits to potencies < 50 nM (**11**, EC$_{50}$ = 47 nM, maximum response = 98%). The activity of all our analogues was further tested in cAMP-response assays against RXFP2 and also counter-screened against AVPR1B. Cytotoxicity was also evaluated by measuring cellular ATP levels 72 h after treatment. Most of the analogues were inactive against RXFP2 and AVPR1B and had low cytotoxicity. These analogues also show a remarkable rodent and human microsomal stability, especially important in light of the poor metabolic stability of the recombinant hormone[26], with intrinsic half-lives > 100 min and at least 100-fold potency separation between RXFP1 activities and cytotoxicity in the same cells, measured by overall ATP cellular levels as an indicator of cell growth and viability (Table 1). In addition, no activity with RXFP3, another member of the relaxin family of receptors, was detected for compound **8** (R. Bathgate, personal communication).

The cAMP EC$_{50}$ of the molecules decreases only by a factor of two between RXFP1-transfected HEK293 cells and THP1 cells endogenously expressing this receptor. Differences in EC$_{50}$ among transfected and native cell lines have been previously reported for G-protein-coupled receptors and explained as function of receptor reserve, which is a measurement of the receptor occupancy required to mediate the response and amplification of the signal[27]. Transfected cell lines, with an elevated number of receptor transcripts, produce a higher expression of the receptor on the cell surface and might require less amount of compound to elicit an equivalent functional signal. Moreover, transfection efficiency is cell type dependent. Thus, differences in EC$_{50}$ depend on the cell type and expression of the receptor in transfected cells.

Although *VEGF* stimulation seems to be dependent on cAMP activation[23], some differences in compound activity were observed between assays measuring cAMP elevation and *VEGF* stimulation. The strongest effect on *VEGF* activation was obtained after treatment with compounds **7** and **8**. In addition to cAMP elevation, RXFP1 activation by relaxin hormone is known to stimulate other pathways including protein kinase A, protein kinase C and extracellular signal-regulated protein kinases 1 and 2[28]. These other pathways might also contribute to the modulation of *VEGF* transcriptional activation. Differences in functional selectivity between members of our series or between relaxin hormone and our compounds might have an impact on *VEGF* expression. Our group has previously described significant differences in functional selectivity with compounds belonging to a specific chemical class for other G-protein-coupled receptors[29]. As a further confirmation that the compound effects were RXFP1 dependent, we recapitulated previous work showing that RXFP1 activation by compound **8** increases the cell impedance of transfected cells[25].

Balancing the potency, efficacy and *in vitro* metabolic stability properties of our analogues, we chose compound **8** for full mouse *in vivo* pharmacokinetic (PK) studies investigating its levels in plasma and heart upon drug administration. Upon a single intraperitoneal dose of compound **8** at $30\,mg\,kg^{-1}$ in male C57BL/6 mice, the concentration of compound **8** in heart reached $28.6\,\mu mol\,kg^{-1}$ (C_{max}) within 1 h, and concentrations above its EC_{50} of 200 nM in THP1 cells was maintained for a period of 12 h in plasma and more than 24 h in heart. Oral gavage and intravenous administration recapitulate the overall PK properties of compound **8** (Supplementary Table S6), indicating good metabolic stability with an extended exposure, and preferential distribution towards the heart. The oral bioavailability was low ($F \approx 14\%$), which we attribute to poor solubility and suboptimal formulation. Nevertheless, excellent exposure was observed at this dose. Additional formulation studies or introducing solubilizing moieties into the molecule might further improve oral bioavailability.

According to the two-domain model of relaxin binding to RXFP1, the native hormone first interacts with leucine-rich repeats of extracellular domain, and then with the extracellular loops of the transmembrane domain, most probably with ECL2[30-32]. This follows by an effect on the intracellular N terminus located at low-density lipoprotein class A domain that is necessary for the activation of the RXFP1 signalling. Receptors without this domain or with a mutated domain including both mutations at the calcium-binding asparagine or substituted with glutamic acid ($D_{58}E$) bind relaxin normally but do not signal[33]. Surprisingly, compound **8** can still induce cAMP production with this latter $D_{58}E$ mutant, indicating that the receptor activation by the small molecule does not require a functional lipoprotein domain (Supplementary Fig. S3). The evaluation of compound **8** up to a concentration of 30 μM was unable to displace the binding of [^{125}I]-human relaxin to human RXFP1 (Supplementary Table S7). This data, in addition to our mutagenesis studies, suggest that our small-molecule agonists likely interact with an allosteric site at the ECL3 loop and act non-competitively with the natural hormone to activate RXFP1.

In summary, we present the first synthetic small-molecule alternative to relaxin hormone. The described molecules show good potency, selectivity and functional activity in cell-based assays. Our structural studies show that our agonists appear to function through a novel allosteric mechanism. Optimized compounds display excellent *in vitro* ADME properties and *in vivo* PK properties with high levels of exposure for extended period of time. These molecules represent the first bioavailable small-molecule agonists of human RXFP1 and a promising series to further investigate relaxin biology and evaluate the therapeutic benefits of RXFP1 activation in chronic settings.

Methods

General methods for chemistry. Full experimental details and characterization data for all new compounds are included in the Supplementary Methods.

Measurements of cAMP concentration. cAMP assay was performed using HTRF cAMP HiRange kit (CisBio, Bedford, MA, USA). The THP1 and HEK293 cells (ATCC, Manassas, VA, USA) stably[7,34] or transiently transfected with human RXFP1, RXFP2 or AVPR1B receptor were stimulated with relaxin, the compounds or forskolin for 30 min at 37 °C, 5% CO_2, after which, 8 μl per well of each HTRF detection reagent (diluted according to assay kit directions in HTRF lysis buffer) was added. The plates were incubated for 30 min at room temperature, and the signal was read on a ViewLux (PerkinElmer, Waltham, MA, USA) or a FLUOstar Omega (BMG Labtech, Cary, NC, USA) plate readers. Nonlinear regressions to the

Hill equation were performed using Prism software (GraphPad Software, San Diego, CA, USA).

ATP cytotoxicity assay in HEK293-RXFP1 cells. A cytotoxicity assay to measure the effect of compounds on cell viability was performed by measuring ATP levels (ATPLite; Promega, Madison, WI, USA). Cells were incubated with compounds for 72 h in growth media (DMEM 10% FBS, $1 \times$ Pen/Strep, $0.5\,mg\,ml^{-1}$ of G418) in 384-well format. After compound incubation, the levels of ATP in each well were measured with the addition of the ATPLite assay reagent. Nonlinear regressions to the Hill equation were performed using Prism software.

Aqueous solubility and metabolic stability measurement. Kinetic solubility analysis in PBS solution was performed via a fee-for-service type of contract at Analiza based upon quantitative nitrogen detection as described (www.analiza.com). One sample was supplied as a dimethylsulphoxide (DMSO)-dissolved stock (10 mM). A final DMSO concentration of 2.0% and maximum theoretical compound concentration of 200 μM was achieved by diluting a 6 μl aliquot of DMSO stock with 294 μl of $1 \times$ PBS using Hamilton Starlet liquid handling and incubated directly in a Millipore solubility filter plate. Following 24 h incubation at ambient temperature (22.0–23.0 °C), the sample was vacuum filtered. The filtrate was injected into the nitrogen detector for quantification on Analiza's Automated Discovery Workstation. The results are reported in both μM and $\mu g\,ml^{-1}$. Three separate on-board performance indicating standards were assayed in triplicate with supplied compounds, and the results were within the acceptable range. Mouse liver microsomal stability analysis was performed via a fee-for-service type of contract by Pharmaron (www.pharmaron.com). The detailed protocols can be found in the Supplementary Table S2.

***VEGF* expression analysis.** The *VEGF* stimulation in THP1 cells was analysed by quantitative real-time PCR. A total of 400,000 THP1 cells (0.4 ml at 1×10^6 cells per ml) in test media (RPMI-1640 without phenol red, 0.5% FBS, $1 \times$ Pen/Strep and 0.05 mM of 2-mercaptoethanol) were seeded in each well on a 24-well plate. After 24 h at 37 °C, 5% CO_2, relaxin, compounds or vehicle were added for 2 h. The cells were collected and RNA was extracted using Trizol reagent (Invitrogen, Carlsbad, CA, USA) according to the manufacturer's instructions. cDNA was synthesized using Verso cDNA kit (Thermo Scientific, Waltham, MA, USA) according to the manufacturer's protocol. The *VEGF* and *GAPDH* gene expression were analysed using Roche LightCycler 480 (Roche Diagnostics) with the appropriate set of primers and probes spanning different exons. The relative fold change in *VEGF* mRNA level was calculated by the comparative C_t ($2^{-\Delta\Delta C_t}$) method using *GAPDH* expression for normalization. The experiments were repeated three times in quadruplicates. The data were analysed by Student's *t*-test.

Cell impedance assay in HEK293-RXFP1 cells. The cell line stably transfected with *RXFP1* receptor and the parental HEK293 cells were used for the cell impedance assay. Cellular impedance was measured using a Roche DP RCTA xCELLigence Analyzer (Roche Diagnostics) on E-Plates as described before[35]. Delta cellular indices were calculated as the change of impedance at a given time t, from the time of compound addition ($CI_{compound}$): $\Delta CI_t = CI_t - CI_{compound}$. Impedance at each time point was then normalized to the average of quadruplicate CI of cells treated with vehicle (V1, V2, V3 and V4), to calculate normalized delta cell index $N\Delta CI = (CI_t - CI_{compound})/average\,[\Delta CI_{V1}, \Delta CI_{V2}, \Delta CI_{V3}, \Delta CI_{V4}]$. A total of 20,000 cells were added per well in a volume of 100 μl test media and allowed to sediment at room temperature for 30 min. The plate was placed into xCELLigence RTCA DP Instrument in the CO_2 incubator overnight to allow the cells to attach. Relaxin (10 ng ml^{-1}; 1.66 nM), vehicle or compound at different concentrations (250, 500 and 750 nM) were added to the wells, and the cellular impedance was measured every 30 s for 30 min. The graphs depicted in this manuscript were prepared in Prizm software using a subset of data points acquired by the xCELLigence software. The data were analysed by two-tailed, Student's *t*-test using Prism software.

Study of chimeric and site-specific mutant receptors. Full-length human *RXFP1* in pCR3.1 was used for production of site-specific and chimeric constructs. Mouse *RXFP1* cDNA clone was a kind gift from Dr R. A. D. Bathgate (Howard Florey Institute, Melbourne, Australia). Chimeric receptors containing parts of mouse or human sequence were generated using overlap PCR. Site-specific human and mouse mutant receptors were generated by conventional method with long-range PCR with overlapping primers containing mutated nucleotide sites, then digested by DpnI and transformed into competent cells. The cDNA inserts of the resulted clones were completely sequenced to confirm the correct substitutions. Transient transfections of HEK293 cells were performed using Lipofectamine 2000 transfection reagent (Invitrogen) according to the manufacturer's instructions. Cells transiently expressing the receptors were used within 48 h of transfection in cAMP assay as described above. Cells expressing each construct were treated with different concentrations of relaxin or compound **8** in the same experiment in quadruplicates. Each construct was tested at least three times.

References

1. Roger, V. L. et al. Executive summary: heart disease and stroke statistics—2011 update. Circulation 123, 459–463 (2011).
2. Hisaw, F. L. Experimental relaxation of the pubic ligament of the guinea pig. Exp. Biol. Med. 23, 661–663 (1926).
3. Fevold, H. L., Hisaw, F. L. & Meyer, R. K. The relaxative hormone of the corpus luteum. Its purification and concnetration. J. Am. Chem. Soc. 52, 3340–3348 (1930).
4. Baylis, C. Relaxin may be the "elusive" renal vasodilatory agent of normal pregnancy. Am. J. Kidney Dis. 34, 1142–1144 (1999).
5. Jeyabalan, A., Shroff, S. G., Novak, J. & Conrad, K. P. The vascular actions of relaxin. Adv. Exp. Med. Biol. 612, 65–87 (2007).
6. Bathgate, R. A. et al. Relaxin family peptides and their receptors. Physiol. Rev. 93, 405–480 (2013).
7. Kern, A., Hubbard, D., Amano, A. & Bryant-Greenwood, G. D. Cloning, expression, and functional characterization of relaxin receptor (leucine-rich repeat-containing g protein-coupled receptor 7) splice variants from human fetal membranes. Endocrinology 149, 1277–1294 (2008).
8. Van Der Westhuizen, E. T., Summers, R. J., Halls, M. L., Bathgate, R. A. D. & Sexton, P. M. Relaxin receptors - new drug targets for multiple disease states. Curr. Drug Targets 8, 91–104 (2007).
9. Teerlink, J. R. et al. Serelaxin, recombinant human relaxin-2, for treatment of acute heart failure (RELAX-AHF): a randomised, placebo-controlled trial. Lancet 381, 29–39 (2013).
10. Metra, M. et al. Effect of serelaxin on cardiac, renal, and hepatic biomarkers in the relaxin in acute heart failure (RELAX-AHF) development program: correlation with outcomes. J. Am. Coll. Cardiol. 61, 196–206 (2013).
11. Unemori, E., Sibai, B. & Teichman, S. L. Scientific rationale and design of a phase I safety study of relaxin in women with severe preeclampsia. Ann. N. Y. Acad. Sci. 1160, 381–384 (2009).
12. Tozzi, C. A. et al. Recombinant human relaxin reduces hypoxic pulmonary hypertension in the rat. Pulm. Pharmacol. Ther. 18, 346–353 (2005).
13. Yoshida, T. et al. Relaxin ameliorates salt-sensitive hypertension and renal fibrosis. Nephrol. Dial. Transplant. 27, 2190–2197 (2012).
14. Samuel, C. S. et al. Relaxin remodels fibrotic healing following myocardial infarction. Lab. Invest. 91, 675–690 (2011).
15. Du, X.-J., Bathgate, R. A. D., Samuel, C. S., Dart, A. M. & Summers, R. J. Cardiovascular effects of relaxin: from basic science to clinical therapy. Nat. Rev. Cardiol. 7, 48–58 (2010).
16. Teichman, S. L., Unemori, E., Teerlink, J. R., Cotter, G. & Metra, M. Relaxin: review of biology and potential role in treating heart failure. Curr. Heart Failure Rep. 7, 75–82 (2010).
17. Teerlink, J. R. et al. Relaxin for the treatment of patients with acute heart failure (Pre-RELAX-AHF): a multicenter, randomized, placebo-controlled, parallel-group, dose-finding phase IIb study. Lancet 373, 1429–1439 (2009).
18. Segal, M. S. et al. Relaxin increases human endothelial progenitor cell NO and migration and vasculogenesis in mice. Blood 119, 629–636 (2012).
19. Austin, C. P., Brady, L. S., Insel, T. R. & Collins, F. S. NIH molecular libraries initiative. Science 306, 1138–1139 (2004).
20. Inglese, J. et al. Quantitative high-throughput screening: a titration-based approach that efficiently identifies biological activities in large chemical libraries. Proc. Natl Acad. Sci. USA 103, 11473–11478 (2006).
21. Chen, C. Z. et al. Identification of small-molecule agonists of human relaxin family receptor 1 (RXFP1) by using a homogenous cell-based cAMP assay. J. Biomol. Screen. doi:10.1177/1087057112469406 (2013).
22. Hansch, C. et al. Aromatic substituent constants for structure-activity correlations. J. Med. Chem. 16, 1207–1216 (1973).
23. Unemori, E. N. et al. Relaxin stimulates expression of vascular endothelial growth factor in normal human endometrial cells in vitro and is associated with menometrorrhagia in women. Hum. Reprod. 14, 800–806 (1999).
24. Unemori, E. N. et al. Relaxin induces vascular endothelial growth factor expression and angiogenesis selectively at wound sites. Wound. Repair. Regen. 8, 361–370 (2000).
25. Shemesh, R. et al. Activation of relaxin-related receptors by short, linear peptides derived from a collagen-containing precursor. Ann. N. Y. Acad. Sci. 1160, 78–86 (2009).
26. Dschietzig, T., Bartsch, C., Baumann, G. & Stangl, K. Relaxin-a pleiotropic hormone and its emerging role for experimental and clinical therapeutics. Pharmacol. Ther. 112, 38–56 (2006).
27. Wilson, C. N. & Mustafa, S. J. (ed) in Handb. Exp. Pharmacol. (Springer GmbH, 2009).
28. Summers, R. J., Halls, M. L. & van der Westhuizen, E. T. in Encyclopedia of Signalling Molecules Ch. 362 (ed. Choi, S.) 1635–1643 (Springer, 2012).
29. McCoy, J. G. et al. Selective modulation of Gq/Gs pathways by naphtho pyrano pyrimidines as antagonists of the neuropeptide s receptor. ACS Chem. Neurosci. 1, 559–574 (2010).
30. Sudo, S. et al. H3 relaxin is a specific ligand for LGR7 and activates the receptor by interacting with both the ectodomain and the exoloop 2. J. Biol. Chem. 278, 7855–7862 (2003).
31. Halls, M. L. et al. Multiple binding sites revealed by interaction of relaxin family peptides with native and chimeric relaxin family peptide receptors 1 and 2 (LGR7 and LGR8). J. Pharmacol. Exp. Ther. 313, 677–687 (2005).
32. Halls, M. L. et al. Identification of binding sites with differing affinity and potency for relaxin analogues on LGR7 and LGR8 receptors. Annu. N.Y. Acad. Sci. 1041, 17–21 (2005).
33. Kern, A., Agoulnik, A. I. & Bryant-Greenwood, G. D. The low-density lipoprotein class A module of the relaxin receptor (leucine-rich repeat containing G-protein coupled receptor 7): its role in signalling and trafficking to the cell membrane. Endocrinology 148, 1181–1194 (2007).
34. Hsu, S. Y. et al. Activation of orphan receptors by the hormone relaxin. Science 295, 671–674 (2002).
35. Hodgson, M. C. et al. Decreased expression and androgen regulation of the tumor suppressor gene INPP4B in prostate cancer. Cancer Res. 71, 572–582 (2011).

Acknowledgements

We acknowledge Dr O. D. Sherwood at the University of Illinois at Urbana-Champaign for providing porcine relaxin; Dr G. D. Bryant-Greenwood at the University of Hawaii and Dr A. Kern at the Scripps Research Institute, Florida, for providing HEK293 cells stably transfected with RXFP1, Dr S. Y. Hsu at Stanford University for HEK293 cells stably transfected with RXFP2; and Dr R. A. D. Bathgate at Howard Florey Institute, Melbourne, for the mouse RXFP1 construct and RXFP3 data. We also thank Drs X. Xu and A. Wang at NCATS for assessment of oral bioavailability in mice, and Dr A. L. Rheingold at the UCSD for the X-ray analysis of compound 8. This research was supported by the Molecular Libraries Initiative of the NIH Roadmap for Medical Research (U54MH084681 and R03MH085705 to A.I.A.), the Intramural Research Program of the National Human Genome Research Institute (NHGRI) and National Center for Advancing Translational Sciences (NCATS), National Institutes of Health (NIH) and the Faculty Research Support Program of the Florida International University.

Author contributions

J.X. designed, synthesized and characterized all new compounds. Z.H. and I.U.A. performed secondary assays and structural mutagenesis studies. C.Z.C., R.E.J., M.F. and W.Z. adapted the assay and conducted the quantitative high-throughput screening and confirmatory assays. N.S. and X.H. provided data analysis and model docking study support. A.I.A. and J.J.M. guided the design and proposed follow-up experimentation. J.X., N.S., A.I.A. and J.J.M. drafted the manuscript. All authors discussed the results, analysed the data and commented on the manuscript.

Additional information

Accession codes: The X-ray crystallographic coordinates for structure reported in this article have been deposited at the Cambridge Crystallographic Data Centre (CCDC), under deposition number CCDC 933133. These data can be obtained free of charge from the Cambridge Crystallographic Data Centre via www.ccdc.cam.ac.uk/data_request/cif

17

Structural basis for drug-induced allosteric changes to human β-cardiac myosin motor activity

Donald A. Winkelmann[1], Eva Forgacs[2], Matthew T. Miller[3] & Ann M. Stock[3,4]

Omecamtiv Mecarbil (OM) is a small molecule allosteric effector of cardiac myosin that is in clinical trials for treatment of systolic heart failure. A detailed kinetic analysis of cardiac myosin has shown that the drug accelerates phosphate release by shifting the equilibrium of the hydrolysis step towards products, leading to a faster transition from weak to strong actin-bound states. The structure of the human β-cardiac motor domain (cMD) with OM bound reveals a single OM-binding site nestled in a narrow cleft separating two domains of the human cMD where it interacts with the key residues that couple lever arm movement to the nucleotide state. In addition, OM induces allosteric changes in three strands of the β-sheet that provides the communication link between the actin-binding interface and the nucleotide pocket. The OM-binding interactions and allosteric changes form the structural basis for the kinetic and mechanical tuning of cardiac myosin.

[1] Department of Pathology and Laboratory Medicine, Robert Wood Johnson Medical School, Rutgers University, Piscataway, New Jersey 08854, USA.
[2] Department of Physiological Sciences, Eastern Virginia Medical School, Norfolk, Virginia 23507, USA. [3] Center for Advanced Biotechnology and Medicine, Robert Wood Johnson Medical School, Rutgers University, Piscataway, New Jersey 08854, USA. [4] Department of Biochemistry and Molecular Biology, Robert Wood Johnson Medical School, Rutgers University, Piscataway, New Jersey 08854, USA. Correspondence and requests for materials should be addressed to D.A.W. (email: winkelma@rwjms.rutgers.edu).

Heart failure is a common human disease with a significant lifetime risk that increases with age[1]. In its most common manifestation, heart failure is marked by a decrease in cardiac contractility culminating in systolic heart failure. Recently, a novel approach to the treatment of systolic heart failure has been developed on the basis of pharmacologic agents called 'cardiac myosin activators' that bind directly to myosin and target the kinetic mechanism driving contraction[2]. Directly targeting the contractile mechanism of cardiac myosin could theoretically improve heart performance without altering intracellular cAMP or calcium transients. A large, high-throughput, drug screen of a biochemically reconstituted contractile system identified a series of potential cardiac myosin activators[3]. Omecamtiv Mecarbil (OM) is one such small molecule effector of cardiac myosin that is in clinical trials for treatment of systolic heart failure. Initial characterization of OM with bovine cardiac myosin shows that it binds directly to the myosin catalytic domain and operates by an allosteric mechanism to increase the transition rate of weak to strong bound actin states and enhance force generation[4]. In animal models, OM increases cardiac muscle function by extending the duration of systolic ejection without altering the heart rate[4,5].

We have elucidated the precise action of OM on steady state and transient kinetics of the actomyosin mechanism and motor activity of porcine ventricular heavy meromyosin (HMM)[6]. We find that OM shifts the equilibrium of the hydrolysis step of the myosin ATPase towards products, and this accelerates the flux through the product dissociation steps of the actomyosin mechanical cycle without altering the ADP dissociation rate, the key step that regulates the maximum shortening velocity[7]. The subtle changes in the kinetic mechanism lead to an increase in the transition rate of weak to strong bound actin states, resulting in increased number of force-producing crossbridges and, paradoxically, a dramatic reduction in the unloaded shortening velocity measured in vitro[6,8]. These fascinating kinetic results led to an intense effort to determine the drug-binding site and define the structural interactions within the human β-cardiac myosin motor domain that alter the motor activity.

Purification of human cardiac myosin was not an option for accomplishing this objective because of limited availability and poor stability of clinical specimens. The alternative, expression and purification of recombinant cardiac muscle myosin, had been technically unfeasible until we showed that the principal obstacle for the expression of vertebrate striated muscle myosin was that motor domain folding follows a regulated pathway that is unique to striated muscle cells[9-12]. To demonstrate this principle, we designed a striated muscle myosin motor domain (MD)::green fluorescent protein (GFP) chimeric protein and expressed it in muscle cells using adenovirus-mediated expression vectors[9]. This unique single-chain motor design is functionally active, fluorescent and ideally suited for structural studies.

Here we present the structure of the human β-cardiac motor domain (cMD) fused to GFP determined without drug (Apo structure) and with OM bound (OM + structure). OM binds in a narrow cleft that separates the N-terminal 25-K domain from the lower portion of the 50-K domain of the cMD. The drug interacts with the key residues involved in coupling structural elements that are linked to the rotation of the lever arm into the pre-power stroke conformation. Strong binding to actin triggers the reversal of the rotation, leading to the power stroke and force production. Surprisingly, OM binding induces an allosteric change in the conformation of three strands of a β-sheet that are crucial to communication between the nucleotide pocket and actin-binding interface[13]. Together, these interactions form the basis of the kinetic and mechanical effects of the drug. This structural analysis characterizes a highly significant binding cleft for drugs designed to modulate myosin motor activity.

Results

Human β-cardiac myosin motor domain design. The human β-cardiac myosin motor domain was expressed as a single-chain fusion protein with GFP. The protein design was based on a single-chain embryonic skeletal muscle MD::GFP chimera that was used to analyse motor domain folding[9,10]. The lever arm α-helix projecting from the myosin MD is truncated within the IQ motif that forms the essential light-chain-binding site and joined to a short amino terminal α-helix of GFP. This corresponds to residues 1–787 of the human β-cardiac myosin fused to residues 5–238 of Aequorea victoria GFP. The chimeric gene was cloned into a replication-deficient adenovirus expression vehicle, and high-titre adenovirus stocks were used to infect post-mitotic C2C12 myocytes. The brightly fluorescent cardiac MD::GFP protein was harvested from the myotubes and purified for crystallization. Nucleotide-free crystals of the β-cardiac MD::GFP were grown in hanging drops without OM (Apo structure) and with 125 µM OM (OM + structure). SDS–polyacrylamide gel electrophoresis (SDS–PAGE) and tandem mass spectrometry (MS/MS) spectroscopy of the crystallized protein established that the full-length 117-kDa cMD::GFP chimera was crystallized (Supplementary Fig. 1).

Structure of the Apo and OM + cMD. The structure of the cardiac MD::GFP chimera (cMD) was determined to a resolution of 3.2 Å for the Apo and 2.25 Å for the OM + crystals (Table 1). The drug-free Apo cMD crystallized in space group P1, and with OM bound, the protein crystallized in space group P2₁. There are two molecules (A and B chains) in the asymmetric unit in both crystal forms, and the overall conformation of the A and B chains in each structure is very similar, independent of drug. The protein was crystallized without nucleotide and is in the extended, near-rigour conformation. The folding pattern and domain structure of the Apo and OM + cMD structures are typical of the striated myosin II from chicken skeletal muscle root-mean-square deviation (r.m.s.d.) = 0.70 Å for 558 Cα atoms), scallop striated muscle (r.m.s.d. = 0.64 Å for 544 Cα atoms) and human β-cardiac myosin with AMPPNP bound (0.45 Å for 608 Cα atoms)[14-16]. The domains and features of the cMD structure are illustrated for the A chain of the OM + structure in Fig. 1. The model is colour-coded to highlight the various regions of the structure associated with motor activity[15,17,18].

The bound OM is nestled in a cleft and is just visible in the space-filling model (Fig. 1). The OM is more apparent in the ribbon diagram nestled between the 25-K domain and the lower portion of the 50-K domain. The N-terminal 25-K domain (blue) forms one face of the OM-binding cleft. About 35 Å removed from the drug cleft the 25-K domain also forms one face of the nucleotide-binding pocket. The lower 50-K domain (red) includes major elements of the actin-binding surface and forms the other face of the OM-binding cleft. The upper 50-K domain (orange) includes additional elements of the actin-binding surface that are separated by a deep cleft from the lower 50-K domain. The upper 50-K domain forms the other surface of the nucleotide pocket. The converter domain (yellow) abuts the OM-binding cleft and couples the motor domain to the lever arm helix (LAH).

In all myosin II molecules, including β-cardiac myosin, the LAH forms the light-chain-binding domain; however, in this chimeric protein the helix was truncated in the centre of the essential light-chain IQ-binding motif and fused to a short N-terminal helix of GFP (residues 791–1026; green). As a consequence, the GFP domain is positioned by design in the

Table 1 | Data collection and refinement statistics.

	Apo cMD (4P7H)[*]	OM + cMD (4PA0)[†]
Data collection		
Space group	P1	P2$_1$
Cell dimensions		
a, b, c (Å)	59.6, 97.7, 118.1	100.2, 88.9, 137.8
α, β, γ (°)	71.0, 82.4, 75.0	90.0, 93.9, 90.0
Resolution (Å)	25.0-3.2 (3.3–3.2)[‡]	46.0-2.25 (2.33-2.25)
R_{merge}	0.352 (1.299)	0.258 (1.367)
$I/\sigma(I)$	9.0 (2.0)[§]	9.0 (1.1)[§]
Completeness (%)	99.5 (98.0)	93.3 (84.1)
Redundancy	11.3 (10.2)	7.4 (3.3)
Refinement		
Resolution (Å)	3.2	2.25
No. of reflections	39,840 (3,966)	107,033 (9,608)
R_{work}/R_{free}	0.191/0.265	0.201/0.246
No. of atoms		
Protein	14,882	14,533
Ligand/ion	54	118
Water	5	306
B-factors		
Protein	49.0	46.0
Ligand/ion	59.8	62.3
Water	24.2	33.8
R.m.s.d.		
Bond lengths (Å)	0.007	0.011
Bond angles (°)	1.08	1.35

cMD, β-cardiac motor domain; OM, Omecamtiv Mecarbil; r.m.s.d., root-mean-square deviation.
[*]Data collected from three crystals.
[†]Data collected from a single crystal
[‡]Values in parentheses are for the highest-resolution shell.
[§]The Apo data set was truncated at 3.2 Å with the mean $(I/\sigma(I)) = 2$ and a CC* > 0.88 for the highest-resolution shell[61]. The CC* statistic for the OM + 2.33-2.25 Å resolution shell is > 0.73, supporting the inclusion of the full data range in determination of the model[62,63]. Applying traditional cutoff criteria of the mean $(I/\sigma(I)) \geq 2$ would make this a nominal 2.40-Å-resolution structure.

space normally occupied by the light chains[9]. The GFP chromophore occupies a cavity in the centre of the GFP β-barrel.

Effect of OM on cardiac myosin motor activity. The GFP domain substitutes a rigid β-barrel for the myosin light chains and provides a convenient handle for assaying the effect of drug binding on cMD motor activity by using anti-GFP to immobilize the cMD on surfaces[9]. The unloaded shortening velocity was measured using the *in vitro* motility assay (Fig. 2). The cMD::GFP chimera supports sliding actin filament velocities of 0.8 µm s^{-1}, equivalent to the human β-cardiac HMM (cHMM) and comparable to the velocity measured for porcine ventricular HMM (0.96 µm s^{-1})[6]. Addition of OM to the assay dramatically slows the filament velocity (15–20-fold) powered by both the cMD and cHMM. This is identical to what was found with porcine ventricular HMM and is explained by a drug-induced increase in crossbridges interacting with the actin filaments that impose an internal load on the sliding filament movement[6,8]. The K_i for OM inhibition of the sliding velocity powered by the cMD is 100 nM, indicating a high affinity for the intermediates of the mechanochemical cycle. The sliding filament velocity powered by a fast skeletal muscle myosin is much faster (6.3 µm s^{-1}) than the cMD, as is expected, but is virtually unaffected by the drug, consistent with the report that OM does not bind to skeletal muscle myosin[4].

OM modulates the steady-state ATPase of the cMD, decreasing the V_{max} from 5.3 to 1.9 s^{-1} but also lowering the K_{ATPase} for actin activation fourfold from 22.5 to 5.4 µM (Supplementary Fig. 2). This is consistent with the effect of OM on the porcine ventricular HMM ATPase activity. The effects of OM on the cMD motor activity and ATPase activity and the 100-nM K_i for

modulating the activity corroborate the specificity of the binding site observed in the crystal structure.

OM-binding site and the coupling region. The drug, OM, is tightly nestled in a narrow cleft separating the lower 50-K domain from the N-terminal 25-K domain (Fig. 3 and Supplementary Fig. 3). OM is in an extended conformation that lies along the SH1 helix (698–707) and is adjacent to C705 (SH1) on one side and extends to and interacts with the first strand (711–713) of the three-stranded β-sheet of the converter domain. The drug packs against and wraps around two loops from the 25-K domain. OM binding involves extensive interaction with at least six residues from the 25-K domain (A91, M92, L96, S118, G119 and F121), two from the relay helix (M493 and E497), four from the SH1 helix (V698, G701, I702 and C705) and four from the β-sheets of the converter domain (P710, N711, R712 and L770; Supplementary Table 1). There are four potential hydrogen-bonding interactions between the protein and drug that involve A91, M92, S118 and N711. The N711 H-bond to the OM methyl-pyridine ring is of interest because this residue is a serine in fast skeletal muscle myosin and is one of only three sequence differences in the binding cleft that might account for the selectivity of the drug for modulating the activity of cardiac myosin but not skeletal myosin (Supplementary Table 2). The same interactions are found in the protein–drug-binding site of the A and B chains of the OM + structure, although the conformation of the drug and binding cleft is slightly different in the two molecules. The A chain-binding site is depicted in Fig. 3.

The conformation of the main chain and the side-chain rotamers of residues lining the drug-binding cleft are essentially the same in the Apo and OM + structures, indicating that drug

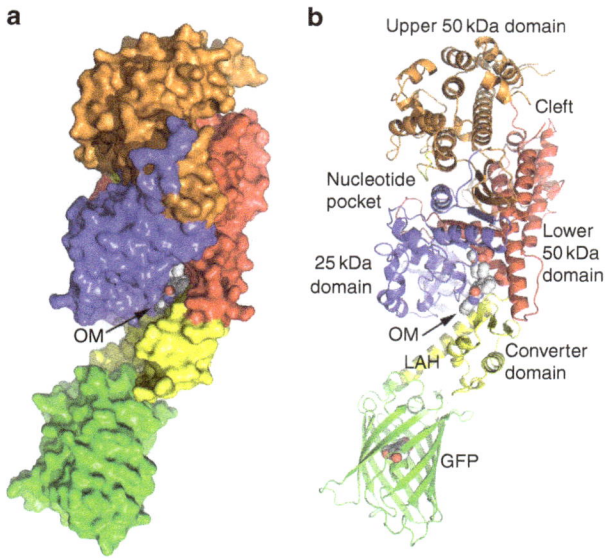

Figure 1 | The structural organization of the human β-cardiac MD with bound OM. (**a**) Space-filling model of the A chain of the OM + structure showing the buried OM-binding site nestled between the N-terminal 25-K domain (residues 2-204; blue) and the lower 50-K domain (residues 471-708; red). The upper 50-K domain (211-470; orange) is separated by the 'Cleft' from the lower 50-K domain. There is no nucleotide in this structure, the cleft is 'open' and the lever arm is extended consistent with the near-rigour conformation. The converter domain (residues 709-777) and LAH (residues 778-787) are in yellow and the GFP domain is in green. (**b**) Ribbon diagram of the same orientation to show the OM-binding site bound deeply in a narrow cleft between the 25-K and lower 50-K domains. The LAH linking the converter domain to the GFP domain is labelled. The conformation of the Apo cMD structure is very similar to the OM + structure shown here with an r.m.s.d. = 1.14 Å for all 962 Cα atoms.

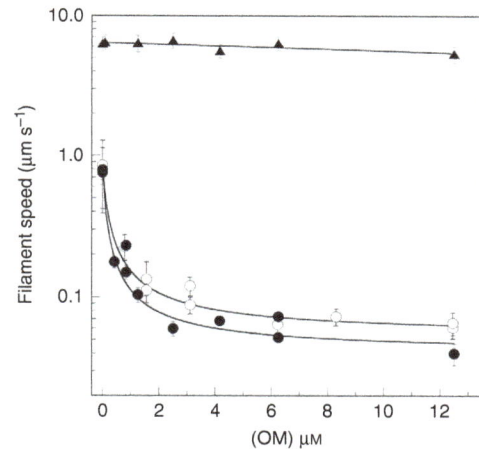

Figure 2 | The unloaded shortening velocity of cMD is inhibited by OM. Titration of the effect of OM on the unloaded shortening velocity measured with the *in vitro* motility assay. The cMD was bound indirectly to surfaces through an anti-GFP monoclonal antibody (●) and compared with the human β-cardiac HMM (○) bound directly to the nitrocellulose surface. In the absence of the drug, both cardiac myosin fragments support actin filament velocities of $0.8\,\mu m\,s^{-1}$. Titration with OM from 0.42 to 12.5 μM dramatically slowed the velocity of filament movement by 15-20-fold. The apparent K_i for OM binding is 100-150 nM for the human cMD and cHMM. Adult fast skeletal muscle myosin (▲) moves actin filaments at $6.3\,\mu m\,s^{-1}$, and even the highest concentration of OM tested has little effect on filament velocity. Assays were conducted at 32 °C. The cardiac motor activity was fit to the hyperbolic inhibition curve: $v_o = \frac{V_{max} - (V_{max} - V_i) \times [OM]}{K_i + [OM]}$, where, v_o is the observed velocity, V_{max} is the unloaded shortening velocity, V_i is the maximum inhibited velocity and [OM] is the concentration of drug. The mean velocity ± s.d. of the velocity distribution for hundreds of filaments is plotted.

binds to an existing cleft and does not induce significant local perturbation of the cMD conformation. However, analysis of the protein–drug interface indicates that OM binding results in extensive solvent shielding of residues that couple the structural elements that are central to the conformation changes of the recovery stroke: the SH1 helix, the relay helix and the converter domain. Photo-crosslinking of a benzonphenone derivative of OM had identified this cleft as the potential OM-binding site[4]. The drug-binding site is consistent with that crosslinking experiment; however, the drug is deeper in the cleft than previously imagined.

The recovery stroke involves the priming of the lever arm at the start of the mechanical cycle resulting in the rotation of the converter domain and LAH through ~65°. The priming step is a conformational equilibrium driven by the nucleotide bound in the active site. The nucleotide state is transmitted via the relay helix to a coupling region that links the SH1 helix, relay helix and converter domain together. The packing of the drug against the SH1 helix, relay helix and converter domain shields these elements from solvent and enhances interactions among them[19]. For example, OM buries the only solvent-accessible surface of the E497-R712 salt bridge that links the relay helix to the converter domain, thereby fortifying the bond. It also shields the M493-C705 H-bond that links the relay helix to the SH1 helix (Fig. 3).

Converter domain–LAH–GFP rotation. There are two distinct molecules in the unit cell (A and B) of both the Apo and OM + structures. In both structures the core motor domains (residues

2–708) are packed tightly together in the crystal lattice with extensive non-crystallographic symmetry between them. The conformation of the core motor domain is very similar in the two molecules of the Apo (r.m.s.d. = 0.305 Å for 567 Cα atoms) and the two molecules of the OM + (r.m.s.d. = 0.311 Å for 550 Cα atoms) structures. The similarity is shared between corresponding core motor domains of the Apo and OM + in pairwise comparison (Apo-A to OM-A r.m.s.d. = 0.33 Å; Apo-B to OM-B r.m.s.d. = 0.36 Å). The organization of the converter domains, the position of the GFP domains and the LAH linking the two are markedly different between the A and B chains in the asymmetric unit of both crystal structures. There is an ~15° rotation of the converter domain–LAH–GFP domain as a unit between the two molecules in the unit cell of both crystal structures (Fig. 4). The apparent 15° rotation of the LAH from the A to the B position is in the same direction as a much larger LAH rotation during the recovery stroke (~65°). The conformation change involves movement of the relay helix and a portion of the N-terminal 25-K region called the SH3 domain in addition to the converter domain–LAH. The hinge point for the rotation is G708 of the cMD, adjacent to the OM-binding cleft. As a consequence, the conformation of the drug-binding cleft is different between the OM + A and B chains.

OM moves with the rotation of the converter domain. The changes in the drug cleft as a consequence of the 15° rotation of the converter domain–LAH in the two molecules of the OM + structure (OM-A and OM-B) are shown in Fig. 5. To accommodate changes in the position of the converter domain, there is

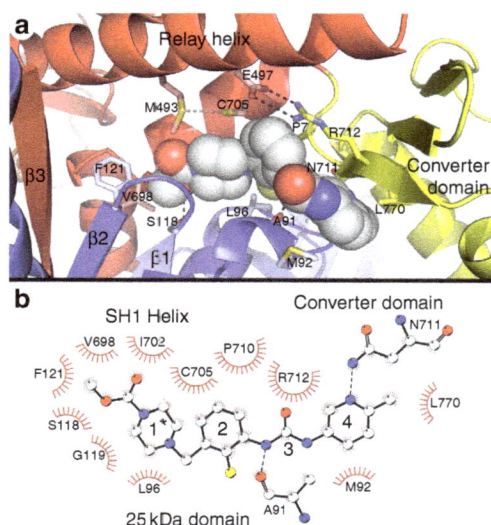

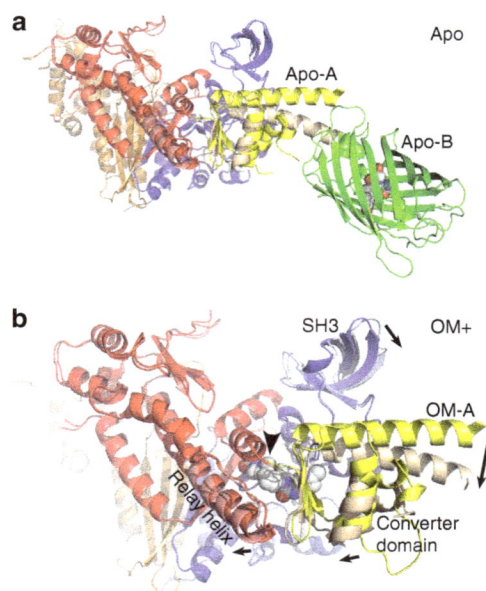

Figure 3 | OM-binding site on the human β-cardiac MD. (**a**) A ribbon diagram of the A chain of the OM + structure is shown with OM (space-filling model) nestled in a narrow cleft separating the 25-K domain (blue) from the lower 50-K domain (red), and interacting with residues from these domains and the converter domain (yellow). The drug is in an extended conformation with the carboxymethyl-piperazine group buried deeply in the cleft. One surface of this ring and the fluoro-benzene ring of OM make extensive packing interactions with residues along one face of the SH1 helix including C705 (SH1). The drug bridges the gap from the SH1 helix to the first strand (N711-I713) of the three-stranded β-sheet of the converter domain. In bridging the gap, OM buries a bi-dentate salt bridge, E497-R712, beneath the fluoro-benzene ring. The amido group of N711 forms a H-bond with the nitrogen of the OM methyl-pyridinyl ring. The other surface of OM wraps around a turn (A91-L96) of the 25-K domain and interacts with the first two strands (β1–β2) and connecting loop of the seven-stranded β-sheet of the cMD. The 25-K domain residues S118, A91 and M92 form likely H-bonds with OM (shown with dotted lines), and there are at least 12 packing and hydrophobic interactions as well[19]. (**b**) A protein-drug interaction diagram[64] summarizing the most extensive interactions in the binding cleft. Hydrogen bonds involving A91 and N711 are indicated in the diagram; however, two additional H-bonds between OM and M92 and S118 are not drawn in the diagram for clarity. All of the interactions between OM and the binding cleft residues are summarized in Supplementary Table 1. *Numbers associated with the drug are added to identify the subregions of the molecule: (1) carboxymethyl-piperazine ring; (2) fluoro-benzine ring; (3) amino-carbamoyl linker; and (4) methyl-pyridinyl ring. The drug-binding interactions and the accessible and buried surface areas of the residues in the binding cleft were analysed with PISA (Protein Interfaces, Surfaces and Assemblies)[19].

Figure 4 | The two cardiac MD::GFP molecules in the asymmetric unit for both the Apo and the OM + structures differ in the rotation of the LAH and GFP. In both structures, the B chain converter domains, LAH and GFP, are rotated ~15° from the near-rigour configuration towards the pre-power stroke state. (**a**) The core MD (residues 2–708) of the Apo-A and B chains is aligned to show the rotation of the B chain converter domain and LAH (coloured tan). The A chain GFP domain is not shown for clarity. (**b**) The A and B chains of OM + structure are similarly aligned and enlarged to show the rotation of the LAH. The A chain OM molecule is shown as a space-filling model in the centre of the image. The B chain converter domain and LAH are coloured tan. The arrows indicate the direction of rotation of the SH3-like domain, the LAH, the converter domain and the relay helix of the B chain relative to the A chain. The point of rotation in both structures is G708, immediately above OM and marked by an arrowhead in **b**. Perhaps as a consequence of the rotation, the B chain converter domains, LAH and GFP, are less well defined in both structures with higher crystallographic atomic displacement parameters.

rotation of the fluoro-benzene and methyl-pyridinyl rings and the amino-carbamoyl linker of OM. These changes mirror the shift in position of the residues interacting with the drug. In particular, the bond distance for the H-bond with N711 remains constant despite significant movement of the β-strands of the converter domain. OM follows the linkage between the SH1 helix and converter domain–LAH elements in the two molecules (OM-A and OM-B). The carboxymethyl-piperazine ring of OM is most deeply buried in the drug-binding cleft and changes very little between the two conformations of the cleft. This OM ring interacts with residues of strands β1 and β2 of the central seven-stranded β-sheet of the cMD structure. Comparison of the Apo and OM + structures reveals subtle changes in the seven-stranded β-sheet that propagate out from the drug-binding cleft, perhaps arising from the interaction with these first two strands.

The transducer region. Twisting and distortion of the last three strands (β5, β6 and β7) of the seven-stranded β-sheet of the myosin MD is essential for rearrangements within the nucleotide-binding pocket depending on the nucleotide state and forms the structural basis for communication between the actin-binding interface, the nucleotide pocket and the converter domain[13,20]. The structural elements have been called collectively 'The Transducer' and include Loop 1 (204–210), the β-bulge (252–259) connecting strands β6 and β7 and the loop-linking helix O (HO) to the β5-strand (448–455). The β5-strand leads directly into Switch II (SW-II): the γ-phosphate-sensing loop in the nucleotide pocket. Switch II in turn leads into the relay helix, the coupling region and the drug-binding cleft.

OM interactions within the binding cleft include residues of the strands β1 and β2 of the central seven-stranded β-sheet. Comparison of the Apo and OM + structures reveals changes in the β-sheet that propagates out from the drug-binding cleft and results in a twist of the final three strands (β5, β6 and β7) of the sheet affecting the β-bulge and the HO-β5 loop, key elements of the Transducer region (Fig. 6). The conformations of the two molecules in the OM + structure (OM-A and OM-B) are not identical to one another in this region (Fig. 6a,b). The OM-B conformation has a greater twist, an extension of the β6 and β7 strands of the sheet into the β-bulge, and displacements of 1–3 Å in the Cα positions for residues of the β-bulge and the HO-β5

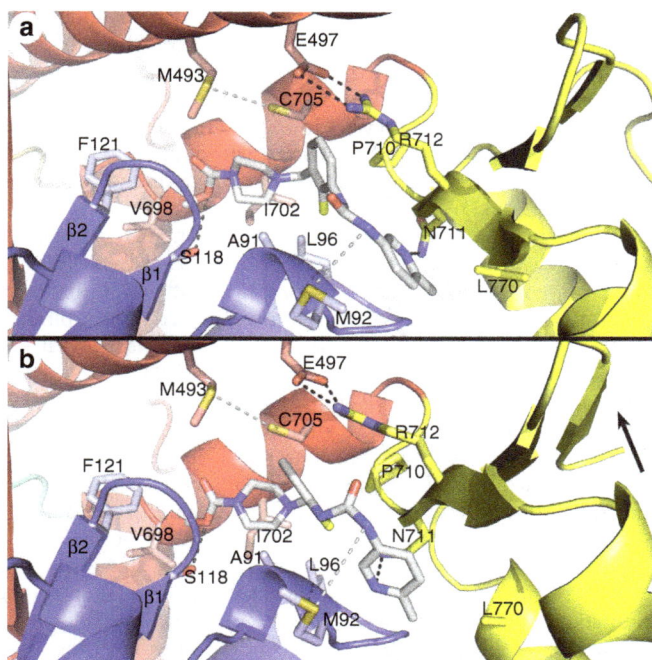

Figure 5 | The differences in the drug-binding cleft between the two molecules in the OM + structure. (**a**) The A chain conformation of the drug-binding site showing the interacting residues. (**b**) The B chain conformation of the drug-binding site. OM interacts with the same set of residues in both conformations of the binding cleft. The principal change between OM-A and OM-B is the rotation of the converter domain indicated by the arrow in **b**. In this view the converter domain moves up and towards the viewer, shifting the position of both N711 and R712. The fluoro-benzyl and methy-pyidinyl rings of OM rotate between OM-A and OM-B conformations as does the amino-carbamoyl group linking them. This maintains the H-bond to N711 and the shielding of the E497-R712 salt bridge. The carboxymethyl-piperazine is buried deep in the cleft and interacts with S118 and F121 of the β1 and β2 strands of the seven-stranded β-sheet.

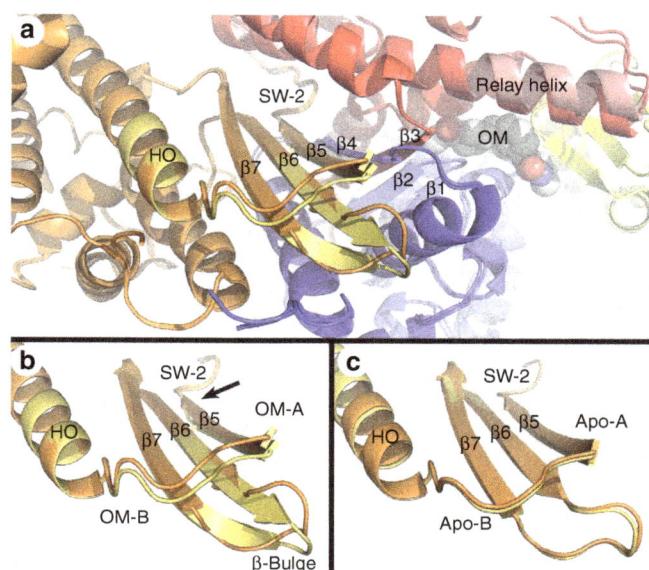

Figure 6 | Conformational changes in the Transducer region in the OM + structure. (**a**) The core cMD (2–708) of the OM-A and OM-B chains were aligned. Overall, the conformations of the two chains are nearly identical (r.m.s.d. = 0.31 Å); however, strands β5, β6 and β7 of the β-sheet and the elements of the Transducer region (the β-bulge and HO-β5 loop) are significantly different. The OM-A chain in this region is coloured orange and the OM-B chain is yellow-orange. Displacement of the relay helix as a result of LAH rotation is also highlighted. Note that OM (space-filling model) in the binding cleft is 35 Å from the Transducer elements. (**b**) Comparison of the isolated Transducer elements of OM-A (orange) and OM-B (yellow-orange) showing an increased twist, a downward shift of the HO-β5 loop and extension of the β6 and β7 strands of the sheet into the β-bulge. The arrow highlights the changes in β5 to SW-II link. These differences are between the two molecules in the same unit cell. (**c**) In contrast, the Apo-A (orange) and Apo-B (yellow-orange) transducer elements superimpose. The Transducer region changes shown here are not as large as those reported for cleft closure as seen in myosin V (Supplementary Fig. 4b) but are following the same trajectory.

loop. There also is subtle shift at the transition of β5-strand into SW-II (arrow in Fig. 6b). The conformations of these elements in both molecules of the Apo structure are essentially identical and differ from both molecules in the OM + structure (Fig. 6c). The nucleotide-free conformation of the Transducer region of the OM-B molecule is in fact more similar to that in the cardiac myosin MD with AMPPNP bound[14] than either Apo structure or the OM-A molecule in the same unit cell (Supplementary Fig. 4b).

The crystallographic packing between the two molecules of the Apo and the OM + structures is essentially identical and does not involve the elements of the Transducer region, suggesting that crystal packing is not the source of this highly localized conformational change. In addition, this region of the structure is well defined in both the Apo and OM + structures with B-factors that are about half of the average for the protein as a whole. All of these changes are ∼35 Å distant from the OM-binding site and thus are allosteric changes affecting a link in the communication between the nucleotide pocket and the actin-binding interface.

We conclude that the stabilization of the coupling between the SH1 helix, relay helix and converter domain within the drug-binding cleft and the allosteric distortion of the β-sheet in the Transducer region are the principal structural changes associated with drug binding. These changes may be sufficient

to account for the shift in the hydrolysis equilibrium in the nucleotide pocket and the accelerated rate of γ-phosphate release contributing to the measured kinetic effects of drug binding on cardiac myosin[6].

Discussion

Here we report the structural basis for the allosteric mechanism of the novel cardiac myosin-specific drug, OM. The drug binds to the human β-cardiac myosin motor domain in a narrow cleft between the N-terminal 25-K domain and the lower portion of the 50-K domain. Within the binding cleft the drug is intimately involved with the key elements of the recovery stroke. In addition, OM binding induces allosteric changes distant from the binding cleft that affect the twist of the central seven-stranded β-sheet of the motor domain. These interactions help explain how the drug modulates cardiac myosin motor activity.

In addition to OM, there are several other reversible allosteric effectors of myosin activity that bind to the motor domain including blebbistatin, halogenated pseudilins and EMD 57033. Blebbistatin binds at the apex of the myosin cleft separating the upper and lower 50-K domains blocking the myosin in a product complex with low actin affinity[21,22]. The halogenated pseudilins are a class of myosin inhibitors with activity similar to blebbistatin that also bind in the cleft but at a site that is ∼7.5 Å from the blebbistatin site[23,24]. EMD 57033 is a thiadiazinone derivative that stabilizes myosin against thermal denaturation and is an allosteric activator of β-cardiac myosin ATPase and myofilament contraction[25]. *In silico* docking studies suggest that it binds in a pocket near the N-terminal SH3 domain. None of these other allosteric effectors bind in or near the OM cleft or are under consideration for therapeutic potential.

The key to the actomyosin mechanochemical cycle is the ability of the myosin motor domain to couple small changes in the catalytic ATPase site to large conformational changes in both the actin-binding and force-generating domains[26]. This pathway is summarized in the actomyosin kinetic scheme in Fig. 7. The nucleotide bound in the active site (ATP, ADP·P$_i$ or ADP) defines the conformation of the MD and its affinity for actin. This requires a communication pathway to amplify changes in the nucleotide pocket and couple them to domain movements. OM acts along this pathway as a traditional allosteric effector binding ∼35 Å from the nucleotide pocket and altering the ATP hydrolysis mechanism and motor activity of cardiac myosin[4,6,27]. A detailed analysis of the transient kinetics of porcine ventricular HMM reveals that OM does not activate of the actomyosin ATPase activity as was originally suspected[4] and instead inhibits the V_{max} by two- to threefold[6]. This was shown here for the human β-cardiac myosin as well. The principal effect of OM on the myosin kinetic mechanism is a shift in the equilibrium for ATP hydrolysis in the active site towards product formation (M↑·ADP·P$_i$) that is coupled to an increase in the rate of the fast phase of phosphate release. These changes produce an increase in

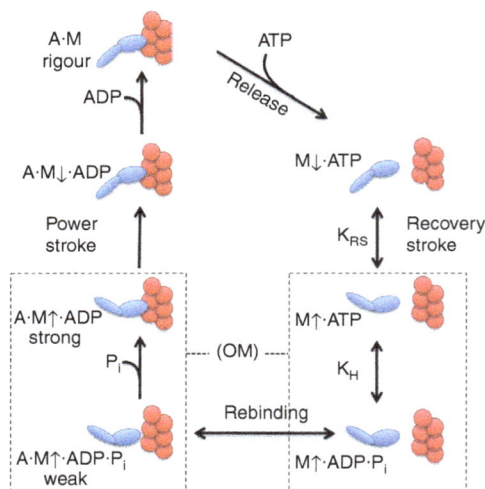

Figure 7 | A general kinetic scheme for the actomyosin ATPase cycle. The myosin motor domain (M, blue) is shown at the top left at the end of the cycle, tightly bound to actin (A, red) in the nucleotide-free rigour state (A·M). ATP binds rapidly and releases the MD from actin. The MD then undergoes a conformational equilibrium before ATP hydrolysis between two states designated as M↓ and M↑. These states correspond to the near-rigour (M↓) and pre-power stroke (M↑) conformations. The arrows indicate the down position of the LAH (M↓) and the up position in the pre-power stroke state (M↑) and correlate with intrinsic fluorescent states. The 'Recovery Stroke' is the rapid equilibrium (K$_{RS}$) between these states. The hydrolysis equilibrium (K$_H$) is coupled to this transition before binding to actin[6]. On rebinding to actin the weak to strong transition is coupled to γ-phosphate (P$_i$) release. This results in a conformation change triggering rotation of the LAH producing the 'Power Stroke' and force production. Rapid ADP dissociation follows, completing the cycle. OM influences the hydrolysis equilibrium (K$_H$), and it accelerates P$_i$ release associated with the weak to strong actin-binding transition[6]. These steps are boxed with dotted lines.

the flux of the intermediates through the actomyosin mechanochemical pathway leading to a faster transition of weak to strong bound actin states. In the kinetic assays, we measured the unloaded rate of ADP dissociation from actomyosin ADP at the end of the contractile cycle and showed that OM does not affect this step. Faster phosphate release without a change in ADP dissociation leads to a higher fraction of myosin bound to actin in a strong A·M↑·ADP state[6].

OM produces a large (15–20-fold) reduction in the unloaded shortening velocity measured in the *in vitro* motility assay (Fig. 2). The reported K_i reflects the apparent affinity of OM for a composite of steps in the kinetic pathway rather than a binding constant for any single step. Specifically, OM affects both the hydrolysis equilibrium (M↑·ATP to M↑·ADP·P$_i$) and P$_i$ release (AM↑·ADP·P$_i$ to AM↑·ADP transitions). Thus, the measured K_i reflects the interaction of OM with an ensemble of states. The effect on the motility assay is likely a result of the recruitment of crossbridges to the actin filament as a consequence of the faster transition from weak to strong bound actin states, resulting in a higher fraction of cMDs tightly bound to actin producing an internal drag on filament movement. Although this slows the velocity of filament movement, it also leads to more force production per filament, a favourable outcome for improving cardiac systolic function. A strain-dependent slowing of the ADP dissociation rate has recently been reported for porcine β-cardiac myosin, and this additional mechanism could contribute to the decrease in filament velocity[28]. A strain-dependent step would extend the duration of systole as is reported in animal models of heart failure treated with OM[5]. An increase in strongly attached crossbridges induced by OM also could facilitate systolic Ca^{2+} activation in the heart by triggering movement of the Tpm-Tn switch out of the inhibitory state. However, the significance of this activation mechanism under physiological conditions in heart muscle has been questioned recently[29,30].

The communication pathway linking the ATPase state to the rotation of the lever arm has been delineated by crystal structures of non-cardiac myosin motor domains with different bound ATP analogues[13,18,31,32]. These structures reveal distinct orientations of the converter domain that lead to an ∼65° rotation of the LAH. On the basis of these known structural states, mutational analyses and molecular dynamics simulations, it has been proposed that with ATP bound the myosin motor domain exists in two alternative conformations, the pre-recovery M↓ state (down state) and post-recovery M↑ state (up state with rotated LAH)[33–37]. The transition between these myosin conformations is controlled by the myosin nucleotide interaction and is called the recovery stroke. The pre-recovery state (M↓) has nucleotide bound with SW-II in the open position. In the M↑ state the SW-II loop closes and a glycine in the loop makes a hydrogen bond with the nucleotide γ-phosphate. This small change is transmitted to the coupling region where concerted domain movements result in the rotation of the LAH into the primed, pre-power stroke conformation. In myosin, ATP hydrolysis is a reversible equilibrium in the active site that occurs predominantly in the post-recovery M↑·ATP state[38]. This prevents unproductive release of hydrolysis products from a pre-recovery state (M↓·ATP). We have shown that OM specifically shifts the hydrolysis equilibrium towards products (ADP·P$_i$). This in turn shifts the coupled equilibria (K$_{RS}$ and K$_H$, Fig. 7) towards the primed LAH conformation (M↑·ADP·P$_i$) for rebinding to actin[6].

The SW-II loop is contiguous with N terminus of the relay helix providing a link from the nucleotide pocket to the SH1 helix and the converter domain. A defining feature of the M↑ primed conformation is a kink in the relay helix around F489 of the human cMD. On the transition from M↓ to M↑, the bend in the relay helix is strongly coupled to the position of the SH1 helix and the converter domain[13,33,37,39]. The converter domain remains anchored to the relay helix as the converter–LAH undergoes its sweeping rotation. OM binds in the centre of the region that couples the SH1 helix, relay helix and converter domain and involves the key residues linking the SH1 helix to the relay helix (M493-C705 sulfhydryl H-bond) and the relay helix to the converter domain (E497-R712 salt bridge). OM binding shields these interactions from solvent and strengthens the links responsible for the concerted domain movement of the recovery stroke.

An extensive hydrophobic cluster involving Y501, I506, W508, F510, I511, F513, F709 and F764 is also involved in coupling the relay helix and loop with the SH1 helix and the converter domain[33]. The E497-R712 salt bridge lies immediately below this aromatic cluster and is shielded from solvent on three sides by it; thus, OM binding completes the burial of the salt bridge in a hydrophobic pocket. This salt bridge is found in both the near-rigour and pre-power stroke conformation of the scallop myosin II MD structure, suggesting that it is essential to the coupling mechanism[31]. We have shown here that the drug-binding interactions are maintained through a 15° rotation of the converter domain and LAH ($\sim$25% of the recovery stroke), suggesting that the drug may stabilize this coupling region throughout the recovery stroke.

Both E497 and R712 have been identified as sites of cardiomyopathy-associated mutations: an E497D mutation results in a benign hypertrophic cardiomyopathy (HCM) and a R712L mutation is associated with a severe HCM phenotype and sudden cardiac death[40,41]. Three of the eight aromatic residues involved in the hydrophobic cluster are also sites associated with HCM (Y501, F513) and DCM (F764) mutations. Five of the sixteen residues that form the drug-binding cleft and interact with OM (M493, E497, V698, P710 and R712) are sites of missense mutations associated with human cardiac pathology. The clustering of cardiomyopathic mutations in this region correlates with the importance of these links to the communication pathway between the nucleotide state and priming of the LAH.

The Transducer is a structural element of the motor domain near the nucleotide-binding site that includes the last three strands of the central seven-stranded β-sheet of the MD[13]. Distortion of the β-sheet is essential for the domain movements needed to accommodate closure of the cleft between the upper and lower portions of the 50-K domain on strong binding to actin[13,20]. That in turn reverses the rotation of the LAH leading to the power stroke (Fig. 7). The movements involve a twist of the last three strands (β5, β6 and β7) of the β-sheet, changes in the loops linking β6 to β7 (β-bulge) and the HO helix to β5, and Loop 1 (204–210). It has been suggested that the twist provides the structural basis for communication between the actin interface and the nucleotide pocket and may be involved in the γ-phosphate release[13,20,39,42]. We have found that OM binding alters the conformation of the β-bulge and HO-β5 loop and the twist of the β5, β6 and β7 strands when compared with the Apo structure and between the two cMD conformations within the OM+ structure. These structural changes are consistent with a mechanism, whereby OM accelerates the rate of P_i release and the weak to strong actin-binding transition by facilitating β-sheet distortion.

We conclude that OM binding acts to stabilize the interactions within the coupling region. This region is central to the recovery stroke and the priming of the cMD for a productive contractile cycle. In addition, drug binding shifts the conformational equilibrium of the Transducer region to favour phosphate release. Together, these subtle changes alter the mechanical tuning of β-cardiac myosin producing changes in activity that in cardiac muscle will increase force production at the expense of speed of contraction. The candidate drugs from which OM was developed were originally identified by a high-throughput screen of a biochemically reconstituted contractile system[3]. That screen and subsequent selection of OM has identified a fundamentally important site for fine-tuning the motor activity of myosin.

Methods

Construction of the β-cardiac myosin MD expression vector. A cDNA encoding the human β-cardiac muscle myosin HMM was kindly provided by James Sellers (National Heart, Lung, and Blood Institute (NHLBI)) from a clone isolated by Giovanni Cuda and Neil Epstein (NHLBI). Construction of the β-cardiac MD::GFP chimera is based on the skeletal muscle MD::GFP chimera (S1$_{795}$GFP) described in detail elsewhere[9]. A cDNA encoding residues 1–787 of the cardiac myosin motor domain was amplified with PCR using primers to insert a unique NotI site at the 5′ end of the open reading frame and a unique MluI site at the 3′ end. The cardiac MD sequence then replaced the skeletal muscle myosin MD in the shuttle vector pSH-S1$_{795}$GFP (ref. 9). A four-residue linker (788–791) forms the fusion site to the GFP-coding sequence that comprise residues 5–238 of A. victoria GFP. The complete coding region was confirmed by sequencing. A FLAG-tagged variant of chimeric protein was prepared by mutating the C-terminal-coding sequence of the GFP domain from DELYK to DYKDHD. This minimal FLAG tag sequence added a single additional residue to the protein, with no effect on protein activity or crystallization conditions[43].

Adenovirus manipulation. Recombinant adenovirus DNA was prepared by homologous recombination of pSH-CaMD::GFP with the pAdEasy1 vector in E. coli strain BJ5183 (refs 9,12,44). Colonies were selected for kanamycin resistance and plasmid DNA was characterized by restriction digestion. The recombinant virus DNA was transformed into E. coli DH10B cells, and the purified pAdCaMD DNA was linearized by digestion with PacI and transfected into human 293 cells (CRL 1573; American Type Culture Collection, Rockville, MD) for adenovirus packaging and amplification[44]. The human 293 cells are maintained in growth medium containing DMEM with 10% fetal bovine serum (FBS), 1 mM sodium pyruvate and 0.5% gentamycin at 37 °C and 5% CO_2. Cells were monitored using fluorescence microscopy for expression of the cMD::GFP fusion protein. The original human β-cardiac HMM clone encodes residues 1–1,138 of the MYH7 gene with a FLAG tag added on the C terminus (1,139–1,146) of the S2 domain. The cHMM cDNA was cloned into the pShuttle-IRES-hrGFP-1 vector (Stratagene, LaJolla CA), and an AdcHMM-Flag virus was prepared and amplified for expression and purification of the cHMM protein in C2C12 cells. The virus was expanded by infection of a large number of plates of confluent 293 cells at an multiplicity of infection of 3–5. The virus was harvested from the cells by cycles of freeze-thaw, and then it was purified by CsCl density sedimentation yielding final virus titres of 10^{10}–10^{11} plaque-forming units per ml (p.f.u. ml^{-1}).

Muscle cell expression and purification of β-cardiac MD::GFP. Myoblasts of the mouse C2C12 cell line (CRL 1772; American Type Culture Collection) are maintained by seeding the cells at an initial density of 7.5×10^4 cells cm^{-2} in 90% DMEM, 10% FBS and passaging the cells at less than 60% confluence[9,12,45]. Confluent C2C12 myoblasts are infected with replication-defective recombinant adenovirus (Ad-CaMD::GFP) at 5×10^8 p.f.u. ml^{-1} in fusion medium (89% DMEM, 10% horse serum, 1% FBS) to induce differentiation. Expression of recombinant cMD::GFP is monitored by accumulation of GFP fluorescence in infected cells. Myocyte differentiation and fluorescence accumulation are monitored for the next 120–144 h when the cells are harvested. Cells are chilled, media is removed and the cell layer is rinsed with cold PBS. The cells are scraped into 0.5 ml per dish of Triton extraction buffer: 100 mM NaCl, 0.5% Triton X-100, 10 mM imidazole pH 7.0, 1 mM dithiothreitol (DTT), 5 mM MgATP and Protease Inhibitor cocktail (Sigma, St Louis). The cell suspension is collected in an ice-cold Dounce homogenizer and lysed with 15 strokes of the A pestle. The cell debris in the whole-cell lysate is pelleted by centrifugation at 17,000g for 15 min at 4 °C. The Triton-soluble extract is fractionated by ammonium sulfate precipitation using two sequential steps of 0–30% saturation and 30–60% saturation. The CaMD::GFP precipitates between 30 and 60% saturation of ammonium sulfate.

The recovered pellet is dissolved in 1/10 the original volume of buffer and dialysed against 25 mM imidazole, pH 7.0, 1 mM DTT for anion exchange chromatography of the cMD lacking the FLAG tag sequence, or into the same buffer without DTT for affinity purification of the FLAG-tagged cMD on M2 monoclonal antibody-Sepharose beads (Sigma). Anion exchange chromatography on a HR 5/5 Mono-Q column at 23 °C (Pharmacia Biotech, Piscataway, NJ) was carried out as previously described[9]. The FLAG-tagged cMD was bound to an M2-Sepharose column, washed and eluted with 0.1 mg ml^{-1} FLAG peptide (Sigma). The FLAG-tagged human cHMM was purified in the same manner as the tagged cMD. Protein was concentrated and buffer-exchanged on Amicon Ultracel-10 K centrifugal filters (Millipore; Darmstadt, Germany), checked by SDS–PAGE (Supplementary Fig. 1), aliquoted and stored at −80 °C.

Motility and ATPase assays. An anti-GFP monoclonal antibody (3E6; Molecular Probes; Grand Island, NY) was bound to freshly prepared nitrocellulose-coated glass coverslips[9]. The cMD at 25 µg ml^{-1} was incubated with the surface and bound via the GFP domain as previously described. Skeletal muscle myosin was bound to the surfaces via an anti-S2 monoclonal antibody[46,47]. Recombinant human β-cardiac HMM at 40 µg ml^{-1} was bound directly to fresh nitrocellulose surfaces as described[6,46]. The surfaces were blocked with 1% bovine serum albumin in PBS for 5 min. Motility is measured in a 12-µl assay chamber in motility buffer (25 mM Imidazole, 25 mM KCl, 4 mM MgCl$_2$, 7.5 mM Mg^{2+} ATP, 0.5% methyl cellulose, 0.1 mg ml^{-1} glucose oxidase, 0.018 mg ml^{-1} catalase, 2.3 mg ml^{-1} glucose and 5 mM 2-mercaptoethanol, pH 7.6) containing 1 nM phalloidin-rhodamine-labelled actin. OM (CK-1827452) was purchased from Selleckchem.com (Boston, MA). To titrate the effect of the drug on motility, a 2.5-mM stock of OM in dimethylsulphoxide (DMSO) was serially diluted with DMSO before a final 1/200 dilution into motility buffer with the rhodamine-labelled actin. The final 0.5% DMSO in the assay buffer had no effect on motility in the absence of drug. The chamber is observed with a temperature-controlled stage and objective set at 32 °C on an upright microscope with an image-intensified charge-coupled device camera capturing data to an acquisition computer at 5–30 f.p.s. dependent on assay parameters. Movement of actin filaments from 500 to 1,000 frames of continuous imaging is analysed with semiautomated filament tracking programmes[12,46,48]. The trajectory of every filament with a lifetime of at least 10 frames is determined; the instantaneous velocity of the filament moving along the trajectory, the filament length, the distance of continuous motion and the duration of pauses are tabulated. A weighted probability of the actin filament velocity for hundreds of events is fit to a Gaussian distribution and reported as a mean velocity and s.d. for each experimental condition.

Steady-state ATPase activity was measured as described previously[49]. Experiments were carried out in a buffer containing 4 mM MOPS, 2 mM MgCl$_2$ with or without 100 µM OM (0.5% DMSO), pH 7.2. The cMD at 0.06 µM was used to measure the ATPase activity over a range of actin (0–100 µM). The ATPase activity of the actin filaments alone was subtracted from the actomyosin data.

Crystallization and structure determination. Human β-cardiac MD::GFP protein (1.5–2.0 mg ml^{-1}) in 25 mM HEPES pH 7.0, 5 mM TCEP (Sigma) was screened against four Hampton Research (Aliso Viejo, CA) high-throughput crystallization screens using 0.2 µl protein and 0.2 µl mother liquor (ML) per drop equilibrated against 60 µl of ML at room temperature. Five drops containing brightly fluorescent birefringent crystals were found. These initial conditions were refined and single crystals without drug (Apo) were grown from 10% Tacsimate, pH 6.0, 14–15% PEG 3350, 10% glycerol, 0.2 mM MgCl$_2$ and 5 mM TCEP. Crystals with OM (OM +) were grown in essentially the same condition with 125 µM OM added to the protein drop (0.5% DMSO). The crystallization conditions proved to be a suitable cryoprotectant; therefore, crystals taken directly from the ML were fast-cooled in liquid nitrogen for X-ray analysis.

Single-crystal diffraction data for the Apo structure were collected on a Rigaku rotating anode X-ray generator ($\lambda = 1.542$ Å) with a Raxis IV + + detector at 100 °K. The OM + crystal diffraction data were collected at Brookhaven National Laboratory NSLS beamline X29A ($\lambda = 1.075$ Å) with an ADSC QUANTUM 315 detector at 100 °K. Reflections were indexed, integrated and scaled with iMosflm and Aimless from the ccp4 package[50,51]. The Apo structure was determined first by molecular replacement with Phaser[52] using residues 4–780 of chicken skeletal muscle myosin subfragment 1 structure, PDB ID: 2MYS[15], together with the structure of GFP, PDB ID: 2QLE[53], as the search ensemble. The molecular replacement map clearly identified two motor domains associated with one GFP per domain. The helix linking the MD to the GFP was not included in the search models; however, new density corresponding to the helix was apparent in the initial maps. After building the linking helix into the density and joining the MD and GFP domains, the cMD and GFP sequence were built into the model with PHENIX Autobuild[54]. The structure was refined with PHENIX refine[55] and iterative model building in Coot[56]. Only a very limited number of well-defined water molecules and two sulfate anions in the cMD β-phosphate-binding loop were included in the structure at this resolution. The statistics for favoured, allowed and outlier Ramachandran angles are 93.4%, 6.1% and 0.5%, respectively. The Molprobity score for the refined structure is 2.16 and the coordinates are deposited as PDB ID: 4P7H[57,58].

The OM + structure was solved by molecular replacement using the motor domain (2–708) of the Apo structure A chain and the helix–GFP domain as separate models in the search ensemble followed by PHENIX Autobuild. After limited initial refinement, unassigned density likely coming from the ligand was apparent. PHENIX LigandFit was used to search and dock OM into the map using Resolve[59]. Ligand restraints for refinement were generated with eLBoW[60]. The structure was refined as with the Apo structure. The statistics for favoured, allowed and outlier Ramachandran angles are 95.3%, 4.2% and 0.5%, respectively. The Molprobity score for the refined structure is 1.87.

The Karplus and Diederichs CC* data and model quality-assessment tool were applied to both models and data sets to assess the high-resolution cutoff[61]. The Apo data set was truncated at 3.2 Å, with mean ($I/\sigma(I)$) = 2 and a CC* > 0.88 for the highest-resolution shell (3.3–3.2 Å). The CC* statistic for the OM + data is > 0.73 for the highest-resolution shell (2.33–2.25 Å), supporting the inclusion of the full data range in determination of the model[62,63]. Alternatively, applying

traditional cutoff criteria of the mean ($I/\sigma(I)$) ≥ 2 to the OM + data would make this a nominal 2.40-Å resolution structure. The coordinates for the OM + structure are deposited as PDB entry 4PA0 (ref. 57). Data collection and refinement statistics are summarized in Table 1.

References

1. Lloyd-Jones, D. et al. Executive summary: heart disease and stroke statistics--2010 update: a report from the American Heart Association. *Circulation* **121**, 948–954 (2010).
2. Teerlink, J. R. A novel approach to improve cardiac performance: cardiac myosin activators. *Heart Fail. Rev.* **14**, 289–298 (2009).
3. Morgan, B. P. et al. Discovery of omecamtiv mecarbil the first, selective, small molecule activator of cardiac Myosin. *ACS Med. Chem. Lett.* **1**, 472–477 (2010).
4. Malik, F. I. et al. Cardiac myosin activation: a potential therapeutic approach for systolic heart failure. *Science* **331**, 1439–1443 (2011).
5. Shen, Y. T. et al. Improvement of cardiac function by a cardiac Myosin activator in conscious dogs with systolic heart failure. *Circ. Heart Fail.* **3**, 522–527 (2010).
6. Liu, Y., White, H. D., Belknap, B., Winkelmann, D. A. & Forgacs, E. Omecamtiv Mecarbil modulates the kinetic and motile properties of porcine beta-cardiac myosin. *Biochemistry* **54**, 1963–1975 (2015).
7. Siemankowski, R. F., Wiseman, M. O. & White, H. D. ADP dissociation from actomyosin subfragment 1 is sufficiently slow to limit the unloaded shortening velocity in vertebrate muscle. *Proc. Natl Acad. Sci. USA* **82**, 658–662 (1985).
8. Wang, Y., Ajtai, K. & Burghardt, T. P. Analytical comparison of natural and pharmaceutical ventricular myosin activators. *Biochemistry* **53**, 5298–5306 (2014).
9. Chow, D., Srikakulam, R., Chen, Y. & Winkelmann, D. A. Folding of the striated muscle myosin motor domain. *J. Biol. Chem.* **277**, 36799–36807 (2002).
10. Liu, L., Srikakulam, R. & Winkelmann, D. A. Unc45 activates Hsp90-dependent folding of the myosin motor domain. *J. Biol. Chem.* **283**, 13185–13193 (2008).
11. Srikakulam, R. & Winkelmann, D. A. Chaperone-mediated folding and assembly of myosin in striated muscle. *J. Cell Sci.* **117**, 641–652 (2004).
12. Wang, Q., Moncman, C. L. & Winkelmann, D. A. Mutations in the motor domain modulate myosin activity and myofibril organization. *J. Cell Sci.* **116**, 4227–4238 (2003).
13. Coureux, P. D., Sweeney, H. L. & Houdusse, A. Three myosin V structures delineate essential features of chemo-mechanical transduction. *EMBO J.* **23**, 4527–4537 (2004).
14. Klenchin, V., Deacon, J., Combs, A., Leinwand, L. & Rayment, I. Cardiac human myosin S1dc, beta isofrom complexed with Mn-AMPPNP. *PDB ID: 4DB1. 10.2210/pdb4db1/pdb* (2012).
15. Rayment, I. et al. Three-dimensional structure of myosin subfragment-1: a molecular motor. *Science* **261**, 50–58 (1993).
16. Risal, D., Gourinath, S., Himmel, D. M., Szent-Gyorgyi, A. G. & Cohen, C. Myosin subfragment 1 structures reveal a partially bound nucleotide and a complex salt bridge that helps couple nucleotide and actin binding. *Proc. Natl Acad. Sci. USA* **101**, 8930–8935 (2004).
17. Dominguez, R., Freyzon, Y., Trybus, K. M. & Cohen, C. Crystal structure of a vertebrate smooth muscle myosin motor domain and its complex with the essential light chain: visualization of the pre-power stroke state. *Cell* **94**, 559–571 (1998).
18. Houdusse, A., Kalabokis, V. N., Himmel, D., Szent-Gyorgyi, A. G. & Cohen, C. Atomic structure of scallop myosin subfragment S1 complexed with MgADP: a novel conformation of the myosin head. *Cell* **97**, 459–470 (1999).
19. Krissinel, E. & Henrick, K. Inference of macromolecular assemblies from crystalline state. *J. Mol. Biol.* **372**, 774–797 (2007).
20. Behrmann, E. et al. Structure of the rigor actin-tropomyosin-myosin complex. *Cell* **150**, 327–338 (2012).
21. Allingham, J. S., Smith, R. & Rayment, I. The structural basis of blebbistatin inhibition and specificity for myosin II. *Nat. Struct. Mol. Biol.* **12**, 378–379 (2005).
22. Kovacs, M., Toth, J., Hetenyi, C., Malnasi-Csizmadia, A. & Sellers, J. R. Mechanism of blebbistatin inhibition of myosin II. *J. Biol. Chem.* **279**, 35557–35563 (2004).
23. Fedorov, R. et al. The mechanism of pentabromopseudilin inhibition of myosin motor activity. *Nat. Struct. Mol. Biol.* **16**, 80–88 (2009).
24. Preller, M., Chinthalapudi, K., Martin, R., Knolker, H. J. & Manstein, D. J. Inhibition of Myosin ATPase activity by halogenated pseudilins: a structure-activity study. *J. Med. Chem.* **54**, 3675–3685 (2011).
25. Radke, M. B. et al. Small molecule-mediated refolding and activation of myosin motor function. *Elife* **3**, e01603 (2014).
26. Sweeney, H. L. & Houdusse, A. Structural and functional insights into the Myosin motor mechanism. *Annu. Rev. Biophys.* **39**, 539–557 (2010).
27. Changeux, J. P. 50 years of allosteric interactions: the twists and turns of the models. *Nat. Rev. Mol. Cell Biol.* **14**, 819–829 (2013).
28. Greenberg, M. J., Shuman, H. & Ostap, E. M. Inherent force-dependent properties of beta-cardiac myosin contribute to the force-velocity relationship of cardiac muscle. *Biophys. J.* **107**, L41–L44 (2014).

29. Spudich, J. A. Hypertrophic and dilated cardiomyopathy: four decades of basic research on muscle lead to potential therapeutic approaches to these devastating genetic diseases. *Biophys. J.* **106**, 1236–1249 (2014).

30. Sun, Y. B., Lou, F. & Irving, M. Calcium- and myosin-dependent changes in troponin structure during activation of heart muscle. *J. Physiol.* **587**, 155–163 (2009).

31. Gourinath, S. *et al.* Crystal structure of scallop myosin S1 in the pre-power stroke state to 2.6 a resolution: flexibility and function in the head. *Structure* **11**, 1621–1627 (2003).

32. Gulick, A. M., Bauer, C. B., Thoden, J. B. & Rayment, I. X-ray structures of the MgADP, MgATPgammaS, and MgAMPPNP complexes of the Dictyostelium discoideum myosin motor domain. *Biochemistry* **36**, 11619–11628 (1997).

33. Baumketner, A. The mechanism of the converter domain rotation in the recovery stroke of myosin motor protein. *Proteins* **80**, 2701–2710 (2012).

34. Fischer, S., Windshugel, B., Horak, D., Holmes, K. C. & Smith, J. C. Structural mechanism of the recovery stroke in the myosin molecular motor. *Proc. Natl Acad. Sci. USA* **102**, 6873–6878 (2005).

35. Furch, M., Fujita-Becker, S., Geeves, M. A., Holmes, K. C. & Manstein, D. J. Role of the salt-bridge between switch-1 and switch-2 of Dictyostelium myosin. *J. Mol. Biol.* **290**, 797–809 (1999).

36. Kintses, B., Yang, Z. & Malnasi-Csizmadia, A. Experimental investigation of the seesaw mechanism of the relay region that moves the myosin lever arm. *J. Biol. Chem.* **283**, 34121–34128 (2008).

37. Koppole, S., Smith, J. C. & Fischer, S. The structural coupling between ATPase activation and recovery stroke in the myosin II motor. *Structure* **15**, 825–837 (2007).

38. Malnasi-Csizmadia, A. *et al.* Kinetic resolution of a conformational transition and the ATP hydrolysis step using relaxation methods with a Dictyostelium myosin II mutant containing a single tryptophan residue. *Biochemistry* **40**, 12727–12737 (2001).

39. Sweeney, H. L. & Houdusse, A. The motor mechanism of myosin V: insights for muscle contraction. *Philos. Trans. R Soc. Lond. B Biol. Sci.* **359**, 1829–1841 (2004).

40. Arad, M. *et al.* Gene mutations in apical hypertrophic cardiomyopathy. *Circulation* **112**, 2805–2811 (2005).

41. Sakthivel, S., Joseph, P. K., Tharakan, J. M., Vosberg, H. P. & Rajamanickam, C. A novel missense mutation (R712L) adjacent to the 'active thiol' region of the cardiac beta-myosin heavy chain gene causing hypertrophic cardiomyopathy in an Indian family. *Hum. Mutat.* **15**, 298–299 (2000).

42. Holmes, K. C., Schroder, R. R., Sweeney, H. L. & Houdusse, A. The structure of the rigor complex and its implications for the power stroke. *Philos. Trans. R Soc. Lond. B Biol. Sci.* **359**, 1819–1828 (2004).

43. Roosild, T. P., Castronovo, S. & Choe, S. Structure of anti-FLAG M2 Fab domain and its use in the stabilization of engineered membrane proteins. *Acta Crystallogr. Sect. F Struct. Biol. Cryst. Commun.* **62**, 835–839 (2006).

44. He, T. C. *et al.* A simplified system for generating recombinant adenoviruses. *Proc. Natl Acad. Sci. USA* **95**, 2509–2514 (1998).

45. Kinose, F., Wang, S. X., Kidambi, U. S., Moncman, C. L. & Winkelmann, D. A. Glycine 699 is pivotal for the motor activity of skeletal muscle myosin. *J. Cell Biol.* **134**, 895–909 (1996).

46. Barua, B., Winkelmann, D. A., White, H. D. & Hitchcock-DeGregori, S. E. Regulation of actin-myosin interaction by conserved periodic sites of tropomyosin. *Proc. Natl Acad. Sci. USA* **109**, 18425–18430 (2012).

47. Winkelmann, D. A., Bourdieu, L., Ott, A., Kinose, F. & Libchaber, A. Flexibility of myosin attachment to surfaces influences F-actin motion. *Biophys. J.* **68**, 2444–2453 (1995).

48. Bourdieu, L., Magnasco, M. O., Winkelmann, D. A. & Libchaber, A. Actin filaments on myosin beds: The velocity distribution. *Phys. Rev. E* **52**, 6573–6579 (1995).

49. Forgacs, E. *et al.* Switch 1 mutation S217A converts myosin V into a low duty ratio motor. *J. Biol. Chem.* **284**, 2138–2149 (2009).

50. Potterton, E., Briggs, P., Turkenburg, M. & Dodson, E. A graphical user interface to the CCP4 program suite. *Acta Crystallogr. D Biol. Crystallogr.* **59**, 1131–1137 (2003).

51. Evans, P. R. & Murshudov, G. N. How good are my data and what is the resolution? *Acta Crystallogr. D Biol. Crystallogr.* **69**, 1204–1214 (2013).

52. Adams, P. D. *et al.* PHENIX: a comprehensive Python-based system for macromolecular structure solution. *Acta Crystallogr. D Biol. Crystallogr.* **66**, 213–221 (2010).

53. Shu, X. *et al.* An alternative excited-state proton transfer pathway in green fluorescent protein variant S205V. *Protein Sci.* **16**, 2703–2710 (2007).

54. Terwilliger, T. C. *et al.* Iterative model building, structure refinement and density modification with the PHENIX AutoBuild wizard. *Acta Crystallogr. D Biol. Crystallogr.* **64**, 61–69 (2008).

55. Afonine, P. V. *et al.* Towards automated crystallographic structure refinement with phenix.refine. *Acta Crystallogr. D Biol. Crystallogr.* **68**, 352–367 (2012).

56. Emsley, P., Lohkamp, B., Scott, W. G. & Cowtan, K. Features and development of Coot. *Acta Crystallogr. D Biol. Crystallogr.* **66**, 486–501 (2010).

57. Berman, H. M. *et al.* The Protein Data Bank. *Nucleic Acids Res.* **28**, 235–242 (2000).

58. Chen, V. B. *et al.* MolProbity: all-atom structure validation for macromolecular crystallography. *Acta Crystallogr. D Biol. Crystallogr.* **66**, 12–21 (2010).

59. Terwilliger, T. C., Klei, H., Adams, P. D., Moriarty, N. W. & Cohn, J. D. Automated ligand fitting by core-fragment fitting and extension into density. *Acta Crystallogr. D Biol. Crystallogr.* **62**, 915–922 (2006).

60. Moriarty, N. W., Grosse-Kunstleve, R. W. & Adams, P. D. electronic Ligand Builder and Optimization Workbench (eLBOW): a tool for ligand coordinate and restraint generation. *Acta Crystallogr. D Biol. Crystallogr.* **65**, 1074–1080 (2009).

61. Karplus, P. A. & Diederichs, K. Linking crystallographic model and data quality. *Science* **336**, 1030–1033 (2012).

62. Diederichs, K. & Karplus, P. A. Better models by discarding data? *Acta Crystallogr. D Biol. Crystallogr.* **69**, 1215–1222 (2013).

63. Wang, J. & Wing, R. A. Diamonds in the rough: a strong case for the inclusion of weak-intensity X-ray diffraction data. *Acta Crystallogr. D Biol. Crystallogr.* **70**, 1491–1497 (2014).

64. Laskowski, R. A. & Swindells, M. B. LigPlot + : multiple ligand-protein interaction diagrams for drug discovery. *J. Chem. Inf. Model* **51**, 2778–2786 (2011).

Acknowledgements

We want to thank Lily Liu for technical assistance during the early stages of the work and Howard White for many helpful discussions on the interpretation of the results. We appreciate the assistance of Robert Sweet and Howard Robinson of Brookhaven National Laboratory NSLS beamline X29A. This work was supported by funding from the AHA (10GRNT4300022; 12BGIA12030120) and the NIH (1R56HL124284-01).

Author contributions

D.A.W. designed experiments, carried out the majority of the experimental work including the crystallography and wrote the manuscript. E.F. contributed to the kinetic assays, interpretation and integration of the kinetic data. M.T.M. and A.M.S. provided advice and guidance with the crystallography, and A.M.S. provided access to the X-ray sources and detectors. All authors discussed the results and contributed to the manuscript.

Additional information

Accession codes: Coordinates and structure factors for Apo cMD and OM + cMD have been deposited in the Protein Data Bank under accession codes 4P7H and 4PA0 respectively.

18

Ultraflexible organic amplifier with biocompatible gel electrodes

Tsuyoshi Sekitani[1,2], Tomoyuki Yokota[1], Kazunori Kuribara[3,†], Martin Kaltenbrunner[1,4], Takanori Fukushima[5], Yusuke Inoue[1], Masaki Sekino[1], Takashi Isoyama[6], Yusuke Abe[6], Hiroshi Onodera[1,7] & Takao Someya[1,3,7]

In vivo electronic monitoring systems are promising technology to obtain biosignals with high spatiotemporal resolution and sensitivity. Here we demonstrate the fabrication of a biocompatible highly conductive gel composite comprising multi-walled carbon nanotube-dispersed sheet with an aqueous hydrogel. This gel composite exhibits admittance of 100 mS cm^{-2} and maintains high admittance even in a low-frequency range. On implantation into a living hypodermal tissue for 4 weeks, it showed a small foreign-body reaction compared with widely used metal electrodes. Capitalizing on the multi-functional gel composite, we fabricated an ultrathin and mechanically flexible organic active matrix amplifier on a 1.2-μm-thick polyethylene-naphthalate film to amplify (amplification factor: ~200) weak biosignals. The composite was integrated to the amplifier to realize a direct lead epicardial electrocardiography that is easily spread over an uneven heart tissue.

[1] Department of Electrical and Electronic Engineering, The University of Tokyo, 7-3-1 Hongo Bunkyo-ku, Tokyo 113-8656, Japan. [2] The Institute of Scientific and Industrial Research, Osaka University, 8-1, Mihogaoka, Ibaraki, Osaka 567-0047, Japan. [3] Department of Applied Physics, The University of Tokyo, 7-3-1 Hongo, Bunkyo-ku, Tokyo 113-8656, Japan. [4] Soft Matter Physics, Linz Institute of Technology LIT, Johannes Kepler University Linz, Altenbergerstrasse 69, Linz 4040, Austria. [5] Chemical Resource Laboratory, Tokyo Institute of Technology, 4259R1-1, Nagatsuda, Midoriku, Yokohama, Kanagawa 226-8503, Japan. [6] Department of Biomedical Engineering, Graduate School of Medicine, The University of Tokyo, 7-3-1 Hongo, Bunkyo-ku, Tokyo 113-8656, Japan. [7] Photon Science Center, The University of Tokyo, 7-3-1 Hongo, Bunkyo-ku, Tokyo 113-8656, Japan. † Present address: Flexible Electronics Research Center, Central 5, The National Institute of Advanced Industrial Science and Technology (AIST), 1-1-1 Higashi, Tsukuba, Ibaraki 305-856, Japan. Correspondence and requests for materials should be addressed to T.So. (email: someya@ee.t.u-tokyo.ac.jp).

An implantable electronic system that monitors *in vivo* biological signals is expected to play an important role in realizing next-generation medical electronics and in deeply understanding biological systems. By using non-invasive medical instruments such as magnetic resonance imaging, ultrasound and X-ray systems, various types of biological information can be obtained from outside the body. However, by going inside the body (*in vivo*), abundant biological information can be measured with higher spatial and temporal resolution and sensitivity. One of the ultimate goals of *in vivo* monitoring systems is to elucidate biological activities at the organ level, such as in the brain and heart, with high spatial and temporal resolution over a large area.

Long-term stability and reliability are among the biggest challenges for *in vivo* electronic systems. In fact, realizing long-term *in vivo* monitoring is very difficult, because monitoring biosignals requires sensitivity on the order of microvolts to millivolts, which is made further difficult because of the inherently wet and deformable surfaces of biological tissues. Although a pacemaker for heart stimulation and a probe of deep brain stimulation for supressing epilepsy have a lifetime exceeding 10 years in the body, they simply apply high voltages (typically ~5 V) to stimulate heartbeats and neural networks, respectively, and do not perform detection. To increase *in vivo* monitoring periods with microvolt sensitivity, improving the long-term stability, reliability (especially the signal-to-noise ratio (SNR)) and biocompatibility of electrodes used in electric probes that directly touch the surface of biological tissues is important. Replacing conventional hard metal electrodes with soft conducting biocompatible materials is a promising solution to obtain reliable large-area mechanical and electrical contacts at the bioelectrode interfaces. Furthermore, integration of soft conductive biocompatible materials with ultraflexible electronic amplifier is indispensable in realizing *in vivo* monitoring periods with sensitivity on the order of microvolts to millivolts.

Here we demonstrate the fabrication of a biocompatible, ultraflexible and thin-film organic amplifier using biocompatible highly conductive gel electrodes with organic transistor-based circuits. The gel electrodes comprise multi-walled carbon nanotube (CNT)-dispersed sheet with an aqueous hydrogel. This gel electrode exhibits admittance of $100 \, mS \, cm^{-2}$ and maintains high admittance even in a low-frequency range. On implantation into a living hypodermal tissue for 4 weeks, it showed a small foreign-body reaction compared with widely used metal electrodes. Capitalizing on the multi-functional gel composite, we fabricated an ultrathin and mechanically flexible organic active matrix amplifier on a 1.2-μm-thick polyethylene-naphthalate (PEN) film to amplify (amplification factor: ~200) weak biosignals. The composite was integrated to the amplifier, to realize a direct lead epicardial electrocardiography that is easily spread over an uneven heart tissue.

A biocompatible, ultraflexible and thin-film organic amplifier was realized with a biocompatible highly conductive hydrogel-based electrode that comprises a multi-walled CNT sheet and a stretchable elastic aqueous polyrotaxane-based gel with a movable cross-linker (cyclodextrin/polyethylene), which is known as a 'slide-ring gel' or a 'topological gel'. The entire CNT surface is uniformly coated with aqueous polyrotaxane-based gel using a hydrophilic ionic liquid. This structure has an increased effective surface ratio (electrode area) and it exhibits an admittance of $100 \, mS \, cm^{-2}$ without sacrificing softness, which is a characteristic of gels. Furthermore, the admittance does not change even in the low-frequency range and its value is two or three orders of magnitude larger than that of conventional gel electrodes. The gel composite is chemically stable and mechanically flexible and stretchable, showing Young's modulus of approximately on the

order of 10 kPa. When the gel composite was implanted in the hypodermal tissue of a living body for 4 weeks, the foreign-body reaction of the tissue was smaller than those using existing metal electrodes. Furthermore, by combining the gel composite with an organic-transistor-based mechanically compliant waterproof amplifier manufactured on a 1.2-μm-thick ultraflexible polymeric substrate, we demonstrated a sheet-type ultraflexible electrocardiograph measurement system that can be fully spread over the uneven surface of the heart of a living body. These organic-transistor-based amplifiers have extreme flexibility, whose critical bending radii are much less than 500 μm. The soft and biocompatible gel composite, as well as the amplifiers, enables the sensor system to detect a very small electronic potential; a 1-mV signal coming from a rat heart was amplified by a factor of 200 by the organic amplifiers, thus enabling ultra-sensitivity without any noise related to signal cross-talk and interference.

Results

Biocompatible gel electrode. A biocompatible gel composite is formed by a uniformly dispersed multi-walled CNT composite sheet (CNT sheet) (length: > 100 μm and diameter: 5 nm, unless otherwise noted) and a stretchable, soft, elastic and aqueous polyrotaxane-based gel with a movable cross-linker (cyclodextrin/polyethylene)[1] (Fig. 1 and Supplementary Figs 1–6). Thick CNT bundles (50 mg) were mixed with *N,N*-diethyl-*N*-methyl-*N*-(2-methoxyethyl)ammonium tetrafluoroborate (DEMEBF$_4$; 100 mg), which is a hydrophilic ionic liquid. Through the above process, the thick CNT bundles were untangled into thin bundles and the CNT surface was then coated with the ionic liquid by self-assembly (Fig. 1b). The resulting suspension with CNTs and ion liquid DEMEBF$_4$ was subjected to an automatic grinding system for 6 h to form a black substance, referred to as 'bucky gel.' The bucky gel (150 mg) was successively added to deionized water (10 ml) and a microfibrillar cellulose (200 mg of water solution containing 10% cellulose, Celish, Daicel Chemical Industries, Ltd, referred to as microcellulose in this study). The mixture was stirred at 25 °C (1 h) and sonicated (UH-50, SMT Co., Ltd) at 30 °C (10 min). The resulting swollen gel was poured onto a polytetrafluoroethylene plate by drop casting and air dried for 24 h to produce a CNT sheet, as shown in Fig. 1c.

A 50- to 150-μm-thick conductive CNT sheet was prepared, followed by a 1-mm-thick polyrotaxane-gel precursor comprising a photo-cross-linking agent (1.0 mg; Irgacure 2959, Nagase & Co., Ltd). In addition, an adamantine-polyrotaxane-based xerogel[1] (1 g; Advanced Materials Ltd) without CNT was cast to form a bilayer composite comprising a CNT sheet and a polyrotaxane gel. After cross-linking using 365-nm ultraviolet irradiation for 5 min, the bilayer CNT-sheet/gel composite was formed (Fig. 1e,f). This polyrotaxane gel can be easily patterned to form microstructures with a spatial resolution of ~50 μm via photo-cross-linking using an ultrafine digital ultraviolet exposure system (Supplementary Figs 1–5).

Figure 1a,b,d show the high-resolution cross-sectional electron microscopy images of a single CNT, an ionic-liquid-coated CNT, and a CNT/polyrotaxane gel composite, respectively. The transmission electron microscopy (TEM) (80-kV HF-2000 Cold-FE TEM, Hitachi High-Technologies Corp.) images of the specimen after being dried in vacuum clearly show the polyrotaxane-based gels coated on the multi-walled CNTs with a diameter of 5–10 nm (Fig. 1d). Owing to the hydrophilic ion-based ionic liquids, an aqueous polyrotaxane-based gel (slide-ring gel) was formed around the CNT. Energy-dispersive X-ray (EDX) spectrometry (Genesis APEX2, EDAX Corp.) clearly shows aqueous polyrotaxane-based gels around the CNTs (Supplementary Fig. 6).

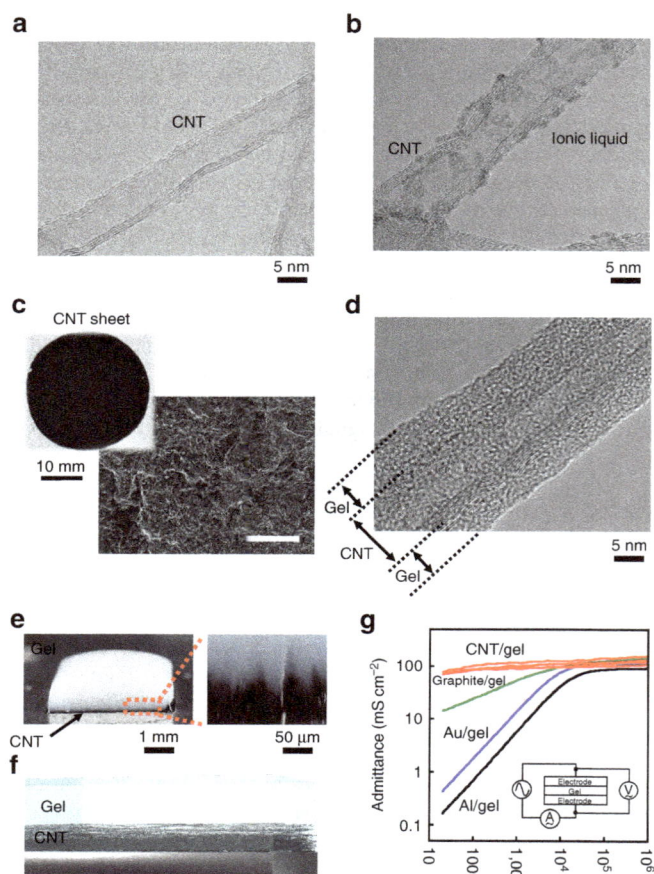

Figure 1 | Conductive gel. High-resolution cross-sectional electron microscopy image of (**a**) stand-alone multiwalled CNT and (**b**) ionic-liquid-coated CNT. The specimen was dried in vacuum and imaged by TEM (80 kV). (**c**) Conductive CNT sheet and magnified picture of the surface. The scale of the SEM image is 100 µm. (**d**) High-resolution cross-sectional electron microscopy image of the CNT/polyrotaxane composite. (**e**) Cross-sectional picture of the CNT/polyrotaxane composite comprising a 50- to 100-µm-thick CNT gel layer and a 1-mm-thick polyrotaxane-gel layer. A magnified picture of the CNT/polyrotaxane interface is also shown. (**f**) Schematic cross-section of the conductive gel where a concentration gradient of CNT is formed in the gel. (**g**) Admittance (mS cm^{-2}) of CNT/polyrotaxane gel in the vertical direction as a function of frequency, represented as red line. The admittance values of a polyrotaxane gel with different conductive layers are also shown for comparison. Polyrotaxane gel with (red) CNT, (green) graphite sheet, (blue) Au-coated film and (black) Al-coated film. The admittance was derived by subtracting the parasitic resistance in the experimental setup as open/short error compensation.

As shown in Fig. 1g, the bilayer gel composite had an admittance of 100 mS cm^{-2} even in the low-frequency range, which, to the best of our knowledge, is the highest among CNT-based conductive gels[2–4]. The admittance of the CNT/polyrotaxane gel composite was evaluated through AC measurements, as shown in Fig. 1g. Polyrotaxane-based gels with different conductive layers, such as the graphite sheet, Au-coated film and Al-coated film, are also shown for comparison. The CNT-sheet/gel composite showed the highest admittance in the low-frequency range, owing to the large surface ratio of the CNT-based conductive electrodes, whose admittance was two or three orders of magnitude larger than that of metal/gel-based composite electrodes. In fact, the CNT/gel interface formed a

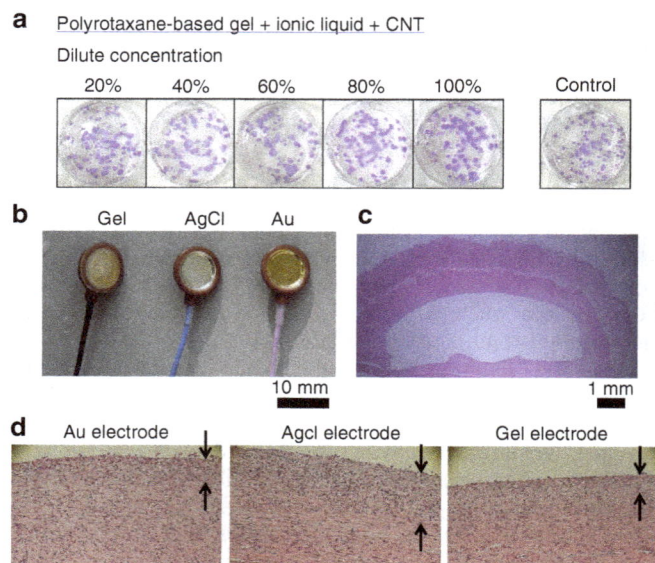

Figure 2 | Biocompatibility test 1. (**a**) Colony-forming assay for cytotoxic evaluation. (**b**) Implant assay in living body to evaluate long-term foreign-body response. Three probes that can change the surfaces of the electrodes were used for implantation into the hypodermal tissue of living rats for 4 weeks. (**c**) Pathology graft after explanting the probes and staining. (**d**) Magnified pictures of the surfaces of the pathology grafts. The arrows represent the depth of inflammation reaction.

highly capacitive electronic double layer whose capacitance exceeded 140 µF cm^{-2}. The CNT-sheet/gel bilayer electrode was chemically stable and mechanically flexible and stretchable, showing Young's modulus below 100 kPa.

Biocompatible tests. The biocompatibility was examined through a four-step test. We organized all the biocompatibility tests throughout under a rule described by an internationally standardized procedure, namely colony-forming assay (ISO10993-5) and implant assay (ISO10993-6). First, in a colony-forming assay (ISO10993-5), hamster fibroblasts (V79) were cultivated for cytotoxic evaluation. The conductive gels were finely cut and sterilized by autoclaving (121 °C for 20 min). Next, extraction liquid was extracted at 37 °C for 24 h, which corresponds to an undiluted sample. This liquid was diluted to 20, 40, 60, 80 and 100%. Each diluted liquid was cast on V79 (100 cells per well) and cultivated at 37 °C for 6 days in 5% CO$_2$ atmosphere. The number of cells per well was counted after fixing and staining the cells. The number of cells did not change after casting the extraction liquid and the cell state was similar to that of the negative control, which showed that the conductive gels are not cytotoxic (Fig. 2a and Supplementary Figs 7 and 8).

Second, in an implant assay (ISO10993-6), the gel composites were implanted into the hypodermal tissues of living rabbits for 4 weeks. Indeed, 4 weeks is one of the examination periods for ISO10993-6. The degree of foreign-body reaction was quantified based on ISO 10993-6:2007 in terms of the cell type. The irritant ranking score was averaged in four populations, compared them with that of the negative control and classified them into four categories: non-, slight, moderate and severe irritant (Table 1).

Three subcutaneously implanted electrodes whose surfaces were coated with the gel composite, AgCl and Au were used in this experiment, as shown in Fig. 2b and Supplementary Fig. 8. Figure 2c shows the cross-sectional images of a subcutaneous tissue after an electrode was explanted. Figure 2d and

Table 1 | Average irritant ranking score, comparison with negative control and degree of irritant for six samples.

Sample (four-week implantation)	Average irritant ranking score	Δ Between test sample and control	Non-irritant (0.0–2.9) Slight irritant (3.0–8.9) Moderate irritant (9.0–15.0) Severe irritant (>15)
Negative control	4.0	—	—
Gel	18.0	14.0	Moderate irritant
Gel + IL	15.5	11.5	Moderate irritant
Gel + CNT	18.3	14.3	Moderate irritant
Gel + IL + CNT	15.3	11.3	Moderate irritant
Au	22.0	18.0	Severe irritant

CNT, carbon nanotube; gel, polyrotaxane-based gel with movable cross-linker (cyclodextrin/polyethylene); IL, ionic liquid; Negative control, high-density polyethylene sheet. The assays were quantified based on ISO 10993-6:2007, Biological Evaluation of Medical Devices—Part 6: Tests for Local Effects After Implantation.

Supplementary Fig. 9 show the magnified images of graft pathology after staining. The top surfaces of the grafts were exposed to the three electrodes. Fibrosing cell infiltration was observed near the surface, whose thickness represented the amount of inflammation (indicated as arrows in Fig. 2d). Table 1 lists the implant assays for six samples. The gel composite shows an irritant ranking score of 15.3, which is smaller than that of conventional Au implant electrodes (ranking score: 22). Each irritant ranking score was averaged in four populations and a dominant difference was observed even if we considered the error, indicating that the gels exhibited smaller foreign-body reaction.

Third, optical cleaning process was carried out on the above three pathology grafts to evaluate the biocompatibility. Several tissue-cleaning methods have been reported by other groups and used as new analysis techniques for living tissues[5–8]. The transparent tissues enabled us to observe an internal haemorrhage with inflammation. We found remarkable inflammation from the AgCl electrodes, as shown in Fig. 3a. Therefore, as a result of the laboratory procedure for the three pathology grafts described above, the gel electrode is more compatible with a living tissue.

We have evaluated not only the above three biological assays but also the biocompatibility viewed from the electrical characteristic perspective. The technical details of the result are presented in the Supplementary Information. Figure 3b shows the admittance between each electrode pair through the subcutaneous tissue as a function of the implanted time, where the admittance values were average values obtained from more than three samples. We verified that the gel electrode exhibited stable conductance equal to the conventional metal electrode typically used in biomedical applications, demonstrating the excellent feasibility of the gel electrodes from the viewpoint of electrical performance, mechanical flexibility and biocompatibility.

Ultraflexible organic amplifier. To detect weak biosignals, a two-dimensional array of organic amplifiers was directly fabricated on a 1.2-μm-thick ultraflexible PEN substrate (Fig. 4a). The schematic cross-sectional diagram is shown in Fig. 4b. The amplifier was formed using an inverter with a pseudo-complementary metal-oxide semiconductor (CMOS) layout[9] comprising four p-channel organic transistors with semiconducting dinaphtho[2,3-b:2′,3′-f]thieno[3,2-b]thiophene[10] and an organic self-assembled monolayer (SAM) gate dielectric[11–13], a capacitor and a resistor (Supplementary Fig. 13). A waterproof hybrid encapsulation stack comprising a 200-nm-thick Au layer sandwiched between a 100-nm- and 1.2-μm-thick parylene layer was deposited on the transistors to serve as a passivation layer against oxygen diffusion, humidity and

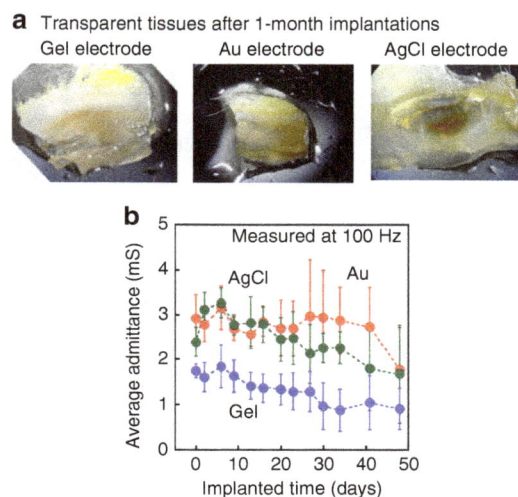

a Transparent tissues after 1-month implantations
Gel electrode   Au electrode   AgCl electrode

b Average admittance (mS) vs Implanted time (days). Measured at 100 Hz. Curves labelled AgCl, Au, Gel.

Figure 3 | Biocompatibility test 2. (**a**) Samples (pathology grafts) are transferred to the final clearing solution (LUCID: nine parts thiodiethanol and one part glycerol) at room temperature. The cleaned tissues are evaluated using microscopy. Internal haemorrhage is observed in the pathology grafts where the AgCl electrode is explanted. (**b**) Averaged conductance of electrodes subcutaneously implanted in living rats, whose details can be seen in Supplementary Fig. 9.

mechanical attrition *in vivo*, and as an overcoat layer to enhance mechanical flexibility and durability, because the organic semiconducting layer was located at the neutral strain position[13], leading to the reduction in the effective strain at the thin-film transistor (TFT) plane. Figure 4c,d show the schematic cross-section and TEM image of one transistor on a 1.2-μm-thick ultraflexible PEN and the manufacturing details and electrical performance are described in the Supplementary Information (Supplementary Figs 12–21). The ultrathin transistors exhibited high mechanical flexibility whose performance did not change even after a 50-μm bending radius, as shown in Fig. 4e and Supplementary Fig. 18.

Figure 5a shows the circuit diagram and a photograph of the organic amplifier comprising a pseudo-CMOS inverter on a 1.2-μm-thick ultraflexible PEN with organic circuits, CNT-gel composite (CNT-gel), input capacitor (C) and resistance (R). The input impedance and power requirements for the amplifiers were 100 kΩ and 10 μW, respectively. The pseudo-CMOS inverter has five electrical terminals: input, output, power source voltage V_{DD}, tuning voltage V_{SS} and ground (GND). It can operate within 2 V with a signal gain exceeding 400 (Fig. 5c and Supplementary

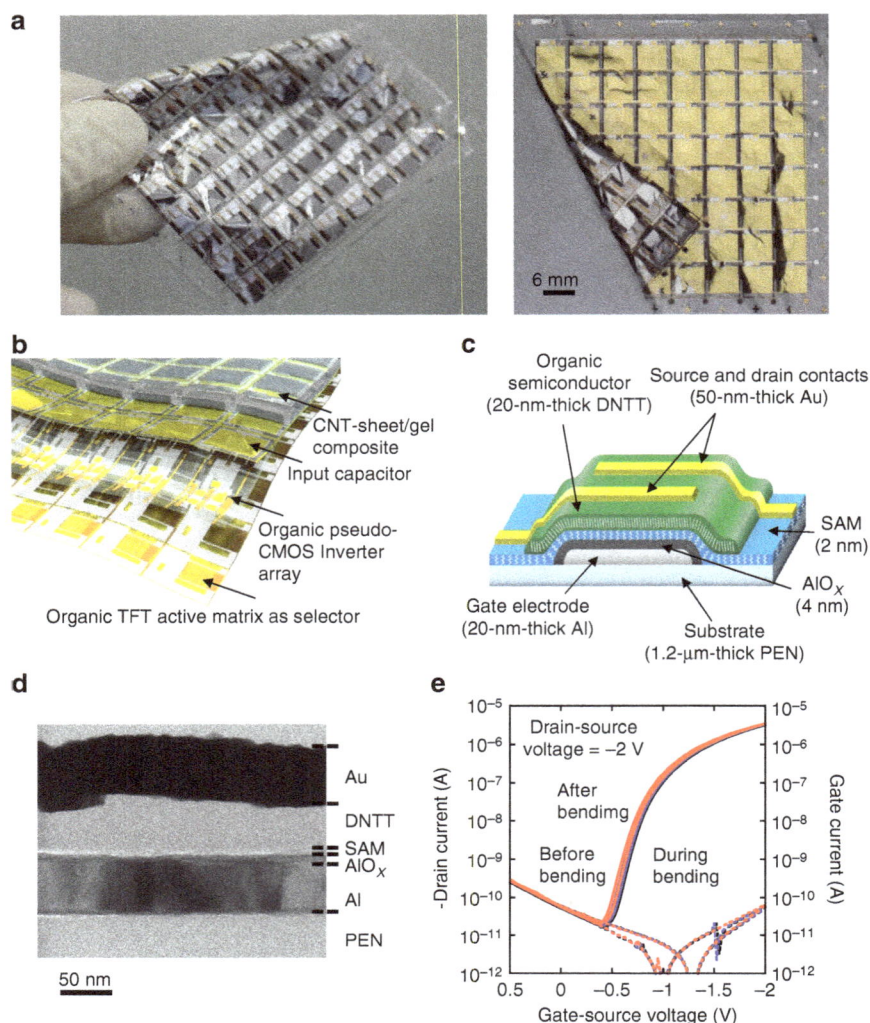

Figure 4 | Ultraflexible organic integrated circuits. (**a**) Picture and (**b**) schematic illustration of the 1.2-μm-thick ultraflexible amplifier array comprising organic transistors. (**c**) Cross-sectional image and (**d**) high-resolution cross-sectional electron microscopy image of an organic transistor on a 1.2-μm-thick plastic substrate. (**e**) Electrical characteristics of an organic transistor before, during and after bending to a radius of 50 μm. The transistor is fabricated on a 1.2-μm-thick PEN substrate and 1.3-μm-thick parylene encapsulation stack. The transistor channel is located at the neutral strain position. The transistor characteristics confirm that the devices are not damaged when bent to a radius of 50 μm.

Fig. 21) and it can maintain this electrical performance even when bent at a bending radius of 50 μm. The propagation delay per stage of the transistors was 23.4 μs at 2 V, which corresponds to the frequency response of 42.7 kHz on a single transistor, as shown in the Supplementary Information (Supplementary Fig. 20)[9]. The excellent electrical and mechanical performance of the inverter was demonstrated by evaluating its characteristics before and after being used to coat a rat heart; the change in the characteristics was negligible (<1%) (Fig. 5b,c).

Figure 5d shows the amplifier gain obtained from the organic amplifier for this experiment. The frequency responses of the gain were similar at frequencies exceeding 10 Hz. However, the amplifier with larger capacitance (C) showed higher gain even below 10 Hz. This result indicates that the input capacitor should be carefully chosen in accordance with the required monitoring frequency.

Electrocardiogram monitoring. Next, a direct epicardial electrocardiogram was obtained using self-feedback-type organic

amplifiers by combining the inverter, a conductive gel sheet, a resistor made of conductive carbon paste ($R = 2.1$ MΩ) and a capacitor formed using SAM/AlO$_x$ dielectrics sandwiched by Au electrodes ($C = 670$ nF) (Fig. 5a and Supplementary Fig. 13). The gel composite was placed on the rat heart and interconnected to an organic amplifier sheet using electrical wirings. A 1.2-mV input signal obtained from the heart was amplified to a 220-mV output signal using the amplifier (signal gain: ~200) (Fig. 5e,f). Here we note that a high amplifier gain exceeding 100 was obtained, owing to a large capacitor of 670 nF and an internal resistance of 10–50 kΩ, whose gain is consistent with the theoretical estimation. The input SNR of 0.53 was increased to 64 after amplification, which is the first demonstration of amplification of *in vivo* biosignals from a hypodermal tissue using organic circuits. The amplifier gain exceeded 10 at below 1 kHz and 100 at below 100 Hz (Supplementary Fig. 21). The frequency dependence did not affect the measurement accuracy and the amplifier gain was sufficiently large, considering that important heart signals lie within 1 kHz (ref. 14). The low-frequency gain can be increased by optimizing the passive components (resistance and capacitance) of the organic amplifier, as shown in Fig. 5d.

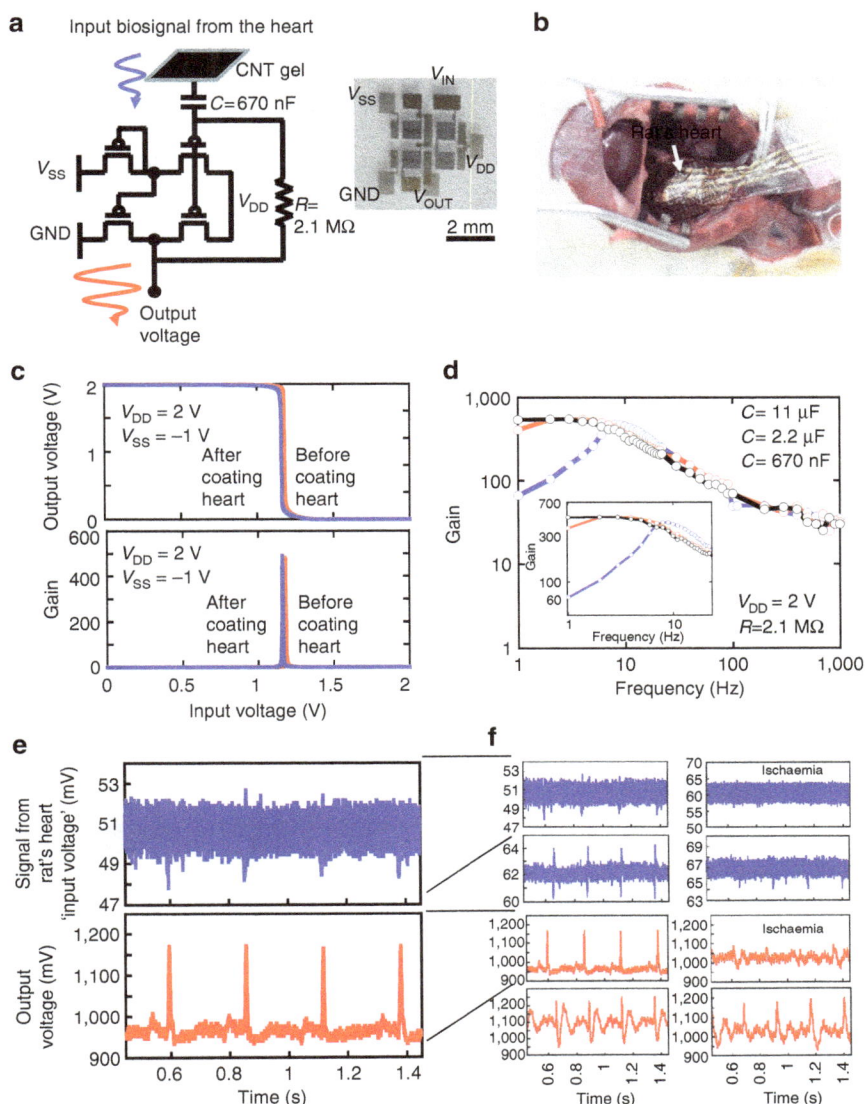

Figure 5 | Electrocardiogram using conductive gel probes and ultraflexible organic circuit. (a) Circuit diagram of one cell of an organic amplifier with a conductive gel for *in vivo* electrocardiograph comprising an organic pseudo-CMOS inverter that works as an amplifier, where V_{DD} is the power source voltage, V_{SS} is the tuning voltage, L is the channel length and W is the channel width. Photograph of an organic pseudo-CMOS inverter is also shown. **(b)** Photograph of ultraflexible circuits (pseudo-CMOS inverter) on the rat heart. **(c)** Characteristics of the pseudo-CMOS inverter before and after coating the rat heart. The electrical performance does not change after coating. **(d)** Frequency responses of the gain of an organic amplifier by varying the input capacitor (c) from 0.67 to 2.2, to 11 μF. **(e)** Amplification performance and **(f)** the magnified characteristics of the organic amplifier. (Blue line) Input signal is directly obtained from the heart where CNT conductive gel is used for the electronic interface. (Red line) Output signal is amplified using an organic amplifier. An input signal of 1.2 mV is amplified to a 220-mV output signal. A series of electrocardiograms is also shown in the right. An ischaemia-induced myocardial infarction is clearly observed. The total thickness of the cardiac electrodes is ~1 mm, while the size is 6 mm × 6 mm, which was determined by the size of a pixel of an organic amplifier (Fig. 5 and Supplementary Fig. 16).

Discussion

One of the ultimate goals of *in vivo* monitoring systems is to elucidate biological activities at the organ level, such as in the brain and in the heart, with high spatial and temporal resolution over a large area. From this viewpoint, flexible electronic devices[13,15–18] have been intensively studied, because they can be applied on complex curved surfaces with a large area coverage. In recent times, flexible *in vivo* neural interfaces have been demonstrated using silicon nanomembrane TFT active matrices to electrically monitor neural activities in a cat brain with high spatial and temporal resolution[18], and to investigate the mapping of neural circuits in acute brain slices[19]. Organic TFTs[20–22] and related structures[23–25] have been investigated to further improve mechanical flexibility.

Long-term stability and reliability are the biggest challenges for *in vivo* electronic systems. Realizing long-term *in vivo* monitoring is very difficult, because monitoring biosignals requires sensitivity on the order of microvolts to millivolts. Furthermore, the inherently wet and deformable surfaces of biological tissues result in further difficulty in monitoring very small biosignals. We have demonstrated fabrication of smart stress-absorbing electronic devices that can adhere to wet and complex tissue surfaces for reliable and long-term electronic measurements of vital signals[26]. Combining the adhesive gel technology with the biocompatible active amplifier proposed in the work, more precise measurement can be realized *in vivo* for a long time.

Highly conformable conducting poly(3,4-ethylenedioxythiophene) poly(styrenesulfonate) electrodes have been reported for *in vivo* electrocorticography[27,28]. Au-coated poly(dimethylsiloxane) has been demonstrated for stretchable *in vivo* neural interfaces[29]. However, the biocompatibility of these soft electrodes in contact with the tissues for a long duration has not yet been evaluated. Furthermore, an electronic system combined with soft electrodes has not yet been demonstrated. Replacing conventional metal electrodes with soft conducting materials is a promising solution to obtain reliable large-area mechanical and electrical contacts at the bio/electrode interfaces. Moreover, integration of soft conductive gels with ultraflexible electronic amplifier is indispensable in realizing *in vivo* monitoring periods with sensitivity on the order of microvolts to millivolts.

Flexible silicon nanomembrane transistors have been manufactured for buffering biological signals and multiplexing electrodes to record the spatial properties of a cat brain activity *in vivo*, demonstrating the excellent feasibility of flexible electronic systems[18]. In our work, an organic-based transistor with an ultraflexible PEN substrate, instead of inorganic-based transistors with silicon membranes, was found to improve mechanical flexibility. Furthermore, the use of a biocompatible conductive gel as an electrode enabled long-term sustainable *in vivo* circuits. The use of organic amplifiers near a living tissue enabled high-resolution, high-sensitivity and multi-channel monitoring with improved SNR.

A previous report regarding organic-transistor-based implantable electronic systems was presented by Feili *et al.*[30], who manufactured a stimulation array to a heart using organic-transistor active matrices. Moreover, the cytotoxicity of the transistors was evaluated with respect to the potential effects on cell viability[30]. Huang *et al.*[31] have demonstrated implantable electrocardiogram monitors using single-probe ultrasonic apparatus, which had already been actually used in clinical practices[32]. However, the novelty of our works lies in the complete system of an ultrathin electronic amplifier sheet with ultrasoft and biocompatible gel. To the best of our knowledge, this technique is the first integration of an ultrathin active matrix amplifier array with biocompatible gels and the first demonstration of electrocardiogram measurement of a heart of a living rat. Furthermore, we have successfully monitored ischaemia-induced myocardial infarction on a living heart, which was amplified using the ultrathin organic amplifier. Owing to the ultraflexible, ultrathin and ultralightweight thin-film amplifier, it can conform to dynamic motion such as that in a living heart. It can reduce the burden of long-term monitoring. Furthermore, we will no longer be concerned of the lifetime of organic circuits.

In conclusion, by using novel gelatinous composite as a biocompatible electrode for implantable electronics, we have succeeded in reducing foreign-body reaction compared with the widely used metal electrodes, whereas the new material maintains extraordinarily high AC admittance of $100\,\mathrm{mS\,cm^{-2}}$ even in the low-frequency range. Intensely viewed from multiple perspectives, this gel composite was quantitatively evaluated by four different types of biocompatibility tests. Both standard *in vitro* and *in vivo* biocompatibility tests, namely colony-forming assay (ISO10993-5) and implant assay (ISO10993-6) using hypodermal tissues of living rabbits for 4 weeks, clearly demonstrated that the implantable gel composite electrodes show minor foreign-body reaction compared with the widely used metal electrodes. This result is also consistent with the *in vivo* impedance measurements of our gel electrode implanted for 48 days. Furthermore, one of the highlights in the manuscript is that the newly developed 'tissue-cleaning method' was used for the first time, to the best of our knowledge, to characterize biocompatibility. The new three-dimensional imaging using the tissue-cleaning method has unambiguously established that no internal haemorrhage with inflammation was observed

using the gel electrode, whereas the AgCl and other metal electrodes exhibited remarkable inflammation. This study is a very important step towards realizing long-term implantable monitoring systems.

Furthermore, the abovementioned gel composites were integrated with a two-dimensional array of ultrathin, ultraflexible organic amplifiers to make the interfaces between the bio tissues and electrodes of the electronics biocompatible. The world's thinnest ultrathin organic amplifier system was directly laminated over a complex and dynamically moving surface of a living heart, while minimizing the mechanical interference due to motions. The feasibility of the system is demonstrated by the direct measurement of epicardial electrocardiogram signals at an amplification factor of 200, which, to the best of our knowledge, is the largest among flexible amplifier circuits. Furthermore, we have successfully monitored ischaemia-induced myocardial infarction on a living heart. The combination of biocompatible gel composites and ultrathin organic electronics can reduce the burden of long-term monitoring of bio-signals and, therefore, it will broaden the potential application of flexible biomedical electronics from disposable flexible electronics used only during medical surgery to long-term implantable monitoring systems.

Methods

Approval for animal testing. The protocols for the animal experiments were approved by the Institutional Animal Care and Use Committee of the University of Tokyo (Approval numbers: KA12-1 and P08-020). The cytotoxic evaluation of gel composite was performed based on a colony-forming assay using hamster fibroblasts (V79, unauthenticated) obtained from the Health Science Research Resources Bank, Japan Health Sciences Foundation. Mycoplasma contamination was not detected in an inspection using a dedicated test kit (MP Biomedicals, LLC). The implant assay of gel composites was performed using male JW/csk rabbits whose weights ranged from 2.9 to 3.6 kg. These colony-forming assay and implant assay were carried out by Kamakura Techno-science Co., Ltd, Japan, according to the internationally standardized procedures ISO10993-5 and ISO10993-6. The evaluation of gel electrode characteristics and the recordings of electrocardiogram were carried out using 12-week-old male Wistar rats. The implant tolerance test of organic transistors was performed using a 4-year-old female Saanen goat.

Water dispersibility of CNTs. The water dispersibility of five CNT samples was tested—all samples were first stirred in deionized water at 25 °C using a magnetic stirrer (>700 r.p.m.) for a week and pictures were taken after the stirring was stopped—(1) CNT (30 mg); (2) mixture of CNT (30 mg) and DEMEBF$_4$ (60 mg); (3) CNT (30 mg) subsequently processed on a high-pressure jet-milling homogenizer (60 MPa; Nano-jet Pal, JN10, Jokoh); (4) mixture of CNT (30 mg) and DEMEBF$_4$ (60 mg) subsequently processed on the homogenizer; and (5) mixture of CNT (30 mg), DEMEBF$_4$ (60 mg) and microfibrillar cellulose (100 mg water solution containing 10% cellulose; Celish, Daicel Chemical Industries, Ltd) subsequently processed on the homogenizer (see Supplementary Fig. 1A). Samples (4) and (5) showed excellent dispersibility of CNT in water. High-resolution scanning electron microscope (SEM) images of Samples (1–4) were collected (Supplementary Fig. 1B) showing the dispersibility of CNTs. The specimens were dried in air before the SEM observation. The high-pressure jet-milling homogenizer can effectively untangle the CNT bundles, as observed in Sample (3).

Manufacturing process of CNT composite sheet. Supplementary Fig. 2A shows the schematic of the fabrication process. Fabrication of the conductive CNT sheet was realized, because the ultrafine bundles of the CNT could be uniformly distributed in microfibrillar cellulose using room-temperature, aliphatic-system hydrophilic ion-based ionic liquids. CNTs (with purity of $>99.98\%$) were used as highly conductive and chemically stable dopant. The CNTs (50 mg) were mixed with 100 mg of hydrophilic ionic liquid DEMEBF$_4$ and the resulting suspension was subjected to automatic grinding for 1 h to form a black substance, referred to as 'bucky gel.' The gel (150 mg) was successively added to deionized water (10 ml) and processed on a high-pressure jet-milling homogenizer (60 MPa; Nano-jet Pal, JN10, Jokoh). The mixture was stirred at 25 °C (1 h) and added to microfibrillar cellulose (200 mg of water solution containing 10% cellulose, Celish, Daicel Chemical Industries, Ltd, referred to as microcellulose in this study). The resulting swollen gel was poured onto a polytetrafluoroethylene plate by drop casting and air-dried for 24 h to produce a CNT sheet. The fabricated CNT sheet had a surface with highly uniform entanglement between the CNT and cellulose, resulting in a large surface ratio (large capacitance when dielectric materials are deposited on the surface). Supplementary Fig. 2B shows the SEM images of the CNT sheet as a function of the cellulose content. With the increase in the cellulose content, the surface became rough.

Supplementary Fig. 3A shows that the conductivity of the conductive CNT sheet strongly depends on the cellulose content. In the CNT sheet, the cellulose content was changed from 5 to 65 wt%, whereas the amounts of CNT and DEMEBF$_4$ were 50 and 100 mg, respectively. When the cellulose content was >40 wt%, the CNT sheet was thick and porous; when it was <10 wt%, the CNT sheet became porous and fragile. We found that the highest conductivity could be obtained when the cellulose content was ~12 wt% and the mixing ratio of CNT and DEMEBF$_4$ was 1:2. The CNT easily formed strongly entangled bundles because of the strong covalent bonds, thus resulting in a well-developed entanglement from an unfavourable re-aggregation in the polymer matrix or other base materials. However, ionic liquids can prevent the entanglement of CNT. The high conductivity of the sheet is mainly due to the uniform dispersion of CNT as conductive dopants into the cellulose using ionic liquids.

Supplementary Fig. 3B shows that the conductive paper looks and feels like a regular paper. Moreover, it is used as wiring to transmit power from a battery to a light-emitting diode, demonstrating the very high conductivity of the CNT sheet (Supplementary Fig. 3C). The AC admittance of the CNT/gel electrodes can be observed in Supplementary Fig. 3, obtained from four different samples. The magnified image is also shown in the inset.

Another manufacturing process of CNT/gel composite. Using the above-described water-dispersed CNTs, a CNT/gel composite was fabricated (see Supplementary Figs 4 and 5). The CNTs were swollen and uniformly dispersed in water by stirring with a hydrophilic ionic liquid followed by homogenization by high-pressure jet milling. The resulting paste containing dispersed CNT was easily mixed with a photo-cross-linking agent (Irgacure 2959, Nagase & Co., Ltd) and an aqueous cyclodextrin/polyethylene-based polyrotaxane (Advanced Materials Ltd) to form an aqueous CNT/polyrotaxane composite, which is a precursor of CNT conductive gels. The composite was then cast onto a glass plate and was covered with a glass plate. The thickness was controlled using a spacing sheet (50 µm in this experiment). Next, 365-nm ultraviolet light was irradiated on the composite to obtain a 50-µm-thick CNT conductive gel sheet. The swelling ratio is ~2,000 and the volume content of water is 90% in the gel/composite.

A digital ultraviolet exposure system (PMT Corporation, Japan) can create a very fine ultraviolet source with a linewidth of <1 µm. In this experiment, we used a linewidth of 50 µm. The minimum linewidth of the gel depends not only on the spot size of the ultraviolet exposure but also on the thickness of the gel and its adhesive characteristic to the substrates.

The gel/CNT sheet containing microfibrillar cellulose has an adhesive characteristic and easily adheres to the electrodes of an active matrix amplifier. Furthermore, our gel layer can be patterned using a photolithographic process. After the fabrication of the active matrix amplifier, it is coated with the gel precursor and then exposed to light, to pattern the gel on the electrodes of the amplifier.

Young's modulus of the composite gel is ~10 kPa, which is almost the same as that of a brain (the softest region in living creatures), which means that a softness of 10 kPa or less is good enough for electrodes to measure biological signals. Young's modulus was measured using conventional compression and resonance methods.

TEM observation of CNT/rotaxane composite. High-resolution cross-sectional electron microscopy images of three samples were obtained, as shown in Supplementary Fig. 6: (A) multi-walled CNT, (B) CNT/polyrotaxane composite without ionic liquid ((rotaxane (100 mg) and jet-milled CNT (30 mg) mixture was stirred in water) and (C) CNT/polyrotaxane composite with ionic liquid (as described in the main text). The specimens were dried in air and imaged by TEM (80-kV HF-2000 Cold-FE TEM, Hitachi High-Technologies Corp.). Sample A showed a multi-walled CNT structure with three to four walls. Sample B showed a multi-walled CNT structure and a heterogeneous incrustation on the surface, which could be a rotaxane. Sample C showed a very uniform incrustation on the CNT surface. We believe that DEMEBF$_4$ coated the CNT surface owing to its large surface energy and then promoted adhesion of hydrophilic polyrotaxane. Elementary characterization by EDX spectrometry is also shown. Aqueous polyrotaxane-based gels were detected around the CNT, as shown in the figure.

Colony-forming assay for cytotoxic evaluation. Supplementary Fig. 7A shows the procedure of the colony-forming assay with results summarized in Supplementary Table 1. This assay was performed in a certified independent evaluation organization with the Good Laboratory Practice (Kamakura Techno-science Co., Ltd.) according to the guidelines for preclinical biological evaluation of medical materials and devices (Ministry of Health, Labour and Welfare, Japan, memorandum, JIMURENRAKU Iryokiki-Shinsa, 36, 2003 and ISO 10993-5:2009: the Biological Evaluation of Medical Devices—Part 5: Tests for In Vitro Cytotoxicity).

We cultivated 100 Chinese hamster fibroblasts (V79) in a well seeding. First, the CNT/gel composites were finely cut and sterilized by autoclaving (121 °C for 20 min). Then, the extraction liquid was extracted using extraction culture media (non-essential amine acid containing minimum essential medium with 5% fetal

bovine serum: MO5) at 37 °C for 24 h, which corresponds to an undiluted sample, with an extraction ratio of 0.1 g ml^{-1}. The extraction liquid was diluted to 20, 40, 60, 80 and 100%. Each diluted liquid was cast on V79 (100 cells per well) and cultivated at 37 °C for 6 days in 5% CO$_2$ atmosphere. Next, the cells were fixed using methanol for 15 min and dyed using 5% Giemsa stain for 15 min, and the number of cells was counted. A negative control (high-density polyethylene sheet), positive control A with moderate cytotoxicity (0.1% zinc diethyldithiocarbamate (ZDBC)-containing polyurethane film) and positive control B with mild cytotoxicity (0.25% ZDBC-containing polyurethane film) were processed to guarantee the extraction operation. An additional positive control (ZDBC) was also processed to guarantee the sensitivity of the V79 cells.

Supplementary Fig. 7B shows the results of the assay. The polyrotaxane-based gel and CNT/polyrotaxane gel composite without ionic liquid showed no changes in the number of colonies even after the extraction liquid was cast and the cell state was similar to that of the negative control. The CNT/polyrotaxane gel composite with ionic liquid also showed no changes. These results suggest that the CNT conductive gels are not cytotoxic. Supplementary Fig. 8 shows additional details about the counting of the number of cells and the results.

Implant assay for biocompatibility evaluation. The assay was performed in a certified independent evaluation organization in Good Laboratory Practice (Kamakura Techno-science Co., Ltd) according to ISO 10993-6:2007: Biological Evaluation of Medical Devices—Part 6: Tests for Local Effects After Implantation.

For this experiment, three types of bioprobes were prepared, as shown in Supplementary Fig. 8A. The surfaces of the electrodes in these probes were coated with Ag/AgCl (commercially available) (Type1), Ag/AgCl/Au (50 nm) (Type2) and Ag/AgCl/Au/Gel (Type3). The detailed structure of Type3 can be seen in the right figure, which is indispensable for fixing the gel to the electrode. These three electrode types were implanted into the hypodermal tissues of living rabbits for 34 days. The position of the electrodes and the population for the implantation test are shown in Supplementary Fig. 8B. We measured the impedance between the electrodes at daily intervals using an LCR meter (E4980, Agilent), whose current is <0.1 mA, to avoid inflammation by continuous impedance measurements. The average impedance was calculated in terms of the admittance, as shown in Fig. 3b.

Supplementary Fig. 9 shows the magnified cross-sectional images of the raft pathology by staining a subcutaneous tissue after an electrode was explanted (this is the same experiment shown in Fig. 2b–d, for reference). The top surfaces of the grafts were exposed to the three electrodes. Fibrosing cell infiltration was observed near the surface.

Reproductive experiment under different conditions. CNT conductive gels (size: 1×1 cm^2) were implanted into the hypodermal tissues of living rabbits for 1 and 4 weeks. Next, pathology grafts with samples were dyed and analysed by a certified pathological specialist. The degree of foreign-body reaction was quantified based on ISO 10993-6:2007 in terms of the cell type (polymorphonuclear cells, lymphocytes, plasma cells, macrophages and giant cells), necrosis and response (neovascularization, fibrosis and fatty infiltrate). We averaged the irritant ranking scores of the four populations, compared them with those of the negative control and classified them into four categories: non-, slight, moderate and severe irritants.

Supplementary Fig. 10 shows the graft pathologies of the four different samples after implantation for 4 weeks: (A) high-density polyethylene sheet as negative control sample, (B) 200-nm-thick Au layer on 75-µm-thick polyimide substrate as a conventional metal electrode, (C) polyrotaxane-based gel with ionic liquid and (D) CNT/polyrotaxane gel composite with ionic liquid. All graft pathologies, except for the negative control sample, showed fibrosing cell infiltration at the sample interface. Here, the Au electrode caused much larger cell infiltration than the gel-based materials. Supplementary Tables 2 and 3 show more quantitative data analysed from the pathology grafts and a summary of the results. The results clearly indicate the good biocompatibility of the CNT/polyrotaxane gel composite.

Tissue-cleaning method. After explanting the above (Type1), (Type2) and (Type3) electrodes, the animals were transcardially perfused with PBS followed by 4% paraformaldehyde (Sigma-Aldrich, St Louis, MO) in PBS. To label the blood vessel wall, Texas Red-labelled lectin from Lycopersicon esculentum (700 µg lectin for rats, Vector Laboratories, Inc.) was intravenously administered before the perfusion fixation. Hypodermal tissues with implanted gels were postfixed in paraformaldehyde at 4 °C for 24 h. To optically clean the tissues, the tissue blocks were washed in water for 3–16 h at 4 °C and incubated in pretreatment solution 1 (two parts thiodiethanol, four parts glycerol and four parts 30% sucrose solution) for 24 h at room temperature and solution 2 (five parts thiodiethanol and five parts glycerol) for 24 h at room temperature. The samples were then transferred to the final clearing solution (LUCID: nine parts thiodiethanol and one part glycerol) at room temperature. For accurate adjustment of the refractive index of the solutions, the samples were moved to a fresh LUCID solution the next day and were stored at 4 °C until the scheduled multi-photon microscopic observation. All washes and incubations were done in a light-resistant container by constant and gentle shaking. Two days after immersion in LUCID, a satisfactory cleaning effect was achieved. For multiphoton microscopy, excitation was achieved using Chameleon Vision II with a laser oscillator at 860 nm (Coherent, Santa Clara,

CA) or Spectra-Physics MaiTai DeepSee with a laser oscillator at 860 nm (Newport, Santa Clara, CA). A Nikon A1RMP-only Ti GaAsP two-photon microscope (Nikon, Tokyo, Japan) was used (step size, 3 μm) with objective lenses Nikon CFI LWD × 16 (numerical aperture, 0.8; working distance, 3 mm) and Nikon CFI75 APO 25 × W MP (numerical aperture, 1.1; working distance, 2 mm). The images were processed using NIS-Elements C and AR (Nikon). Tiled images were obtained with 20% overlap. Second-harmonic generation was obtained at 436 nm/20 nm (central wavelength/bandwidth). Texas Red and DyLight595 fluorescence were obtained at 629 nm/53 nm (the images are shown in Supplementary Fig. 11).

Organic transistors in ultrathin polymeric substrates. We manufactured a two-dimensional array of organic amplifiers comprising four organic transistors on a 1.2-μm-thick PEN substrate (Fig. 4). Transistor gate electrodes were prepared on the surface of a 1-μm-thick PEN substrate by evaporating a 30-nm-thick Al layer through a shadow mask. A 4-nm-thick (AlO_x) layer was then formed on the Al surface by oxygen plasma treatment (5 min, 300 W). The substrate was then immersed in a 2-propanol solution of n-octadecylphosphonic acid, to create a densely packed 2-nm-thick organic SAM on the oxidized Al surface. The total dielectric gate thickness was therefore 6 nm and it had a capacitance per unit area of 0.6–0.65 μF cm^{-2}. Some 50-nm-thick layers of dinaphtho[2,3-b:2',3'-f]thieno [3,2-b]thiophene (DNTT), an organic semiconductor, for the p-channel TFTs were then deposited by vacuum sublimation through shadow masks. The source and drain contacts were prepared on top of the organic semiconductors by evaporating Au to a thickness of 50 nm through a shadow mask.

***In vivo* implant tolerance of organic transistors.** Organic transistors must show *in vivo* implant tolerance, in addition to biocompatibility. The encapsulation stack comprised 100-nm-thick parylene (diX-SR, Daisankasei Co., Ltd), 200-nm-thick Au and 1.2-μm-thick parylene layers on organic transistors. The entire organic transistor sheet was coated with polyrotaxane-based gel, immersed in saline and then sterilized by autoclaving at 121 °C for 20 min. The technical details of encapsulation and thermal resistance of the organic transistors can be seen in refs 33,34. The electrical mobility changed by 3.2% and the threshold voltage shift was − 0.35 V after high-temperature sterilization (Supplementary Fig. 12B). The sterilized organic transistor sheet was implanted into a hypodermal tissue of a goat (Supplementary Fig. 12A). Although the off-currents of the transistors were one order of magnitude larger than those before implantation, the on/off ratio exceeded 10^4. Furthermore, the average mobility changed by <4.3% and the average threshold voltage (V_{th}) was − 0.13 V (Supplementary Fig. 12C). This result indicates that the organic transistors maintain their electronic performance owing to their excellent encapsulation, enabling the design of sophisticated *in vivo* integrated circuits.

Integration methods for 1.2-μm-thick organic circuits. Supplementary Fig. 13A shows an array of ultraflexible organic pseudo-CMOS inverters on a 1.2-μm-thick PEN substrate. These circuits comprised an ultrathin substrate, enabling them to be spread over arbitrary curved surfaces (Supplementary Fig. 13B). The ultraflexible amplifier comprised the pseudo-CMOS inverter with a transistor active matrix, capacitors and resistors. The contact holes of each layer were produced using CO_2 laser and/or green laser, depending on the materials and the size required for contact holes. The matrix, manufactured at the bottom of the pseudo-CMOS inverter substrate, was used to address the pixel position. Supplementary Fig. 13C shows the circuit diagram of the active matrix amplifier array. The active matrix amplifier system comprising organic transistors (selector TFT) enables random-access readout with high spatiotemporal resolution and sensitivity. Supplementary Fig. 13D shows a pseudo-CMOS inverter comprising four p-type transistors. The channel widths and lengths of the transistors were precisely designed to detect and amplify weak biosignals. M_1 has a channel width and length of 2,000 and 20 μm or 1,000 and 10 μm, respectively, whereas M_2, M_{UP} and M_{DP} have a channel width and length of 6,000 and 20 μm or 3,000 and 10 μm, respectively. An input capacitor array is also shown.

The conductive CNT-sheet/gel composites were manually integrated to an ultrathin-film amplifier array. The gel/CNT-sheet composite containing microfibrillar cellulose has an adhesive characteristic and easily adheres to the electrodes of the active matrix amplifier, although it strongly depends on the degree of the content of the microfibrillar cellulose. Furthermore, our gel layer can be patterned using a photolithographic process. After the fabrication of the active matrix amplifier, the gel composites are placed on the input electrodes of the amplifier array. Owing to the parylene encapsulation layers, active matrix amplifier and the input electrodes maintain their electrical performance *in vivo*. These layers, manufactured independently, were laminated and integrated using anisotropic conductive films (ANISOLM, Hitachi Chemical Co., Ltd).

Material profiling and cross-sectional imaging of the organic transistors on a 1.2-μm-thick substrate was performed using ultrahigh resolution scanning TEM (STEM) and EDX analysis system. Supplementary Fig. 14A shows a cross-sectional image of the organic transistors on a 1.2-μm-thick substrate using ultrahigh resolution STEM (200-kV HD-2700 Cs-corrected STEM, Hitachi High-Technologies Corp.). The cross-section shows four layers. Supplementary Fig. 14B shows the characterization by EDX spectrometry. The spectra show that only a few nanoscale metal and molecule

structures can be formed on very thin plastic substrates. Supplementary Fig. 15 shows other cross-sectional images and profiles of the constituent materials of the organic transistors. These spectra validate the feasibility of our manufacturing process.

Morphology of DNTT on SAM. The morphology of DNTT was determined by atomic force microscopy. We prepared two different samples: DNTT manufactured on SAM dielectric gate with SiO_2 wafer and that with a 1.2-μm-thick PEN substrate; the other layers were identical. The average mobility of DNTT on the respective surfaces was 2.3 and 1.0 cm^2 V^{-1} s^{-1}. The lower mobility on the PEN substrate might be due to the slightly rough surface of the SAM dielectric gate layer affected by the substrate roughness. The smoothness of the respective surfaces was ~0.18 and 2–3 nm RMS. The grain size of DNTT on the PEN substrate was slightly smaller than that on the SiO_2 wafer, which might also be due to the substrate roughness (Supplementary Fig. 16).

Manufacturing process on a 1-μm-thick substrate. Supplementary Fig. 17A shows the drain current as a function of the drain-source voltage of a DNTT transistor (V_{GS} in steps of 0.5 V). Supplementary Fig. 17B shows the drain and gate current as a function of the gate-source voltage for a DNTT transistor (V_{DS}: − 2 V). The transfer characteristics of the ten transistors were plotted to show the variation. Because of the small thickness of the gate dielectric (6 nm), the operating voltage was ~2 V. The average field-effect mobility was 1 cm^2 V^{-1} s^{-1} from the transfer characteristics. The channel width and length of the transistors were 500 and 50 μm, respectively.

The manufacturing process, especially the oxygen plasma treatment, affects the electrical performance of organic transistors. Supplementary Fig. 17C shows the mobility, on/off ratio and saturation current of four different organic transistors under various plasma process conditions: (A) 100 W for 10 min, (B) 150 W for 5 min, (C) 150 W for 10 min, (D) 300 W for 5 min and (E) 300 W for 10 min; the other manufacturing conditions were fixed. Condition (D) produces the best mobility of 1 cm V^{-1} s^{-1} and large on/off ratio exceeding 10^5. The other conditions result in lower mobilities mainly because of the rougher surface in condition (E) and the lower packing density of the SAMs on the AlO_x layer due to insufficient plasma exposure.

Bending test. Supplementary Fig. 18 shows the experimental setup for the bending test of the organic transistors. Bending stresses were applied to the flexible circuits fixed on the stage and push plate using a numerically controlled mechanical stage. The bending radii were precisely measured using a digital microscope (Keyence) from the side of the flexible circuits. All measurements were performed in ambient air. The transistor characteristics were measured using a semiconductor parameter analyser (B1500A, Agilent) with manual probes.

Design of organic transistor for higher amplifier gain. To obtain high amplifier gain and large power to amplify weak biosignals, the dimensions of the four organic transistors, especially the channel width (W) and length (L), should be carefully designed. Typically, we design organic transistors with $W = 6,000$ μm and $L = 20$ μm, which can produce large currents exceeding 100 μA and leakage current on the order of nanoamperes, owing to the excellent insulating characteristics of the SAM dielectric gate layer (Supplementary Fig. 19). The mobility was 0.9 cm V^{-1} s^{-1}. Depending on the frequency response required for the applications, we also designed organic transistors with $W = 3,000$ μm and $L = 10$ μm, which is much faster than those with $W = 6,000$ μm and $L = 20$ μm, as described below.

Pseudo-CMOS inverter. Although the pseudo-CMOS inverter comprises four p-type transistors (Supplementary Fig. 20A), the inverter characteristics are superior to those of the organic unipolar inverters and conventional organic CMOS inverters. Supplementary Fig. 20B shows the output voltage and gain as a function of the input voltage, where V_{SS} is − 1 V and V_{DD} varies from 2 to 0.5 V. This inverter can operate within 2 V and the signal gain exceeds 400 even at $V_{DD} = 0.5$ V. Thus, excellent inverter characteristics are exhibited even at a 2-V operation.

Supplementary Fig. 20C shows the oscillation frequency of a five-stage ring oscillator comprising five pseudo-CMOS inverters, which was cited in our previous report[9]. From the result, the operating speed of the single transistor was 42.7 kHz and the propagation delay per stage was 23.4 μs. This temporal resolution is sufficiently fast; thus, the system can measure the biological signals, which are within 1 kHz.

Signal gain and frequency response of organic amplifiers. Supplementary Fig. 21A shows the circuit diagram of an organic amplifier with a CNT gel. Supplementary Fig. 21B shows the output signal voltage and amplifier gain as a function of the input signal voltage. The former is proportional to the latter and the gain is almost constant (~100 at input exceeding 2 mV). Here we should note that the high amplifier gain exceeding 100 was obtained, owing to the large capacitor of 670 nF and internal resistance of 10–50 kΩ, whose gain is consistent with the theoretical estimation indicated below.

Supplementary Fig. 21C shows the frequency response of the amplifier gain. The same frequency response was obtained for repeated experiments, demonstrating excellent reproducibility. The frequency response of the amplifier gain strongly depends on the input capacitor (C). To evaluate the effect of C, we constructed three different amplifiers with C values of 0.67, 2.2 and 11 µF.

The spatial resolution of the amplifier array was determined by the input capacitance of the amplifier, whose size was 6 mm × 6 mm. The periodicity of the circuit was 7 mm. The temporal resolution was determined by two operating speeds: one was the operating speed of the amplifier, which corresponded to the recording speed; the other was the operating speed of the pseudo-CMOS inverter in the amplifier, which corresponded to the addressing speed in the active matrix amplifier. Figure 5d in the main text and in Supplementary Figs 20C and 21C show the operating speed of the amplifier (recording time) whose amplifier gains were 550 in the frequency range from 1 to 30 Hz, 71 at 100 Hz and 30.9 at 1 kHz.

Detection of ischaemic state due to myocardial infarction. Supplementary Fig. 22 shows a picture of the ischaemic state of a rat heart due to myocardial infarction. A coronary artery was ligated to induce a myocardial infarction in the right half of the heart. Figure 5f shows the input signal voltage of the abnormal rat heart and the amplified output signal voltage from the organic amplifier.

Effects of the CNT-sheet/gel-composite electrode. To evaluate the conductive-gel sheet, body surface electrocardiographs were obtained using two different gel probes (size: $1 \times 1\ cm^2$, thickness: 1 mm) for comparison. One is a commercially available conductive gel comprising a graphite-sheet electrode with acrylamide gel (Supplementary Fig. 23A) and the other is a sheet (Supplementary Fig. 23B). In this experiment, we used a conventional amplifier system marketed for medical use (Neuropack µ, MEB-9104; Nihon Kohden Co., Ltd, Tokyo, Japan; gain: 3,000) to evaluate the stand-alone CNT-sheet/gel-composite electrodes. Body-surface electrocardiographs were clearly detected by both gel probes.

Admittance measurement. Figure 1g shows the comparison of the admittance among the materials in a wide frequency range. We used electrodes made of CNT/gel, graphite/gel, Au/gel and Al/gel to compare the admittance of the materials in the vertical direction. To prepare CNT/gel electrode, we formed hydrogel on our conductive CNT sheet. Graphite/gel electrode was made of graphite electrode, which was typically used in medical practice(Vitrode V, Nihon Kohden). Commercial-type hydrogel on this graphite electrode was removed by swelling in pure water. Next, we formed hydrogel on bare graphite electrode. Au/gel and Al/gel electrode was prepared on polyimmide substrate. By the same way, hydrogel was formed. We measured the impedance between the electrodes using an LCR meter (E4980, Agilent), to avoid damages of the electrodes by continuous impedance measurements. The conductive gel-composite electrode is used as the interface between the electronic amplifier and an adjacent cell or tissue. In this instance, admittance in the vertical direction is important rather than that in the traverse direction.

In the structure of the CNT/gel electrodes, large capacitance is generated because of the electronic double layer phenomenon. Reactance X is determined by the following equation: $X = \frac{1}{j2\pi fC}$, where C is the capacitance and f is the frequency. A large C leads to small reactance (large admittance: admittance is defined as the reciprocal of reactance). Therefore, owing to the large C, large admittance can be maintained even in the low-frequency range, as shown in Fig. 1g.

A large capacitance in the system results in a resistance-capacitance (RC) time constant, thus leading to a signal propagation delay. On the other hand, the biological signals from a living body are within 1 kHz. Therefore, the propagation delay originating from a large RC does not affect the detection of biosignals. The AC admittance of the CNT/gel electrodes can be observed in Supplementary Fig. 3, obtained from four different samples. The magnified image is also shown in the inset.

References

1. Ito, K. Novel cross-linking concept of polymer network: synthesis, structure, and properties of slide-ring gels with freely movable junctions. *Polym. J.* **39**, 489–499 (2007).
2. Kishi, R. *et al.* Electro-conductive double-network hydrogels. *J. Polym. Sci. B. Polym. Phys.* **50**, 790–796 (2012).
3. Matsumoto, K., Sogabe, S. & Endo, T. Conductive networked polymer gel electrolytes composed of poly(meth)acrylate, lithium salt, and ionic liquid. *J. Polym. Sci. A. Polym. Chem.* **50**, 1317–1324 (2012).
4. Mei, X. & Ouyang, J. Highly conductive and transparent single-walled carbon nanotube thin films fabricated by gel coating. *J. Mater. Chem.* **21**, 17842–17849 (2011).
5. Chung, K. *et al.* Structural and molecular interrogation of intact biological systems. *Nature* **497**, 332–337 (2013).
6. Hama, H. *et al.* Scale: a chemical approach for fluorescence imaging and reconstruction of transparent mouse brain. *Nat. Neurosci.* **14**, 1481–1488 (2011).
7. Ke, M.-T., Fujimoto, S. & Imai, T. SeeDB: a simple and morphology-preserving optical clearing agent for neuronal circuit reconstruction. *Nat. Neurosci.* **16**, 1154–1161 (2013).
8. Chung, K. & Deisseroth, K. CLARITY for mapping the nervous system. *Nat. Methods* **10**, 508–513 (2013).
9. Fukuda, K. *et al.* Organic pseudo-CMOS circuits for low-voltage large-gain high-speed operation. *IEEE Electron. Device Lett.* **32**, 1448–1450 (2011).
10. Yamamoto, T. & Takimiya, K. Facile synthesis of highly π-extended heteroarenes, dinaphtho[2,3-b:2′,3′-f]chalcogenopheno[3,2-b]chalcogenophenes, and their application in field-effect transistors. *J. Am. Chem. Soc.* **129**, 2224–2225 (2007).
11. Klauk, H., Zschieschang, U., Pflaum, J. & Halik, M. Ultralow-power organic complementary circuits. *Nature* **445**, 745–748 (2007).
12. Yokota, T. *et al.* Sheet-type flexible organic active matrix amplifier system using pseudo-CMOS circuits with floating-gate structure. *IEEE Trans. Electron. Devices* **59**, 3434–3441 (2012).
13. Sekitani, T., Zschieschang, U., Klauk, H. & Someya, T. Flexible organic transistors and circuits with extreme bending stability. *Nat. Mater.* **9**, 1015–1022 (2010).
14. Vanhatalo, S., Voipio, J. & Kaila, K. Full-band EEG (FbEEG): an emerging standard in electroencephalography. *Clin. Neurophysiol.* **116**, 1–8 (2005).
15. Garnier, F., Hajlaoui, R., Yassar, A. & Srivastava, P. All-polymer field-effect transistor realized by printing techniques. *Science* **265**, 1684–1686 (1994).
16. Forrest, S. R. The path to ubiquitous and low-cost organic electronic appliances on plastic. *Nature* **428**, 911–918 (2004).
17. Kim, D. H. *et al.* Stretchable and foldable silicon integrated circuits. *Science* **320**, 507–511 (2008).
18. Viventi, J. *et al.* Flexible, foldable, actively multiplexed, high-density electrode array for mapping brain activity in vivo. *Nat. Neurosci.* **14**, 1599–1605 (2011).
19. Qing, Q. *et al.* Nanowire transistor arrays for mapping neural circuits in acute brain slices. *Proc. Natl Acad. Sci. USA* **107**, 1882–1887 (2010).
20. Mannsfeld, S. C. B. *et al.* Highly sensitive flexible pressure sensors with microstructured rubber dielectric layers. *Nat. Mater.* **9**, 859–864 (2010).
21. Hsu, Y. J., Jia, Z. & Kymissis, I. A locally amplified strain sensor based on a piezoelectric polymer and organic field-effect transistors. *IEEE Trans. Electron. Devices* **58**, 910–917 (2011).
22. Angione, M. D. *et al.* Interfacial electronic effects in functional biolayers integrated into organic field-effect transistors. *Proc. Natl Acad. Sci. USA* **109**, 6429–6434 (2012).
23. Berggren, M. & Richter-Dahlfors, A. Organic bioelectronics. *Adv. Mater.* **19**, 3201–3213 (2007).
24. Cicoira, F. *et al.* Influence of device geometry on sensor characteristics of planar organic electrochemical transistors. *Adv. Mater.* **22**, 1012–1016 (2010).
25. Khodagholy, D. *et al.* Organic electrochemical transistor incorporating an ionogel as a solid state electrolyte for lactate sensing. *J. Mater. Chem.* **22**, 4440–4443 (2012).
26. Lee, S. *et al.* A strain-absorbing design for tissue–machine interfaces using a tunable adhesive gel. *Nat. Commun.* **5**, 5898 (2014).
27. Khodagholy, D. *et al.* Highly conformable conducting polymer electrodes for in vivo recordings. *Adv. Mater.* **23**, H268–H272 (2011).
28. Khodagholy, D. *et al.* High transconductance organic electrochemical transistors. *Nat. Commun.* **4**, 2133 (2013).
29. Graudejus, O., Morrison, III B., Goletiani, C., Yu, Z. & Wagner, S. Encapsulating elastically stretchable neural interfaces: yield, resolution, and recording/stimulation of neural activity. *Adv. Funct. Mater.* **22**, 640–651 (2012).
30. Feili, D., Schuettler, M. & Stieglitz, T. Matrix-addressable, active electrode arrays for neural stimulation using organic semiconductors—cytotoxicity and pilot experiments in vivo. *J. Neural Eng.* **5**, 68–74 (2008).
31. Huang, J., Dupont, P. E., Undurti, A., Triedman, J. K. & Cleveland, R. O. Producing diffuse ultrasound reflections from medical instruments using a quadratic residue diffuser. *Ultrasound Med. Biol.* **32**, 721–727 (2006).
32. Hopenfeld, B. & Ashikaga, H. Abstract 2681: mechanism of electrocardiographic U wave body surface potential distributions: A 3-D modeling study. *Circulation* **120**, S678–S679 (2009).
33. Sekitani, T. & Someya, T. Air-stable operation of organic field-effect transistors on plastic films using organic/metallic hybrid passivation layers. *Jpn J. Appl. Phys.* **46**, 4300–4305 (2007).
34. Kuribara, K. *et al.* Organic transistors with high thermal stability for medical applications. *Nat. Commun.* **3**, 723 (2012).

Acknowledgements

We thank Professor Takayasu Sakurai and Professor Makoto Takamiya of the University of Tokyo for the valuable discussions. We also thank Daisankasei Co., Ltd, for the high-purity parylene (diX-SR). The biocompatible assay was performed in a certified independent evaluation organization with the Good Laboratory Practice (Kamakura Techno-science Co., Ltd) according to the guidelines for preclinical biological evaluation of medical materials and devices (Ministry of Health, Labour and Welfare, Japan, memorandum, JIMURENRAKJ Iryokiki-Shinsa, 36, 2003 and ISO 10993-5:2009: the Biological Evaluation of Medical Devices—Part 5: Tests for *In Vitro* Cytotoxicity).

Author contributions

T.Se., T.Y., K.K., M.K. and T. Someya designed, fabricated and characterized the transistors and active matrices. T.Y., K.K., M.K., Y.I., M.S. and T.I. performed device fabrication and characterization for animal experiments. Y.I., M.S., T.I., Y.A. and H.O. analysed data from a medical point of view. T.F. analysed data from a synthetic chemistry point of view. All the authors prepared figures and wrote the manuscript.

Additional information

Competing financial interests: The authors declare no competing financial interests.

19

Toxic tau oligomer formation blocked by capping of cysteine residues with 1,2-dihydroxybenzene groups

Yoshiyuki Soeda[1,†], Misato Yoshikawa[1], Osborne F.X. Almeida[2], Akio Sumioka[1], Sumihiro Maeda[3], Hiroyuki Osada[4,5], Yasumitsu Kondoh[4,5], Akiko Saito[6], Tomohiro Miyasaka[7], Tetsuya Kimura[1], Masaaki Suzuki[8], Hiroko Koyama[9], Yuji Yoshiike[10], Hachiro Sugimoto[11], Yasuo Ihara[7,12] & Akihiko Takashima[1]

Neurofibrillary tangles, composed of hyperphosphorylated tau fibrils, are a pathological hallmark of Alzheimer's disease; the neurofibrillary tangle load correlates strongly with clinical progression of the disease. A growing body of evidence indicates that tau oligomer formation precedes the appearance of neurofibrillary tangles and contributes to neuronal loss. Here we show that tau oligomer formation can be inhibited by compounds whose chemical backbone includes 1,2-dihydroxybenzene. Specifically, we demonstrate that 1,2-dihydroxybenzene-containing compounds bind to and cap cysteine residues of tau and prevent its aggregation by hindering interactions between tau molecules. Further, we show that orally administered DL-isoproterenol, an adrenergic receptor agonist whose skeleton includes 1,2-dihydroxybenzene and which penetrates the brain, reduces the levels of detergent-insoluble tau, neuronal loss and reverses neurofibrillary tangle-associated brain dysfunction. Thus, compounds that target the cysteine residues of tau may prove useful in halting the progression of Alzheimer's disease and other tauopathies.

[1] Department of Aging Neurobiology, National Center for Geriatrics and Gerontology, Obu, Aichi 474-8511, Japan. [2] Department of Stress Neurology and Neurogenesis, Max Planck Institute of Psychiatry, Kraepelinstrasse, 2-10, Munich 80804, Germany. [3] Gladstone Institute of Neurological Disease, University of California, San Francisco, California 94158-2261, USA. [4] Chemical Biology Research Group, RIKEN Center for Sustainable Resource Science (CSRS), RIKEN, Wako, Saitama 351-0198, Japan. [5] Antibiotics Laboratory, Advanced Science Institute, RIKEN, Wako, Saitama 351-0198, Japan. [6] Graduate School of Engineering, Osaka Electro-communication University (OECU), 18-8 Hatsu-cho, Osaka 572-8530, Japan. [7] Department of Neuropathology, Faculty of Life and Medical Sciences, Doshisha University, Kyotanabe, Kyoto 610-0394, Japan. [8] Department of Clinical and Experimental Neuroimaging, Center for Development of Advanced Medicine for Dementia, National Center for Geriatrics and Gerontology, Obu, Aichi 474-8511, Japan. [9] Division of Regeneration and Advanced Medical Science, Gifu University Graduate School of Medicine, Gifu 501-1194, Japan. [10] Alzheimer's Disease Project Team, National Center for Geriatrics and Gerontology, Obu, Aichi 474-8511, Japan. [11] Laboratory of Structural Neuropathology, Graduate School of Brain Science, Doshisha University, Kizugawa, Kyoto 619-0225, Japan. [12] Laboratory of Cognition and Aging, Doshisha University, Kizugawa, Kyoto 619-0225, Japan. † Present address: Study Promotion Strategy Section/Clinical Research Center, Fukushima Medical University, Hikarigaoka 1, Fukushima 960-1295, Japan. Correspondence and requests for materials should be addressed to A.T. (email: kenneth@ncgg.go.jp).

Alzheimer's disease (AD) is a progressive neurodegenerative disease, initially characterized by impaired episodic memory and eventually, severe cognitive decline. Since age is the most important risk factor for AD development, the present increase in lifespan across all demographics prioritizes the search for ameliorative and preventative treatments for the disease. Currently, cholinesterase inhibitors and N-methyl-D-aspartate receptor antagonists are used to treat AD symptoms with limited success; the current consensus view is that stopping disease progression will require the development of disease-modifying therapies based on defined pathogenic mechanisms[1].

Deposition of amyloid β (Aβ) peptide in the extracellular space and formation of senile plaques, as well as the intracellular accumulation of tau protein that gives rise to neurofibrillary tangles (NFTs), with contemporaneous neuronal loss are the key pathological hallmarks of AD[2]. The amyloid hypothesis of AD posits that Aβ is the primary cause of dementia owing to its ability to induce the formation of NFT and synaptic and neuronal loss in the neocortex[3-7]. Tau tangle formation occurs downstream from Aβ deposition and appears to be essential for the establishment of AD; the latter view is supported by studies showing that tau depletion prevents Aβ-induced memory impairment in various lines of human amyloid precursor protein-overexpressing mice[8,9].

To date, Aβ-targeted therapies (for example, immunotherapy) have failed for a variety of reasons, including failure to hamper neurodegeneration and cognitive dysfunction in patients with AD[10,11]. The focus of AD drug discovery research has recently shifted towards tau[12] because, in contrast to Aβ load, tau pathology correlates with the degree of cognitive impairment[13,14] and neuronal loss[15,16]. Tau is an attractive target because patients with frontotemporal dementia and Parkinsonism-linked to chromosome-17 (FTDP-17) carry a mutation in the tau gene and display NFT and neuronal loss in the absence of Aβ deposition[17-19]. Moreover, mice overexpressing mutant tau exhibit NFTs, neuronal loss and behavioural abnormalities[20-24]. Several lines of evidence, based on the results of experiments involving expression of the human P301L transgene in mice[25,26] or the human FTDP17 mutation in fruit flies[27], link neuronal death to the tau aggregation process, rather than to NFT formation.

Tau protein in NFTs is highly phosphorylayed, reflecting an imbalance in the activities of various kinases and phosphatases[28,29]. Although the role of phosphorylation in the Tau aggregation process is still debated (for example, in vitro evidence suggests Tau phosphorylation inhibits[30] or has no role on tau aggregation[31]), hyperphosphorylated and/or mutated tau is suggested to adopt an alternative structure that promotes interactions between individual tau molecules. For example, our own in vitro experiments have proposed that tau aggregation occurs in a step-wise manner: initially, tau molecules bind to each other, through disulfide binding of their Cys residues[32], to form soluble tau oligomers[32,33]; in a second step, these oligomers, comprised of ~40 tau molecules, grow and precipitate as granular tau oligomers with a β-sheet structure; last, the granular tau oligomers bind to each other and form tau fibrils[33].

Granular tau oligomers are detectable in the prefrontal cortex at Braak stage I, whereas NFT appear much later (Braak stage V)[34], indicating that their formation represents a crucial early pathogenic event. Observations that neuronal death is strongly associated with the presence of Sarkosyl-insoluble tau[26], imply that granular tau oligomers with a β-sheet structure are a major toxic species of tau and that prevention of their formation could be a promising therapeutic strategy[35]. Following this rationale, we screened a small-molecule library for compounds with the potential to inhibit the formation of granular tau oligomers. We report here that compounds containing 1,2-dihydroxybenzene inhibit granular tau oligomer formation by modifying the Cys residues of tau, thereby reducing Sarkosyl-insoluble tau levels, neuronal death and brain dysfunction in P301L tau-transgenic mice.

Results

Chemical array screening for tau aggregation inhibitors. To find an inhibitor of granular tau oligomer formation, we screened a series of tau-binding compounds, using a small-molecule array consisting of 6,788 compounds in the RIKEN Natural Products Depository (NPDepo). This initial screen led to the identification of 86 compounds displayed the potential to associate with tau. These compounds were subsequently assayed for thioflavin T (ThT) binding, with the exclusion of false positives using a pelleting assay in which tau was quantified in pellets derived from ultracentrifugation of a mixture of tau aggregates. Three compounds, epinephrine (Fig. 1a), pyrocatechol violet (Fig. 1b) and lobaric acid (Fig. 1c), markedly decreased ThT binding (Fig. 1d–f) and insoluble (aggregated) tau in the pellet fraction (Fig. 1g–i). As the chemical backbones of epinephrine and pyrocatechol violet consist of 1,2-dihydroxybenzene (Fig. 1a,b), we hypothesized that 1,2-dihydroxybenzene endows these compounds with the ability to inhibit tau aggregation.

Inhibition of tau aggregation by 1,2-dihydroxybenzene. Supporting our hypothesis, we observed dose-dependent reductions in heparin-induced ThT fluorescence when cell-free preparations containing recombinant wild-type 2N4R tau were exposed to a series of 1,2-dihydroxybenzene-containing compounds. Results are shown for L-3,4-dihydroxyphenylalanine (Fig. 2a), dopamine (Fig. 2b), norepinephrine (Fig. 2c), epinephrine (Fig. 2d) and isoproterenol (ISO; Fig. 2e); adrenochrome, an oxidized form of epinephrine (Fig. 2f), also reduced ThT fluorescence. Octopamine, a compound with a 1-dihydroxybenzene structure, and 3-methoxytyramine, a catechol-O-methyltransferase-mediated metabolite of dopamine, did not alter ThT fluorescence (Fig. 2g,h), verifying the specificity of the effects produced by the compounds with a 1,2-dihydroxybenzene skeleton. This set of data showed that compounds with a 1,2-dihydroxybenzene skeleton can inhibit tau aggregation independently of their oxidation state. Subsequent investigations focused on ISO, a β1/2 adrenergic receptor agonist that can cross the blood–brain barrier (BBB)[36,37]; ISO is indicated for a number of medical conditions and neither interferes with neurotransmission nor induces major adverse effects. ISO treatment of Neuro2A cells engineered to stably express P301L tau[38] results in dose-dependent reductions of SDS-insoluble tau levels in the absence of alterations in the levels of soluble tau (Fig. 3a). Importantly, the inhibitory actions of ISO on tau aggregation were not blocked by pretreatment of P301L tau-expressing Neuro2A cells with propranolol (1–10 μM), a competitive antagonist of the β adrenergic receptor (Fig. 3b), indicating that the inhibitory action of ISO on tau aggregation is not mediated through β adrenergic receptors.

We subsequently made a detailed examination of heparin-induced tau aggregates to gain further insight into the mechanism of action of ISO. Sucrose density gradient centrifugation demonstrated the absence of filamentous tau in ISO-treated (100 μM) tau aggregate mixtures (fractions 4–6; Fig. 4a). This analysis also showed that ISO markedly reduced granular tau oligomer levels (fraction 3) while increasing the levels of tau in fractions 1–2 (Fig. 4a). Analysis of heparin-induced tau aggregates by atomic force microscopy

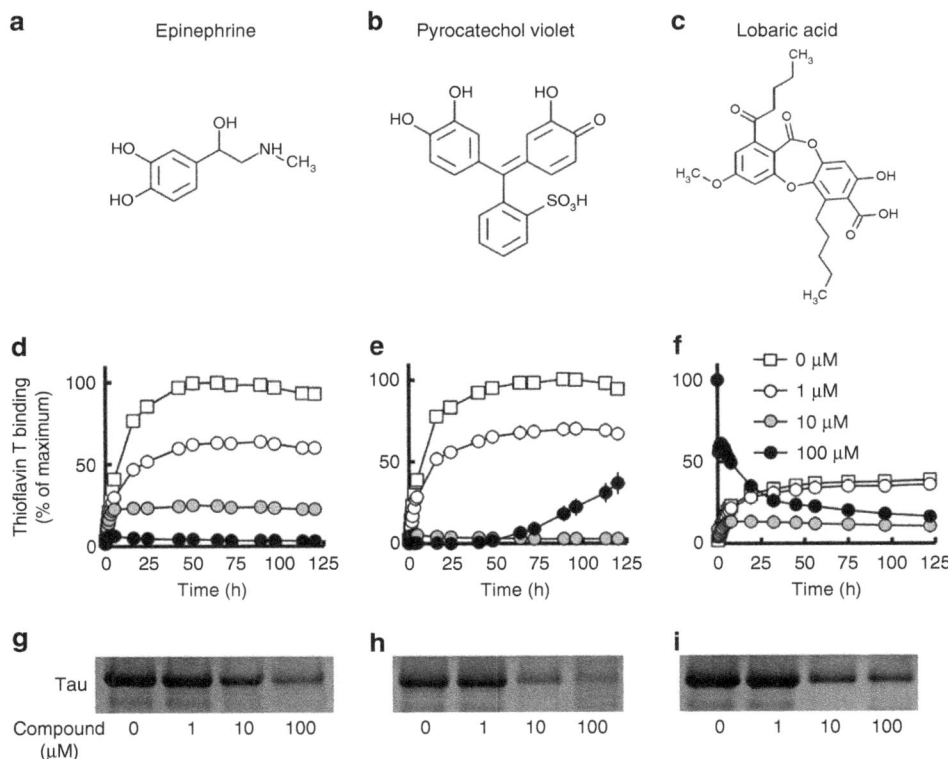

Figure 1 | Identification of tau aggregation inhibitor. Epinephrine (**a,d,g**), pyrocatechol violet (**b,e,h**) and lobaric acid (**c,f,i**) were screened as tau aggregation inhibitors. Inhibitory effects of tau aggregation were determined by fluorescence of thioflavin T (**d,e,f**) and pelleting assay (**g,h,i**) of heparin-induced tau polymerization incubated with various concentrations of compounds (1, 10 and 100 μM). Dimethyl sulfoxide was used as the vehicle. Thioflavin T fluorescence was measured at the indicated time, and results were represented as percentage of maximum thioflavin T fluorescence (**d,e,f**; mean ± s.d. of triplicate experiments; $n = 3$).

(AFM) revealed that ISO treatment leads to a significant reduction of the number of tau filaments and granular tau oligomers and an increase in the number of small tau granules (Fig. 4b). These observations suggest that ISO maintains tau in a soluble form or limits its conversion to small, amorphous granules. This interpretation is consistent with our finding that, under non-reducing conditions, ISO prevents tau molecules from forming soluble oligomers (Fig. 4c).

Inhibitory mechanism of 1,2-dihydroxybenzene. ISO-coated magnetic FG (Functional magnetic) beads (Supplementary Fig. 1) were used to identify the binding site of 1,2-dihydroxybenzene compounds to tau; for this, FG beads were incubated with tau in the presence (+) or absence (−) of ISO before elution with either 1 M KCl or sample buffer (SB). As shown in Fig. 5a, tau-ISO complexes could be efficiently ut not KCl, indicating that the protein–drug interaction depends on non-ionic bonding. Further, we observed that ISO bound monomeric, dimeric, trimeric and tetrameric forms of tau. Compared with when ISO was not included in the incubation mixture, FG beads bound monomeric tau more strongly (14.1-fold) than dimeric tau (2.2-fold) in the presence of ISO, whereas the amounts of trimeric and tetrameric tau bonding to the FG beads were not influenced by ISO (Fig. 5b). Thus, these results demonstrate that ISO primarily associates with monomeric species of tau.

The site at which ISO binds to tau was further explored by comparing the binding of the drug to wild-type tau and a mutant form of tau that lacks the microtubule-binding region (ΔMTBR). As tau could only be eluted (recovered) when wild-type tau was used (Fig. 5c), we conclude that ISO binding to tau depends on

the presence of MTBR. More precise information regarding the ISO-MTBR site of interaction was obtained by pre-treating FG beads with peptides corresponding to each of the four repeats of tau (R1–R4) before the addition of the drug and subsequent recovery of ISO-tau complexes. Such recovery was only possible from beads that had been pre-treated with vehicle or R1 and R4 peptides (Fig. 5d), indicating that ISO binds to sites localized in the R2 and/or R3 regions of tau.

The R2 and R3 regions of tau are characterized by cysteine residues (positions 291 and 322) and hexapeptides (positions 275–280 in PHF6*; positions 306–311 in PHF6); these regions are critical for tau fibril formation[39–41]. By testing the ability of ISO to bind to deletion mutants of tau (ΔPHF6- and ΔPHF6*-2N4R tau) and in mutant forms of tau in which Cys was substituted by Ala (C291, 322A-2N4R and C322A-2N3R tau), we observed associations between ISO, ΔPHF6- and ΔPHF6*-2N4R tau, but not C291, 322A-2N4R and C322A-2N3R tau (Fig. 5e); this demonstrated that ISO binds Cys residues in tau. Based on this and other results reported above, we propose that 1,2-dihydroxybenzene non-ionically binds Cys residues in the MTBR and thus inhibits the formation of tau oligomers by occluding intermolecular tau interactions. We next used mass spectrometry to confirm that 1,2-dihydroxybenzene binds Cys residues in tau; for this, a partial Cys-containing peptide of tau, R3' (skvtskcgslgn; molecular weight (MW) = 1,180.3), was analysed after incubation with either the vehicle or the 1,2-dihydroxybenzene-containing compounds, ISO (MW = 211.3) and pyrocatechol (MW = 110.1). Incubation of the R3' peptide with the vehicle yielded two peaks ($m/z = 1,180.5$ and $2,358.0$), corresponding to peptide monomers and dimers (Fig. 6a); incubation with ISO resulted in a distinct peak ($m/z = 1,389.7$),

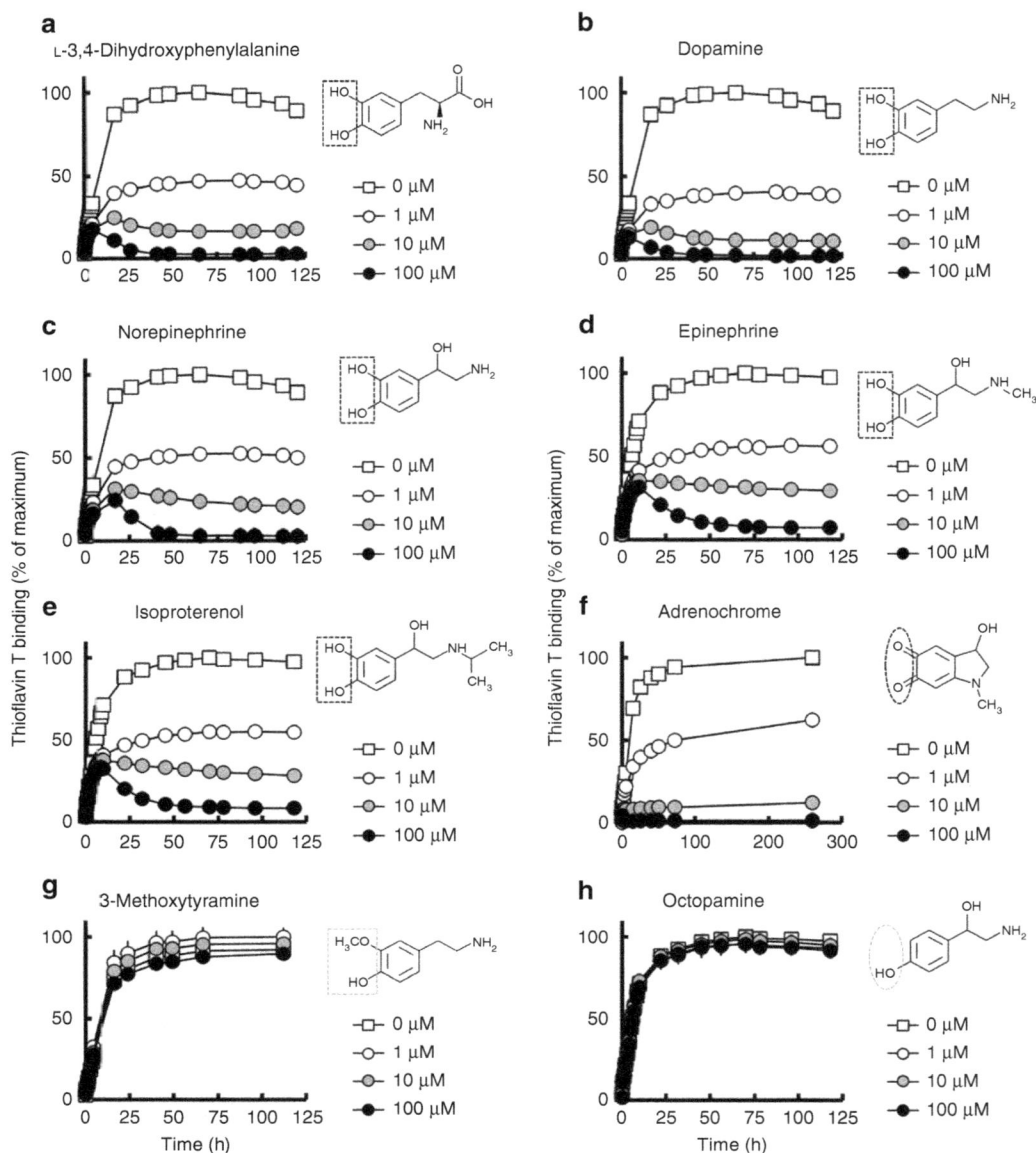

Figure 2 | Inhibitory effects of 1,2-dihydroxybenzene-containing compounds and their derivative compounds on tau aggregation. Thioflavin T-binding activity was dose-dependently inhibited by L-3,4-dihydroxyphenylalanine (**a**), dopamine (**b**), norepinephrine (**c**), epinephrine (**d**) and isoproterenol (**e**) (1,2-dihydroxybenezene; black dotted square), and adrenochrome (**f**) (o-quinone; black dotted circle), but not by octopamine (**h**) (1-hydroxybenzene; grey dotted circle) or 3-methoxythylamine (**g**) (1-hydroxy-2-methoxybenzene; grey dotted square). Results are shown as percentage of maximum fluorescence (mean ± s.d. of triplicate experiments; $n = 3$).

as well as peaks corresponding to the R3' peptide monomers and dimers (Fig. 6b and Supplementary Table 1). Peak shifts ($m/z = 1,180.6 \rightarrow 1,288.5$) were also detected after incubation with pyrocatechol (Fig. 6c and Supplementary Table 1), but not with octopamine, a 1-hydroxybenzene containing compound (Fig. 6d). No peak shifts were observed when a mutant Cys → Ala R3' peptide (skvtskagslgn; MW = 1,143.2) was incubated with the vehicle (Fig. 6e), ISO (Fig. 6f), pyrocatechol (Fig. 6g) or octopamine (Fig. 6h). Together, these analyses confirmed that ISO could block tau aggregation through interaction of its 1,2-dihydroxybenzene group with Cys residues in tau.

Effects of ISO in an animal model of tauopathy. To investigate the efficacy of ISO in inhibiting tau aggregation and subsequent neuronal loss in a relevant animal model of tauopathy, we used a transgenic mouse line that expresses a highly aggregating form of tau, encoded by the human P301L tau gene. Studies were performed in aged mice (17–18 months) as the amount of Sarkosyl-insoluble tau aggregate in the brain increases with age[26]. Animals (non-transgenic controls and P301L tau transgenic mice) received DL-ISO in their chow at dose of 1.5 mg g^{-1} chow; food intake and body weight did not change over the duration (3 months) of treatment (Supplementary Fig. 5). The oral DL-ISO regimen did not alter TBS-soluble levels of tau, but significantly reduced the load of Sarkosyl-insoluble tau in the cortex (26.1 ± 14.5%; $n = 12$), $P = 0.01482$ (unpaired Welch's t-test), Fig. 7a) and hippocampus (36.7 ± 28.3% ($n = 8$), $P = 0.03174$ (unpaired Student's t-test) Fig. 7b), as compared with mice fed the control diet. Appropriate drug dosage was established in pilot studies in wild-type mice; following administration of ISO at 1.5 mg g^{-1} chow for 2 weeks, their blood and brain levels of ISO were 257 and 40 nM,

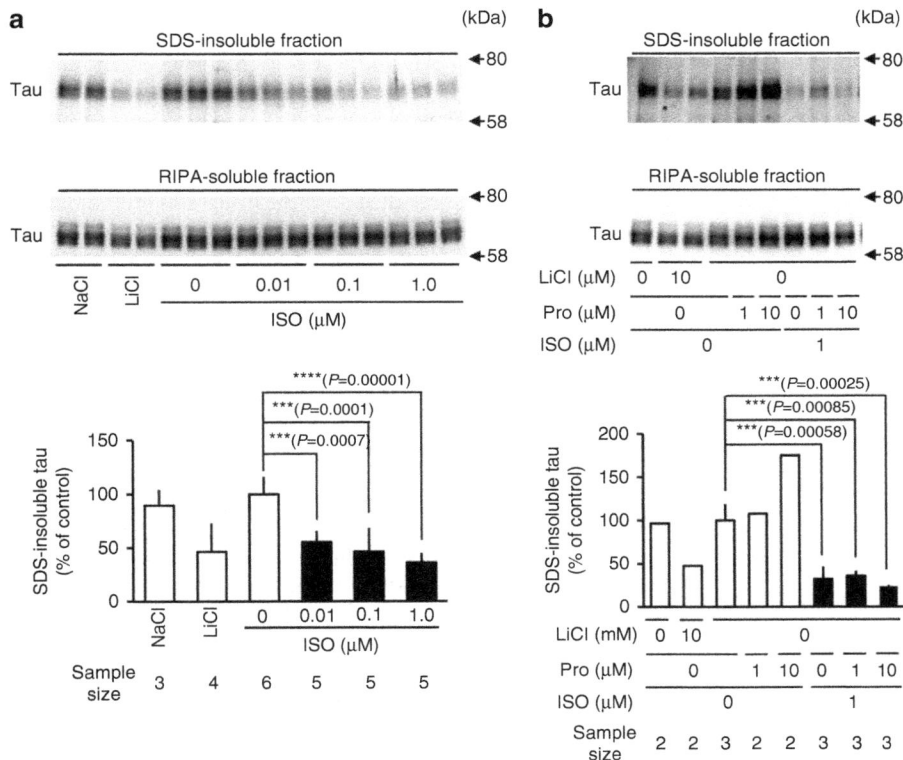

Figure 3 | Isoproterenol inhibits tau aggregation independent of β adrenergic stimulation in cultured cells. Neuro-2a cells expressing human 2N4R tau (P301L) were treated with 0 (milliQ water), 0.01, 0.1 and 1 μM isoproterenol, 10 mM lithium chloride as a positive control as an inhibitor of glycogen synthase kinase and 10 mM sodium chloride as a negative control for 48 h. SDS-insoluble (**a**, upper part of panel) and RIPA-soluble fractions (**a**, middle part of panel) were obtained from the cell homogenates and were subjected to immunoblot analysis with JM antibody that recognized total tau. Immunoreactivity was quantified (**a**, lower part of panel), and levels of SDS-insoluble tau were normalized by corresponding RIPA-soluble tau. Results are represented as percentage of control (mean ± s.d. of 3–6 experiments; 10 mM sodium chloride ($n=3$), 10 mM lithium chloride ($n=4$), vehicle ($n=6$), 0.01 μM isoproterenol ($n=5$), 0.1 μM isoproterenol ($n=5$), 1 μM isoproterenol ($n=5$)). ***$P<0.001$; ****$P<0.0001$ (one-way analysis of variance (ANOVA), with Tukey's multiple comparisons test). (**b**) Neuro-2a cells expressing human 2N4R tau (P301L) were pretreated with 0, 1 and 10 μM propranolol 30 min before treatment with 0 (milliQ water), 1 μM isoproterenol, 10 mM lithium chloride and 10 mM sodium chloride for 48 h. SDS-insoluble (**b**, upper part of panel) and RIPA-soluble (**b**, middle part of panel) fractions were obtained and subjected to immunoblot using JM antibody. Immunoreactivity was quantified (**b**, lower part of panel) and levels of SDS-insoluble tau were normalized to corresponding RIPA-soluble tau. Results are represented as percentage of control (mean ± s.d. of 2–3 experiments; 10 mM sodium chloride ($n=2$), 10 mM lithium chloride ($n=2$), vehicle ($n=3$), 1 μM propranolol ($n=2$), 10 μM propranolol ($n=2$), 1 μM isoproterenol ($n=3$), 1 μM propranolol/1 μM isoproterenol ($n=3$), 10 μM propranolol/1 μM isoproterenol ($n=3$)). ***$P<0.001$ (one-way ANOVA, with Tukey's multiple comparisons test). ISO, isoproterenol; Pro, propranolol.

respectively. Potential mediation of the actions of ISO by β1/2 adrenergic receptors was precluded because similar reductions of Sarkosyl-insoluble tau were observed in both cerebral cortex (Fig. 7c) and hippocampus (Fig. 7d) when P301L tau-transgenic mice were fed for 3 months with the D-isomer of the drug (1.5 mg g^{-1} chow), which lacks adrenergic activity (cf. Fig. 7a,b, respectively). In addition, administration of the inactive isomer of ISO for 2 months resulted in dose-dependent reductions of Sarkosyl-insoluble tau (Fig. 7e). The latter two observations indicate that the ability of D/DL-ISO to inhibit tau aggregation are dose- and time-dependent.

Our previous observations that aged P301L tau-transgenic mice display neuronal loss in the entorhinal cortex, temporal lobe and amygdala[26] were reproduced in the present study (Fig. 7f–h). Having previously attributed these effects to the increased levels of insoluble Sarkosyl-insoluble (aggregated) tau in the brains of aged P301L tau-transgenic mice[26], we hypothesized that ISO would promote neuronal survival by reducing tau aggregation. Our hypothesis was supported by the results depicted in Fig. 7f–h, where ISO (1.5 mg g^{-1} chow for 3 months) is seen to prevent age-related reductions in neuron numbers in the entorhinal cortex, temporal lobe and basolateral amygdala of aged P301L tau-

transgenic mice; the drug did not influence neuron numbers in any of these areas in non-transgenic mice.

On the basis of above findings, we suggest that inhibition of tau aggregation via ISO-capping of Cys residues of tau prevents the aggregation of toxic tau and therefore, neuronal loss. Such a mechanism is supported by the observation that D-ISO (15 mg g^{-1} chow) reduces Sarkosyl-insoluble tau and blocks neuronal loss in the hippocampus of PS19 mice (a model of tauopathy which also displays severe hippocampal neuronal loss[20]); the latter conclusion is supported by the magnetic resonance imaging data presented in Supplementary Fig. 2. Although the neuronal loss observed in P301L tau-transgenic mice was not accompanied by significantly impaired spatial memory in the Morris water maze test[26], they displayed significantly reduced locomotor activity during the first minute of placement in an open field arena (Fig. 7i). On the other hand, their locomotor activity over 30 min in the open field arena did not differ from that observed in non-transgenic mice (Fig. 7j); these observations suggest that P301L tau-transgenic mice exhibit emotional disturbance without any change in overall motor activity. Interestingly, ISO alleviated the emotional disturbance in aged P301L tau-transgenic mice (Fig. 7i).

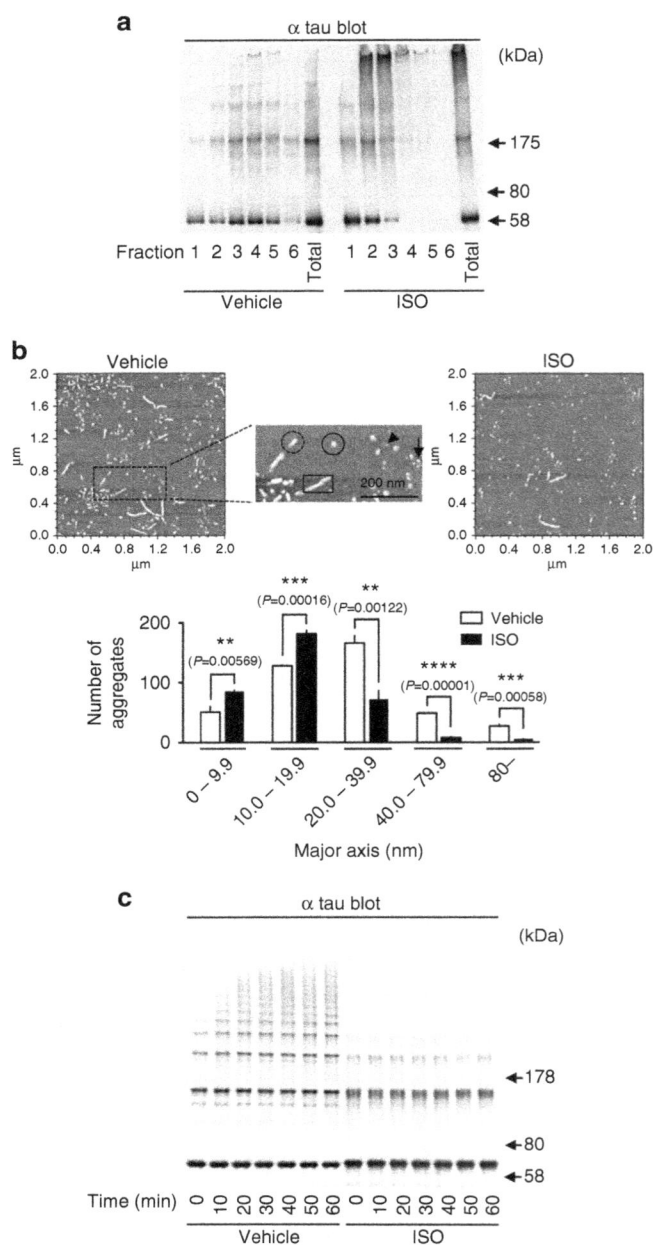

Figure 4 | Inhibition of tau oligomer formation by isoproterenol.
Heparin-induced tau aggregation mixture (120 h incubation) was
subjected to sucrose density gradient centrifugation (**a**) and AFM
observation (**b**). Tau aggregation mixture was separated into six fractions,
and levels of tau in each fraction were analysed by western blot using
tau5 antibody that recognized total tau. In AFM observation, three
images were obtained from different areas ($2 \times 2\,\mu m^2$) of the mica and the
number and size of tau aggregates was quantitated using the image
analysis programme, Matlab. Sizes of tau aggregates are 0–9.9 nm
(arrowhead), 10.0–19.9 nm (arrow), 20.0–39.9 nm (black solid circle),
40.0–79.9 nm (black dotted circle) and not less than 80 nm (black
solid square). Results represented as mean ± s.d. of three experiments
($n = 3$; **b**, lower panel). $**P<0.01$; $***P<0.001$; $****P<0.0001$ (unpaired
Student's t-test). In first 60 min of heparin-induced tau aggregation, higher
order tau oligomer was formed in soluble fraction with longer incubation
time (**c**, vehicle), but growth of tau oligomer was not seen in the presence
of isoproterenol (**c**, ISO). Tau oligomer in soluble fraction was detected by
non-reducing condition using tau5 antibody.

Discussion

Growing evidence for the key role of aggregates of tau protein in
AD and FTDP-17 has spurred efforts to explore pharmacological
means to maintain tau in its soluble form and thus, to prevent its
aggregation.

ISO was identified as a potential inhibitor of tau aggregation
after screening a library of small molecules. Detailed analysis
revealed that the drug acts by binding Cys residues in tau that
prevent tau oligomerization and formation of insoluble tau
aggregates. This property of ISO is attributed to the two phenolic
hydroxyl groups in the 1,2-dihydroxybenzene backbone, as other
compounds sharing this structure (L-3,4-dihydroxyphenylalanine,
dopamine, norepinephrine, epinephrine, and ISO), as well as
1,2-dihydroxybenzene itself, also inhibit tau aggregation, albeit
to lesser extents and/or ability to easily traverse the BBB. The prerequisite role of the 1,2-dihydroxybenzene backbone structure is
illustrated by the inability of octopamine and 3-methoxytyramine
or 3-methoxy-4-hydroxyphenethylamine, whose chemical backbones include 1-hydroxybenzene, to inhibit tau aggregation. Given
that ISO is subject to oxidation, our finding that o-quinone
(adrenochrome) inhibit tau aggregation as effectively as
epinephrine (its non-oxidized parent molecule) is important
because it demonstrates that the inhibitory actions of
1,2-dihydroxybenzene-containing compounds on tau aggregation
do not depend on their oxidative status. Interestingly, previous
work demonstrated nucleophilic covalent attachment of the
o-quinone in 1,2-dihydroxybenzene compounds to the
sulfate group in Cys[42,43]; consistent with this finding. It would
therefore appear that oxidized 1,2-dihydroxybenzene-containing
compounds and their o-quinone forms bind covalently to the
sulfate group of Cys; this view is plausible because we found that
the ISO-bound tau bond cannot be broken eluted by 1 M KCl. The
site of chemical reaction between Cys residue of tau and
o-quinone would be regulated by steric and electronic
interactions of these two compounds. Further, MS analysis
revealed that complexes comprised of a partial tau R3' peptide
and ISO include two phenolic hydroxyl groups, but not
o-quinone. As shown in the schema in Supplementary Fig. 3,
quinone binding to the sulfate group of Cys in tau will be followed
by electron transfer to quinone and its back-conversion into ISO
(personal communication, M.S. and H.K.)[44]. Oxidation during tau
aggregation leads to increased disulfide bonding between Cys
residues in tau[45,46]; however, substitution of Cys to Ala in tau
(C291, 322A-2N4R tau) can induce tau aggregation, suggesting
that capping of Cys residues of tau by 1,2-dihydroxybenzene
precludes the formation of toxic tau aggregates by hindering
disulfide bonding and formation of tau oligomers (Supplementary
Fig. 4a,b). The aggregation of wild-type tau was significantly
attenuated by both 10 and 100 μM of ISO, whereas that of C291,
322A-2N4R tau was only inhibited by the higher dose of ISO
(Supplementary Fig. 4c). Besides showing that ISO binds the Cys
residue of tau, this observation indicates that ISO also affects
PHF6((306) VQIVYK(311))[41,47] binding, and thus increasing the
propensity to form β-sheets and inhibiting the formation of seeds
for the aggregation of toxic tau.

It deserves mention that, although NFTs themselves do not
exert toxic actions[25], the degree of dementia correlates well with
NFT number and the extent of neuronal loss[13,14]. Accordingly,
the irreversible brain dysfunction observed in dementia may be
ascribed to the neuronal loss that follows the aggregation of toxic
tau. Support for this view comes from our finding that ISO
reverses emotional disturbances associated with the expression of
P301L tau (Fig. 7i) and stimulates neural activity in the prelimbic
frontal cortex (Supplementary Fig. 6a); the latter is accompanied
by contemporaneous reductions in the levels of Sarkosyl-
insoluble tau in the prelimbic cortex (Supplementary Fig. 6b).

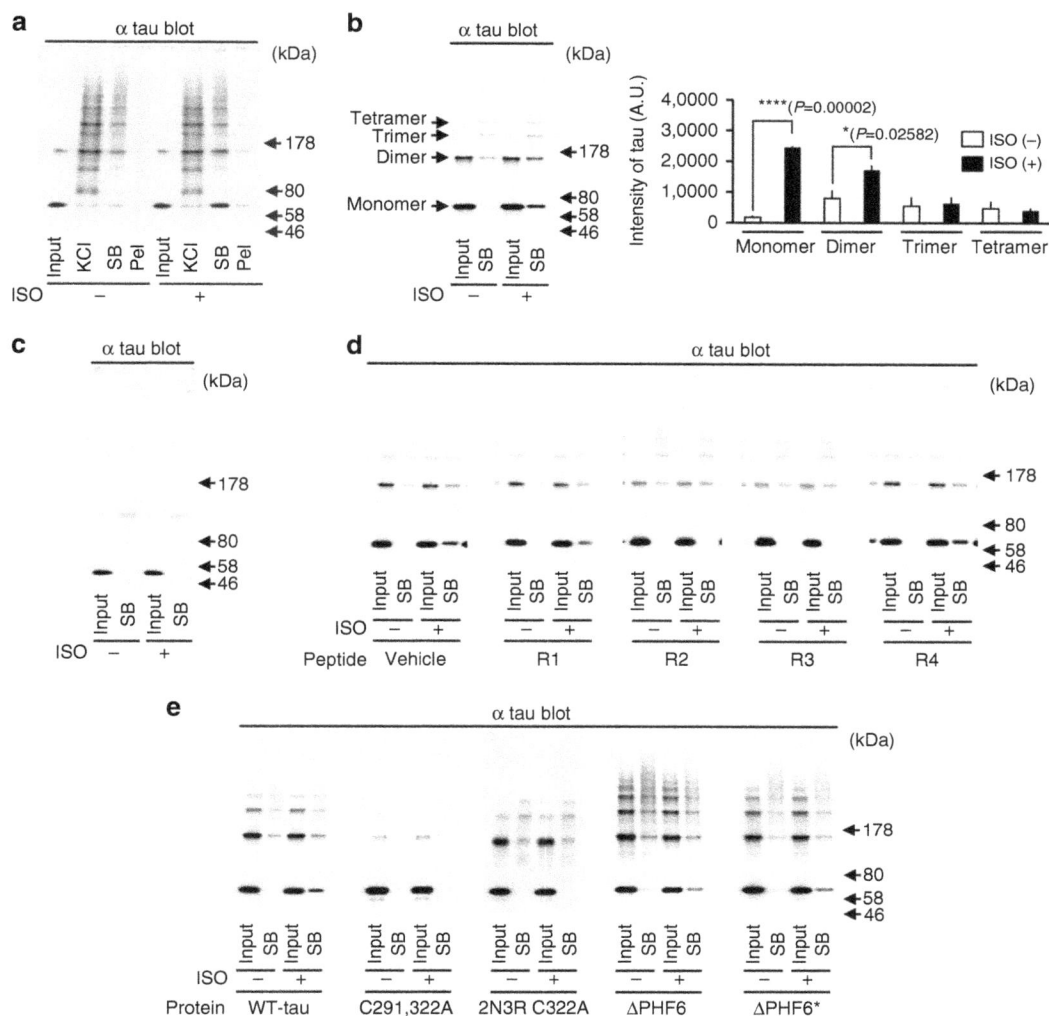

Figure 5 | Identification of isoproterenol (ISO)-binding site on tau. ISO and tau binding were performed according to the protocol described in Supplementary Fig. 1 and ISO-bound tau was recovered in KCl, SB and Pel. Each fraction was subjected to immunoblot analysis with tau5 antibody (**a**). In SB fraction, tau monomer and oligomer were detected from an eluate of FG beads with ISO (ISO (+)) and without ISO (ISO (−); **b**, left part of panel). Levels of tau monomer and oligomer were quantified (**b**, right part of panel) and shown as mean ± s.d. (triplicate experiments; $n = 3$). *$P < 0.05$; ****$P < 0.0001$ (unpaired Student's t-test). FG beads with ISO (ISO (+)) and without ISO (ISO (−)) were reacted with ΔMTBR-tau. Tau was not recovered in SB fraction (**c**). Pretreated ISO with R1 (tapvpmpdlknvkskigstenlkhqpgggk), R2 (vqiinkkldlsnvqskcgskdnikhvpgggs), R3 (vqivykpvdlskvtskcgslgnihhkpgggq) and R4 (vevksekldfkdrvqskigsldnithvpgggn) peptides was incubated with wild-type (WT) 2N4R tau. Pretreated ISO with R2 and R3 could not bind to tau, but R1 and R4 pretreatment could bind (**d**). C291, 322A-2N4R tau and C322A-2N3R tau did not show tau band as well as tau incubating beads without ISO, ISO (+), but WT 2N4R tau, ΔPHF6-tau and ΔPHF6*-tau showed tau band as ISO-bound tau (**e**). MTBR, microtubule-binding domain repeat.

In summary, we have demonstrated that ISO, a drug that penetrates the BBB, efficiently inhibits the formation of Sarkosyl-insoluble tau in a mouse line carrying an aggressive mutant form of tau (P301L); the P301L mutation is responsible for FTDP-17, and mice expressing it are very prone to tau aggregation and neuronal death. Our results point to the potential of 1,2-dihydroxybenzene-based compounds to prevent and delay tauopathies such as FTDP-17 and AD by preventing neuronal dysfunction and loss restoring behavioural homeostasis. Using a variety of analytical approaches, we propose that the therapeutic efficacy of 1,2-dihydroxybenzene-containing compounds hinges on their ability to hinder intermolecular interactions between tau molecules by binding to the Cys residues of tau. No untowards reactions to chronic (3 month) ISO exposure were observed in this study; further, oral administration of the pharmaceutical PROTERENOL S (0.25 mg kg^{-1}) to cynomologus monkeys for 8 weeks was not accompanied by adverse effects (unpublished observations). Nevertheless, the caveat that toxicity might result

from covalent modification of Cys residues in other proteins must be considered during subsequent development of ISO-related compounds for therapeutic use. On the other hand, it should be noted that ISO is commonly prescribed for conditions such as asthma and bradycardia, with the therapeutic dosages in humans being almost fivefold those that we found to be effective in disrupting tau aggregation in mice[48]. The present work suggests a promising novel therapeutic target in the management of tauopathies; its screening strategy and description of a series of compounds that display nucleophilie for Cys residues in tau[49], provide an important lead in this respect.

Methods

Materials. Six-thousand seven-hundred eighty-eight small molecular compounds were obtained from the RIKEN Natural Products Depository (NPDepo) and dissolved in dimethyl sulfoxide to obtain a stock solution (10 mM or 10 mg ml^{-1}). The polyclonal anti-total tau antibody (JM) was prepared as previously described[50]. The monoclonal anti-total tau antibody (tau5) was purchased from

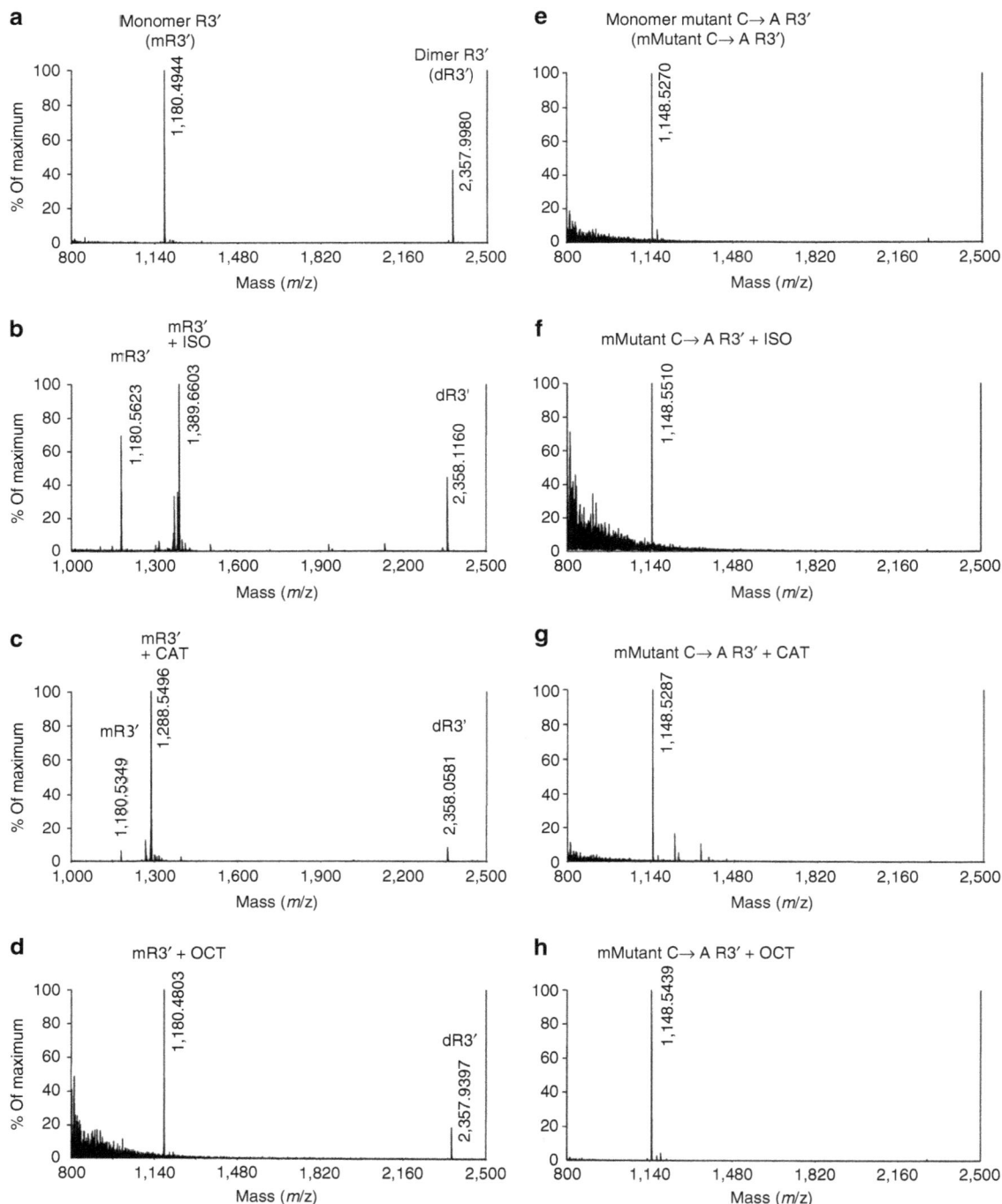

Figure 6 | Binding of 1,2-dihydroxybenzene-containing compounds with Cys residue of tau by mass spectrometry analysis. Vehicle (milliQ water; **a**) and 1-hydroxybenzene-containing octopamine (OCT; MW = 153.2; **d**) were used as negative controls. Compounds containing 1,2-dihydroxybenzene isoproterenol (ISO; MW = 211.3; **b**) and pyrocatechol (CAT; MW = 110.1; **c**) incubated with tau R3 partial peptide, R3' (skvtskcgslgn; MW = 1,180.3) showed ISO/R3' and CAT/R3 signal in mass spectrum (**b,c**). Mutant C → A R3' peptide (skvtskagslgn; MW = 1,148.2; **e–h**) incubated with vehicle (**e**), ISO (**f**), CAT (**g**) and OCT (**h**) only showed mutant R3' signal. Data are normalized to the each maximum mass spectrometry signal.

Invitrogen. All other reagents were of analytical grade and purchased from Nacalai Tesque Inc., Sigma-Aldrich Corp. and WAKO Pure Chemical Industries.

Chemical array screening. The method is based on identification of associations between a protein of interest with a library of candidate chemicals. In this study, the array consisted of 6,788 small-molecule compounds (RIKEN Natural Products Depository, *NPDepo*) immobilized under ultraviolet radiation on to photo-affinity linker-coated glass slides; the assay was performed using a previously reported method[51–53] with slight modifications. Briefly, after blocking with 1% skimmed

milk in 10 mM HEPES/100 mM NaCl for 1 h at room temperature, the slides were treated with recombinant tau protein in 10 mM HEPES/100 mM NaCl/0.05% Tween for 16 h at 4 °C. The slides were then probed with anti-tau antibody (JM) for 4 h, followed by incubation with a Alexa 633-labelled secondary antibody for 1 h at room temperature. Signal detection was performed with a GenePix 4100A microarray scanner (Molecular Devices), equipped with a 635-nm laser and 655–695 nm band-pass emission filter. When Fraction 1 (soluble tau) was used as bait, 86 out of 6,788 compounds showed potential association with tau. In contrast, none of the compounds tested showed associations either Fraction 3 (granular tau oligomer) or Fraction 6 (fibrilar tau).

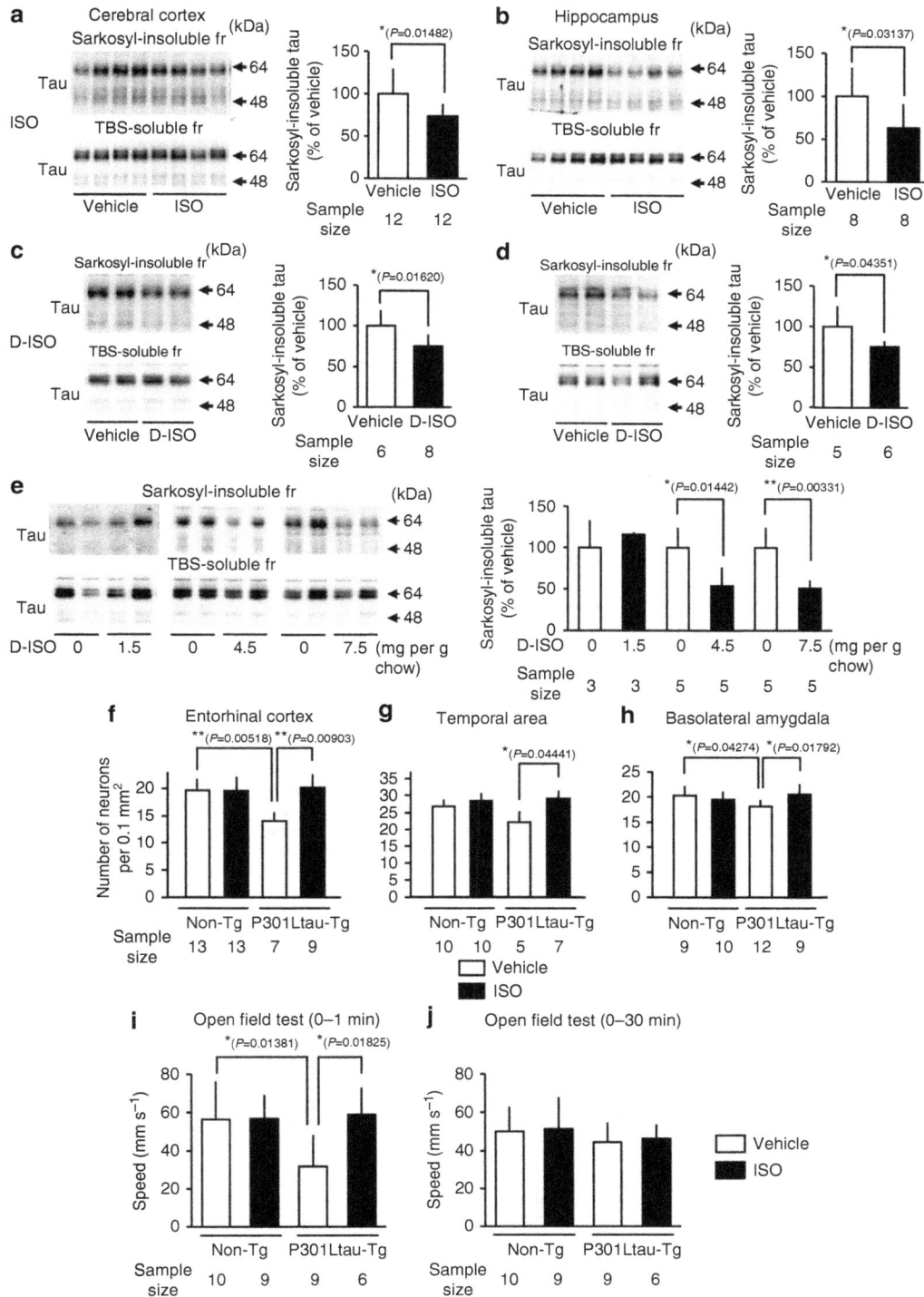

Figure 7 | Inhibition of tau aggregation and neuronal loss by isoproterenol (ISO) *in vivo*. Mice expressing human 2N4R tau (P301L) and non-transgenic (Tg) littermate were administrated with vehicle, 1.5 mg ISO (**a,b,f-j**) and D-ISO (**c,d**) per g chow for 3 months. The mice were treated with 1.5–7.5 mg D-ISO per g chow for 2 months (**e**). In the cerebral cortex (**a,c**) and hippocampus (**b,d,e**), levels of Sarkosyl-insoluble and TBS-soluble tau were analysed by western blot and quantified. JM antibody that recognized total tau was used for detection. Densitometry of tau immunoreactivity was quantified and intensity levels of Sarkosyl-insoluble tau normalized to that of TBS-soluble tau. Results are shown as percentage of control (mean ± s.d. of 3–12 samples from 3–8 mice from three repeated independent experiments). *$P < 0.05$; **$P < 0.01$ (unpaired Welch's (**a**) and Student's *t*-tests (**b-e**)). Coronal sections (4-µm) of mice administrated the vehicle and ISO for 3 months were stained with cresyl violet. The number of neurons in entorhinal cortex (**f**), temporal area (**g**) and basolateral amygdala (**h**) were counted under a microscope assisted with the Neurolucida tracing system. Results are shown as mean ± s.d. of 5–13 samples from 3–5 mice from two independent experiments. *$P < 0.05$; **$P < 0.01$ (one-way analysis of variance (ANOVA), with Tukey's multiple comparisons test). Locomotor activity in ISO-treated and untreated mice was monitored in an open field arena ($50 \times 50 \times 40\ cm^3$) as described in the Methods. Velocity over the 1st minute (**i**) or 30th minute of testing (**j**) was determined by computing the time intervals between sequential positions of the mice in each video frame. Results are shown as mean ± s.d. of 6–10 mice. *$P < 0.05$ (one-way ANOVA, with Tukey's multiple comparisons test). Sample sizes in each experiment are presented in each figure, and mice numbers are described in Supplementary Table 2. fr, fraction.

Preparation of recombinant tau protein. Various human tau cDNA was constructed in a pRK172 vector based on the longest form of human wild-type tau encoded 441 amino acid (2N4R); deletion of amino acids at positions 252 to 376 (ΔMTBR), positions 306 to 311 (ΔPHF6), positions 275 to 280 (ΔPHF6*) and with substitutions at C291A and C322A (C291, 322A). A construct that encoded 2N3R tau with a mutation at C322A (2N3R-C322A) was produced. Each recombinant tau was expressed in *Escherichia coli* BL21 (DE3) and purified by modified method reported previously[33]. After *E. coli* expressing tau was sonicated and boiled, recombinant tau proteins in the heat-stable fraction was purified by ion-exchange chromatography (P11; GE Healthcare, or Cellufine Phosphate; JNC Corp.), ammonium sulfate fractionation, gel filtration chromatography (NAP10 column; GE Healthcare) and reverse phase-HPLC (COSMOSIL Protein-R Waters; Nacalai Tesque Inc.). After freeze-drying, recombinant tau proteins were dissolved in milliQ water and stored at −80 °C as a stock solution.

ThT assay. ThT binding was measured with modified method reported previously[33]. Recombinant wild-type 2N4R tau (10 μM), compounds (indicated concentration) and ThT (10 μM) were mixed in the HEPES buffer (10 mM HEPES, pH = 7.4; 100 mM NaCl), and incubated with heparin (0.06 mg ml^{-1}; Acros Organics) at 37 °C. At specific time points, fluorescence generated by the binding of ThT to tau aggregates was measured (excitation wavelength: 444 nm; emission wavelength: 485 nm). The tau aggregation mixture was collected 120 h after incubation, and analysed with a pelleting assay, sucrose density gradient centrifugation or AFM.

Sucrose density gradient centrifugation. Sucrose density gradient centrifugation was performed as described previously[33]. Tau aggregation mixture (1 ml) was layered on top of sucrose step gradients (each 1 ml of 10, 20, 30, 40 and 50% sucrose in HEPES buffer (pH = 7.4)) was centrifuged (50,000 r.p.m., 2 h) in a MLS50 rotor (Beckman Coulter) and separated into fractions. Pellet (Pel; Fraction 6) was suspended in 1 ml of buffer containing HEPES buffer, and the recovered tau in each fraction was evaluated with western blotting.

Pelleting assay. Pelleting assay was performed by modified method reported previously[54]. After ThT assay, samples including tau aggregates were centrifuged (70,000 r.p.m., 2 h) in TLA100.4 or TLA110 rotors (Beckman Coulter) and separated into supernatant and pellet. After the pellet was suspended and sonicated in Laemmli SB including 2-mercaptoethanol, they were boiled for 5 min.

Cell culture. Neuro2A cell line stably expressing myc-tagged tau (P301L) was established according to a previously described method[38]. Cells were cultured in Dulbecco's Modified Eagle's medium supplemented with 10% fetal bovine serum, 50 μg ml^{-1} gentamicin, 5 μg ml^{-1} puromycin and 1 mg ml^{-1} G418 at 37 °C under 5% CO$_2$. Cells at 80–90% confluency were plated in mediums without puromycin and G418. Cells were treated with ISO (0.01, 0.1 and 1 μM), lithium chloride (10 mM) as a positive control that is a glycogen synthase kinase inhibitor, or sodium chloride (10 mM) as a negative control. To confirm the relationship between tau aggregation with β adrenergic effect by ISO, cells were treated with 1 μM ISO, 30 min after pretreating with or without 1 or 10 μM propranolol, which is a competitive adrenergic β blocker. Cells were sonicated in modified RIPA buffer containing 50 mM Tris (pH = 7.4), 1% NP-40, 0.25% sodium deoxycholate, 150 mM NaCl, 1 mM ethylene glycol tetraacetic acid (EGTA), protease inhibitors (5 μg ml^{-1} pepstatin, 5 μg ml^{-1} leupeptin, 2 μg ml^{-1} aprotinin and 0.5 mM 4-(2-aminoethyl)benzenesulfonyl fluoride hydrochloride) and phosphatase inhibitors (1 mM okadaic acid, 1 mM Na$_3$VO$_4$ and 1 mM NaF) 48 h after treatment. The lysates (1 ml) were layered onto 0.32 M sucrose containing 10 mM Tris (pH = 7.4), 0.8 M NaCl and 1 mM EGTA, and centrifuged (15,000 r.p.m., 10 min, 4 °C) in an ARO15–24 rotor (Tomy Seiko). The upper part (1 ml) was transferred to 1.5-ml tubes (357448; Beckman Coulter), centrifuged (50,000 r.p.m., 30 min, 4 °C) in a TLA55 rotor (Beckman Coulter) and separated into supernatant (RIPA-soluble fraction) and pellet. After the pellets were sonicated in 1% SDS/RIPA and 1% SDS/TBS buffers, they were centrifuged (50,000 r.p.m., 1 h, 4 °C) in a TLA55 rotor and separated into supernatant and pellet. Pel (SDS-insoluble fraction) was dissolved in 70% formic acid and air-dried. Samples from RIPA-soluble and SDS-insoluble fractions were dissolved in Laemmli SB including 2-mercaptoethanol, and then boiled for 5 min.

AFM observation. Morphology of the recombinant tau aggregate was observed under AFM[33]. After ThT assay, samples including tau aggregates were loaded to mica and incubated at room temperature for 30 min in a moist box. The mica was washed with milliQ water and then cantilever (OMCL-TR400PSA; Olympus) detected tau aggregate with 3D-Stand Alone AFM (Asylum Research) under the tapping mode. Major and minor axis of tau aggregates and the number of tau aggregates were determined by image analysis using Matlab-based software (MathWorks Co. Ltd.).

Tau oligomerization assay. After recombinant wild-type 2N4R tau protein (10 μM), and ISO (100 μM) or methylene blue (100 μM) mixing with buffer containing HEPES (10 mM, pH = 7.4) and NaCl (100 mM), heparin sulfate (0.06 mg ml^{-1}) was added, and incubated at 37 °C. In each time point 10–60 min, tau aggregation mixture were collected and dissolved in Laemmli SB without 2-mercaptoethanol. Tau protein in the samples was separated in SDS–polyacrylamide gel electrophoresis gel without dithiothreitol buffer and visualized in western blotting (Figs 4c and 5).

Binding assay with FG beads. To determine binding of tau and ISO, we prepared Streptavidin FG beads (5 mg ml^{-1}; Tamagawa Seiki) reacted with biotinylated ISO (62.5 μM; Supplementary Fig. 1A), and Streptavidin FG beads (5 mg ml^{-1}) reacted with biotin (62.5 μM) as a negative control. Avidin-biotin complexes were formed by incubation for 1 h at 4 °C. After recombinant wild-type 2N4R tau (0.6 μM; input) was reacted with the complexes by rotation (4 h at 4 °C), they were centrifuged and separated into pellet and supernatant. After washing the pellet with 100 mM KCl buffer (pH 7.4) thrice, the pellet was suspended and incubated in 1 M KCl solution for 5 min on ice. The suspension was centrifuged, the supernatant (KCl) was analysed, or the pellet was suspended in Laemmli SB without 2-mercaptoethanol, incubated for 15 min at 60 °C and separated into Pel and supernatant (SB; Supplementary Fig. 1b). The Input, KCl and Pel were solubilized or resuspended in Laemmli SB. Tau protein in the samples was detected with western blotting. To determine binding region, R1 (tapvpmpdlknvkskigstenlkhqpgggk), R2 (vqiinkkldlsnvqskcgskdnikhvpgggs), R3 (vqivykpvdlskvtskcgslgnihhkpgggq) or R4 (vevksekldfkdrvqskigsldnithvpgggn) peptides (120 μM) were pretreated with the avidin-biotin complexes before incubation with recombinant wild-type 2N4R tau.

MASS spectrometry. Recombinant R3' (skvtskcgslgn) and mutant Cys→ Ala R3' (skvtskagslgn) peptides (10 μM) were incubated with compounds (100 μM) for 5 days at 37 °C. The samples were diluted 20 times with milliQ water and loaded to spot under presence of α-Cyano-4-hydroxycinnamic acid (10 mg ml^{-1}). After drying, the samples were analysed using 4800 plus MALDI Tof/Tof analyzer (Applied Biosystems).

Animals. Transgenic mice expressing 2N4R tau (P301L) with myc- and flag-tag at N- and C-terminal under CaM kinase II promoter was created previously[26]. Male P301L tau-transgenic mice 17- to 18-month old were treated with ISO or D-ISO (1.5–7.5 mg g^{-1} chow) for 2 or 3 months. The numbers of animals used in each experiment are indicating in Supplementary Table 2. All experimental procedures used in this study were approved by the Committee of Animal Experiments at the National Center for Geriatrics and Gerontology.

Tissue extraction. P301L tau-transgenic mice were anaesthetized and killed after treatment with the compounds; the hippocampus and cerebral cortex were collected. The tissues were homogenized in TBS buffer containing 50 mM Tris (pH = 7.4), 150 mM NaCl, 1 mM EGTA, 1 mM EDTA, protease inhibitors and phosphatase inhibitors. The homogenates were centrifuged (23,000 r.p.m., 15 min, 4 °C) in a TLA55 rotor and separated into supernatant (TBS-soluble fraction) and pellet. Pellets were resuspended in 0.32 M sucrose containing 10 mM Tris (pH 7.4), 0.8 M NaCl and 1 mM EGTA and centrifuged (23,000 r.p.m., 15 min, 4 °C) in a TLA55 rotor. Supernatants were collected and treated with 1% Sarkosyl for 1 h at 37 °C. They were centrifuged (60,000 r.p.m., 1 h, 4 °C) in a TLA100.4 or 110 rotors and separated into supernatant and pellet (Sarkosyl-insoluble fraction). Samples from TBS-soluble and Sarkosyl-insoluble fractions were dissolved in Laemmli SB including 2-mercaptoethanol, and then boiled for 5 min.

Count of neuronal cells. Number of neuronal cells in the brain was measured with modified method reported previously[26]. After P301L tau-transgenic mice were anaesthetized and transcardially perfused with 10% formalin, brains were fixed in 10% formalin solutions for 48 h. Coronal sections (4 μm) were produced from brains embedded by paraffin, and stained with cresyl violet. We counted the number of neuronal cells in the sections using microscope linked to a Neurolucida tracing system (MicroBrightField Inc.).

Western blotting. Samples dissolved in Laemmli SB were separated by Novex 3–8% Tris-Acetate Gel (binding assay and tau oligomerization assay; Invitrogen) or SuperSep Ace 5–20% gel (other assays; WAKO Pure Chemical Industries) and transferred onto membranes with semi-dry transfer systems (Bio-Rad Laboratory). The membrane was blocked with 5% milk in PBS-T for 1 h at room temperature. They were probed with antibodies overnight at 4 °C. After washing the membrane with PBS-T, blots were incubated with horseradish peroxidase-linked second antibodies and then examined by enhanced chemiluminescence detection on Las3000 or Las4000 (GE Healthcare).

Open field test. Mice were placed in the centre of an open field apparatus (50 × 50 × 40 cm^3; O'Hara Co., Ltd.), and their locomotor activity was monitored with a CCD camera; digital data of real-time images were recorded using the public domain NIH Image J software (http://rsb.info.nih.gov/nih-image/). Images were sampled at 2 Hz. Data were analysed using customized Matlab-based software, using an image analysis tool box (Mathworks Co. Ltd.). During testing, the sequential position of the mouse was determined in each video frame from which locomotor speed was calculated.

Mn-enhanced magnetic resonance imaging. Mn-enhanced MRI was performed as previously described[55]. Mice were given an intraperitoneal injection of 30 mM $MnCl_2$ (100 µmol kg^{-1}) and returned to their home cages. After 1 h, mice were exposed successively to three different novel places separated by a small (diameter, 30 cm; height, 30 cm) and big (diameter, 60 cm; height, 30 cm) transparent plastic wall and was allowed to explore for 120 min. Thereafter, mice were returned to their home cages for 1 h before being anaesthetized with isoflurane (0.5–1.5% in air) and placement in a Bruker 3T MR scanner; during scanning, breathing and depth of anaesthesia was continuously monitored, with breathing rate maintained at 80–100 breaths per min. Mn-enhanced MRI images were visualized with open-source Osirix software (version 2.5) that allowed navigation through multidimensional DICOM images; relative regional brain activity was determined by measuring MR signal intensities, normalized to the mean signal intensity in the dorsal striatum.

Measurement of ISO levels in the blood and brain. Male C57BL/6J mice ($n = 7$) were administered ISO (1.5 mg g^{-1} chow) for 2 weeks before sacrifice when blood plasma and whole brain were collected. The samples were deproteinized using acetonitrile before determination of ISO concentrations using an LC-MS instrument (UPLC/Quattro Premier XE; Waters).

Statistical analysis. Data are expressed as means ± s.d. The significance of differences between two groups was assessed by Student's or Welch's t-tests, and differences between multiple groups were assessed by one-way analysis of variance and Tukey's multiple comparisons test, using PRISM4 (GraphPad Software Inc.). $P < 0.05$ was considered statistically significant.

References

1. Schirmer, R. H., Adler, H., Pickhardt, M. & Mandelkow, E. "Lest we forget you--methylene blue...". *Neurobiol. Aging* **32**, 2325.e2327–2316 (2011).
2. Selkoe, D. J. Alzheimer disease: mechanistic understanding predicts novel therapies. *Ann. Intern. Med.* **140**, 627–638 (2004).
3. Desai, A. K. & Chand, P. Tau-based therapies for Alzheimer's disease: wave of the future. *Primary Psychiatry* **16**, 40–46 (2009).
4. Hardy, J. & Selkoe, D. J. The amyloid hypothesis of Alzheimer's disease: progress and problems on the road to therapeutics. *Science* **297**, 353–356 (2002).
5. Kosik, K. S. Traveling the tau pathway: a personal account. *J. Alzheimers Dis.* **9**, 251–256 (2006).
6. Liu, J. *et al.* Amyloid-beta induces caspase-dependent loss of PSD-95 and synaptophysin through NMDA receptors. *J. Alzheimers Dis.* **22**, 541–556 (2010).
7. Roselli, F. *et al.* Soluble beta-amyloid1-40 induces NMDA-dependent degradation of postsynaptic density-95 at glutamatergic synapses. *J. Neurosci.* **25**, 11061–11070 (2005).
8. Ittner, L. M. *et al.* Dendritic function of tau mediates amyloid-beta toxicity in Alzheimer's disease mouse models. *Cell* **142**, 387–397 (2010).
9. Roberson, E. D. *et al.* Reducing endogenous tau ameliorates amyloid beta-induced deficits in an Alzheimer's disease mouse model. *Science* **316**, 750–754 (2007).
10. Holmes, C. *et al.* Long-term effects of Abeta42 immunisation in Alzheimer's disease: follow-up of a randomised, placebo-controlled phase I trial. *Lancet* **372**, 216–223 (2008).
11. Rosenblum, W. I. Why Alzheimer trials fail: removing soluble oligomeric beta amyloid is essential, inconsistent, and difficult. *Neurobiol. Aging* **35**, 969–974 (2014).
12. Giacobini, E. & Gold, G. Alzheimer disease therapy--moving from amyloid-beta to tau. *Nat. Rev. Neurol.* **9**, 677–686 (2013).
13. Guillozet, A. L., Weintraub, S., Mash, D. C. & Mesulam, M. M. Neurofibrillary tangles, amyloid, and memory in aging and mild cognitive impairment. *Arch. Neurol.* **60**, 729–736 (2003).
14. Gomez-Isla, T. *et al.* Clinical and pathological correlates of apolipoprotein E epsilon 4 in Alzheimer's disease. *Ann. Neurol.* **39**, 62–70 (1996).
15. Bondareff, W., Mountjoy, C. Q., Roth, M. & Hauser, D. L. Neurofibrillary degeneration and neuronal loss in Alzheimer's disease. *Neurobiol. Aging* **10**, 709–715 (1989).
16. Bobinski, M. *et al.* Neurofibrillary pathology--correlation with hippocampal formation atrophy in Alzheimer disease. *Neurobiol. Aging* **17**, 909–919 (1996).
17. Hutton, M. *et al.* Association of missense and 5'-splice-site mutations in tau with the inherited dementia FTDP-17. *Nature* **393**, 702–705 (1998).
18. Poorkaj, P. *et al.* Tau is a candidate gene for chromosome 17 frontotemporal dementia. *Ann. Neurol.* **43**, 815–825 (1998).
19. Spillantini, M. G. *et al.* Mutation in the tau gene in familial multiple system tauopathy with presenile dementia. *Proc. Natl Acad. Sci. USA* **95**, 7737–7741 (1998).
20. Yoshiyama, Y. *et al.* Synapse loss and microglial activation precede tangles in a P301S tauopathy mouse model. *Neuron* **53**, 337–351 (2007).
21. Allen, B. *et al.* Abundant tau filaments and nonapoptotic neurodegeneration in transgenic mice expressing human P301S tau protein. *J. Neurosci.* **22**, 9340–9351 (2002).
22. Lewis, J. *et al.* Neurofibrillary tangles, amyotrophy and progressive motor disturbance in mice expressing mutant (P301L) tau protein. *Nat. Genet.* **25**, 402–405 (2000).
23. Tanemura, K. *et al.* Neurodegeneration with tau accumulation in a transgenic mouse expressing V337M human tau. *J. Neurosci.* **22**, 133–141 (2002).
24. Tatebayashi, Y. *et al.* Tau filament formation and associative memory deficit in aged mice expressing mutant (R406W) human tau. *Proc. Natl Acad. Sci. USA* **99**, 13896–13901 (2002).
25. Santacruz, K. *et al.* Tau suppression in a neurodegenerative mouse model improves memory function. *Science* **309**, 476–481 (2005).
26. Kimura, T. *et al.* Aggregation of detergent-insoluble tau is involved in neuronal loss but not in synaptic loss. *J. Biol. Chem.* **285**, 38692–38699 (2010).
27. Cowan, C. M. *et al.* Modelling tauopathies in *Drosophila*: insights from the fruit fly. *Int. J. Alzheimers Dis.* **2011**, 598157 (2011).
28. Bretteville, A. *et al.* Hypothermia-induced hyperphosphorylation: a new model to study tau kinase inhibitors. *Sci. Rep.* **2**, 480 (2012).
29. Gong, C. X. *et al.* Phosphorylation of microtubule-associated protein tau is regulated by protein phosphatase 2A in mammalian brain. Implications for neurofibrillary degeneration in Alzheimer's disease. *J. Biol. Chem.* **275**, 5535–5544 (2000).
30. Schneider, A., Biernat, J., von Bergen, M., Mandelkow, E. & Mandelkow, E. M. Phosphorylation that detaches tau protein from microtubules (Ser262, Ser214) also protects it against aggregation into Alzheimer paired helical filaments. *Biochemistry* **38**, 3549–3558 (1999).
31. Wang, Y. P., Biernat, J., Pickhardt, M., Mandelkow, E. & Mandelkow, E. M. Stepwise proteolysis liberates tau fragments that nucleate the Alzheimer-like aggregation of full-length tau in a neuronal cell model. *Proc. Natl Acad. Sci. USA* **104**, 10252–10257 (2007).
32. Sahara, N. *et al.* Assembly of two distinct dimers and higher-order oligomers from full-length tau. *Eur. J. Neurosci.* **25**, 3020–3029 (2007).
33. Maeda, S. *et al.* Granular tau oligomers as intermediates of tau filaments. *Biochemistry* **46**, 3856–3861 (2007).
34. Maeda, S. *et al.* Increased levels of granular tau oligomers: an early sign of brain aging and Alzheimer's disease. *Neurosci. Res.* **54**, 197–201 (2006).
35. Takashima, A. Tauopathies and tau oligomers. *J. Alzheimers Dis.* **37**, 565–568 (2013).
36. Chi, O. Z., Wang, G., Chang, Q. & Weiss, H. R. Effects of isoproterenol on blood-brain barrier permeability in rats. *Neurol. Res.* **20**, 259–264 (1998).
37. Eriksson, T. & Carlsson, A. Isoprenaline increases brain concentrations of administered L-dopa and L-tryptophan in the rat. *Psychopharmacology (Berl)* **77**, 98–100 (1982).
38. Hatakeyama, S. *et al.* U-box protein carboxyl terminus of Hsc70-interacting protein (CHIP) mediates poly-ubiquitylation preferentially on four-repeat Tau and is involved in neurodegeneration of tauopathy. *J. Neurochem.* **91**, 299–307 (2004).
39. Bhattacharya, K., Rank, K. B., Evans, D. B. & Sharma, S. K. Role of cysteine-291 and cysteine-322 in the polymerization of human tau into Alzheimer-like filaments. *Biochem. Biophys. Res. Commun.* **285**, 20–26 (2001).
40. von Bergen, M. *et al.* Assembly of tau protein into Alzheimer paired helical filaments depends on a local sequence motif ((306)VQIVYK(311)) forming beta structure. *Proc. Natl Acad. Sci. USA* **97**, 5129–5134 (2000).
41. von Bergen, M. *et al.* Mutations of tau protein in frontotemporal dementia promote aggregation of paired helical filaments by enhancing local beta-structure. *J. Biol. Chem.* **276**, 48165–48174 (2001).
42. Jagoe, C. T., Kreifels, S. E. & Li, J. Covalent binding of catechols to Src family SH2 domains. *Bioorganic Med. Chem. Lett.* **7**, 113–116 (1997).
43. Lipton, S. A. Pathologically activated therapeutics for neuroprotection. *Nat. Rev. Neurosci.* **8**, 803–808 (2007).
44. Guin, P. S., Das, S. & Mandal, P. Electrochemical reduction of quinones in different media: a review. *Int. J. Electrochem.* **2011**, 816202 (2011).
45. Nakashima, H. *et al.* Effects of alpha-tocopherol on an animal model of tauopathies. *Free Radic. Biol. Med.* **37**, 176–186 (2004).
46. Dias-Santagata, D., Fulga, T. A., Duttaroy, A. & Feany, M. B. Oxidative stress mediates tau-induced neurodegeneration in *Drosophila*. *J. Clin. Invest.* **117**, 236–245 (2007).
47. Gruning, C. S. *et al.* Alternative conformations of the Tau repeat domain in complex with an engineered binding protein. *J. Biol. Chem.* **289**, 23209–23218 (2014).

48. Conolly, M. E. *et al.* Metabolism of isoprenaline in dog and man. *Br. J. Pharmac.* **46**, 458–472 (1972).

49. Singh, J. *et al.* Structure-based design of a potent, selective, and irreversible inhibitor of the catalytic domain of the erbB receptor subfamily of protein tyrosine kinases. *J. Med. Chem.* **40**, 1130–1135 (1997).

50. Takashima, A. *et al.* Presenilin 1 associates with glycogen synthase kinase-3beta and its substrate tau. *Proc. Natl Acad. Sci. USA* **95**, 9637–9641 (1998).

51. Hagiwara, K. *et al.* Discovery of novel antiviral agents directed against the influenza A virus nucleoprotein using photo-cross-linked chemical arrays. *Biochem. Biophys. Res. Commun.* **394**, 721–727 (2010).

52. Kanoh, N. *et al.* Photo-cross-linked small-molecule microarrays as chemical genomic tools for dissecting protein-ligand interactions. *Chem. Asian J.* **1**, 789–797 (2006).

53. Miyazaki, I., Simizu, S., Ichimiya, H., Kawatani, M. & Osada, H. Robust and systematic drug screening method using chemical arrays and the protein library: identification of novel inhibitors of carbonic anhydrase II. *Biosci. Biotechnol. Biochem.* **72**, 2739–2749 (2008).

54. Pickhardt, M. *et al.* Screening for inhibitors of tau polymerization. *Curr. Alzheimer Res.* **2**, 219–226 (2005).

55. Kimura, T. *et al.* Hyperphosphorylated tau in parahippocampal cortex impairs place learning in aged mice expressing wild-type human tau. *EMBO J.* **26**, 5143–5152 (2007).

Acknowledgements

We thank Drs Tamio Saito and Aya Asami (RIKEN, Wako, Japan) for kindly providing 6,788 test compounds; Dr Toshihide Hashimoto (Eisai Co., Ltd., Tukuba, Japan) for kindly providing biotinylated ISO; Ms. Miyuki Murayama (RIKEN, Wako, Japan) and Mr Shunji Yamashita (O'HARA & Co., Ltd., Tokyo Japan) for valuable technical advice; and Ms Midori Yamamoto (National Center for Geriatrics and Gerontology, Obu, Japan) and Mr Tatsuya Mizoroki (Institute of Immunology Co., Ltd., Utsunomiya, Japan) for assistance in the maintenance of mice.

This work was supported by JSPS KAKENHI Grant Number 23790313 (to Y.S.), Mext Grant-in-aid project, Scientific Research on Innovation Area (Brain Protein Aging and Dementia control (to A.T.), Brain environment (to A.T.)) and Strategic Research Program for Brain Science ('Integrated Research on Neuropsychiatric Disorders') from Japan Agency for Medical Research and development, AMED (to Y.I., A.T. and H.S.) and Intramural grant of NCGG (to A.T.).

Author contributions

M.Y. and A.Su. performed in vivo experiments. O.F.X.A. provided critical suggestions during writing of the manuscript. S.M., H.O., Y.K. and A.Sa. performed the chemical array screening and evaluated the data. T.M. and Y.I. performed MS analysis. T.K. calculated major axis and number of tau aggregates in images obtained by AFM using Matlab. M.S. and H.K. analysed chemical data. H.S. synthesized and purified D-ISO. Y.Y. provided critical techniques for ThT assay and cultured cell analysis. Y.S. and A.T. designed the experiment, and evaluated all data. Y.S. and A.T. wrote the manuscript. A.T. supervised the study.

Additional information

20

Drug design from the cryptic inhibitor envelope

Chul-Jin Lee[1,*], Xiaofei Liang[2,*], Qinglin Wu[1,*], Javaria Najeeb[1,*], Jinshi Zhao[1], Ramesh Gopalaswamy[2], Marie Titecat[3], Florent Sebbane[3], Nadine Lemaitre[3], Eric J. Toone[1,2] & Pei Zhou[1,2]

Conformational dynamics plays an important role in enzyme catalysis, allosteric regulation of protein functions and assembly of macromolecular complexes. Despite these well-established roles, such information has yet to be exploited for drug design. Here we show by nuclear magnetic resonance spectroscopy that inhibitors of LpxC—an essential enzyme of the lipid A biosynthetic pathway in Gram-negative bacteria and a validated novel antibiotic target—access alternative, minor population states in solution in addition to the ligand conformation observed in crystal structures. These conformations collectively delineate an inhibitor envelope that is invisible to crystallography, but is dynamically accessible by small molecules in solution. Drug design exploiting such a hidden inhibitor envelope has led to the development of potent antibiotics with inhibition constants in the single-digit picomolar range. The principle of the cryptic inhibitor envelope approach may be broadly applicable to other lead optimization campaigns to yield improved therapeutics.

[1] Department of Biochemistry, Duke University Medical Center, Durham, North Carolina 27710, USA. [2] Department of Chemistry, Duke University, Durham, North Carolina 27708, USA. [3] Inserm, Univ. Lille, CHU Lille, Institut Pasteur de Lille, CNRS, U1019-UMR 8204-CIIL-Center for Infection and Immunity of Lille, F-59000 Lille, France. * These authors contributed equally to this work. Correspondence and requests for materials should be addressed to P.Z. (email: peizhou@biochem.duke.edu).

The availability of high-resolution crystal structures of protein-inhibitor complexes has revolutionized the drug development process, enabling structure-aided design of improved therapeutics based on visual inspection of receptor-ligand interactions. However, it is increasingly recognized that high-resolution structures of protein-inhibitor complexes do not necessarily enable a successful lead optimization campaign, as the static structural models often fail to capture the conformational flexibility of receptors or their bound inhibitors[1,2]. In contrast to the largely static view of protein structures provided by crystallography, the discovery of ring flipping events of buried aromatic residues of the basic pancreatic trypsin inhibitor by NMR (ref. 3) has heralded the widespread observation of molecular motions within macromolecules in solution. Conformational dynamics involving side-chain rearrangement, domain reorganization and binding-induced structural remodelling has been shown to play important roles in enzyme catalysis[4-7], allosteric regulation[8] and nucleic acid function[9]. Molecular recognition of small molecules likewise alters protein dynamics[10]. Despite the extensive demonstration of conformational dynamics of macromolecules in solution, the application of such information to drug development has remained an unmet challenge.

In this study, we used solution NMR to investigate the conformational states of small-molecule inhibitors bound to LpxC, an essential metalloamidase that catalyses the deacetylation of UDP-(3-O-acyl)-N-acetylglucosamine during the biosynthesis of lipid A in Gram-negative bacteria[11,12]. We show that these enzyme-bound inhibitors dynamically access alternative, minor conformations in solution in addition to the ligand state observed in the crystal structure. Furthermore, we demonstrate that these ligand conformational states collectively define a cryptic inhibitor envelope that can be exploited for optimization of lead compounds.

Results

A cryptic inhibitor envelope invisible in crystal structures. We chose *Aquifex aeolicus* LpxC (AaLpxC) in the lipid A biosynthetic pathway (Supplementary Fig. 1) for structural and dynamics investigation due to its exceptional thermostability, which has enabled both NMR measurements and crystallographic studies (for example, refs 13–16). *Pseudomonas aeruginosa* LpxC (PaLpxC) was exploited when co-crystal structures of the desired AaLpxC-inhibitor complexes could not be obtained. As a starting point, we investigated the conformations of CHIR-090 and LPC-011 bound to AaLpxC, two inhibitors that share the same threonyl-hydroxamate head group, but differ in their tail groups (Supplementary Fig. 1, Supplementary Table 1). CHIR-090 features a substituted biphenyl acetylene tail group that competes with the acyl chain of the LpxC substrate to occupy the hydrophobic substrate passage of the enzyme[14]. Replacing the tail group of CHIR-090 with a substituted biphenyl diacetylene group generated LPC-011 with improved antibiotic activity due to minimization of vdW clashes with the substrate-binding passage[16,17]. To provide a direct comparison with solution NMR investigations, we determined the crystal structure of AaLpxC in complex with LPC-011 (Fig. 1a, Supplementary Table 2). This structure reveals a single conformation of the threonyl-hydroxamate head group in the active site, with the threonyl Cγ2 methyl group packing against an invariant phenylalanine residue (F180 in AaLpxC) and the Oγ1 hydroxyl group forming a hydrogen bond with the catalytically important lysine residue (K227 in AaLpxC). The threonyl side chain of the inhibitor features a *trans* configuration with a χ^1 angle of 180°, a rotameric state that is less energetically favourable

(7% population of all threonine side chains in proteins) compared with the alternative rotameric states of *gauche-* ($\chi^1 = -60°$) and *gauche+* ($\chi^1 = 60°$) collectively accounting for 92% of the observed threonine side-chain conformations[18]. Since the observed ligand conformation in the crystal structure represents an unfavourable χ^1 rotameric state of the threonyl head group, we investigated whether this group could access alternative ligand conformations in solution.

Database analysis of high-resolution protein structures has indicated that amino acid side-chains adopt specific rotameric conformations[18], and side-chain motions can be approximated as conformational hopping between rotameric states[19]. Such motions occur over a wide range of timescales, from ns movement of surface exposed residues to µs-ms timescale ring flipping in protein cores. To determine rotameric populations of the ligand threonyl side chain over a wide timescale, we synthesized isotopically labelled CHIR-090 and LPC-011 and measured the scalar couplings $^3J_{NC\gamma2}$ and $^3J_{C'C\gamma2}$ that are dependent on the χ^1 angle of the threonyl side chain (Supplementary Fig. 2 and Supplementary Table 3). Specifically, a large $^3J_{NC\gamma2}$ value of ~1.9 Hz is consistent with a $trans^{NC\gamma2}$ relationship between the amide nitrogen and the Cγ2 methyl group of the threonyl head group, corresponding to a χ^1 angle of $-60°$ (*gauche-* χ^1), whereas a small value of ~0.2 Hz reflects a $gauche^{NC\gamma2}$ relationship (*gauche+* $^{NC\gamma2}$ or *gauche-* $^{NC\gamma2}$), corresponding to χ^1 angles of 180° (*trans* χ^1) or 60° (*gauche+* χ^1), respectively. An intermediate value reflects a population-weighted average between the $trans^{NC\gamma2}$ and $gauche^{NC\gamma2}$ states[20]. A similar relation is noted for the $^3J_{C'C\gamma2}$ coupling[20]. Thus simultaneous measurements of the $^3J_{NC\gamma2}$ and $^3J_{C'C\gamma2}$ scalar couplings enable the determination of the populations of all three rotameric states of the threonyl side chain[19]. Measurements of LPC-011 yielded a $^3J_{NC\gamma2}$ coupling of 0.58 ± 0.05 Hz and a $^3J_{C'C\gamma2}$ coupling of 0.77 ± 0.04 Hz, corresponding to a predominant *trans* χ^1 configuration with a population of 0.65 ± 0.03 (Fig. 1b, Supplementary Table 3). Such an observation is consistent with the ligand conformation in the AaLpxC/LPC-011 crystal structure (Fig. 1a). However, the measurements also revealed that the threonyl side chain of LPC-011 can readily access alternative, minor conformational states with a population of 0.23 ± 0.03 for the *gauche-* χ^1 conformation and a population of 0.12 ± 0.01 for the *gauche+* χ^1 conformation (Fig. 1b). Measurements of CHIR-090 yielded a similar result, with a $^3J_{NC\gamma2}$ coupling of 0.45 ± 0.07 Hz and a $^3J_{C'C\gamma2}$ coupling of 0.67 ± 0.04 Hz, corresponding to populations of 0.77 ± 0.04 for the *trans* χ^1 configuration, 0.14 ± 0.04 for the *gauche-* χ^1 configuration and 0.09 ± 0.01 for the *gauche+* χ^1 configuration (Fig. 1b, Supplementary Table 3). Modelling of the threonyl side chain in the second-most-populated *gauche-* χ^1 state indicates that the Cγ2 methyl group would experience vdW interactions with the hydrophobic component of the K227 side chain with the Oγ1 hydroxyl group oriented towards solvent, leaving a cavity against the F180 side chain of AaLpxC (Fig. 1c). Although the protein-ligand interactions in the *gauche-* χ^1 rotameric conformation are less favourable than those in the ground state of the *trans* χ^1 rotamer, the lack of optimal interactions is partially compensated by the intrinsic free energy difference of the rotameric states of the threonyl side chain that favours the *gauche-* χ^1 rotamer over the *trans* χ^1 rotamer in the unbound ligand. Taken together, these solution measurement-derived rotamers collectively portray an inhibitor envelope that can accommodate three substitutions at the Cβ position of the threonyl head group (Fig. 1c).

To test this prediction, we merged the two conformations of the threonyl head group and generated Cβ-di-methyl substituted compounds with the third Cβ-substitution containing either a hydroxyl group (LPC-037) or an amino group (LPC-040)

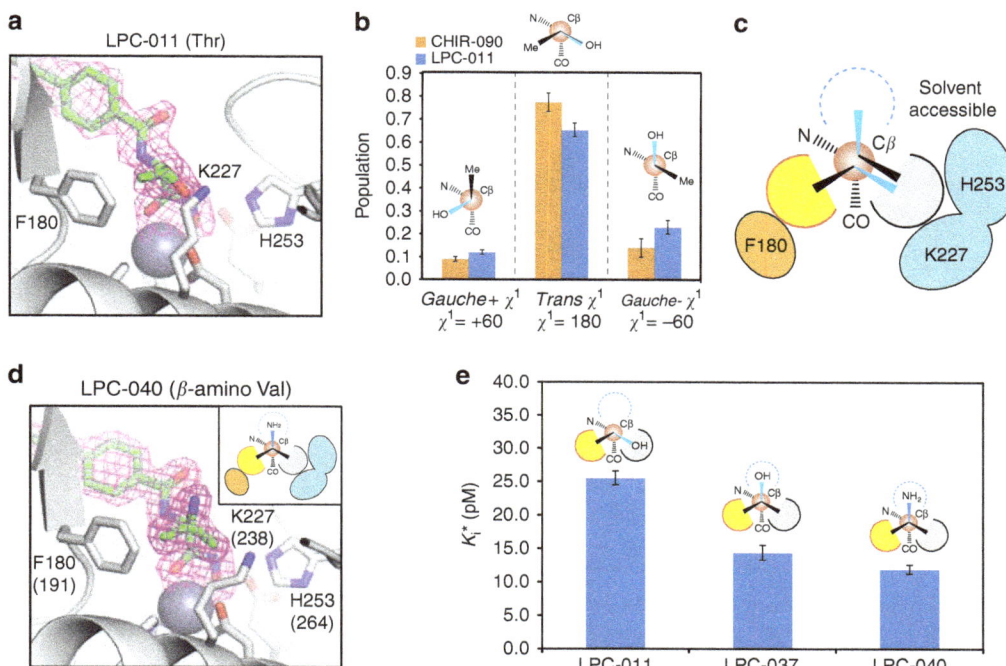

Figure 1 | Dynamic access of minor conformational states of LpxC inhibitors containing the threonyl head group. (**a**) Crystal structure of the AaLpxC/LPC-011 complex, showing a single *trans* χ^1 rotamer of the threonyl side chain of the inhibitor. AaLpxC is shown in the cartoon model and catalytically important residues in the stick model. LPC-011 is shown in the stick model, with the purple mesh representing the inhibitor omit map (2mFo-DFc) contoured at 1.0σ. (**b**) NMR measurements of scalar couplings ($^3J_{NC\gamma2}$ and $^3J_{C'C\gamma2}$) of the threonyl-head-group-containing LpxC inhibitors CHIR-090 (orange) and LPC-011 (blue) reveal a dynamic distribution of all three rotameric χ^1 states. (**c**) Combining the two most-populated ligand states creates a dynamically accessible inhibitor envelope around the $C\beta$ atom of the threonyl head group. The binding pockets near F180 and H253/K227 are coloured in yellow and grey, respectively, and a third binding pocket accessible to solvent is denoted by an open dashed circle in blue. (**d**) The $C\beta$-triply substituted compound LPC-040 occupies all three pockets within the inhibitor envelope. PaLpxC is shown in the cartoon model, with catalytically important residues shown in the stick model. Residue numbering reflects the corresponding residues in AaLpxC, with PaLpxC residue numbers shown in parentheses. LPC-040 is shown in the stick model, with the purple mesh representing the inhibitor omit map (2mFo-DFc) contoured at 1.0σ. (**e**) Inhibition constants (K_i^*) of LpxC inhibitors. Chemical substitutions at the $C\beta$-position of the inhibitors and their observed (LPC-011 and LPC-040) and predicted (LPC-037) binding modes within the inhibitor envelope are labelled.

(Supplementary Table 1). Structural analysis of LPC-040 in complex with PaLpxC indeed revealed the anticipated ligand conformation (Fig. 1d; Supplementary Table 2) with the two $C\beta$-substituted methyl groups forming hydrophobic interactions with F180 (F191^{PaLpxC}) and the stem of K227 (K238^{PaLpxC}) and the amino group directed towards solvent accessible space to form a water-mediated hydrogen bond with the backbone carbonyl of F180 (F191^{PaLpxC}).

We next investigated whether these compounds show enhanced LpxC inhibition in enzymatic assays. *Escherichia coli* LpxC inhibition by CHIR-090 and LPC-011 both displayed slow-binding kinetics consistent with the transition from a rapid-forming initial encounter complex (enzyme-inhibitor complex (EI)) to the stable complex (EI*; Supplementary Fig. 3). Therefore, we focused enzymatic assays on the stable EI* complex. CHIR-090 and LPC-011 are potent LpxC inhibitors with K_i^* values of $153 \pm 8\,pM$ and $26 \pm 1\,pM$, respectively. Excitingly, the $C\beta$-triply substituted compounds LPC-037 and LPC-040 both showed enhanced LpxC inhibition, displaying K_i^* values of $14 \pm 1\,pM$ and $12 \pm 1\,pM$, respectively (Fig. 1e; Supplementary Table 4).

Drug design from the expanded inhibitor envelope. Having delineated the hidden inhibitor envelope at the $C\beta$ position of the threonyl head group, we next examined whether the dynamically accessible envelope of LpxC inhibitors can be further expanded at

the γ position. The molecule that fits this purpose is LPC-023 bearing an isoleucine-hydroxamate head group (Supplementary Table 1). Isoleucine shares a basic molecular scaffold with threonine, and its $C\gamma1$-$C\delta1$ group can be viewed as a substitution of the $O\gamma1$ group of threonine near the conserved lysine (K227^{AaLpxC}; K238^{PaLpxC}) and histidine (H253^{AaLpxC}; H264^{PaLpxC}) residues. The isoleucine analogue was crystallized with AaLpxC (Supplementary Table 2), and two copies of the LpxC-inhibitor complexes were found in the asymmetric unit. Among the two protomers of LpxC, the second protomer (chain B) displayed a distorted active site with the catalytic H253 flipped out of the active site in a configuration that has not been observed in any of the previously reported LpxC structures. We reasoned that this would likely reflect a crystallization artifact and consequently focused our analysis on the first LpxC protomer (chain A) in complex with the isoleucine analogue, LPC-023 (Fig. 2a). In this protomer, the isoleucine head group displays a *trans* χ^1 configuration, consistent with the predominant rotameric state observed in the threonyl group of CHIR-090 and LPC-011. The $C\delta1$ methyl group adopts a *gauche*+ χ^2 conformation with regard to the $C\alpha$ atom. In such a configuration, the $C\delta1$ methyl group is closest to and potentially forms vdW interactions with the nearby imidazole ring of the catalytic H253. This observation is somewhat surprising as the *gauche*+ χ^2 angle is rarely observed for isoleucine in protein structures and contributes to <5% of the observed χ^2 rotamers, indicating that such a rotamer represents a high-energy state of the free ligand.

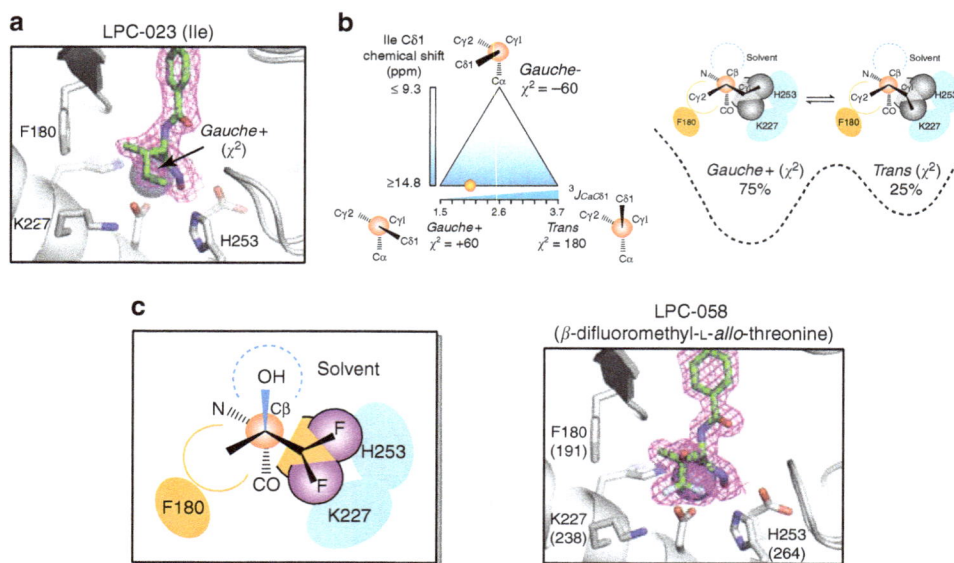

Figure 2 | Expanded inhibitor envelope enables the design of a potent inhibitor, LPC-058. (a) Crystal structure of AaLpxC in complex with LPC-023, an isoleucine derivative, reveals a *gauche+* χ^2 rotamer conformation of the inhibitor. AaLpxC is shown in the cartoon model, with the catalytically important residues in the stick model. LPC-023 is shown in the stick model, with the purple mesh representing the inhibitor omit map (2mFo-DFc) contoured at 1.0σ. (b) Combined measurements of the Cδ1 chemical shift and the $^3J_{C\alpha C\delta 1}$ coupling of LPC-023 in the protein-bound complex reveal a dynamic equilibrium between *gauche+* and *trans* χ^2 rotameric states, with the *gauche+* state being the predominant conformation ($\sim$75% population) and the *trans* state being the minor conformation ($\sim$25%). (c) Design and structural validation of LPC-058 that optimally occupies the inhibitor envelope. PaLpxC is shown in the cartoon model, with the catalytically important residues in the stick model. Residue numbering reflects the corresponding residues of AaLpxC, with PaLpxC numbers shown in parentheses. LPC-058 is shown in the stick model, with the purple mesh representing the inhibitor omit map (2mFo-DFc) contoured at 1.1σ.

We thus investigated whether the Cδ1 methyl group of the isoleucine analogue LPC-023 can access alternative χ^2 rotameric states in solution using the isotopically labelled compound.

The isoleucine Cδ1 chemical shift is sensitive to its χ^2 dihedral angle[21]. For the *gauche+* and *trans* χ^2 rotamers, isoleucine Cδ1 methyl groups display downfield shifted chemical shifts of >14.8 p.p.m., whereas upfield shifted Cδ1 chemical shifts of <9.3 p.p.m. indicate a *gauche-* χ^2 conformation. The unbound LPC-023 compound has a Cδ1 chemical shift of 12.8 p.p.m. (Supplementary Fig. 4), consistent with rotameric averaging between a *gauche-* χ^2 romateric state and the *trans/gauche+* states. In contrast, the LpxC-bound LPC-023 displays a Cδ1 chemical shift of 15.2 p.p.m. (Supplementary Fig. 4), indicating that the χ^2 conformation resides entirely in the *trans* or *gauche+* rotameric states or switches between these two states, but has no detectable population in the *gauche-* state (Fig. 2b, Supplementary Table 5). We next measured the ^3J coupling between the Cδ1 and Cα atoms (Supplementary Fig. 4). A *trans* configuration between Cα and Cδ1 would yield a large scalar coupling of $\sim$3.7 Hz, whereas a *gauche* configuration would yield a small coupling of $\sim$1.5 Hz (ref. 21). Our measurements yielded a $^3J_{C\alpha C\delta 1}$ coupling of 2.05 ± 0.04 Hz, corresponding to $75 \pm 2\%$ population in the *gauche+* χ^2 state with the Cδ1 methyl group located adjacent to H253 and $25 \pm 2\%$ population in the *trans* χ^2 state with the same methyl group oriented towards K227 (Fig. 2b, Supplementary Table 5). Although the predominant *gauche+* χ^2 rotameric state is consistent with the crystallographically observed inhibitor conformation, our NMR measurements support the notion that both the *gauche+* and *trans* states of the χ^2 rotamers are conformationally populated and they collectively expand the inhibitor envelope at the γ-position, whereas the *gauche-* χ^2 rotamer is energetically occluded and dynamically inaccessible in solution.

The delineation of two additional pockets that can accommodate methyl-sized functional groups to interact with side chains of the catalytically important histidine and lysine residues suggests fluorine as an attractive functional group for substitution. Fluorine has a slightly smaller size compared with the methyl group[22], and the fluorine atom is both strongly electronegative and lipophilic[23]. This renders the fluorine group well-suited for forming hydrophobic interactions with the deprotonated histidine side chain and the stem of the lysine group, or forming electrostatic interactions with a protonated histidine imidazolium and a positively charged lysine terminal ammonium group.

Based on this analysis, we introduced difluoro substitution to the pro-R methyl group of LPC-037 to yield LPC-058. Structural analysis of LPC-058 with PaLpxC indeed revealed the anticipated ligand conformation (Fig. 2c; Supplementary Table 2), with the β-methyl group occupying the hydrophobic pocket next to F180 (F191^{PaLpxC}) for vdW contacts, the β-hydroxyl group residing in the solvent pocket to form a water-mediated hydrogen bond with the backbone of F180 (F191^{PaLpxC}), and finally with the difluoromethyl group oriented towards H253 (H264^{PaLpxC}) and K227 (K238^{PaLpxC}). One of the fluorine atoms adopts a *gauche+* configuration with respect to Cα and forms a hydrogen bond with Nϵ1 atom of the protonated H253 (H264^{PaLpxC}), while the second fluorine atom adopts a *trans* configuration with respect to Cα and forms an electrostatic interaction with the ammonium group of K227 (K238^{PaLpxC}).

Excitingly, LPC-058 is an exceptionally potent inhibitor. It displayed slow-binding kinetics consistent with the rapid formation of an initial encounter complex (EI) followed by slow transition to the stable EI* complex (Supplementary Fig. 5). Accordingly, k_{obs} increased hyperbolically over the inhibitor concentration[24]. Steady-state kinetics analysis of the stable EI*

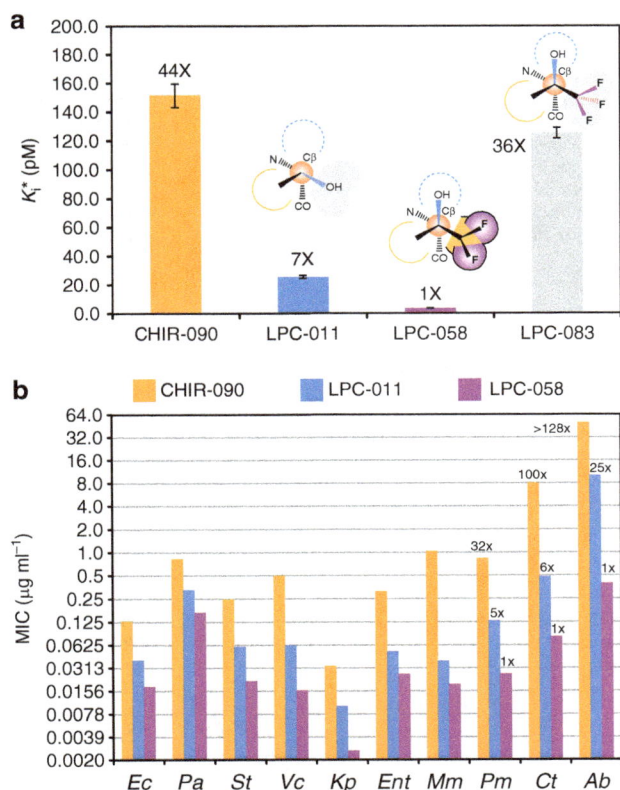

Figure 3 | LPC-058 is a superior inhibitor compared with the parent compounds LPC-011 and CHIR-090. (a) Inhibition constants of CHIR-090, LPC-011, LPC-058 and LPC-083. The head group of each compound and its conformation within the inhibitor envelope is denoted. (b) LPC-058 is a potent antibiotic and displays enhanced activity over LPC-011 and CHIR-090 against a diverse array of Gram-negative pathogens. MIC enhancement of >4-fold over LPC-011 and ≥32-fold over CHIR-090 is labelled. Tested bacterial species include *E. coli* (Ec), *P. aeruginosa* (Pa), *Salmonella typhimurium* (St), *Vibrio cholerae* (Vc), *Klebsiella pneumoniae* (Kp), *Enterobacter cloacae* (Ent), *Morganella morganii* (Mm), *Proteus mirabilis* (Pm), *Chlamydia trachomatis* (Ct) and *Acinetobacter baumannii* (Ab).

complex revealed an inhibition constant (K_i^*) of 3.5 ± 0.2 pM, a 7-fold enhancement of potency over LPC-011 and a 44-fold enhancement over CHIR-090 (Fig. 3a). Incorporation of the K_i^* value into the analysis of the inhibitor concentration-dependent k_{obs} values enabled accurate determination of the forward rate ($k_5 = 0.39 \pm 0.02$ min^{-1}) and reverse rate ($k_6 = 0.0014 \pm 0.0001$ min^{-1}) from EI to EI* and the inhibition constant of the initial encounter complex EI ($K_i = 973 \pm 128$ pM).

To examine whether LPC-058 designed from the cryptic inhibitor envelope shows improved antibiotic activity over CHIR-090 and LPC-011, we determined its minimum inhibitory concentration (MIC) values against a range of Gram-negative pathogens. LPC-058 showed uniform improvement over CHIR-090 and LPC-011 against all Gram-negative bacterial strains tested (Fig. 3b, Supplementary Table 6). In general, enhanced antibiotic activities of 2- to 4-fold over LPC-011 and 5- to 55-fold over CHIR-090 were observed for *E. coli*, *P. aeruginosa*, *Salmonella typhimurium*, *Vibrio cholerae*, *Klebsiella pneumoniae*, *Enterobacter cloacae* and *Morganella morganii*. More pronounced improvements (5- to 25-fold over LPC-011 and 32- to >128-folds over CHIR-090) were observed for *Proteus mirabilis*, *Chlamydia trachomatis* and *Acinetobacter baumannii*. Of particular importance is the potent antibiotic activity of LPC-058

against *Acinetobacter baumannii* (MIC = 0.39 µg ml^{-1}). To the best of our knowledge, LPC-058 is the first reported LpxC inhibitor with an MIC value below 1 µg ml^{-1} against this clinically important Gram-negative pathogen *in vitro*. The broad-spectrum antibiotic activity of LPC-058 highlights the therapeutic potential of LpxC inhibitors as effective antibiotics against a wide range of Gram-negative infections.

Discussion

It is widely acknowledged that the dynamic interconversion of multiple conformational states is an intrinsic property of proteins and nucleic acids in solution. In comparison, the conformational dynamics of small molecules in their receptor-bound states has rarely been investigated, let alone utilized for drug design. Here we show that small-molecule inhibitors of LpxC dynamically access alternative, minor-state ligand conformations in addition to the predominant conformational state observed in crystal structures. These minor-state ligand conformations, together with that of the major state, collectively delineate a cryptic inhibitor envelope in solution that is invisible to crystallographic studies. Furthermore, we show that such a cryptic inhibitor envelope provides important molecular insights for the design of high-affinity ligands. In the case of LpxC inhibitors, analysis of the inhibitor envelope has led to the development of a potent antibiotic LPC-058. With inclusion of only three additional heavy atoms, the newly designed compound LPC-058 enhanced the inhibitory effect towards *E. coli* LpxC over its parent compound LPC-011 by 7-fold and improved antibiotic activity by 2- to 25-fold against a wide range of Gram-negative pathogens, rendering it the most potent and the most broad-spectrum LpxC inhibitor *in vitro*. Although some features of the LpxC inhibitor envelope, such as the solvent accessible pocket at the Cβ position of the threonyl head group, might have been envisaged based on structural analysis of the LpxC/CHIR-090 complex[14] and LpxC inhibitors bearing similar head groups to LPC-037 and LPC-040, but different tail groups, have been reported[25,26], the precise definition of two accessory pockets at the Oγ1-position of the threonyl head group could not have been predicted by structural analysis alone. In fact, the most widely employed functional substitution of a pro-*R* methyl of LPC-037 is the trifluoromethyl group (CF$_3$), not the difluoromethyl group (CF$_2$) utilized in LPC-058. However, the trifluoromethyl substituted compound LPC-083 compromised the inhibitory effect ($K_i^* = 125 \pm 4$ pM) over its parent compound LPC-037 ($K_i^* = 14 \pm 1$ pM) by nearly ninefold (Supplementary Table 4). Its inhibition constant is worse than LPC-011 by fivefold (Fig. 3a), and it is a less potent antibiotic against *E. coli* (MIC = 0.1 µg ml^{-1}) than LPC-011 (MIC = 0.04 µg ml^{-1}), which would have argued away from development of the synthetically more challenging β-difluoromethyl-*allo*-threonyl compound LPC-058 designed from the dynamic inhibitor envelope.

The work presented here departs from the established paradigm of ligand design from the crystallographically visible, static ligand conformation and highlights the potential of drug development from the 'invisible', dynamically accessible inhibitor envelope in solution, which encompasses the receptor-bound ligand conformations from both major and minor states. The framework presented here should be broadly applicable to lead optimization campaigns for small molecules, peptides and peptidomimetics to yield more effective therapeutics.

Methods

Chemical synthesis. Details of chemical synthesis and characterization are described in Supplementary Methods.

Crystallography structural analysis. Protein samples of AaLpxC and PaLpxC were prepared as described previously[16]. Before crystallization trials, a fourfold molar excess of each compound, dissolved in DMSO, was mixed with 8 mg ml^{-1} AaLpxC (1-275, C181A) in 100 mM potassium chloride, 2 mM dithiothreitol and 25 mM HEPES (pH 7.0) or 12 mg ml^{-1} PaLpxC (1-299, C40S) in 50 mM sodium chloride, 2 mM tris(2-carboxyethyl)phosphine and 25 mM HEPES (pH 7.0), respectively. For PaLpxC, 10 mM zinc sulfate was added as a crystallization additive. The protein-inhibitor mixture was incubated for 30 min at room temperature to obtain a homogenous sample. All of the LpxC-inhibitor complex crystals were obtained by the sitting-drop vapour diffusion method at 20 °C. Initial crystallization screening yielded microcrystals for the AaLpxC/LPC-011 complex in a reservoir solution containing 0.1 M HEPES (pH 7.0) and 15% PEG 8000 and for the AaLpxC/LPC-023 complex in a reservoir solution containing 0.18 M ammonium chloride, 11.8% PEG3350 and 4% 1,3-propanediol. The microcrystals were used to prepare seeding stocks by the Seed-Bead protocol (Hampton Research, HR2-320). Diffraction quality crystals were obtained by the streak-seeding method. The final crystallization reservoirs contained 0.05 M ammonium acetate and 10% PEG3350 for the AaLpxC/LPC-011 complex and 0.18 M ammonium chloride, 11.8% PEG3350 and 10% 1,3-propanediol for the AaLpxC/LPC-023 complex, respectively. High quality crystals of the PaLpxC/LPC-040 and PaLpxC/LPC-058 complexes were obtained in precipitant solutions containing 0.1 M sodium acetate trihydrate (pH 4.8–5.1) and 2.4–2.6 M ammonium nitrate. Crystals were cryoprotected using the corresponding mother liquor solutions containing 30% 2-methyl-2,4-pentanediol (MPD) for the AaLpxC/LPC-011 complex, 30% ethylene glycol for the AaLpxC/LPC-023 complex and 10% glycerol for the PaLpxC/inhibitor complexes, respectively, before flash-freezing for data collection.

Data sets of the PaLpxC/LPC-040 and PaLpxC/LPC-058 complexes were collected in-house using a Rigaku MicroMax-007 HF rotating anode generator and R-Axis IV + + detector. Data sets of the AaLpxC/LPC-011 and AaLpxC/LPC-023 were collected at the SER-CAT 22-ID beamline at the Advanced Photon Source at Argonne National Laboratory. The collected X-ray diffraction data were processed using HKL2000 (ref. 27) or XDS (ref. 28). The crystal structures of LpxC-inhibitor complexes were solved by molecular replacement with the programme PHASER (ref. 29) using PDB entries 3P3O and 3P3E for the AaLpxC-inhibitor complexes and the PaLpxC-inhibitor complexes, respectively. Restraints of the inhibitors were generated by using ELBOW (ref. 30) and edited manually. Iterative model building and refinement was carried out using COOT (ref. 31) and PHENIX (ref. 32). The 2mFo-DFc omit maps[33] were generated using PHENIX[32].

Solution NMR measurements. Deuterated AaLpxC was expressed and purified as described previously[13]. The AaLpxC-inhibitor complexes were prepared by adding individual inhibitors to the purified protein in the presence of 5% deuterated dimethylsulfoxide (DMSO) in a 1:2 protein-inhibitor molar ratio, and incubated initially at room temperature and then at 45 °C to form the complex. Samples were concentrated and exchanged into the NMR buffer containing 25 mM sodium phosphate pH 7.0, 100 mM KCl, 5% deuterated DMSO and 100% D$_2$O. The NMR sample concentration was ∼1 mM.

The scalar couplings of $^3J_{C'C\gamma2}$ and $^3J_{NC\gamma2}$ for the AaLpxC/CHIR-090 and AaLpxC/LPC-011 complexes were measured on a Bruker 700 MHz NMR spectrometer at 45 °C, using J-modulated ^{1}H-^{13}C constant-time HSQC experiments[34,35]. The reference and scalar coupling-modulated CT-HSQC spectra were recorded in an interleaved manner with a constant-time delay (2T) set to 57.4 ms, and the maximum evolution time for the indirect (^{13}C) dimension set 12.1 ms. Data were processed using NMRPIPE (ref. 36) with eightfold zero-filling in the indirect dimension. The peak intensities were measured by SPARKY (ref. 37), and the $^3J_{C'C\gamma2}$ and $^3J_{NC\gamma2}$ couplings were calculated from the ratio of the peak intensities between the reference spectrum (I$_{ref}$) and the J-modulated spectrum (I$_{mod}$) according to equation (1):

$$\frac{I_{mod}}{I_{ref}} = \cos(2\pi JT) \tag{1}$$

Rotameric populations were calculated based on the three-site jump model[19] using values derived from self-consistent parameterization of ^3J couplings[20].

The scalar coupling $^3J_{C\alpha C\delta1}$ for the AaLpxC/LPC-023 complex was measured on an Agilent 800 MHz NMR spectrometer at 37 °C using a J-modulated constant-time ^{13}C HSQC experiment using selective Ile-Cα inversion pulses. The $^3J_{C\alpha C\delta1}$ coupling was calculated from the ratio of the peak intensities between the reference spectrum (I$_{ref}$) and the J-modulated spectrum (I$_{mod}$) according to equation (1). Since the Cδ1 chemical shift of 15.2 p.p.m. of LPC-023 excludes the gauche- χ^2 rotamer[21], populations of the remaining rotamers were calculated from $^3J_{C\alpha C\delta1}$ based on the two-site jump model between the gauche + and trans rotameric states[21].

Enzymatic assays. The radiolabeled substrate for the LpxC enzymatic assays, [α-^{32}P] UDP-3-O-[(R)-3-hydroxymyristoyl]-N-acetylglucosamine, and the unlabelled carrier substrate were prepared as previously described[38]. The assays were performed in a buffer consisting of 25 mM HEPES pH 7.4, 100 mM KCl, 1 mg ml^{-1} BSA, 2 mM dithiothreitol and 5 μM substrate at 30 °C. Serial twofold dilutions of each inhibitor were prepared in DMSO and added to the reaction

mixture with a 10-fold dilution. The assays were initiated by addition of purified LpxC protein into the reaction mix with 1:4 dilution to the final concentration as specified.

The K_M value was determined by varying substrate concentrations from 0.4 to 50 μM with 0.2 nM of LpxC. To study the slow, tight-binding inhibition, LpxC activity was assessed in the presence of varying inhibitor concentrations. The product conversions were determined from 15 s up to 2 h after addition of 0.2 nM enzyme for CHIR-090 and LPC-011 in the presence of 5 μM substrate. Time-dependent inhibition of LPC-058 was assayed in the presence of 30 μM substrate and 0.1 nM enzyme such that k_{obs} can be extracted under the slow, but not tight-binding conditions[39]. The following time-dependent equation was used to fit the data:

$$[P] = v_s t + \frac{v_i - v_s}{k_{obs}} [1 - e^{-k_{obs}t}] + c \tag{2}$$

with v_s representing the steady-state rate, v_i the initial rate, k_{obs} the rate of transition from the initial encounter complex to the final complex and c the baseline.

The K_i^* was determined by analysing the rate of product accumulation after formation of the stable EI* complex. IC$_{50}$ curves for individual compounds were determined in the presence of 20 pM of the enzyme and varying inhibitor concentrations. The Morrison's quadratic equation was used to fit the fractional activity data to determine K_i^{*app}:

$$\frac{v_i}{v_0} = 1 - \frac{[E]_T + [I]_T + K_i^{*app} - \sqrt{([E]_T + [I]_T + K_i^{*app})^2 - 4[E]_T[I]_T}}{2[E]_T} \tag{3}$$

where $[E]_T$ and $[I]_T$ represent the total enzyme and inhibitor concentrations, respectively. The inhibition constant K_i^* is converted from K_i^{*app} according to the following relationship:

$$K_i^* = K_i^{*app}/(1 + \frac{[S]}{K_M}) \tag{4}$$

For two-step slow-binding inhibition, kinetic parameters k_5, k_6 and K_i were extracted from curve fitting of experimental k_{obs} values to inhibitor concentrations based on equations (5 and 6).

$$k_{obs} = k_6 + \frac{k_5[I]}{K_i^{app} + [I]} = k_6 + \frac{k_5[I]}{K_i(1 + [S]/K_M) + [I]} \tag{5}$$

$$K_i = K_i^*(1 + k_5/k_6) \tag{6}$$

Measurements of the minimum inhibitory concentration (MIC). The MIC assay protocol was adapted from methods described in National Committee for Clinical Laboratory Standards (NCCLS) to using 96-well plates[40]. Bacteria were grown in the Mueller–Hinton medium at 37 °C in the presence of varying concentrations of inhibitors and 5% DMSO. To obtain more accurate readings of the MICs, three series of twofold dilutions of inhibitors were used. The starting concentrations of the three series are different by factors of 1.33 and 1.67, respectively. MICs were reported as the lowest compound concentration that inhibited bacterial growth.

References

1. Thanos, C. D., Randal, M. & Wells, J. A. Potent small-molecule binding to a dynamic hot spot on IL-2. J. Am. Chem. Soc. **125**, 15280–15281 (2003).
2. Carlson, H. A. & McCammon, J. A. Accommodating protein flexibility in computational drug design. Mol. Pharmacol. **57**, 213–218 (2000).
3. Wagner, G. & Wuthrich, K. Dynamic model of globular protein conformations based on NMR studies in solution. Nature **275**, 247–248 (1978).
4. Eisenmesser, E. Z. et al. Intrinsic dynamics of an enzyme underlies catalysis. Nature **438**, 117–121 (2005).
5. Whittier, S. K., Hengge, A. C. & Loria, J. P. Conformational motions regulate phosphoryl transfer in related protein tyrosine phosphatases. Science **341**, 899–903 (2013).
6. Bhabha, G. et al. A dynamic knockout reveals that conformational fluctuations influence the chemical step of enzyme catalysis. Science **332**, 234–238 (2011).
7. Boehr, D. D., McElheny, D., Dyson, H. J. & Wright, P. E. The dynamic energy landscape of dihydrofolate reductase catalysis. Science **313**, 1638–1642 (2006).
8. Tzeng, S. R. & Kalodimos, C. G. Dynamic activation of an allosteric regulatory protein. Nature **462**, 368–372 (2009).
9. Kimsey, I. J., Petzold, K., Sathyamoorthy, B., Stein, Z. W. & Al-Hashimi, H. M. Visualizing transient Watson-Crick-like mispairs in DNA and RNA duplexes. Nature **519**, 315–320 (2015).
10. Frederick, K. K., Marlow, M. S., Valentine, K. G. & Wand, A. J. Conformational entropy in molecular recognition by proteins. Nature **448**, 325–329 (2007).
11. Barb, A. W. & Zhou, P. Mechanism and inhibition of LpxC: an essential zinc-dependent deacetylase of bacterial lipid A synthesis. Curr. Pharm. Biotechnol. **9**, 9–15 (2008).

12. Raetz, C. R. H. & Whitfield, C. Lipopolysaccharide endotoxins. *Annu. Rev. Biochem.* **71**, 635–700 (2002).
13. Coggins, B. E. *et al.* Structure of the LpxC deacetylase with a bound substrate-analog inhibitor. *Nat. Struct. Biol.* **10**, 645–651 (2003).
14. Barb, A. W., Jiang, L., Raetz, C. R. & Zhou, P. Structure of the deacetylase LpxC bound to the antibiotic CHIR-090: Time-dependent inhibition and specificity in ligand binding. *Proc. Natl Acad. Sci. USA* **104**, 18433–18438 (2007).
15. Whittington, D. A., Rusche, K. M., Shin, H., Fierke, C. A. & Christianson, D. W. Crystal structure of LpxC, a zinc-dependent deacetylase essential for endotoxin biosynthesis. *Proc. Natl Acad. Sci. USA* **100**, 8146–8150 (2003).
16. Lee, C. J. *et al.* Species-specific and inhibitor-dependent conformations of LpxC: implications for antibiotic design. *Chem. Biol.* **18**, 38–47 (2011).
17. Liang, X. *et al.* Syntheses, structures and antibiotic activities of LpxC inhibitors based on the diacetylene scaffold. *Bioorg. Med. Chem.* **19**, 852–860 (2011).
18. Lovell, S. C., Word, J. M., Richardson, J. S. & Richardson, D. C. The penultimate rotamer library. *Proteins* **40**, 389–408 (2000).
19. Hennig, M. *et al.* Side-chain conformations in an unfolded protein: chi1 distributions in denatured hen lysozyme determined by heteronuclear ^{13}C, ^{15}N NMR spectroscopy. *J. Mol. Biol.* **288**, 705–723 (1999).
20. Perez, C., Lohr, F., Ruterjans, H. & Schmidt, J. M. Self-consistent Karplus parametrization of ^{3}J couplings depending on the polypeptide side-chain torsion chi1. *J. Am. Chem. Soc.* **123**, 7081–7093 (2001).
21. Hansen, D. F., Neudecker, P. & Kay, L. E. Determination of isoleucine side-chain conformations in ground and excited states of proteins from chemical shifts. *J. Am. Chem. Soc.* **132**, 7589–7591 (2010).
22. Meng, H., Clark, G. A. & Kumar, K. in *Fluorine in Medicinal Chemistry and Chemical Biology.* (ed. Ojima, I.) 411–446 (Blackwell Publishing Ltd, 2009).
23. Wang, J. *et al.* Fluorine in pharmaceutical industry: fluorine-containing drugs introduced to the market in the last decade (2001–2011). *Chem. Rev.* **114**, 2432–2506 (2014).
24. Vogt, A. D. & Di Cera, E. Conformational selection or induced fit? A critical appraisal of the kinetic mechanism. *Biochemistry* **51**, 5894–5902 (2012).
25. Mansoor, U. F. *et al.* Design and synthesis of potent Gram-negative specific LpxC inhibitors. *Bioorg. Med. Chem. Lett.* **21**, 1155–1161 (2011).
26. Fei, Z. *et al.* A scalable synthesis of a hydroxamic acid LpxC inhibitor. *Org. Process Res. Dev.* **16**, 1436–1441 (2012).
27. Otwinowski, Z. & Minor, W. Processing of X-ray diffraction data collected in oscillation mode. *Methods Enzymol.* **276**, 307–326 (1997).
28. Kabsch, W. XDS. *Acta Crystallogr. D Biol. Crystallogr.* **66**, 125–132 (2010).
29. McCoy, A. J. *et al.* Phaser crystallographic software. *J. Appl. Crystallogr.* **40**, 658–674 (2007).
30. Moriarty, N. W., Grosse-Kunstleve, R. W. & Adams, P. D. electronic Ligand Builder and Optimization Workbench (eLBOW): a tool for ligand coordinate and restraint generation. *Acta Crystallogr. D Biol. Crystallogr.* **65**, 1074–1080 (2009).
31. Emsley, P. & Cowtan, K. Coot: model-building tools for molecular graphics. *Acta Crystallogr. D Biol. Crystallogr.* **60**, 2126–2132 (2004).
32. Adams, P. D. *et al.* PHENIX: a comprehensive Python-based system for macromolecular structure solution. *Acta Crystallogr. D Biol. Crystallogr.* **66**, 213–221 (2010).
33. Terwilliger, T. C. *et al.* Iterative-build OMIT maps: map improvement by iterative model building and refinement without model bias. *Acta Crystallogr. D Biol. Crystallogr.* **64**, 515–524 (2008).
34. Grzesiek, S., Vuister, G. W. & Bax, A. A simple and sensitive experiment for measurement of JCC couplings between backbone carbonyl and methyl carbons in isotopically enriched proteins. *J. Biomol. NMR* **3**, 487–493 (1993).
35. Vuister, G. W., Wang, A. C. & Bax, A. Measurement of three-bond nitrogen-carbon J couplings in proteins uniformly enriched in ^{15}N and ^{13}C. *J. Am. Chem. Soc.* **115**, 5334–5335 (1993).
36. Delaglio, F. *et al.* NMRPipe: a multidimensional spectral processing system based on UNIX pipes. *J. Biomol. NMR* **6**, 277–293 (1995).
37. Goddard, T. D. & Kneller, D. G. *Sparky 3* (Univeristy of California, 2008).
38. Jackman, J. E., Raetz, C. R. H. & Fierke, C. A. Site-directed mutagenesis of the bacterial metalloamidase UDP-(3-O-acyl)-N-acetylglucosamine deacetylase (LpxC). Identification of the zinc binding site. *Biochemistry* **40**, 514–523 (2001).
39. Zhang, R. & Windsor, W. T. In vitro kinetic profiling of hepatitis C virus NS3 protease inhibitors by progress curve analysis. *Methods Mol. Biol.* **1030**, 59–79 (2013).
40. National Committee for Clinical Laboratory Standards. *Approved Standard M7-A1: Methods For Dilution Antimicrobial Susceptibility Test For Bacteria That Grow Aerobically.* Clinical and Laboratory Standards Institute, Wayne, PA, USA (1997).

Acknowledgements

Diffraction data of LpxC-inhibitor complexes were collected at the Duke Macromolecular X-ray Crystallography Shared Resource and at the Southeast Regional Collaborative Access Team (SER-CAT) 22-ID beamline at the Advanced Photon Source, Argonne National Laboratory, supported by the US Department of Energy, Office of Science and the Office of Basic Energy Sciences under Contract number W-31-109-Eng-38. NMR data were collected at the Duke University NMR Center. This work was supported by National Institutes of Health grants AI055588 and AI094475, and the Duke Bridge Fund awarded to P.Z. The authors would like to acknowledge Drs Bidong D. Nguyen and Raphael Valdivia for providing the MCC (minimal chlamydiacidal concentration) measurements of LpxC inhibitors against *Chlamydia trachomatis*, and Dr Xin Chen for insightful discussions on compound synthesis.

Author contributions

P.Z. conceived the project. C.-J.L. and J.N. determined crystal structures of LpxC-inhibitor complexes; X.L. and R.G. synthesized LpxC inhibitors under the direction of E.J.T.; Q.W. performed NMR studies; J.Z. carried out enzymatic assays; and J.Z., C.-J. L., M.T., F.S. and N.L. determined the antibiotic activities of LpxC inhibitors. P.Z. wrote the manuscript with critical inputs from all authors.

Additional information

Accession codes: The coordinates for the X-ray structures have been deposited to the Protein Data Bank (PDB) with accession codes of 5DRO, 5DRQ, 5DRP and 5DRR for the AaLpxC/LPC-011, PaLpxC/LPC-040, AaLpxC/LPC-023 and PaLpxC/LPC-058 complexes, respectively.

Competing financial interests: P.Z. and E.J.T. declare a competing financial interest. A patent on designed LpxC inhibitors was awarded to P.Z. and E.J.T. The remaining authors declare no competing financial interest.

21

Lysosome triggered near-infrared fluorescence imaging of cellular trafficking processes in real time

Marco Grossi[1], Marina Morgunova[1], Shane Cheung[1,2], Dimitri Scholz[3], Emer Conroy[3], Marta Terrile[3], Angela Panarella[4], Jeremy C. Simpson[4], William M. Gallagher[3] & Donal F. O'Shea[1,2]

Bioresponsive NIR-fluorophores offer the possibility for continual visualization of dynamic cellular processes with added potential for direct translation to *in vivo* imaging. Here we show the design, synthesis and lysosome-responsive emission properties of a new NIR fluorophore. The NIR fluorescent probe design differs from typical amine functionalized lysosomotropic stains with off/on fluorescence switching controlled by a reversible phenol/phenolate interconversion. Emission from the probe is shown to be highly selective for the lysosomes in co-imaging experiments using a HeLa cell line expressing the lysosomal-associated membrane protein 1 fused to green fluorescent protein. The responsive probe is capable of real-time continuous imaging of fundamental cellular processes such as endocytosis, lysosomal trafficking and efflux in 3D and 4D. The advantage of the NIR emission allows for direct translation to *in vivo* tumour imaging, which is successfully demonstrated using an MDA-MB-231 subcutaneous tumour model. This bioresponsive NIR fluorophore offers significant potential for use in live cellular and *in vivo* imaging, for which currently there is a deficit of suitable molecular fluorescent tools.

[1] Department of Pharmaceutical and Medicinal Chemistry, Royal College of Surgeons in Ireland, 123 St Stephen's Green, Dublin 2, Ireland. [2] School of Chemistry and Chemical Biology, Conway Institute, University College Dublin, Belfield, Dublin 4, Ireland. [3] School of Biomolecular and Biomedical Science, Conway Institute of Biomolecular and Biomedical Research, University College Dublin, Belfield, Dublin 4, Ireland. [4] School of Biology and Environmental Science, Conway Institute of Biomolecular and Biomedical Research, University College Dublin, Belfield, Dublin 4, Ireland. Correspondence and requests for materials should be addressed to D.F.O. (email: donalfoshea@rcsi.ie).

Ehrlich's use of synthetic dyes as a means of staining biological samples can be viewed as one of the foundation stones of modern scientific research. A century later, the use of fluorescence imaging as a technique to visualize specific regions of live cellular[1–4] or whole organisms[5,6] is often central to research programmes, with clinical applications such as fluorescence-guided surgery now emerging[7–11].

The major shortcomings of fluorescence imaging using molecular fluorophores are interference from nonspecific background fluorescence outside the region of interest (ROI), insufficient photostability and cytotoxicity. Poor ROI selectivity necessitates a time delay to allow background fluorophore clearance and/or a washing procedure between fluorophore administration and image acquisition. This can limit imaging to fixed cells or static snapshots, without the possibility of continuous data acquisition throughout the experiment. An innovative approach to enhance target-to-background signal ratio is to exploit a mechanism of selective fluorescence quenching in the background areas, while establishing the emitting potential of the fluorophore only in the ROI[12,13]. Continuous recording of dynamic cellular events in real time may become feasible if the on/off fluorescence switching is reversible.

Developing a responsive fluorophore suitable for real-time live-cell imaging poses a series of challenges. Stringent criteria are required, such as near-perfect response selectivity, exceptional photostability and low dark and light toxicities. Obtaining selective fluorescence responses for intracellular analytes is not trivial, as analyte selectivity observed in a controlled homogeneous environment of a cuvette does not necessarily translate to far more complex in vitro or in vivo settings. Continuous live-cell imaging places very high demands on photostability of the fluorophore, as the same cell(s) are repeatedly imaged over time. Fluorophore dark toxicity must be low, so that cell viability is not compromised and normal cellular processes are unperturbed. To minimize light-induced toxicity, it is preferable to use low-energy wavelengths in the near-infrared (NIR) spectral region ($\lambda = 700$–900 nm). For in vivo imaging, the use of NIR fluorophores is essential. This spectral region is required for effective light transmission through body tissue, as there are reduced levels of absorption and scattering at these longer wavelengths and less intrinsic autofluorescence. In addition, if on/off NIR fluorescence switching could be accomplished in vivo, then similar imaging advantages could be gained as for in-vitro cell imaging.

Currently, there is a small yet growing selection of NIR fluorophore classes but they often suffer from insufficient photostability and lack emission wavelengths above 700 nm[14]. Our recent research focus led to the development of BF$_2$-chelated azadipyrromethene class 1 (Fig. 1)[15–18]. This class is relatively straightforward to synthesize, amenable to structural elaboration and exhibits excellent photophysical properties. For example, the derivative 1 (R = Ph) has an absorption/emission λ_{max} at 696 and 727 nm in aqueous solutions, high fluorescence quantum yields (0.3–0.4) and excellent photostability[17]. Yet, in spite of recent progress, a significant need remains for new, more sophisticated intracellularly responsive molecular NIR fluorophores, which can be used to visualize dynamic cellular processes in real time with the potential for in vivo translation.

The goal of our current work was to develop an NIR fluorophore capable of a lysosomal-induced off-to-on fluorescence response, thereby permitting real-time imaging of cellular uptake, trafficking and efflux without perturbing function[19]. Endocytosis, the process through which cells internalize biomolecules, is common to all cells and represents a crucial area of research interest due to the numerous associated biological processes[20,21]. The participating organelles at each stage in the endocytosis pathway maintain a unique intravesicular/localized pH, to provide appropriate conditions for specific biochemical processes. Although the extracellular and cytosolic regions are at pH ~ 7.2, the lysosomes are significantly more acidic. Along the endocytic pathway, the pH lowers from ~ 6.3 in early endosomes through ~ 5.5 in late endosomes, down to ~ 4.5 in lysosomes (Fig. 2)[22]. As such, a difference of almost three orders of magnitude in proton concentration exists between the lysosome interior and the outside of a cell, which is sufficient to establish a selective trigger for fluorescence switching[23–26]. However, a major additional response selectivity challenge still remains, in that pH-responsive molecular fluorophores can also be responsive to micro-environmental polarity, which can compromise their use in cellular experiments (vide infra).

Our novel lysosomal responsive probe design is illustrated in Fig. 1 in which functionalization of the fluorophore core (orange box) with an ortho-nitro phenolic group was chosen to impart the pH-responsive feature of the probe. It would be expected that the electron withdrawing o-nitro group would result in the ionized phenolate dominating at pH 7.2, resulting in fluorescence quenching due to a non-emissive intramolecular charge transfer excited state (Fig. 1, grey box). Following cellular uptake via endocytosis and compartmentalization into acidic organelles such as lysosomes, protonation would occur giving the neutral phenol species and the NIR emission signal would be established (Fig. 1, red box). This approach is a significant departure from other lysosomal stains, which rely on an amine protonation to form a positively charged ammonium salt to concentrate the fluorophore in the acidic compartments[19,22]. An important additional design feature includes a covalently linked polyethylene glycol (PEG) polymer to provide aqueous solubility and promote cellular uptake via endocytic pathways (Fig. 1, blue box)[27].

Results

Synthesis and photophysics. The starting point of the synthesis was the previously reported BF$_2$-chelated bis-phenol azadipyrromethene 3, accessible in three synthetic steps from 1-(4-hydroxyphenyl)-3-phenylpropenone (Fig. 1)[28]. Monoalkylation of 3 was achieved to produce 4 by reaction with t-butyl bromoacetate and CsF in dimethylsulfoxide (DMSO) at 30 °C. After isolation, compound 4 was then subjected to ortho-nitration of the remaining phenol ring with KHSO$_4$/KNO$_3$ to provide 5. Next, hydrolysis of the t-butyl ester of 5 with trifluoroacetic acid (TFA) gave the carboxylic acid 6, which was converted into its activated ester 7 by reaction with N-hydroxysuccinimide and N-(3-dimethylaminopropyl)-N'-ethylcarbodiimide in DMSO. Formation of the activated ester was monitored by ^{1}H NMR via the diagnostic CH$_2$ peaks at 5.48 for 7 and 4.83 p.p.m. for carboxylic acid 6, which showed complete conversion within 2 h (Supplementary Fig. 1). Conjugation of 7 in DMSO with a terminal amine functionalized PEG polymer (average molecular weight of 4,900) was effective, with the final fluorophore 2 obtained in high yield (Fig. 1). Matrix-assisted laser desorption/ionization–time of flight (MALDI–TOF) analysis of 2 showed the expected molecular weight centred at 5,410 Da, indicating that the covalent linkage was effective. Furthermore, ^{1}H NMR was consistent with the product structure and analytical high-performance liquid chromatography (HPLC) showed a single peak for 2 with retention time differing from that of both the acid 6 and ester 7 (Supplementary Fig. 2).

Comparative absorption and fluorescence emission spectra were recorded for the organic soluble fluorophore 5 in chloroform and aqueous soluble 2 in phenol red-free imaging DMEM medium adjusted to pH 2 (Fig. 3a). Only small differences were

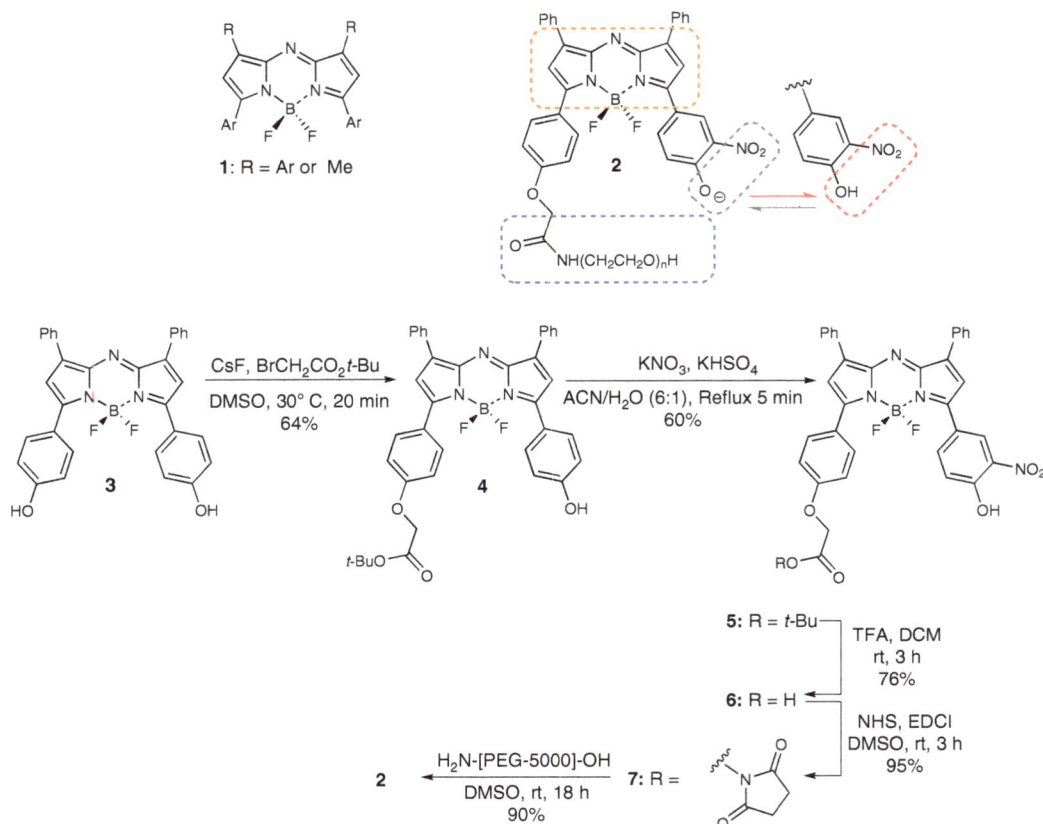

Figure 1 | BF$_2$-azadipyrromethene NIR fluorophores. General structure of BF$_2$-azadipyrromethenes **1**. Design and synthesis of lysosomal responsive BF$_2$-azadipyrromethene NIR fluorophore **2**.

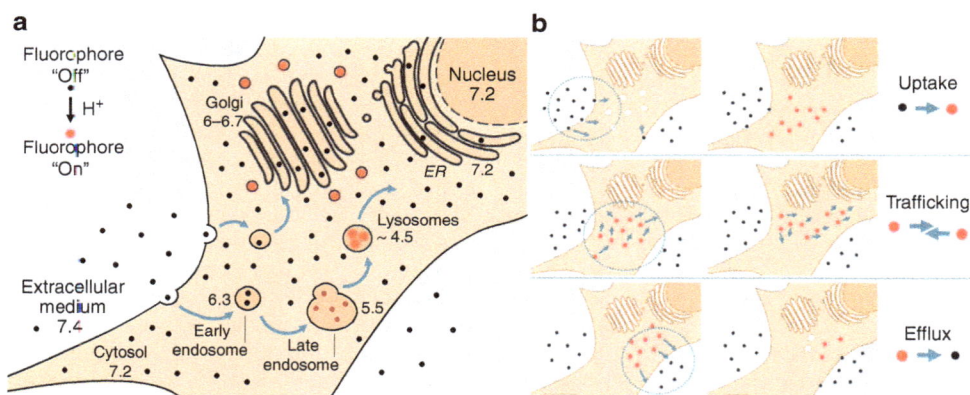

Figure 2 | Cellular uptake responsive NIR-fluorophore. (**a**) Simplified endocytosis of a responsive NIR fluorophore. Numbers represent the approximate pH of the corresponding organelles. (**b**) Three observable stages of the path of the pH-responsive fluorophore in the cellular environment: uptake, trafficking and efflux.

observed between the two fluorophores in the differing organic and aqueous media. Encouragingly, probe **2** had fluorescence λ_{max} at 707 nm with an absorbance λ_{max} at 685 nm. Extinction coefficient and fluorescence quantum yield values for **5** and **2** were similar with polyethylene glycol-substituted **2** having values of 97,000 cm^{-1} M^{-1} and 0.18, respectively (Fig. 3a).

An undesirable feature of some pH-sensitive fluorophores is their strong sensitivity to micro-environmental polarity, which significantly compromises their use in biological settings[29–31]. To test the polarity sensitivity of **2**, its acid/base emission-responsive properties were recorded in toluene, tetrahydrofuran, dimethylformamide and DMSO for both the phenol and phenolate state using 1,8-diazabicyclo[5.4.0]undec-7-ene (DBU)

and TFA to cycle between the two (Fig. 3b). A plot of solvent polarity function (Δf)[32] versus integrated fluorescence intensities in the off states showed highly effective fluorescence quenching as the phenolate irrespective of solvent polarity. A strong fluorescence output was established once protonated to the phenol in all solvents (Fig. 3c). These results predict that the modulation of fluorescence intensity would be selective for pH changes, while remaining unresponsive to differing intracellular micro-environmental polarities, thereby removing the potential for false-positive emissions. An identical study was carried out for fluorophore **5**, giving similar results and indicating that this positive feature is general to the fluorophore class (Supplementary Fig. 3).

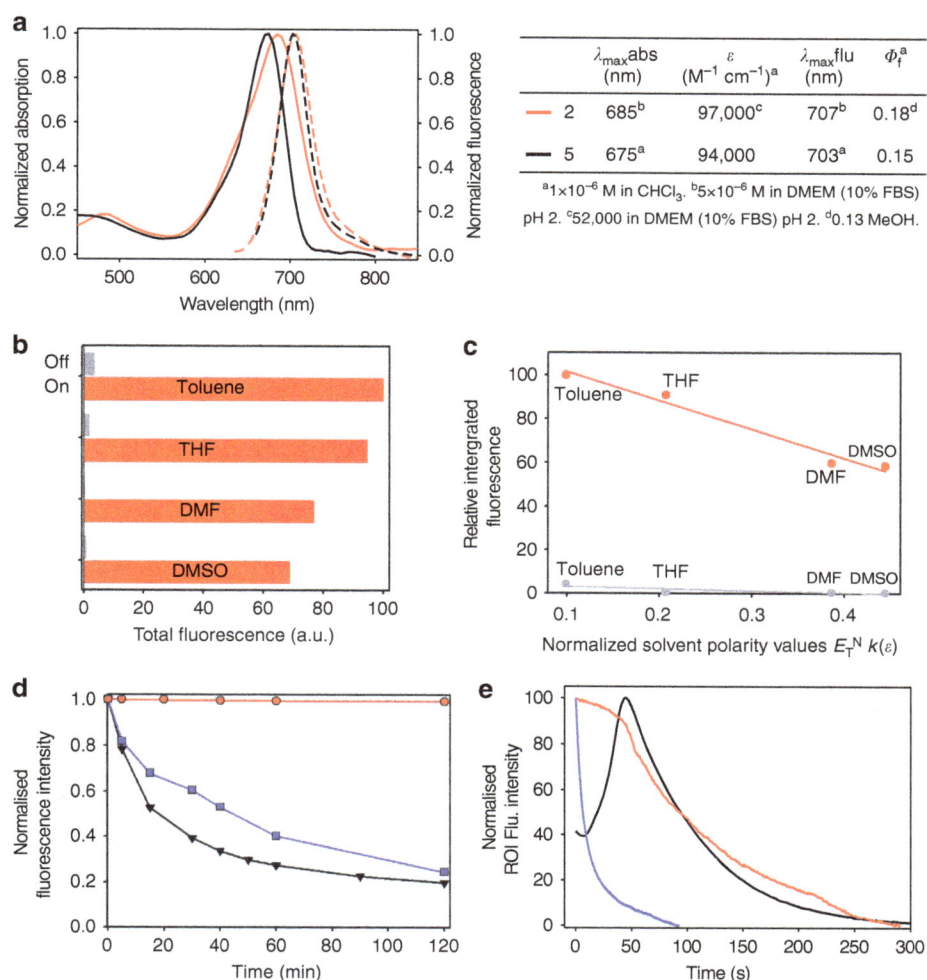

Figure 3 | Photophysical properties of NIR-fluorophores. (a) Light absorption and emission spectra of compounds **2** and **5**, and their photo-physical parameters. (b) Integrated off and on fluorescence states of **2** (5×10^{-6} M) in toluene, tetrahydrofuran (THF), dimethylformamide (DMF) and DMSO with TFA (red bars) and DBU (grey bars). (c) Plot of relative off and on integrated fluorescence versus solvent polarity values for toluene, THF, DMF and DMSO. (d) Comparative photobleaching of 1×10^{-7} M DMEM solutions of **2** (red line), lysotracker red (blue line) and pHrodo red (black line) with 150 W fibre optic delivered light 620(30) nm for **2** and 540(40) nm for lysotracker red and pH-rhodo red at 25 °C. (e) In vitro photobleaching of **2** (red), lysotracker red (blue line) and pHrodo red (black line) with maximum LED power using excitation filter 640(14) nm for **2** and excitation filter 563(9) nm for lysotracker red and pH-rhodo red.

As sufficient photostability is an essential property for prolonged live-cell imaging, a comparative study of the photo-degradation of **2**, lysotracker red and pH-rhodo red was carried out. DMEM solutions of the three fluorophores were illuminated with light of 620(30) nm for **2** and 540(40) nm for lysotracker red and pH-rhodo red for 2 h, and their fluorescence intensity monitored. Encouragingly, no photobleaching for **2** was observed, whereas both other fluorophores were ~80% degraded within that time frame (Fig. 3d). Comparison of their stabilities in HeLa Kyoto cells using illumination from a solid-state light emitting diode (LED) light source was also examined. Cells stained with **2**, lysotracker red or pH-rhodo red were constantly illuminated with LED power set to a maximum, to promote a fast rate of photobleaching. The same excitation filters used for imaging (640(14) nm for **2** and 563(9) nm for lysotracker red and pH-rhodo red) were used, allowing images to be acquired at various time intervals. Graphing the average cell fluorescence intensity versus time showed that **2** was the most photostable with 50% loss of signal in 94 s and lysotracker red being the least photostable with 50% of signal loss in just 6 s (Fig. 3e, Supplementary Fig. 4 and Supplementary Movies 1 and 2). The behaviour of pH-rhodo red was more complex, as its intensity first significantly increased throughout the cell followed by photobleaching (Fig. 3e, Supplementary Fig. 4 and Supplementary Movie 3). This response to irradiation is indicative of a photo-conversion occurring for pH-rhodo red but further studies would be required to fully establish the cause for this. Comparison of these results highlights the distinct advantage of **2** for prolonged live-cell imaging in which fluorophore photostability is an essential parameter.

The pH-responsive properties of **2** were investigated in DMEM containing 10% fetal bovine serum (FBS) before its use in imaging studies. Fluorescence output of **2** was negligible at pH 7.4, but became highly fluorescent at acidic pH with its pKa determined as 4.0 (Fig. 4a). Cy5.5 light filter parameters of 690/50 nm were applied to the emission bands at pH 7.4, 5.5 and 4.5, and the integrated fluorescence intensity differences determined. At pH 5.5, as found in late endosomes, the fluorescence enhancement factor (FEF) was 6-fold, while it reached a remarkable 21-fold at lysosomal pH of 4.5 (Fig. 4b). Taken together, these results predict that at a cellular level **2** would remain non-fluorescent in the extracellular environment and become highly NIR fluorescent on uptake and localization in the lysosomes (Fig. 4c).

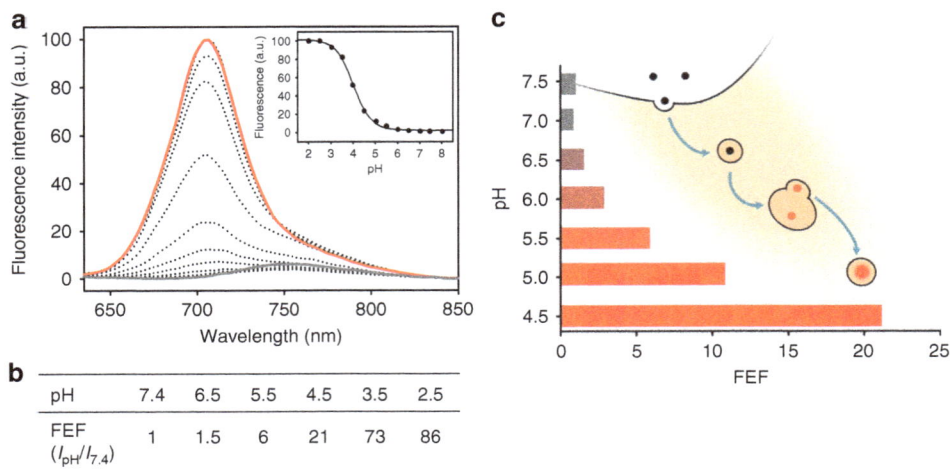

Figure 4 | Cellular uptake responsive NIR-fluorescence. (a) Emission spectra of **2** (5×10^{-6} M) in DMEM (10% FBS) at pH ranging from 8 (grey) to 2 (red). Exc: 625 nm. Inset: fluorescence intensity at $\lambda_{max} = 707$ nm versus pH; sigmoidal plot fit resulted in apparent $pK_a = 4.0$. **(b)** Corresponding FEF values from differing pH solutions applying Cy5.5 filter parameters. **(c)** Diagram represents the pH changes and increasing fluorescence intensity along endocytic path towards lysosomes.

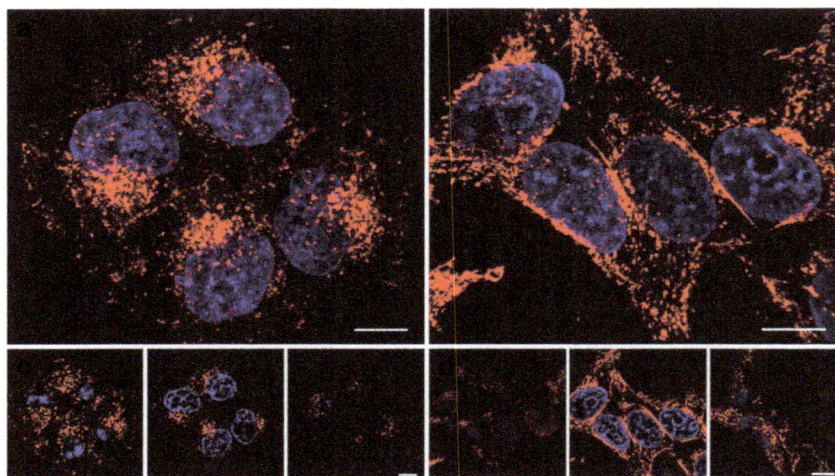

Figure 5 | Intracellular NIR-emission profile. CLSM images showing intracellular localization of pH-responsive compound **2** (10 µM, red) and nuclear counterstain Hoechst 33342 (blue) in fixed **(a,c)** HeLa Kyoto and **(b,d)** HEK293 cell lines. Bottom: three corresponding representative slices of the Z-stack for each cell type. Scale bars, 10 µm.

The difference in emission intensity at pH 5.5 (late endosomes) and 4.5 (lysosomes) suggests that the increased activation of **2** in lysosomes may be sufficient to allow differentiation between these organelles.

***In vitro* fixed and real-time live-cell imaging.** Before testing the imaging capabilities of **2**, its cytotoxicity in HeLa Kyoto (cervical cancer) and HEK (human embryonic kidney) cell lines was determined. Following a 24-h incubation of cells with **2**, an MTT (3-(4,5-dimethylthiazol-2-yl)-2,5-diphenyltetrazolium bromide) assay was performed and EC_{50} values of 0.43 and 0.44 mM, respectively, were obtained (Supplementary Fig. 5). These values were used as the basis to select 10 µM as the concentration for its use in imaging experiments. To establish the ability of **2** to internalize in cells, HeLa Kyoto and HEK293 cells were incubated with **2** for 2 h, followed by fixation, nuclei staining (Hoechst 33342) and imaging with confocal laser scanning microscopy (CLSM) (Fig. 5). These images show that **2** was internalized in both cell lines within 2 h (Supplementary Movie 4). The fluorescence signal was predominately localized in the perinuclear region as would be expected for a lysosomal staining pattern, indicating that the fluorophore had accumulated and become fluorescent in lysosomes[19].

To gain further evidence of selective lysosomal staining, an identical experiment was performed using a HeLa cell line stably expressing the lysosomal-associated membrane protein 1 (LAMP1) fused to green fluorescent protein (GFP)[33]. Following incubation, CLSM-imaged cell images showed very high levels of co-compartmentalization of the red (**2**) and green channel (GFP) emissions to the lysosomes (Fig. 6). Examination of selected focal planes clearly showed a circumferential staining pattern (green) of the LAMP1-GFP in the lysosome membrane and red emission of **2** from within the acidic lumen of the organelles (for Z-stack see Supplementary Movie 5). This ability to resolve the lysosome membrane from the interior is approaching the confocal resolution limit, with ~1 µm being the average diameter of an individual lysosome (for images from an additional independent experiment, see Supplementary Fig. 6). This was achieved due to the high signal-to-noise ratio, as background emission from **2** is not observed, and high red/green contrast with the genetically

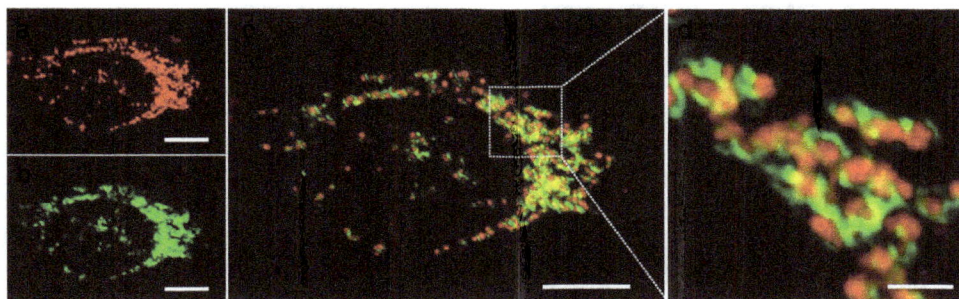

Figure 6 | Identification of subcellular NIR-fluorescent on switch. CLSM fluorescent images showing lysosomal localization of the 'on' state of **2** in LAMP1-GFP-expressing HeLa cells (**a**) Cy5.5 channel; (**b**) GFP channel. (**c**) Three-dimensional image of overlaid Cy5.5 and GFP channels. (**d**) Zoom-in of the dashed box. Scale bars, 10 μm (**a–c**) and 2 μm (**d**).

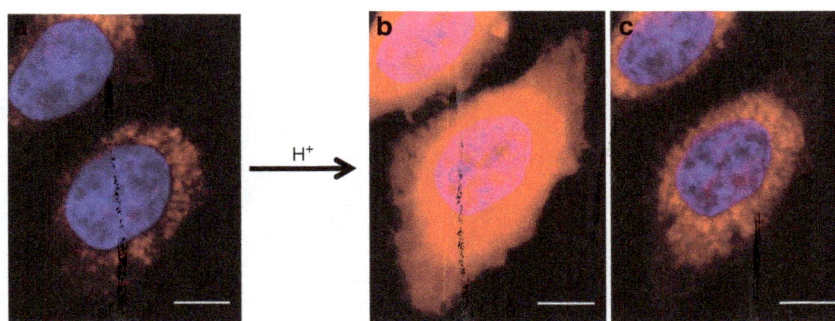

Figure 7 | Illustration of NIR-fluorescence response selectivity. (**a**) CLSM imaging of HeLa Kyoto cells following incubation with **2** (10 μM) for 2 h at 37 °C, DAPI nuclei staining and fixing. (**b**) The same set of cells imaged after buffer changed to pH 4.9, keeping the same laser power and PMT voltage. (**c**) The same set of cells after adjustment of microscope laser power and PMT voltage to obtain a non-saturated image. Red: **2**; blue: DAPI stain. Scale bar, 10 μm.

expressed LAMP1–GFP. Further statistical evidence of co-compartmentalization of the NIR and green emissions was provided by the calculated Manders' coefficients of 0.91 (05) for M_{NIR} and 0.95 (05) for M_{green} and a Pearson's coefficient of 0.79 (09)[34]. The lower Pearson's coefficient value when compared with Manders' may be attributable to the fact that the NIR and green emissions are co-compartmentalized to the lysosomes but not fully co-localized as the green is in the outer membrane and the NIR from within the internal lumen. Golgi co-staining of HeLa cells with **2** showed no significant co-localization (Supplementary Fig. 7, Method 1).

Two possible explanations for the excellent co-compartmentalization of red and green emissions could be envisaged. Either **2** is physically located exclusively in the lysosomes or it is present in other organelles along the endocytic pathway and is only emissive from the lysosomes due to its lower pH, with the remaining **2** being fluorescent silent. To visualize all intracellular **2** in its fluorescent on state, HeLa cells were incubated with **2** in media at pH 7.4 for 2 h, nuclei stained with 4,6-diamidino-2-phenylindole (DAPI) for 15 min, fixed and imaged using CLSM (Fig. 7a and Supplementary Movie 6). The media containing the fixed cells was then changed for media at pH 4.9 (adjusted using HCl), which on penetrating the cell forced on the fluorescence of all **2** within cells not localized in a sufficiently low pH environment. Re-imaging of the same cells (30 min after media change) with identical microscope settings showed a significantly increased fluorescence with saturation of the field of view within the cells (Fig. 7b and Supplementary Movie 7). The mean corrected total fluorescence from the cells (calculated using ImageJ) showed an FEF of 9.5 on lowering of the pH (see Supplementary Fig. 8 for images from additional independent experiment). This clearly illustrates that fluorescence from the majority of **2** was not

switched on by the cells and only **2** localized in the lysosomes was emissive under normal pH conditions. The same field of view was imaged for the third time using adjusted microscope laser power and photomultiplier tube (PMT) voltage and it became clear that the additional fluorescence of **2** was predominantly from other cellular organelles of higher pH (Fig. 7c and Supplementary Movie 8). Unfortunately, the adjustment to lower pH caused a loss of the LAMP1–GFP signal; thus, a comparison of Manders' coefficients was not possible.

To show that fluorophore **2** was internalized in cells via endocytosis and not passive diffusion, HeLa Kyoto cells were incubated at 4 °C for 30 min with **2**. It is known that endocytosis is inhibited at 4 °C, whereas passive diffusion can still occur[35]. Following incubation, cells were imaged, the buffer adjusted to pH 4.9 and re-imaged as described above. In contrast to the result shown in Fig. 7, no fluorescence from **2** was detected before or after changing the buffer to pH 4.9 (Supplementary Fig. 9). From these experiments, it was concluded that **2** was internalized via an energy requiring endocytosis rather than passive diffusion.

For the results outlined above, it was anticipated that cellular uptake of **2** could be continuously imaged in real-time without the need for washing or manipulating cells. The first live-cell imaging experiment involved imaging cells in a single focal plane over a 1.5-h time period. Once in focus, HeLa Kyoto cells were treated with **2** and imaged with an epi-fluorescence live-cell microscope, under optimal conditions of temperature and atmosphere for the cells to remain fully active (37 °C and 5% CO_2 humidified environment). Images were continuously acquired every 30 s for 90 min and then combined to form a movie (Supplementary Movie 9). Representative time-lapse images after 1, 30, 60 and 90 min (in black/white for clarity) are shown below in Fig. 8a with the 90 min time point in red

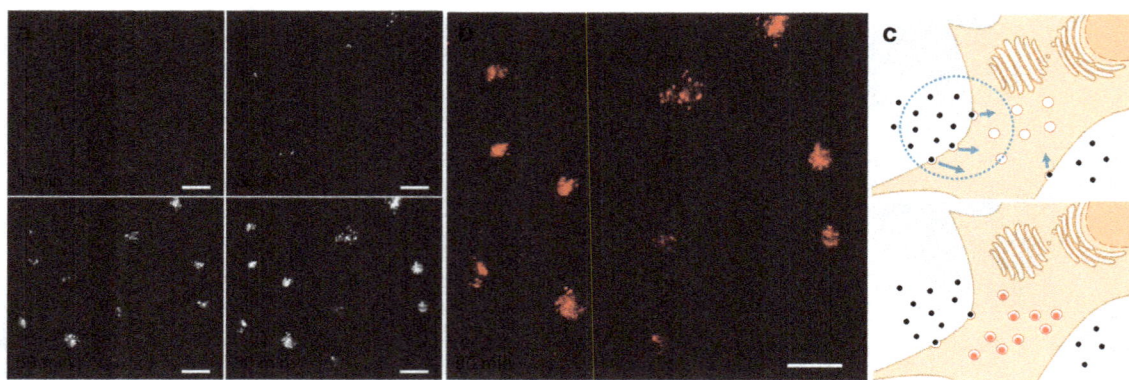

Figure 8 | Widefield live-cell imaging of the uptake of 2 (10 μM) into HeLa Kyoto cells. (**a**) Time-lapse black and white images are shown 1, 30, 60 and 90 min. (**b**) Red-coloured image at 90 min. (**c**) Schematic depiction of the uptake process of responsive fluorophore (**c**). Scale bars, 20 nm.

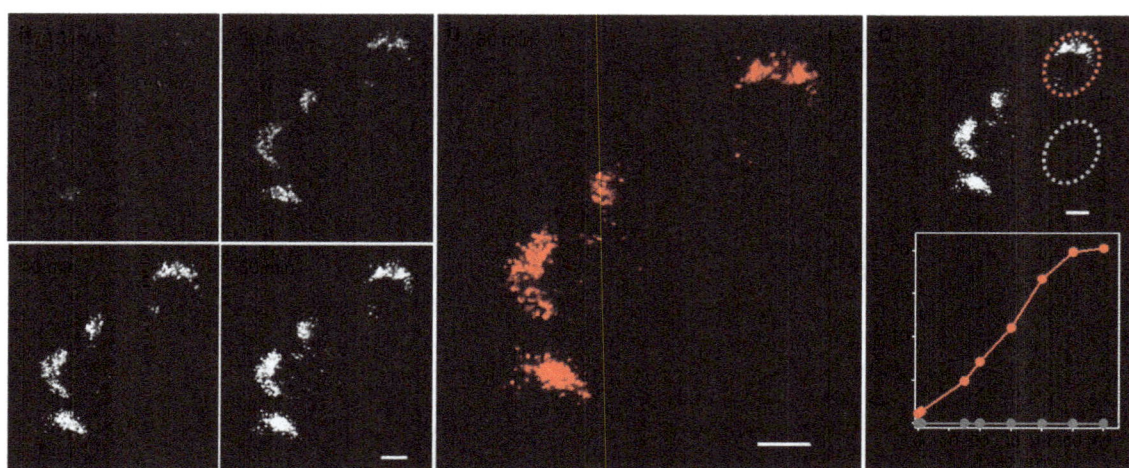

Figure 9 | Z-axis projections of widefield 4D live-cell imaging of the uptake of 2 (10 μM) from HeLa Kyoto cells. Images were acquired in 25 focal planes every 1 min for 60 min. (**a**) Time lapse b/w images are shown for 15, 30, 40 and 60 min. (**b**) Red-coloured image at 60 min. (**c**) Fluorescence intensity quantification in two identical volumes around a selected cell (1) and in the extracellular environment (2). Scale bars, 10 μm.

for comparison (Fig. 8b). The first image acquired at 1 min showed no NIR fluorescence, a signal confirming the effective fluorescence quenching of extracellular **2**. However, over the following 90-min time period, a strong signal arose from point-like organelles as a result of cellular uptake of **2** and transport through the endocytic pathway to the lysosomes (Fig. 8: 60- and 90-min time points). On close inspection, individual lysosomes can be seen emerging into view over the first 30-min time period, following which they increase in intensity and number from 30 to 90 min (Supplementary Movie 9).

The continuous imaging of live cells in the z-axis provides the most realistic method for following the progress of biological events over time and is of particular relevance when imaging small mobile organelles. To generate a three-dimensional (3D) representation of the cell in real time, a z-stack of 25 focal planes through the cell was acquired every minute[36]. This continual recording of cellular 3D volume over a period of time is termed four-dimensional (4D) imaging as the sample is imaged in the x,y,z and time dimensions, from which a time-lapse video of the 3D cellular volume can be created. Using HeLa cells, a 4D data set of the uptake of **2** over a 60-min time period was acquired followed by deconvolution of the data set to correct for motion of fluorescence objects between focal planes during the 1-min time period required to complete a z-stack of the cell. This experiment showed punctuated regions of fluorescence over the 60-min time period starting from a non-fluorescent background at time zero

with individual lysosome movement clearly observable (Fig. 9a,b and Supplementary Movie 10). Quantification of the fluorescence increase was measured by selecting two identical volumes of the imaged area, one overlapping with a chosen cell and the other on the extracellular environment, and applying an image analysis algorithm (ImageJ) to measure the total fluorescence intensity within the volumes (Fig. 9c). A comparative plot of both intensities over time shows how the background remained non-fluorescent, whereas intracellular fluorescence intensity increased over time, reaching a plateau at 60 min at which point a dynamic equilibrium was established between extracellular and intracellular **2**.

This ability to 4D image with **2** provides a tool for tracking lysosomal movements within the cell. Lysosomal staining of HeLa Kyoto cells was achieved by incubation with **2** for 1 h following which they were imaged in 3D for 35 min (without medium replacement) using a widefield microscope. Image analysis software was used to tag individual lysosomes as white spheres to facilitate visualization and the movement of these lysosomes was tracked over the 35-min time period (Fig. 10). The path the lysosome takes through the cell is illustrated by a lengthening white tail, which extends from the lysosome as the video progresses (Fig. 10c,d and Supplementary Movie 11)[37]. Tracking of all lysosomes within a cell (or field of view) was also possible and is shown for Fig. 10 in the Supplementary Information (Supplementary Movie 12).

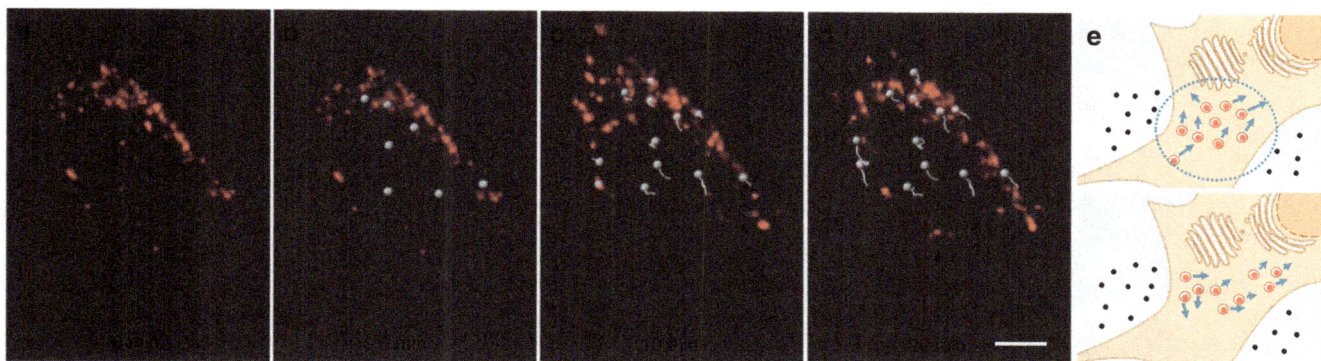

Figure 10 | Lysosome tracking in living HeLa Kyoto cells post 1 h incubation with 2 (10 μM). (**a**) Time-lapse representative snapshot of a single cell chosen for image analysis. (**b**) Lysosome selection at 0 min. (**c,d**) Tracking over time. (**e**) Schematic depiction of tracking intracellular vesicular movements with bioresponsive fluorophore. Scale bar, 5 μm.

Our final *in vitro* experiments with pH-responsive **2** were aimed at studying the efflux of the fluorophore from the cell. HeLa Kyoto cells were pre-treated with **2** for 2 h as previously described, then the medium was replaced with fluorophore-free DMEM. Cells were incubated at 37 °C and imaged at time points of 1, 15, 30 and 120 min using confocal microscopy (Fig. 11). The overall NIR fluorescence detected after 2 h incubation with **2** in the intracellular environment showed to be again arising from point-like organelles (Fig. 11a). The quantity of fluorescent vesicles decreased within 30 min after medium change, with significant clearance of **2** by 120 min (Fig. 11b). Using ImageJ analysis, lysosome number per cell (or field of view) was determined for the different time points and were observed to steadily decrease from time 0 to 120 min (Fig. 11d). In addition, after 60 min cells were fixed and acidified with buffer of pH 4.9 and only a small, 1.6-fold increase in total fluorescence was observed.

***In vivo* imaging.** A distinct advantage of NIR fluorophores is their ability to directly transfer from *in vitro* to *in vivo* imaging due to transparency of biological tissue at these longer wavelengths. To test *in vivo* performance of **2**, the luciferase-expressing human breast cell line MDA-MB-231-luc-D3H1 was chosen to grow subcutaneous tumours of size 100–200 mm^3, which permitted NIR fluorescence imaging with confirmatory bioluminescence. The ability of PEG polymers to act as a drug delivery vehicle has been well established, with several PEGylated drugs in clinical use for over 20 years. PEGylation is known to influence pharmacokinetic properties resulting in prolonged blood circulation times. As such, it was anticipated that the PEG-conjugated **2** may have passive tumour-targeting properties leading to some preferential uptake into tumour cells, thereby generating a distinguishable fluorescent signal. Following an intravenous tail vein injection of **2** (2 mg kg^{-1}), images were acquired at regular intervals over the course of 24 h. A plot of tumour to background NIR fluorescence showed that the fluorescence signal was low in the beginning in both the background and tumour. Emission from the liver peaked at 1 h and subsided over the following 24 h (Fig. 12d dashed red line). In contrast, the tumour fluorescence intensity reached a maximum at 24 h, allowing for good image discrimination at that time point (Fig. 12d solid red line). Bioluminescence and NIR fluorescence imaging at 24 h confirmed that **2** has indeed been taken up into tumour cells and switched on (Fig. 12a–c). No adverse reactions or animal weight loss were observed during or after imaging. These preliminary *in vivo* results represent a unique example of selective NIR *in vivo* tumour imaging using a pH-responsive fluorochrome.

Discussion

Imaging with molecular fluorophores is an indispensable tool for all forms of biological and medical research. Although the full spectrum of colours are available from molecular fluorophores, imaging with lowest energy NIR spectral region offers advantage for prolonged live cellular imaging with the possibility of *in vivo* imaging with the same probe[5,37]. Although most fluorescent markers are permanently fluorescent (unless photobleached), huge imaging advantage can be gained if the fluorescence can be modulated from off to on in a reversible bioresponsive manner[14]. With these goals in mind, we have designed a lysosomal-responsive NIR probe with the potential for real-time visualization of their key cellular operations that can be directly translated for use *in vivo* (Figs 1 and 2). NIR probe **2** is synthesized in five synthetic operations from a bisphenolic substituted member of the BF$_2$-azadipyrromethene fluorophore class (Fig. 1). An *o*-nitro-substituted phenol group on the probe acts as the fluorescent switch with the nitro group tailoring the emission response to the lumen microenvironment of the lysosomes. Photophysical measurements in DMEM shows that **2** remained fluorescent silent at pH 7.2, yet became highly fluorescent in the pH range that corresponds with the acidic micro-environment of the lysosome (Fig. 4). The non-fluorescent state shows little polarity sensitivity, indicating that it could be used in the more complex intracellular environment without resulting in false-positive emissions. Solution and cellular photobleaching experiments indicated high stability, which is an essential feature for imaging over prolonged time periods that is often lacking in both synthetic and genetically expressed probes (Fig. 3).

To illustrate the potential uses of probe **2**, a series of increasingly complex imaging experiments were undertaken in fixed, live cells and *in vivo*. The high fidelity for the switching on of **2** to the lysosomal lumen is observed when imaging with LAMP1-GFP HeLa cells (Fig. 6). We have exploited these responsive emission properties for 3D and 4D real-time live-cell imaging of several fundamental biological events, such as endocytosis, organelle trafficking and efflux. As **2** has extremely low emission in cell media and with fluorescence activated on cellular internalization, a high background-to-noise ratio is achieved, making the continuous acquisition of data as straightforward as just add **2** to cells and image. It could be anticipated that these techniques would be valuable for many types of cellular experiments involving lysosomal response to stimuli.

It is important to note that the mode of action and the use of existing lysosomotropic stains, which are typically amine-functionalized fluorophores to promote retention in acidic

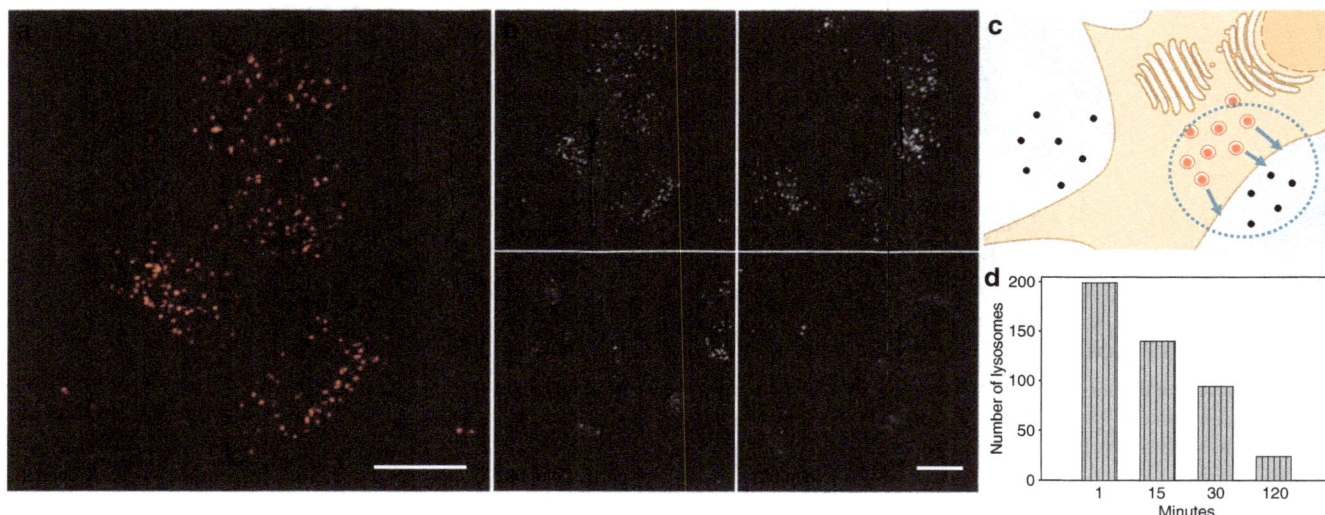

Figure 11 | Imaging of cellular efflux. HeLa Kyoto cells were pre-treated with **2** (10 µM) for 2 h, DMEM replaced with fluorophore-free DMEM and cells fixed at various time points. (**a**) Cells imaged after 2 h incubation. (**b**) Cells imaged after 1, 15, 30 and 120 min post media change. (**c**) Schematic depiction of efflux of bioresponsive fluorophore. (**d**) Decrease in number of NIR fluorescent lysosomes from 1 to 120 min. Scale bars, 20 µm.

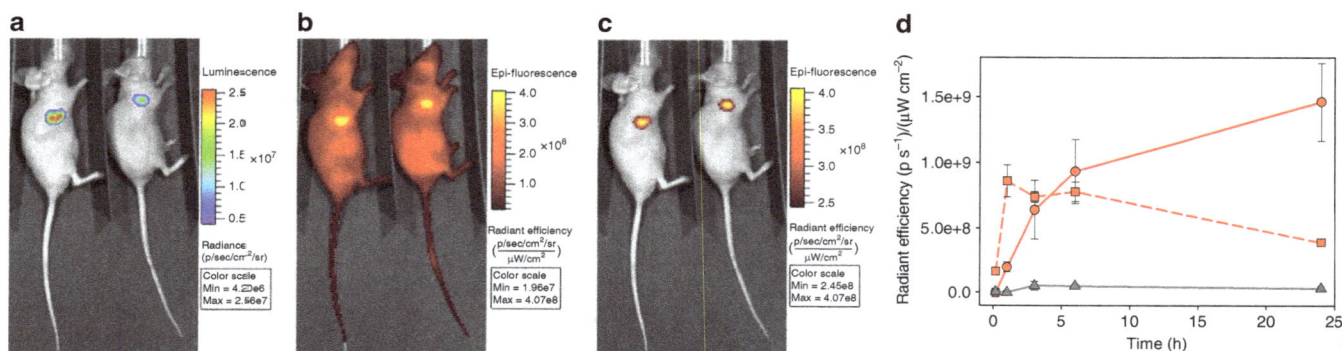

Figure 12 | *In vivo* imaging of 2 using a MDA-MB-231-luc-D3H1 subcutaneous tumour model in two representative mice. (**a**) Bioluminescence imaging confirmation of tumour cells. (**b**) NIR fluorescence imaging 24 h post intravenous (i.v.) administration of **2** (excit. 660–690 nm, emis. 710–730 nm). (**c**) NIR fluorescence imaging 24 h post i.v. administration of **2** with intensity scale adjusted (excit. at 675 nm, emiss. at 720 nm). (**d**) Profile of tumour NIR fluorescence (red solid line) and liver (red dashed line) over time following i.v. tail injection of **2**. Non-injected control tumour NIR fluorescence (grey solid line). Values determined from the same sized ROI from background area and tumour averaged for $n = 3$.

lysosomes on protonation, is significantly different from **2** (refs 38,39). These lysosomotropic fluorophores are pre-incubated for a period of time (typically 30 min), followed by cell washing to remove excess nonspecific fluorophore, before imaging can be carried out for up to a maximum of 1 h (ref. 40). In contrast, **2** in its fluorescent on state is uncharged, showing little cytotoxic effect over long incubation times and no background fluorescence due to the highly selective switching 'on' only in the desired lysosomal ROIs. These characteristics have been demonstrated to be particularly advantageous for continuous real-time live-cell imaging and show significant potential for use in a wider range of complex bio-imaging applications. Overall, the cellular imaging performance, ease of utility and the selectivity for lysosomal staining could be judged as excellent in comparison with the most recently developed probes[41].

To complete the imaging portfolio, we wished to illustrate that the bioresponse of **2** within subcellular compartments could also be visualized at the macroscopic scale of a tumour. This translation to *in vivo* tumour imaging is achievable as shown in

Fig. 12 in which tumour can be clearly distinguished, showing a high potential for targeted responsive fluorescence imaging.

In conclusion, the development of **2** as the first phenol/phenolate controlled molecular NIR lysosome-responsive fluorophore has important implications for the study of intracellular transport mechanisms, lysosome-based diseases and *in vivo* targeting. The use of **2** for further 4D real-time studies of more complex dynamic cell mechanisms involving lysosomes are ongoing. Future studies will include the conjugation of active tumour targeting motifs via **7** (instead of PEG) to the fluorophore, to further broaden the possibilities of *in-vivo* imaging targets with potential applications for fluorescence-guided surgery.

Methods

General information and materials. All commercially available solvents and reagents were used as supplied, unless otherwise stated. All reactions were performed under nitrogen or argon atmosphere in oven-dried glassware. Gel chromatography was performed with Davisil 60 silica (230–400 mesh). On the basis of NMR and reverse-phase HPLC, all final compounds were >95% pure. [1]H and ^{13}C spectra were recorded on 300, 400, 500 or 600 MHz NMR spectrometers and chemical shifts were reported in p.p.m. using solvent residual peak as standard. For spectra of compounds **4**, **5**, **6** and **7**, see Supplementary Figs 10–13, respectively. All ^{19}F NMR chemical shifts are referenced to CFCl$_3$. All ^{11}B NMR chemical shifts are referenced to BF$_3$.Et$_2$O/CDCl$_3$. High-resolution mass spectrometry and tandem mass spectrometry experiments were carried on an electrospray ionisation and MALDI–TOF instruments. Infrared spectra were recorded as a KBr pellet using a Fourier Transform infrared spectrometer. Absorbance spectra were recorded with a Varian Cary 50 Scan ultraviolet–visible spectrometer. Fluorescence spectra were recorded with a Varian Cary Eclipse Fluorescence Spectrometer. Solvents for absorbance and fluorescence experiments were of HPLC quality. SigmaPlot, MestreNova, ChemDraw, Zeiss LSM and ImageJ software were used for data analysis. Phenol red-free imaging DMEM medium was used for all experiments.

Synthesis of compound 4. Compound (ref. 28) (200 mg, 0.38 mmol) and CsF (288 mg, 1.89 mmol) were dissolved in dry DMSO (6 ml) and stirred at 30 °C under a nitrogen atmosphere for 10 min, during which time the colour changed from dark green to dark purple. *t*Butyl bromoacetate (126 mg, 0.64 mmol) was then added via syringe in one go and the solution was stirred at 30 °C for 20 min. The mixture was partitioned between AcOEt (100 ml) and PBS buffer at pH 7 (100 ml). The organic phase was washed with water (3 × 100 ml), brine (50 ml), dried over Na$_2$SO$_4$, filtered and evaporated to dryness. The crude product was purified by silica gel chromatography, eluting with CH$_2$Cl$_2$:AcOEt (99:1 → 90:10) to yield the product **4** as a red metallic solid (151 mg, 64%). mp: 183–187 °C; ^{1}H NMR (400 MHz, DMSO-d_6): δ 10.58 (br s, 1H), 8.19–8.10 (m, 8H), 7.65 (s, 1H), 7.57–7.43 (m, 7H), 7.10 (d, $J = 8.7$ Hz, 2H), 6.95 (d, $J = 8.6$ Hz, 2H), 4.81 (s, 2H), 1.46 (s, 9H); ^{13}C NMR (100 MHz, DMSO-d_6): δ 167.5, 161.5, 160.0, 158.9, 155.7, 145.0, 143.8, 142.6, 141.0, 132.5, 132.0, 131.7, 131.4, 129.6, 129.3, 129.1, 129.0, 128.7, 128.6, 124.1, 121.3, 120.3, 119.1, 116.0, 114.8, 81.6, 65.0, 27.7; ^{11}B NMR (128 MHz, DMSO-d_6) δ: 1.00 (t, $J = 32.6$ Hz); ^{19}F NMR (376 MHz, DMSO-d_6): δ − 130.44 (q, $J = 32.6$ Hz); ultraviolet–visible: λ_{max} (CHCl$_3$): 680 nm (ε: 85,000 cm^{-1} M^{-1}); emission: λ_{max} (CHCl$_3$): 708 nm, Φ_F (CHCl$_3$) = 0.31; high resolution mass spectrometry (HRMS) (m/z): [M-H]$^-$ calcd. for C$_{38}$H$_{31}$BN$_3$O$_4$F$_2$, 642.2376; found, 642.2357.

Synthesis of compound 5. A solution of **4** (300 mg, 0.48 mmol) in acetonitrile (6 ml) was heated under reflux for 5 min. A solution of KNO$_3$ (53 mg, 0.53 mmol) and KHSO$_4$ (130 mg, 0.96 mmol) in water (1 ml) was added and the mixture was heated under reflux for 5 min. The suspension was cooled to room temperature (rt) and partitioned between AcOEt (200 ml) and water (100 ml). The organic phase was washed with water (100 ml), brine (2 × 100 ml), dried over Na$_2$SO$_4$, filtered and evaporated to dryness. The crude was purified by silica gel chromatography, eluting with CH$_2$Cl$_2$:AcOEt (99: 1) to yield the product **5** as a dark red metallic solid (198 mg, 60%). mp: 192–194 °C; ^{1}H NMR (400 MHz, DMSO-d_6): δ 11.88 (br s, 1H), 8.69 (d, $J = 2.0$ Hz, 1H), 8.27 (dd, $J = 8.9$, 2.0, 1H), 8.21 (d, $J = 9.0$ Hz, 2H), 8.19–8.13 (m, 4H), 7.71 (s, 1H), 7.60 (s, 1H), 7.57–7.43 (m, 6H), 7.27 (d, $J = 8.9$ Hz, 1H), 7.12 (d, $J = 9.0$ Hz, 2H), 4.84 (s, 2H), 1.45 (s, 9H); ^{13}C NMR (100 MHz, DMSO-d_6): δ 167.4, 160.9, 159.3, 154.1, 153.9, 145.4, 143.9, 143.3, 141.5, 137.3, 135.6, 132.1, 131.8, 131.5, 129.9, 129.5, 129.2, 129.0, 128.7, 128.6, 123.3, 121.8, 120.8, 119.4, 119.1, 115.0, 81.7, 65.1, 27.7; ^{11}B NMR (128 MHz, DMSO-d_6): δ 0.92 (t, $J = 32.7$ Hz); ^{19}F NMR (376 MHz, DMSO-d_6): δ − 130.31 (q, $J = 32.7$ Hz); ultraviolet–visible: λ_{max} (CHCl$_3$) 675 nm (ε: 94,000 cm^{-1} M^{-1}); emission: λ_{max} (CHCl$_3$) 703 nm, Φ_F (CHCl$_3$) = 0.15; HRMS (m/z): [M-H]$^-$ calcd. for C$_{38}$H$_{30}$BN$_4$O$_6$F$_2$, 687.2226; found, 687.2229.

Synthesis of compound 6. TFA (1 ml) was added dropwise to a solution of **5** (175 mg, 0.25 mmol) in dichloromethane (DCM) (9 ml) and the solution was stirred at rt for 3 h. The solvent was removed under vacuo and the residual TFA was removed azeotropically with serial additions of DCM and subsequent removal under vacuo. The solid was suspended in DCM, filtered and washed with DCM, to yield the product as a dark purple solid (136 mg, 84%). The product was pure enough to proceed to the next synthetic step. To remove the last trace of starting material, the solid was partitioned between AcOEt (90 ml) and Na$_2$CO$_3$ sat. (180 ml). The organic layer was discarded and the water layer was extracted with AcOEt (90 ml), separated, carefully acidified with 5 M HCl and extracted again with AcOEt (180 ml). The organic layer was separated, dried over anhydrous Na$_2$SO$_4$, filtered and evaporated to dryness. The product **6** was obtained as a dark purple solid (122 mg, 76%). mp: 214–219 °C; ^{1}H NMR (400 MHz, DMSO-d_6): δ 13.15 (br s, 1H), 8.68 (d, $J = 2.3$ Hz, 1H), 8.28 (dd, $J = 8.9$, 2.3 Hz, 1H), 8.24–8.13 (m, 6H), 7.71 (s, 1H), 7.60 (s, 1H), 7.57–7.44 (m, 6H), 7.28 (d, $J = 8.9$ Hz, 1H), 7.14 (d, $J = 9.0$ Hz, 2H), 4.87 (s, 2H); ^{13}C NMR (100 MHz, DMSO-d_6): δ 169.7, 161.0, 159.4, 154.1, 153.7, 145.4, 143.9, 143.4, 141.5, 137.3, 135.5, 132.1, 131.9, 131.5, 129.9, 129.5, 129.2, 129.0, 128.7 (2C), 126.6, 123.2, 121.9, 120.8, 119.5, 119.1, 115.1, 64.6; ^{11}B NMR (128 MHz, DMSO-d_6): δ 0.93 (t, $J = 32.8$ Hz); ^{19}F NMR (376 MHz, DMSO-d_6): δ − 130.34 (q, $J = 32.8$ Hz); HRMS (m/z): [M-H]$^-$ calcd. for C$_{34}$H$_{22}$BN$_4$O$_6$F$_2$, 631.1600; found, 631.1603.

^{1}H NMR monitoring of the formation of activated ester 6. A mixture of **5** (45 mg, 0.071 mmol), N-(3-dimethylaminopropyl)-N′-ethylcarbodiimide

hydrochloride (27 mg, 0.14 mmol) and N-hydroxysuccinimide (82 mg, 0.71 mmol) was placed in a sealed dry flask. Anhydrous deuterated DMSO-d_6 (1.2 ml) was added to the mixture and the solution was stirred at rt under N$_2$ atmosphere. Samples (50 µl) were withdrawn at 15, 30, 60, 120 min and 19 h, diluted with DMSO-d_6 in an NMR tube (650 µl) and ^{1}H spectra were recorded at a 600-MHz spectrometer.

Synthesis of compound 7. A mixture of **6** (40 mg, 0.063 mmol), N-(3-dimethylaminopropyl)-N′-ethylcarbodiimide hydrochloride (24 mg, 0.13 mmol) and N-hydroxysuccinimide (73 mg, 0.63 mmol) was dissolved in anhydrous DMSO (1 ml) and stirred at rt for 3 h under N$_2$ atmosphere. The solution was partitioned between with DCM (50 ml) and 0.5 M HCl (50 ml). The organic phase was washed with 0.5 M HCl (50 ml), acidic brine (50 ml), dried over Na$_2$SO$_4$, filtered and evaporated to dryness, keeping the temperature of the bath below 35°C. The product **7** was obtained as a purple metallic solid (44 mg, 95%). m.p.: 177–183 °C; ^{1}H NMR (400 MHz, DMSO-d_6): δ 8.69 (d, $J = 2.2$ Hz, 1H), 8.29 (dd, $J = 8.9$, 2.2 Hz, 1H), 8.23 (d, $J = 8.9$ Hz, 2H), 8.21–8.14 (m, 4H), 7.72 (s, 1H), 7.64 (s, 1H), 7.59–7.45 (m, 6H), 7.28 (d, $J = 8.9$ Hz, 1H), 7.23 (d, $J = 8.9$ Hz, 2H), 5.53 (s, 2H), 2.85 (s, 4H); ^{13}C NMR (100 MHz, DMSO-d_6): δ 169.9, 165.2, 159.8, 158.6, 154.5, 145.2, 144.2, 143.1, 142.0, 137.4, 135.5, 132.0, 131.8, 131.6, 129.8, 129.6, 129.2, 129.1, 128.7, 126.8, 124.1, 121.5, 120.6, 119.6, 119.5, 115.2, 63.0, 25.5; ^{11}B NMR (128 MHz, DMSO-d_6): δ 0.93 (t, $J = 32.8$ Hz); ^{19}F NMR (376 MHz, DMSO-d_6): δ − 130.34 (q, $J = 32.8$ Hz); HRMS (m/z): [M-H]$^-$ calcd. for C$_{38}$H$_{25}$BF$_2$N$_5$O$_8$, 728.1764; found, 728.1730.

Synthesis of compound 2. A mixture of **7** (6.4 mg, 0.0088 mmol) and O-(2-aminoethyl)polyethylene glycol 5000 (CAS 32130–27–1) (40 mg, 0.008 mmol) was dissolved in anhydrous DMSO (0.88 ml) and stirred at rt for 18 h under a N$_2$ atmosphere. The solvent was removed by short-path distillation at rt overnight and the crude was partitioned between DCM (20 ml) and 1 M Na$_2$CO$_3$ (20 ml). The aqueous phase was extracted with DCM (2 × 20 ml). The organic layers were combined, washed with slightly acidic (HCl) water (20 ml), brine (20 ml), dried over anhydrous Na$_2$SO$_4$, filtered and evaporated to dryness. The residue was dissolved in HPLC grade water (8 ml) and the dark solution was passed through a Sep Pak C18 reverse-phase cartridge, then freeze dried. The product **2** was obtained as a dark green solid (40 mg, 90%). mp: 43–45 °C; ^{1}H NMR (400 MHz, DMSO-d_6): δ 8.74–8.72 (m, 1H), 8.28 (dd, $J = 9.0$, 2.3 Hz, 1H), 8.24–8.15 (m, 7H), 7.68 (s, 2H), 7.58–7.52 (m, 4H), 7.52–7.45 (m, 2H), 7.25–7.19 (m, 1H), 7.16 (d, $J = 9.0$ Hz, 2H), 4.66 (s, 2H), 3.70–3.65 (m, 4H), 3.50 (s, 680H); Ultraviolet–visible: λ_{max} (CHCl$_3$) 670 nm, (ε: 97,000 cm^{-1} M^{-1}); emission: λ_{max} (CHCl$_3$) 702 nm, Φ_F (CHCl$_3$) = 0.18; HRMS (m/z): MALDI–TOF distribution maximum centred at 5410.3999 Da.

Fluorescence quantum yields and extinction coefficients. The compound of interest (0.005 mmol) was dissolved in CHCl$_3$ (50 ml) to prepare a stock solution (10^{-4} M). The stock was diluted to concentrations 2, 4, 6, 8 and 10 × 10^{-7} M with CHCl$_3$ and each solution was analysed with an ultraviolet–visible spectrometer and a fluorescence spectrometer against CHCl$_3$ background. Excitation = 640 nm; emission range = 660–900 nm; slit width = 5/5 nm; scan rates = 600 nm min^{-1}. Plots of abs$_{max}$ versus conc and fluorescence area versus abs (640 nm) allowed the calculation of extinction coefficient and fluorescence quantum yield, respectively. Compound **1** (R = Ph, Ar = *p*MeOC$_6$H$_4$) was used as standard for fluorescence quantum yields with Φ_F = 0.36 (refs 17,42).

Fluorescence response of 2 and 5 to addition of DBU/TFA in organic solvents. Compound **2** or **5** was dissolved in toluene, tetrahydrofuran, dimethylformamide and DMSO (25 ml) to a final concentration of 5 µM. A solution of DBU (29.5 mg in 100 ml of CHCl$_3$) was added (64 µl = 1 eq) gradually, and absorbance and fluorescence spectra were recorded before and after each addition. The addition was stopped once spectra remained unchanged. At this stage, an excess of DBU was added and the spectra were recorded. Subsequently, a higher excess of TFA was added and the spectra were recorded. The area below the last two curves was plotted for off/on histogram (shown in Fig. 3). (Note: the toluene solution of **2** contained 1% CHCl$_3$ for solubility).

Fluorescence response of 2 to pH variation in DMEM. Compound **2** (2.8 mg) was dissolved in PBS (500 µl). The stock solution (1 mM) was diluted with DMEM supplemented with 10% FBS to the concentration of 5 µM. The pH of the solution was adjusted with diluted HCl or NaOH, to obtain a range from 8 to 2 at regular intervals, each of which was recorded, and the respective solution analysed by ultraviolet–visible absorption and fluorescence emission. Excitation = 625 nm; emission range = 635–900 nm.

Comparative solution and cellular photobleaching of 2 and lysotracker red and pHrodo red. Entire fluorescence cuvettes contain 1 × 10^{-7} M DMEM solutions at pH 4.0 of **2**; lysotracker red and pH-rodo red were continuously irradiated with light of wavelength 620(30) nm for **2** and 540(40) nm for lysotracker red and pH-rhodo red at 25 °C for 2 h. Filtered light from a 150-W light source used with complete cuvette irradiation via a fibre optic with attached light diffuser. Fluorophore fluorescence intensities were recorded every 20 min. The average fluorescence intensity from three independent experiments were normalized and plotted with sigmaplot 8.

Ten thousand HeLa-Kyoyo cells in DMEM were seeded onto chamber slides and incubated with **2** (20 μM) for 60 min or lysotracker red (150 nM) for 30 min, or pH rhodo red (15 μM) for 30 min. DMEM was replaced with fluorophore-free media and cells constantly irradiated with a Lumencor SPECTRA light engine LED used as the light source set to a maximum power for 400 s. Excitation filter 563/9 nm was used for lysotracker red and pH-rhodo red and excitation filter 640(14) nm was used for **2**. Cells were imaged with the shutter open, a time intervals of either 0.1 or 1.0 or 5 s with exposure of 10 ms and individual frames complied into movie format. The average cellular ROI fluorescence intensities from three independent experiments were plotted. An Olympus × 60 PLANAPO/1.42 objective and Andor iXon 888 ultra were used for signal detection. Acquisition and analysis performed with MetaMorph v7.8.

MTT assay of 2. Compound **2** (4.0 mg) was dissolved in sterile PBS (71 μl) to prepare a stock solution 10 mM. This was serially diluted to prepare samples at 5, 1, 0.5, 0.1 and 0.05 mM. Each of the stock solutions was diluted 1:10 with DMEM medium, which was co-incubated with HeLa or HEK293 cells at 5,000 cells per well on a 96-well plate for 24 h. The solution was removed and substituted with MTT solution (5 mg ml^{-1} in DMEM). The cells were incubated for 3 h. The medium was removed and the wells were treated with DMSO for 10 min. The absorbance of each well was read with a plate reader at 540 nm.

Production and validation of HeLa Kyoto cell line stably expressing LAMP1-GFP fusion protein. An expression plasmid encoding the LAMP1-GFP fusion protein was generated via the complete open-reading frame coded by a I.M.A.G.E. Fully Sequenced cDNA Clone (Source BioScience, I.M.A.G.E. ID: 5019745) of the human LAMP1 (GenBank accession number BC021288) was amplified by PCR using primers designed to append an XhoI site upstream of the translation initiation site and to replace the translation termination site by a segment encoding EcoRI site followed by a linker sequence CTCCTC (single-letter nucleotide code). The PCR product was gel purified and cloned in the XhoI–EcoRI sites of a pEGFP-N1 vector (BD Biosciences Clontech). Constructs were verified by DNA sequencing.

For stable transfection, HeLa cells were grown at 37 °C in complete DMEM supplemented with 10% FBS and 1% glutamine, to 30–40% confluency, and subsequently transfected with the LAMP1–GFP-encoding plasmid using FuGENE 6 (Roche) following the manufacturer's instruction. One day later, 0.6 g l^{-1} G418 was added. The medium was changed every day to remove the G418 non-resistant cells and when the cell number looked stabilized the G418 was lowered to 0.5 g l^{-1}. Cells displaying resistance to G418 and expressing LAMP1-GFP (as judged by fluorescence microscopy) were cloned by limiting dilution and sorted on a BD FACSAria flow cytometer (Becton Dickinson). The clones were validated by immunostaining, by western blotting and by two functional assays (lysotracker uptake and dextran uptake).

Microscopy. Confocal images (Figs 5–7) were acquired using an Olympus Fluoview FV1000 CLSM and × 60/1.35(oil) UPLSAPO objective with a 635-nm laser at 12%, PMT voltage of ∼750 v, pixel dwell time of 4 μs per pixel, pixel size 0.103 μm and image size 1,024 × 1,024. Nuclear staining was performed using Hoe.scht33342 or DAPI. Hoechst33342 signal was imaged using a 405-nm laser at 10% power and PMT voltage of ∼ 700 v. GFP signal was imaged using a 488 nm laser line at 5% power and PMT voltage of ∼600v.

Live-cell images (Figs 8–10) were acquired on a Zeiss AxioVert 200 M epi-fluorescent widefield microscope equipped with a Andor iXon 885 EMCCD, CoolLED pE-2 solid-state LEDs capable of excitation at 445, 488 and 635 nm, and Zeiss Plan-Apochromat × 100/1.40 Oil DIC objective. The microscope was surrounded by an incubation chamber that allowed the temperature and CO$_2$ to be maintained at 37 °C and 5%, respectively. Fluorophore **2** channel was recorded using a 649-nm emission long-pass filter, GFP was imaged using a 520/50 emission bandpass filter.

Fixed cell imaging. Cells were seeded onto an eight-well chambered glass slide and allowed to attach for 24 h. The media was then replaced with 200 μl of **2** (10 μM) in media and incubated for the appropriate time at 37 °C. Cells were counterstained with Hoechst 33342 or DAPI for 15 min. Cells were then washed once with PBS and fixed in 3.7% paraformaldehyde in PBS solution for 3 min and washed thoroughly with PBS. Images were collected by using an Olympus Fluoview 1,000 CLSM. The fluorescence arising from **2** was detected by a Cy5.5 filter. DAPI and GFP channels were used in parallel when cells were counterstained and/or transfected.

Fixed cell imaging at different pH. Cells were seeded onto an eight-well chambered glass slide and allowed to attach for 24 h. The media was then replaced with 200 μl of **2** (10 μM) in media incubated for 2 h at 37 °C. Cells were

counterstained with DAPI for 15 min. Cells were then washed once with PBS and fixed in 3.7% paraformaldehyde in PBS solution for 3 min, and washed thoroughly with PBS. A collection of cell were Z-stack imaged using CLSM (PMT voltage = 782v, laser power 12%) and while maintaining focus of the microscope on the same cells the medium was exchanged with medium acidified to pH 4.9 (by addition of HCl (aq)). After allowing 15 min for equilibration the same cells were re-imaged (PMT voltage = 782v) using the same laser power. Following which the same cells were imaged for the third time following the adjustment of the PMT voltage 512v to obtain a non-saturated image. Mean total cell fluorescence was determined from two independent experiments using ImageJ.

Imaging following 4 °C incubation. Cells seeded onto an 8-well chambered glass slide and allowed to attach for 24 h. The media was then replaced with 200 μl of **2** (10 μM) in media incubated for 30 min at 4 °C. Cells were counterstained with DAPI for 15 min. Cells were then washed once with PBS and fixed in 3.7% paraformaldehyde in PBS solution for 3 min and washed thoroughly with PBS. A collection of cell were imaged using CLSM, and while maintaining focus of the microscope on the same cells the medium was exchanged with medium acidified to pH 4.9 (by addition of HCl (aq)). After allowing 15 min for equilibration, the same cells were re-imaged using the same exposure times and laser power.

Real-time live-cell imaging. HeLa Kyoto cells in Dulbecco's cell growth media containing 10% FBS were seeded onto an eight-well chambered glass slide and incubated for 24 h. The slides were placed on the microscope platform and the microscope was focused on a collection of cells. Next, **2** (final concentration 10 μM) was added and fluorescence images (Cy5.5 filter) were acquired at regular intervals. Images were deconvolved and combined in a video format.

Time-dependant efflux of 2. Cells seeded onto an eight8-well chambered glass slide and allowed to attach for 24 h. The media was then replaced with 200 μl of **2** (10 μM) in media incubated for 2 h at 37 °C. Media was replaced with fresh media and the loss of fluorescence monitored over time. Lysosome counting was carried out at 1, 15, 30 and 120 min using ImageJ.

Image processing. Deconvolution of widefield data sets was performed using AutQuant X3 deconvolution software with ten iterations of adaptive point spread function calculations. Lysosome detection and tracking were performed using Imaris 7.7.1 software (Bitplane Scientific). Background subtraction was applied to all images before lysosome detection. The Spots module of Imaris was used to detect lysosomes with an estimated diameter of 1.27 μm. Detected spots were filtered using the 'quality' algorithm. Only spots with values higher than the set threshold value (>91.76) were analysed. Quality is defined as the intensity at the centre of the spot, Gaussian filtered by the spot radius. The success and accuracy of Spot detection was judged by visual inspection. Tracking lysosome movement over the course of the video was performed using an autoregressive motion algorithm. A maximum search distance of 1 μm was defined to disallow connections between a spot and a candidate match if the distance between the predicted future position of the spot and the candidate position exceeded the maximum distance. A gap-closing algorithm was also implemented to link track segment ends to track segment starts, to recover tracks that were interrupted by the temporary disappearance of particles. The maximum permissible gap length was set equal to three frames. Tracking all the lysosomes in the cell were selected by applying filters, which were based on 'Track Length' (>0.2 μm) and 'Track Duration' (>60 s).

Statistical analysis of cell images. Manders' and Pearson's coefficients used to show co-compartmentalization of LAMP1–GFP and **2** emissions were calculated using the Image J plugin 'Coloc2'. Rolling ball background subtraction (50 pixel diameter) and a Gaussian Filter (1 pixel diameter) were applied to all images before running the 'Coloc2' plugin. The ROI surrounding the cell was selected manually using the freeform drawing tool. Analysis was performed on six cells from two independent experiments.

Corrected total cell fluorescence (CTCF) in Fig. 7 was performed on six cells from two different experiments (Supplementary Fig. 8). Z-stack data acquired on the Olympus FLuoview100 was compressed into a single plane using the 'Sum Slice' function in Image J. Individual cells were selected using the freeform drawing tool to create a ROI (ROI). Selecting the 'Measure' function provided the area, the mean grey value and integrated density of the ROI. The mean background level was obtained by measuring the intensity in three different regions outside the cells and averaging the values obtained. The CTCF for each cell was calculated using the formula: CTCF = Integrated density of cell ROI − (Area of ROI × Mean fluorescence of background). The FEF was calculated by dividing the CTCF value of a cell at pH 7 into the CTCF value of the same cell at pH 4.9.

The number of lysosomes per field of view (Fig. 11) after efflux was counted using Z-stack data acquired on the Olympus Fluoview100, which was compressed into a single plane using the 'Sum Slice' function in Image J. A Max Entropy Threshold 15,000–40,000 was applied to each slice followed by use of the 'Despeckle', 'Erode' and 'Dilate' functions to remove noise. To count the number of lysosomes in each image the 'Analyze Particles' function was used to count objects with a circularity of 0.75–1.00 and size from 0 to 200 pixels.

***In vivo* mouse imaging.** MDA-MB-231-luc-D3H1, a luciferase-expressing human breast adenocarcinoma cell line, was obtained from Caliper Life Sciences. Cells were maintained as a monolayer culture in minimum essential medium containing 10% (v/v) FBS and supplemented with 1% (v/v) L-glutamine, 50 U ml^{-1} penicillin, 50 µl ml^{-1} streptomycin, 1% (v/v) sodium pyruvate and 1% (v/v) non-essential amino acids. All cells were maintained in 5% CO_2 (v/v) and 21% O_2 (v/v) at 37 °C. Balb/C nu/nu mice (Harlan) were housed in the Biomedical Facility (UCD) in individually ventilated cages in temperature and humidity controlled rooms with a 12-h light–dark cycle. Two to five million MDA-MB-231-luc-D3H2LN cells in 100 µl of a DPBS:Matrigel (50:50) solution were injected subcutaneously behind the fore limb of the 5-week-old mice using a 25-g needle. Tumours reached an average diameter of 6 mm before injection. All animal protocols were approved by University College Dublin's local Animal Research Ethics Committee and under the licence from the Department of Health and Children. Animals were split into two groups ($n = 4$) and **2** dissolved in PBS (200 µl) was administered through the lateral tail vein at a concentration of 2 mg kg^{-1}. Optical imaging was performed with an IVIS Spectrum small-animal *in-vivo* imaging system (Caliper LS) with integrated isoflurane anaesthesia. A non-injected control animal was included. Images were acquired at regular intervals post injection of **2** with excitation 675 nm (30 nm band-pass filter) and emission 720 nm (20 nm band-pass filter) narrow band-pass filters and were analysed using Living Image Software v3.0 (Caliper LS).

References

1. Salipalli, S., Singh, P. K. & Borlak, J. Recent advances in live cell imaging of hepatoma cells. *J. BMC Cell Biol.* **15,** 26 (2014).
2. Correa, Jr I. R. Live-cell reporters for fluorescence imaging. *Curr. Opin. Chem. Biol.* **20,** 36–45 (2014).
3. Dean, K. M. & Palmer, A. E. Advances in fluorescence labelling strategies for dynamic cellular imaging. *Nat. Chem. Biol.* **10,** 512–523 (2014).
4. Baker, M. Cellular imaging: taking a long, hard look. *Nature* **466,** 1137–1140 (2010).
5. de Jong, M., Essers, J. & van Weerden, W. M. Imaging preclinical tumour models: improving translational power. *Nat. Rev. Cancer* **14,** 481–493 (2014).
6. Olivo, M., Ho, C. J. H. & Fu, C. Y. Advances in fluorescence diagnosis to track footprints of cancer progression *in vivo*. *Laser Photon. Rev.* **7,** 646–662 (2013).
7. Vahrmeijer, A. L., Hutteman, M., van der Vorst, J. R., van de Velde, C. J. H. & Frangioni, J. V. Image-guided cancer surgery using near-infrared fluorescence. *Nat. Rev. Clin. Oncol.* **10,** 507–518 (2013).
8. Liu, Y. *et al.* Near-infrared fluorescence goggle system with complementary metal-oxide-semiconductor imaging sensor and see-through display. *Biomed. Opt.* **18** 101303 1–10 (2013).
9. Sevick-Muraca, E. M. Translation of near-infrared fluorescence imaging technologies: emerging clinical applications. *Annu. Rev. Med.* **63,** 217–231 (2012).
10. van Dam, G. M. *et al.* Intraoperative tumor-specific fluorescence imaging in ovarian cancer by folate receptor-alpha targeting: first in-human results. *Nat. Med.* **17,** 1315–1319 (2011).
11. Nguyen, Q. T. *et al.* Surgery with molecular fluorescence imaging using activatable cell-penetrating peptides decreases residual cancer and improves survival. *Proc. Natl Acad. Sci. USA* **107,** 4317–4322 (2010).
12. Li, X., Gao, X., Shi, W. & Ma, H. Design strategies for water-soluble small molecular chromogenic and fluorogenic probes. *Chem. Rev.* **114,** 590–659 (2014).
13. Guo, Z., Park, S., Yoon, J. & Shin, I. Recent progress in the development of near-infrared fluorescent probes for bioimaging applications. *Chem. Soc. Rev.* **43,** 16–29 (2014).
14. Yuan, L., Lin, W., Zheng, K., He, L. & Huang, W. Far-red to near infrared analyte-responsive fluorescent probes based on organic fluorophore platforms for fluorescence imaging. *Chem. Soc. Rev.* **42,** 622–661 (2013).
15. Wu, D. & O'Shea, D. F. Synthesis and properties of BF$_2$-3,3'-dimethyldiaryl azadipyrromethene near-infrared fluorophores. *Org. Lett.* **15,** 3392–3395 (2013).
16. Palma, A. *et al.* Cellular uptake mediated off/on responsive near-infrared nanoparticles. *J. Am. Chem. Soc.* **133,** 19618–19621 (2011).
17. Batat, P. *et al.* BF$_2$-azadipyrromethenes: probing the excited-state dynamics of a NIR fluorophore and photodynamic therapy agent. *J. Phys. Chem. A.* **115,** 14034–14039 (2011).
18. Tasior, M. & O'Shea, D. F. BF$_2$-Chelated tetraarylazadipyrromethenes as NIR fluorochromes. *Bioconjugate Chem.* **21,** 1130–1133 (2010).
19. Kilpatrick, B. S., Eden, E. R., Hockey, L. N., Futter, C. E. & Patel, S. Methods for monitoring lysosomal morphology. *Methods Cell Biol.* **126,** 1–19 (2015).
20. Mayor, S. & Pagano, R. E. Pathways of clathrin-independent endocytosis. *Nat. Rev. Mol. Cell Biol.* **8,** 603–612 (2007).
21. Canton, I. & Battaglia, G. Endocytosis at the nanoscale. *Chem. Soc. Rev.* **41,** 2718–2739 (2012).
22. Casey, J. R., Grinstein, S. & Orlowski, J. Sensors and regulators of intracellular pH. *Nat. Rev. Mol. Cell Biol.* **11,** 50–61 (2010).
23. Lee, H. *et al.* Near-infrared pH-activatable fluorescent probes for imaging primary and metastatic breast tumors. *Bioconjugate Chem.* **22,** 777–784 (2011).
24. Han, J. & Burgess, K. Fluorescent indicators for intracellular pH. *Chem. Rev.* **110,** 2709–2728 (2010).
25. Koide, Y., Urano, Y., Hanaoka, K., Terai, T. & Nagano, T. Evolution of group 14 rhodamines as platforms for near-infrared fluorescence probes utilizing photoinduced electron transfer. *ACS Chem. Biol.* **6,** 600–608 (2011).
26. Urano, Y. *et al.* Selective molecular imaging of viable cancer cells with pH-activatable fluorescence probes. *Nat. Med.* **15,** 104–109 (2009).
27. Knop, K., Hoogenboom, R., Fischer, D. & Schubert, U. S. Poly(ethylene glycol) in drug delivery: pros and cons as well as potential alternatives. *Angew. Chem. Int. Ed.* **49,** 6288–6308 (2010).
28. Murtagh, J., Frimannsson, D. O. & O'Shea, D. F. Azide conjugatable and pH responsive near-infrared fluorescent imaging probes. *Org. Lett.* **11,** 5386–5389 (2009).
29. Zhang, X.-X. *et al.* pH-sensitive fluorescent dyes: are they really pH-sensitive in cells? *Mol. Pharm.* **10,** 1910–1917 (2013).
30. Hall, M. J., Allen, L. T. & O'Shea, D. F. PET modulated fluorescent sensing from the BF$_2$ chelated azadipyrromethene platform. *Org. Biomol. Chem.* **4,** 776–780 (2006).
31. Garcia, M. E. D. & Medel, A. S. Dye-surfactant interactions: a review. *Talanta* **33,** 255–264 (1986).
32. Katritzky, A. R., Fara, D. C., Yang, H. & Tamm, K. Quantitative measures of solvent polarity. *Chem. Rev.* **104,** 175–198 (2004).
33. Falcon-Perez, J. M., Nazarian, R., Sabatti, C. & Dell'Angelica, E. C. Distribution and dynamics of Lamp1-containing endocytic organelles in fibroblasts deficient in BLOC-3. *J. Cell Sci.* **118,** 5243–5255 (2005).
34. Bolte, S. & Cordelieres, F. P. A guided tour into subcellular colocalization analysis in light microscopy. *J. Microsc.* **224,** 213–232 (2006).
35. Firdessa, R., Oelschlaeger, T. A. & Moll, H. Identification of multiple cellular uptake pathways of polystyrene nanoparticles and factors affecting the uptake: relevance for drug delivery systems. *Eur. J. Cell Biol.* **93,** 323–337 (2014).
36. De Mey, J. R. *et al.* Fast 4D Microscopy. *Methods Cell Biol.* **85,** 83–112 (2008).
37. Godley, B. F. *et al.* Blue light induces mitochondrial DNA damage and free radical production in epithelial cells. *J. Biol. Chem.* **280,** 21061–21066 (2005).
38. Freundt, E. C., Czapiga, M. & Lenardo, M. J. Photoconversion of lysotracker red to a green fluorescent molecule. *Cell Res.* **17,** 956–958 (2007).
39. Galindo, F. *et al.* Synthetic macrocyclic peptidomimetics as tunable pH probes for the fluorescence imaging of acidic organelles in live cells. *Angew. Chem. Int. Ed.* **44,** 6504–6508 (2005).
40. Chazotte, B. Labeling lysosomes in live cells with lysotracker. *Cold Spring Harb. Protoc.* **2011,** pdb.prot5570 (2011).
41. Zhang, J. *et al.* Near-infrared fluorescent probes based on piperazine-functionalized BODIPY dyes for sensitive detection of lysosomal pH. *J. Mat. Chem. B* **3,** 2173–2184 (2015).
42. Gorman, A. *et al.* In vitro demonstration of the heavy-atom effect for photodynamic therapy. *J. Am. Chem. Soc.* **126,** 10619–10631 (2004).

Acknowledgements

D.O.S. gratefully acknowledges Science Foundation Ireland grant number 11/PI/1071(T) for financial support. E.C. and W.M.G. acknowledge the Irish Cancer Society Collaborative Cancer Research Centre BREAST-PREDICT (CCRC13GAL) for financial support. J.C.S. and A.P. acknowledge Science Foundation Ireland grant 09/IN.1/B2604 for financial support.

Author contributions

M.G. carried out all synthetic chemistry and photophysical measurements. M.M. and S.C. did all fixed and live-cell imaging and imaging analysis. D.S. set up and managed all imaging hardware and software used, and provided expertise advice. E.C. and M.T. conducted the *in vivo* imaging study. A.P. generated LAMP-1 GFP HeLa cells. J.S. provided LAMP-1 GFP HeLa cells and assisted with image and data analysis. W.G. provided expertise on *in vivo* imaging. D.O.S. wrote the manuscript with input from all the co-authors.

Additional information

22

Lipophilic prodrugs of nucleoside triphosphates as biochemical probes and potential antivirals

Tristan Gollnest[1], Thiago Dinis de Oliveira[1], Dominique Schols[2], Jan Balzarini[2] & Chris Meier[1]

The antiviral activity of nucleoside reverse transcriptase inhibitors is often limited by ineffective phosphorylation. We report on a nucleoside triphosphate (NTP) prodrug approach in which the γ-phosphate of NTPs is bioreversibly modified. A series of Tri*PPP*ro-compounds bearing two lipophilic masking units at the γ-phosphate and d4T as a nucleoside analogue are synthesized. Successful delivery of d4TTP is demonstrated in human CD4$^+$ T-lymphocyte cell extracts by an enzyme-triggered mechanism with high selectivity. In antiviral assays, the compounds are potent inhibitors of HIV-1 and HIV-2 in CD4$^+$ T-cell (CEM) cultures. Highly lipophilic acyl residues lead to higher membrane permeability that results in intracellular delivery of phosphorylated metabolites in thymidine kinase-deficient CEM/TK$^-$ cells with higher antiviral activity than the parent nucleoside.

[1] Institute of Organic Chemistry, Department of Chemistry, Faculty of Sciences, University of Hamburg, Martin-Luther-King-Platz 6, D-20146 Hamburg, Germany.
[2] Department of Microbiology and Immunology, Laboratory of Virology and Chemotherapy, Rega Institute for Medical Research, KU Leuven, Minderbroedersstraat 10, B-3000 Leuven, Belgium. Correspondence and requests for materials should be addressed to C.M. (email: chris.meier@chemie.uni-hamburg.de).

Over the last decades, a variety of nucleoside analogues were applied in antitumour and antiviral therapy and still play an important role to combat HIV, herpes virus, hepatitis B and hepatitis C virus infections[1,2]. The target of these nucleoside analogue drugs is the inhibition of the virus-encoded DNA polymerases, such as the HIV reverse transcriptase (RT)[3,4] or the HCV-encoded RNA-dependent RNA-polymerase NS5B (ref. 5), which are the key enzymes in the replication cycle of HIV and HCV, respectively. To date, eight nucleoside analogues have been approved as HIV RT inhibitors (NRTIs)[6]. NRTIs are still used as the backbone of the combined antiretroviral therapy[7]. However, the antiviral efficacy of nucleoside analogues, such as the thymidine analogue 3′-deoxy-2′,3′-didehydrothymidine 1 (d4T) and 3′-deoxy-3′-azidothymidine (AZT), is dependent on the activity of host cell kinases metabolizing these nucleoside analogues into their antivirally active triphosphate forms (nucleoside triphosphates, NTPs)[8–11].

The stepwise transformation via the nucleoside mono- (NMP) and diphosphates (NDP) into the corresponding NTP often occurs insufficiently because of the high substrate specificity of the involved kinases (Supplementary Fig. 1). Furthermore, many nucleoside analogues have limitations such as poor biological half-lives, variable bioavailability after oral administration or selection of drug resistance, which reduce their clinical efficacy[12,13]. To overcome these hurdles, the usage of prodrugs of the phosphorylated metabolites have been explored in the past[14,15].

In the case of d4T 1, the first phosphorylation step to yield its monophosphate form 2 catalysed by the host cell enzyme thymidine kinase (TK) is metabolism-limiting because of the rather modest affinity of d4T 1 to TK as an alternative substrate and because TK activity is S-phase-dependent[11,16,17]. However, to avoid this limitation, it is not possible to apply the charged monophosphorylated metabolite because of the high polarity and thereby extremely poor, if any, membrane permeability. The development of nucleotide prodrugs capable of delivering the monophosphorylated metabolite and thereby bypassing the intracellular activation offered advantages over the use of the corresponding nucleoside analogue[18,19]. Moreover, lipophilic-masked NMPs such as 3 are less vulnerable to degradation by unspecific phosphatases present in the blood. This enhanced not only the plasma half-life but also enables the prodrug to be taken up by cells through passive diffusion[20,21]. A number of successful NMP prodrug strategies were reported in the past that efficiently bypass the nucleoside kinase hurdle. These prodrug forms such as phosphoramidates and cycloSal-phosphate triesters of nucleoside analogues were indeed shown to deliver the NMP either by chemical or enzymatic hydrolysis in the target cells[22–27]. In addition to NMPs also the successful delivery of acyclic nucleoside phosphonates such as cidofovir has been reported[28]. However, all these approaches delivered the monophosphor(n)ylated forms of the nucleosides that subsequently needed further phosphorylation into the triphosphate forms by cellular kinases to inhibit their target polymerase.

However, not in all cases such NMP prodrug strategies were successful. For instance, in the case of AZT the metabolism is limited by the second conversion step, the formation of AZT-diphosphate by thymidylate kinase[10,29]. In this case, a lipophilic prodrug that intracellularly releases the NDP would be desirable. At the same time, this would avoid toxicity caused by the parent nucleoside or the accumulation of the monophosphate form[30]. A further example is 2′,3′-dideoxy-2′,3′-didehydrouridine (d4U). The parent nucleoside proved to be completely inactive against HIV replication in cell cultures. In contrast, the triphosphate form of d4U is one of the most effective inhibitors of the HIV's RT[31].

We reported on NDP prodrugs (DiPPro-approach), which selectively released NDPs not only in phosphate buffer (pH 7.3) but for the first time also in CEM cell extracts[32–35]. These compounds showed very good antiviral activity in TK-deficient CEM/TK⁻ cell cultures infected with HIV, proving the uptake of the compounds and the delivery of at least phosphorylated metabolites, most likely the NDP. The uptake of those compounds was achieved by two acceptor-substituted benzylesters linked to the β-phosphate group of the NDP. The stability of the compounds correlated with the length of the aliphatic residue of the mask[32,33]. However, we have shown that the delivery of the corresponding mono- or diphosphates from prodrug forms (such as the cycloSal- or DiPPro-compounds) did not improve the antiviral activity[34]. Importantly, in the same study we have proven that d4U diphosphate was a very poor substrate for the NDP kinase, the enzyme that is generally accepted to be involved in the conversion of NDPs into their triphosphate forms. Thus, this study showed that the phosphorylation of nucleotide analogues by NDP kinase can be also rate-limiting in the activation process of a nucleoside analogue[34,36]. As a consequence, the development of nucleoside triphosphate prodrugs would be highly interesting and desirable because this would bypass all steps of intracellular phosphorylation and would maximize the intracellular concentration of the ultimately bioactive NTP. Although this has been recognized before[11], it was also claimed that the development of prodrugs of NTP is chemically not feasible because of the low stability of such compounds[37]. For this reason, NTPs were very rarely used as drug platforms because of their expected poor deliverability and their high sensitivity for enzymatic dephosphorylation. Thus, very few reports on potential triphosphate prodrugs have been reported[38,39]. In addition, in the few reported examples the yields in the chemical synthesis were poor, and additionally the compounds proved hydrolytically very unstable. A difficulty that has to be taken into account in the development of NTP prodrugs is related to the energy-rich phosphate anhydride bonds within the triphosphate unit. Under physiological conditions, these linkages are only kinetically stable because of the charges present at that moiety, which prevent nucleophilic reactions that end up in the cleavage of these anhydride bonds but can be enzymatically cleaved. Interestingly, γ-modification of NTPs by esterification or replacement of the γ-phosphate group by a phosphonate moiety led to a marked increase in enzymatic stability of the triphosphate unit[40,41]. On the other hand, complete lipophilic modification and thereby neutralization of the charges would significantly increase the reactivity of the triphosphate unit. For completeness, it should be added that the delivery challenge for NTPs has also been addressed by formulating these compounds with cationic nanogels. However, this approach still requires elaboration with respect to their toxicity, immunogenicity and pharmacokinetics[42,43].

Here we disclose the development of a novel prodrug concept for NTPs that releases directly NTPs with high selectivity by an enzyme-triggered mechanism and thus allows the bypass of all phosphorylation steps normally needed for the activation of a nucleoside analogue (Supplementary Fig. 2). To achieve this goal, the γ-phosphate group of a NTP was modified by esterification with acyloxybenzyl moieties (TriPPPro-compounds). By fine-tuning the lipophilicity through the use of different acyl esters the chemical stability also proved controllable so that the polarity caused by the remaining charges at the α- and β-phosphates could be efficiently compensated.

The cleavage of the prodrug moieties is initiated by an enzymatic hydrolysis of the phenolic acyl-ester. This reaction leads to a spontaneous cleavage of the benzyl C–O bond forming first a monomasked intermediate of the NTPs. This process is repeated for the second mask so that finally the NTP is formed[32]. Lipophilic aliphatic esters have proven to be suitable for prodrugs to allow entering the cell independently of nucleoside transporters but to enable removal of the lipophilic prodrug moieties by cellular esterases/lipases[44]. Moreover, fatty-acid esters are known to be taken up by the mononuclear phagocyte system. These cells are important in the pathogenesis of AIDS and are considered to be reservoirs for HIV particles[45,46].

We report on the synthesis of NTP prodrugs 3 bearing two identical 4-alkanoyloxybenzyl- (a–k), 4-alkoxycarbonyloxybenzyl- (l–n) and 4-aminocarbonyloxybenzyl groups (o–q), their hydrolysis properties in different media, the hydrolysis mechanism, primer extension assays and their anti-HIV activity. In addition, the synthesis of the monomasked (4-alkyloxybenzyl)-d4TTPs 4a,e,j is reported. As a model nucleoside analogue, d4T 1 was used to allow a comparison of the TriPPPro-compounds 3 with the DiPPPro-compounds.

Results

Synthesis of TriPPPro-d4T triphosphate prodrugs 4.

For the synthesis of TriPPPros-d4TTP prodrugs 3 a convergent strategy using a dicyanoimidazol (DCI)-mediated coupling of an appropriate phosphoramidite 5 and d4TDP 6 to form the energetically rich pyrophosphate moiety in the last step was performed (Fig. 1). First, d4T 1 was prepared in good overall yields according to a three-step protocol reported by Horwitz[47]. From that compound, d4TDP 6 was prepared by applying the cycloSal technique (55% yield) because it has been reported that acceptor-substituted cycloSal nucleotides gave access to diphosphorylated compounds by using tetra-n-butylammonium phosphate as a nucleophile[48]. Therefore, the 5-chloro-substituted cycloSal-phosphate triester 7 was synthesized starting from d4T 1 with 5-chlorosaligenylchlorophosphite 8 followed by oxidation with tert-butylhydroperoxide to give the product 7 as a mixture of two diastereomers in high yields.

Despite its very difficult chromatographic properties, the resulting crude (n-Bu)₄N⁺-salt 6 was purified by automatic RP-18 flash chromatography without additional ion exchange.

The hygroscopic tetra-n-butylammonium salt form of d4TDP 6 was co-evaporated in dimethylformamide (DMF) and dried in high vacuum before the coupling reaction to ensure dry reaction conditions. The use of tetra-n-butylammonium counterions afforded a higher reactivity and better solubility in organic solvents. D4TDP 6 was then reacted with a series of phosphoramidites 5 in a very fast DCI-mediated coupling reaction and was oxidized[32,33].

Inspired by recently published biodegradable linear polymers that were degraded by an acid-induced cascade reaction, we also synthesized carbamate derivatives 3o–q (ref. 49). In this case, 4-hydroxybenzyl alcohol 10 was first protected with tert-butyldimethylsilyl chloride to give compound 11 followed by an esterification using 4-nitrophenyl chloroformate. To trap the excess of the chloroformiate, triethylene glycol monomethyl ether was added[49]. The obtained carbonate 12 was then converted with t-Boc-protected dimethylethylenediamine 13 and after acid-catalysed cleavage of both protecting groups the methylcarbamate 14 was isolated in 98% yield. Finally, phenylcarbamates 15 were synthesized starting from 14 in an one-pot reaction including tetramethylsilane (TMS) protection, coupling with the corresponding acyl chloroformiates 16 and desilylation in a yield of up to 59% (Fig. 2).

The 4-hydroxybenzyl alcohols bearing acyl-ester groups at the phenol and the carbamates were converted into phosphoramidites 5 in high yields as published before[32,33]. Finally, d4TDP 6 was mixed with 1.7 equivalents (eq.) of a corresponding phosphoramidite 5 and co-evaporated with acetonitrile. Then, the mixture was dissolved in a minimum of acetonitrile because achieving a high concentration was crucial for the success of the coupling reaction. In case of compounds with long acyl residues ($R \geq C_{11}H_{23}$), tetrahydrofurane (THF) was added to accomplish complete solubility of the reagents. In some cases, the conversion of d4TDP 6 was not complete. In these cases, all volatile components were removed in vacuum, the residue was redissolved and further 1.0 eq. of the phosphoramidite 5 and 0.8 eq. of DCI were added. After another minute of stirring, the reaction mixture was oxidized. After oxidation the quantitative consumption of d4TDP 6 was confirmed using high-performance

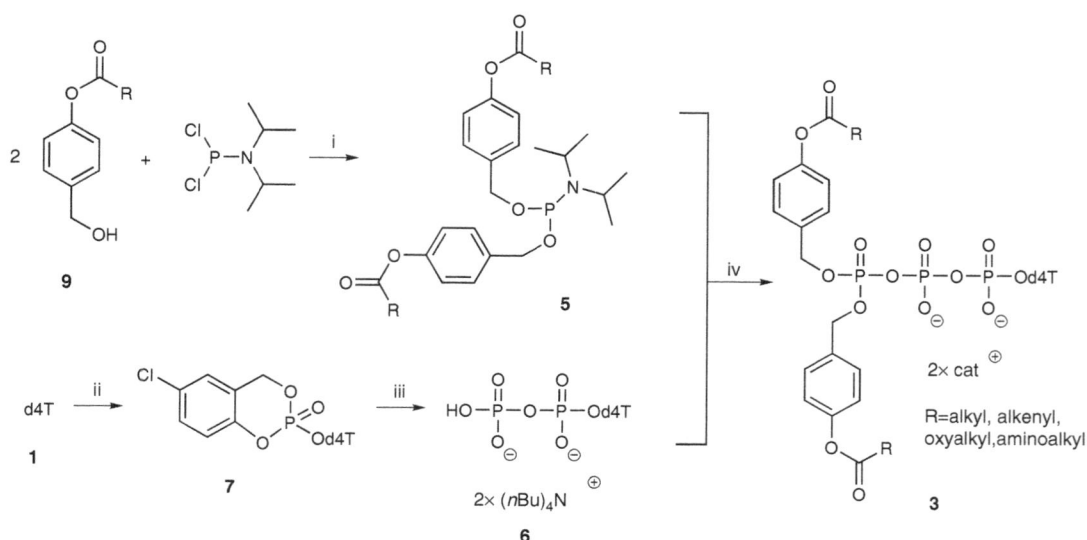

Figure 1 | Reagents and conditions. (i) Triethylamine, THF, 0 °C-rt, 20 h; (ii) **1**. 5-chlorosaligenylchlorophosphite **8**, N,N-diisopropylethylamine, CH₃CN, −20 °C-rt, 3 h, **2**. t-BuOOH in r-decane, 0 °C-rt, 30 min; (iii) (H₂PO₄)Bu₄N, DMF, rt, 20 h; (iv) **1**. DCI, CH₃CN, rt, 1 min, **2**. t-BuOOH in n-decane, 0 °C-rt, 15 min.

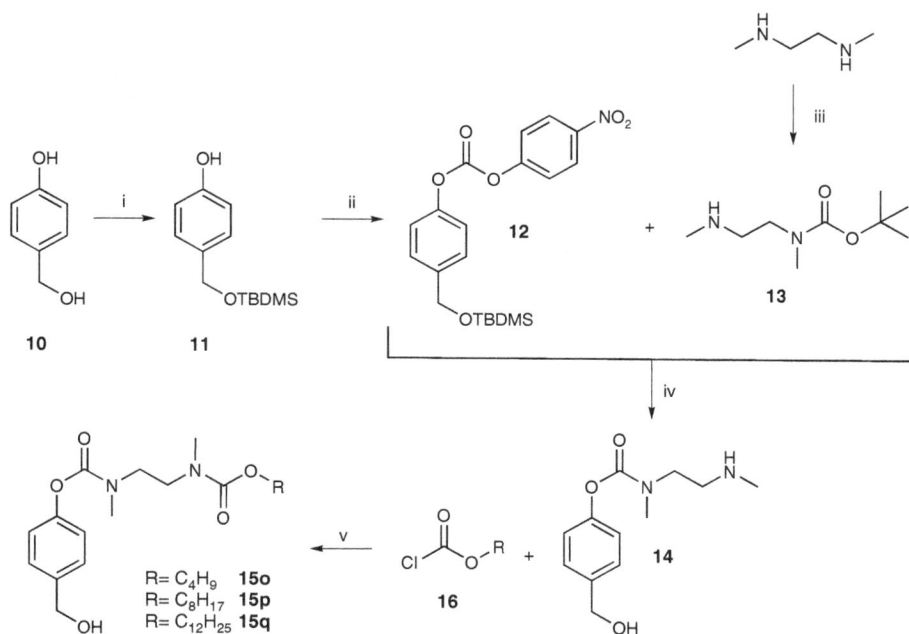

Figure 2 | Reagents and conditions. (i) TBDMSCl, imidazole, CH_2Cl_2, rt, 2 h; (ii) **1**. 4-nitrophenyl chloroformiate, triethylamine, CH_2Cl_2, rt, 16 h, **2**. triethylene glycol monomethyl ether, rt, 20 min; (iii) Boc$_2$O, 0 °C-rt, 20 h; (iv) **1**. 4-DMAP, di*iso*propylethylamine, toluene, rt, 16 h, **2**. TFA/CH_2Cl_2, rt, 0.5 h; (v) **1**. TMSCl, imidazole, THF, 0 °C-rt, 2 h, **2**. triethylamine, 0 °C-rt, 1.5 h, **3**. 1% HCl (12 M) in EtOH, rt, 1 h.

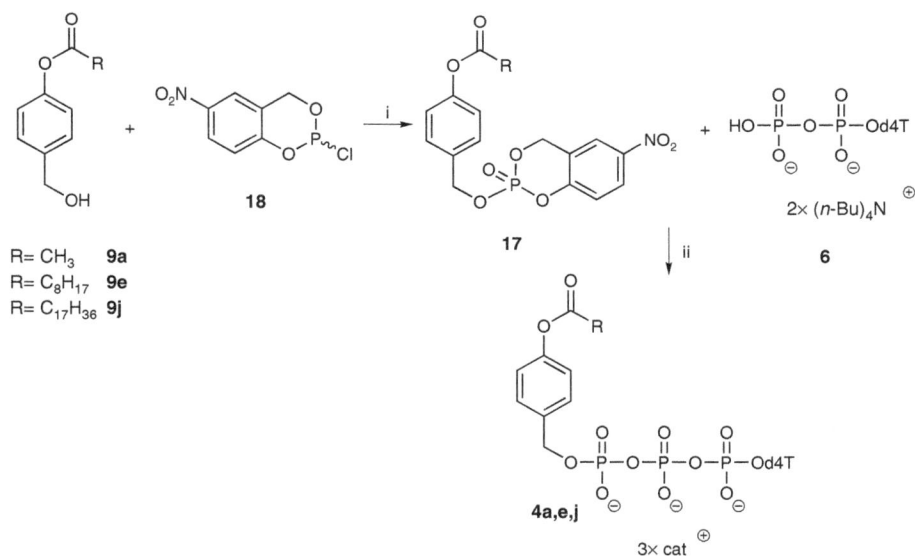

Figure 3 | Reagents and conditions. (i) **1**. di*iso*propylethylamine, CH_3CN, − 20 °C-rt, 1 h, **2**. oxone, H_2O/CH_3CN, rt, 30 min; (ii) bis(tetra-*n*-butyl)ammonium-d4TDP **6**, DMF, rt, 3 h.

liquid chromatography (HPLC; Supplementary Fig. 3). Next, the solvent was removed *in vacuum* and the crude product was purified with RP-18 chromatography using gradients of water/acetonitrile or water/THF as eluents. For compounds **3a–f, l–n, o–q** the tetra-*n*-butylammonium ions were exchanged by ammonium ions using Dowex 50WX8 and the chromatography was repeated.

Synthesis of monomasked triphosphate prodrugs 4. In addition to the Tri*PP*Pro-compounds **3**, the monomasked acyloxybenzyl-NTP derivatives **4** were synthesized as well (Fig. 3). Such

monoesterified substances were described by others as potential triphosphate prodrugs[38,39,50]. Several synthesis routes mainly based on DCC-activated coupling were published. In our recent studies with Di*PP*ro-prodrugs, we isolated such monoesterified compounds by simple hydrolysis[33].

An efficient access to such compounds was developed in this study. The monoesterified NTPs were prepared starting from 4-acyloxybenzyl alcohol **9** and its conversion into the 5-nitro-*cyclo*Sal-triester **17**. Despite the high reactivity of this compound, the purification by preparative thin-layer chromatography (TLC) was successful. The benzyl-(5-nitro-*cyclo*Sal)-phosphate triesters **17** were obtained in high yields (up to

89%). Next, triesters **17** gave the monomasked acyloxybenzyl-d4TTPs **4** in yields of 26–30% by the addition of d4TDP **6**.

Stability studies. The TriPPPros-d4TTP prodrugs **3** and the intermediates **4** were incubated in PBS (25 mM, pH 7.3), or were exposed to pig liver esterase (PLE) in PBS and to human CD_4^+ T-lymphocyte cell extracts to study their stability and the product distribution. The hydrolysis mixtures were analysed by means of analytical RP-18-HPLC. The calculated half-lives (Table 1) were determined for the first removal of one masking unit ($t_{1/2}(1)$) to yield the intermediate **4** and the second hydrolysis step ($t_{1/2}(2)$) to give the triphosphate **19**.

Chemical stability in PBS at pH 7.3. In PBS, the stability of TriPPPro-d4TTP prodrugs **3a–h,l–n** increased with increasing alkyl chain lengths (Table 1). However, the half-lives of more lipophilic compounds **3i–k** decreased because of altered solubility behaviour or micelle formation. The half-lives of the intermediates **4** were always considerably higher than those of their precursors **3** because of the increase in charges leading to repulsive interaction with an incoming nucleophile. Moreover, formation of the three nucleotide forms **2**, **6** and **19** were observed (Supplementary Fig. 4).

Hydrolysis study using esterase. Next, we examined the enzymatic stability of prodrugs **3a–n** by incubation with PLE in PBS, pH 7.3. The cleavage of the masking units for **3b–g** occurred much faster than that in PBS, demonstrating a significant contribution of the enzymatic cleavage (Table 1). As observed in the chemical hydrolysis studies, the cleavage of the second masking group proceeded much slower. According to the substrate specificity of PLE we determined the lowest half-lives for **3c–f** and **3m**. Shorter as well as longer alkyl residues in the ester moiety of the masking group led to increased half-lives. In addition, d4TTP

19 was delivered by enzymatic activation of **3a–n** but was also found to be the sole metabolite from **4a,e,j** as long as the enzymatic cleavage occurred rapidly (Supplementary Fig. 5). The carbamate-functionalized prodrugs **3o–q** were not substrates for PLE, as expected.

To confirm the prodrug concept and thus the direct successful release of the biologically active triphosphate metabolite, the prodrug **3e** was exposed to PLE and the hydrolysis monitored with RP-18-HPLC. After complete consumption of **3e** as well as its intermediate **4e** the solvents were removed. For the template/primer extension assay (Fig. 4a), HIV RT was incubated with the PLE hydrolysate as such (T*) or with the PLE hydrolysate in the additional presence of dCTP (T*, C), or dCTP + dGTP (T*, C, G) or all natural 2′-deoxynucleotides (N*). Interestingly, an immediate DNA chain termination was observed after incorporation of d4TMP **2** (derived from the incoming d4TTP **19** that was released from the prodrug by PLE), while the control reaction containing all four natural NTPs in the absence of the PLE hydrolysate (N) showed full extension of the primer (Fig. 4a). In addition, TriPPPro-TTP **3r** was synthesized (Fig. 5) and also investigated in the same way. As expected, the template/primer extension assay showed efficient DNA elongation (Fig. 4b). The T* lysate resulted in termination of the polymerization because of the lack of the next complementary nucleotide (dCTP; position 26 nt), whereas the reaction proceeded till position 28 nt in the presence of both T* and dCTP (T*, C). The primer could be fully extended till 30 nt when T* was added in the presence of dCTP and dGTP, as also the N* and N samples could.

Hydrolysis in cell extracts. The hydrolysis of the TriPPPro-compounds **3** was further investigated in human CD_4^+ T-lymphocyte CEM cell extracts. Again, the half-lives of the prodrugs **3a–n** correlated well with chain length and were significantly lower than the half-lives in PBS buffer (Table 1). Thus, an enzymatic cleavage reaction took place as described above for the PLE studies. Furthermore, we observed the formation of the corresponding intermediates **4a–n** that had lower half-lives than their parent prodrugs. This assumption was proven by hydrolysis of the synthesized intermediates **4a,e,j**. In contrast to hydrolysis studies with PLE, in addition to d4TTP **19** d4TDP **6** was also detected as a major component in the CEM cell extracts most probably because of the presence of hydrolytic enzymes such as phosphatases and esterases (Supplementary Fig. 6).

The formation of d4TDP **6** was clearly not a result of unselective cleavage of the prodrug **3**. Investigations in cell

Table 1 | Hydrolysis half-lives of TriPPPro-d4TTPs 3 and monoesterified d4TTPs 4 in different media.

Compd	R	PBS, pH = 7.3 (h)		PLE (h)		CEM (h)
		$t_{1/2}(1)$*	$t_{1/2}(2)$†	$t_{1/2}(1)$*	$t_{1/2}(2)$†	$t_{1/2}(1)$*
3a	CH_3	18	75	1.9	71	0.050
3b	C_2H_5	17	150	0.42	33	0.12
3c	C_4H_9	22	270	0.063	7.7	0.43
3d	C_6H_{13}	26	350	0.013	1.6	0.98
3e	C_8H_{17}	52	390	0.013	1.6	2.5
3f	C_9H_{19}	44	350	0.082	3.0	2.8
3g	$C_{11}H_{23}$	68	410	0.95	8.3	2.2
3h	$C_{13}H_{27}$	90	355	30	n.d.‡	4.6
3i	$C_{15}H_{31}$	73	462	33	n.d.‡	5.3
3j	$C_{17}H_{35}$	50	583	37	n.d.‡	13
3k	$C_{17}H_{33}$ (8Z)	27	92	42	n.d.‡	4.3
3l	OCH_3	24	200	3.8	177	0.97
3m	OC_8H_{17}	82	590	0.12	17	2.6
3n	$OC_{11}H_{23}$	99	631	44	n.d.‡	3.0
3o	$NCH_3(C_9H_{19}NO_2)$	27	n.d.‡	n.d.§	n.d.§	n.d.‡
3p	$NCH_3(C_{13}H_{27}NO_2)$	48	n.d.‡	n.d.§	n.d.§	5.6
3q	$NCH_3(C_{17}H_{35}NO_2)$	48	n.d.‡	n.d.§	n.d.§	n.d.‡
4a	CH_3	n.a.‖	95	n.a.‖	108	0.040
4e	C_8H_{17}	n.a.‖	237	n.a.‖	1.5	1.8
4j	$C_{17}H_{35}$	n.a.‖	637	n.a.‖	57	4.6

*Half-lives of **3**.
†Half-lives of **4**.
‡Not determined.
§No substrate for enzyme.
‖Not available.

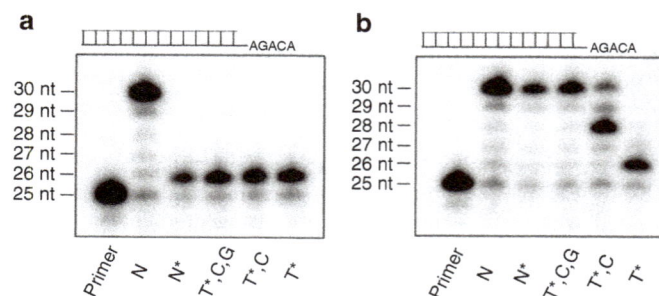

Figure 4 | Primer extension assays with HIV reverse transcriptase. (**a**) PLE hydrolysate based on TriPPPro-d4TTP **3e** (T*); dCTP; dGTP; all natural triphosphates (N); dATP, dCTP, dGTP and the hydrolysate of **3e** (N*). (**b**) PLE hydrolysate based on TriPPPro-compound **3r** (T*); dCTP; dGTP; all natural triphosphates (N); dATP, dCTP, dGTP and the hydrolysate of **3r** (N*). nt: nucleotide, length of primer.

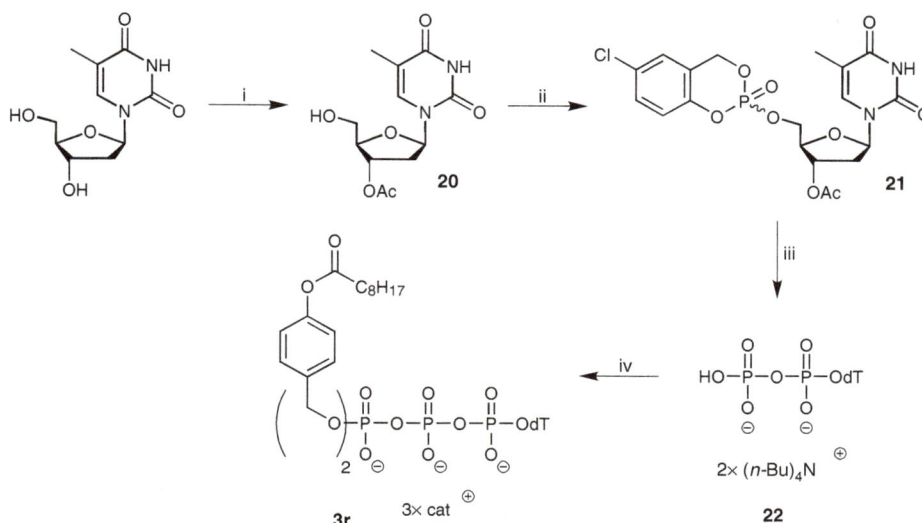

Figure 5 | Reagents and conditions. (i) **1**. TBDMSCl, pyridine, rt, 20 h, **2**. Ac₂O, rt, 5 h, **3**. TBAF, THF, 0 °C, 1.5 h; (ii) **1**. 5-chlorosaligenylchlorophosphite **8**, N,N-diisopropylethylamine, CH₃CN, 0 °C-rt, 3 h, **2**. t-BuOOH in n-decane, 0 °C, 20 min; (iii) **1**. (H₂PO₄)Bu₄N, DMF, rt, 20 h, **2**. MeOH/H₂O/Bu₄NOH (7:3:1), rt, 17 h; (iv) **1**. **5e**, DCI, CH₃CN, rt, 1 min; **2**. t-BuOOH in n-decane, 0 °C-rt, 15 min.

Table 2 | Antiviral activity and cytotoxicity of TriPPPro-d4TTPs 3 in comparison with the parent nucleoside d4T 1.

Compd	EC₅₀ (µM)*			CC₅₀ (µM)†
	CEM		**CEM/TK⁻**	**CEM**
	HIV-1	**HIV-2**	**HIV-2**	
3a	0.43 ± 0.25	0.72 ± 0.16	>10	63 ± 2
3b	0.46 ± 0.21	1.16 ± 0.15	>10	57 ± 6
3c	0.40 ± 0.00	1.05 ± 0.30	>10	58 ± 3
3d	0.36 ± 0.06	0.94 ± 0.16	10 ± 0.00	74 ± 2
3e	0.31 ± 0.01	0.62 ± 0.30	2.26 ± 1.03	52 ± 1
3f	0.25 ± 0.07	0.33 ± 0.03	0.50 ± 0.14	34 ± 5
3g	0.21 ± 0.01	0.27 ± 0.06	0.72 ± 0.16	26 ± 0
3h	0.50 ± 0.14	1.10 ± 0.23	1.63 ± 0.52	28 ± 7
3i	0.62 ± 0.30	0.66 ± 0.08	0.72 ± 0.16	61 ± 3
3j	0.17 ± 0.00	0.31 ± 0.00	0.28 ± 0.04	29 ± 9
3k	0.30 ± 0.01	0.47 ± 0.10	0.93 ± 0.47	25 ± 1
3l	0.40 ± 0.00	0.92 ± 0.12	>10	16 ± 1
3m	0.36 ± 0.06	0.47 ± 0.10	1.26 ± 0.00	51 ± 5
3n	0.50 ± 0.14	0.69 ± 0.21	1.26 ± 0.00	41 ± 12
d4T	0.33 ± 0.11	0.89 ± 0.00	150 ± 9	79 ± 3

*Antiviral activity in CD4⁺ T-lymphocytes: 50% effective concentration; values are the mean ± s.d. of n = 2-3 independent experiments.
†Cytotoxicity: 50% cytostatic concentration or compound concentration required to inhibit CD4⁺ T-cell (CEM) proliferation by 50%; values are the mean ± s.d. of n = 2-3 independent experiments.

extracts starting from d4TTP **19** led to a rapid degradation ($t_{1/2} = 0.63$ h). For this reason d4TDP **6** ($t_{1/2} = 59$ h) accumulated under these conditions. On the other hand, only very small amounts of d4TMP **2** were formed. Nevertheless, it was proven that the triphosphate of d4T **19** was successfully released in biological media such as CD4⁺ T-lymphocyte extracts.

Antiviral evaluation. TriPPPro-compounds **3a–n** were evaluated for their ability to inhibit the replication of HIV. For this purpose, HIV-1- or HIV-2-infected wild-type CEM/0 as well as mutant TK-deficient CEM cell cultures (CEM/TK⁻) were treated with the prodrugs **3**. As can be seen in Table 1, all compounds showed virtually similar activities against HIV-1 and HIV-2 as the parent nucleoside d4T **1**. A somewhat increased antiviral activity with increasing lipophilicity resulting from their advantageous permeability was observed. In addition, all prodrugs with R ≥ C₈H₁₇ were also highly potent in CEM/TK⁻ cells, whereas d4T **1** lacked

relevant anti-HIV activity as expected in this TK-deficient cell model (EC₅₀:150 µM). It should also be noticed that none of the prodrugs **3** were endowed with a significantly higher cytotoxicity than the parent d4T **1** compound (Table 2).

Discussion
We reported on the first successful direct intracellular delivery of NTPs using prodrug technology. D4T triphosphate prodrugs **3a–q** were prepared via a convergent route using phosphoramidite chemistry (Fig. 1). Despite complete and selective conversion, TriPPPro-NTP prodrugs **3** were obtained in yields between 27 and 66%. We assumed that the loss in yield may be the result of a cleavage of the β- and γ-phosphate anhydride bond of the prodrugs during work-up. This assumption was supported by the detection of d4TDP **6** and the bis(benzyl)phosphate diester after chromatography. Alternative purification methods such as extraction and precipitation were investigated but proved to be

inefficient. Nevertheless, by this method a large number of TriPPPro-d4TTPs 3 bearing various acyloxybenzyl-masking units were obtained. Moreover, this synthesis strategy also showed to be applicable to the synthesis of TriPPPro-compounds bearing other pyrimidine or purine nucleoside analogues. In addition, the intermediates 4a,e,j were synthesized using the cycloSal method and were obtained in moderate chemical yields. This method, which is based on the cycloSal strategy, is a reliable method for the synthesis of polyphosphate diesters comprising esters at both ends of the polyphosphate group (Fig. 3)[48,51,52].

In general, three reactions should be considered in the hydrolysis pathways of TriPPPro-nucleotide prodrugs 3. First, the designed pathway yielding the NTP; second, a concurrent reaction that involved a nucleophilic reaction at the γ-phosphate leading to the formation of d4TDP 6; and third, a nucleophilic reaction at the β-phosphate that would lead to d4TMP 2. Figure 6 summarizes all three possible hydrolysis pathways leading to the different phosphorylated nucleotide species. As shown in Fig. 6, to release d4TTP 19 two successive cleavage processes were necessary (path A). Thus, in addition to hydrolysis pathway A, also a reaction at the γ- and β-phosphate groups took place as side-reactions. Owing to the presence of a second energetically rich pyrophosphate bond, but despite its additional negative charge, the half-lives were found to be lower than those published recently for the DiPPPro-d4TDPs[33]. However, the triphosphate 19 was the predominant product formed (Supplementary Fig. 4). Moreover, after the starting material 3e was completely consumed, there was no further increase in the amounts of d4TMP 2 and d4TDP 6, which again points to the fact that the intermediate selectively delivers the triphosphate while the mono- and the diphosphate are formed from the starting

TriPPPro-compounds only. A comparable behaviour has also been observed for the DiPPPro-compounds[33].

In contrast, for the carbamate derivatives 3o–q the cleavage of the masking groups occurred only once leading to the intermediates 4o-q. Therefore, it was concluded that the delivery mechanism should be different as compared with the ester-bearing masking groups. Owing to the highly stable carbamate functions present in the masking group, the first masking group cannot be cleaved by the original mechanism that involves a cleavage within the ester/carbamate residue. To gain more insights into this, a hydrolysis experiment of derivative 3o was conducted in ^{18}O-labelled water to yield 4o. Surprisingly, the ^{18}O-label was found in the cleaved benzyl-alcohol and not at the phosphate, which was convincingly confirmed using mass spectrometry (Supplementary Fig. 7). Two different interpretations are possible for this result: (i) a S_N1-type reaction took place forming a benzyl cation and the monomasked NTP intermediate 4. The cation is then trapped by addition of water or (ii) a S_N2-type reaction took place instead in which the labelled water displaces the monomasked NTP intermediate 4 (Fig. 6, hydrolysis pathway A_2). In addition to hydrolysis in PBS, pH 7.3, 4p was hydrolysed under slightly acidic conditions (pH 6.0), although in comparison with the physiological pH conditions no difference in its hydrolysis behaviour was observed. Because of the very long hydrolysis time periods, a cleavage of the glycosidic bond in d4T 1 resulted in the appearance of the nucleobase thymine. The amount doubles every 63 h; however, this aspect has not been further considered in these investigations because it was irrelevant in the enzyme or cell extract incubations and in the case of other nucleoside analogues.

Finally, a very important result from the studies conducted with the monomasked intermediates 4a,e,j was the finding that exclusively d4TTP 19 was formed from these compounds. In addition, the hydrolysis studies conducted in the presence of PLE clearly led to the selective formation of two different NTPs (d4TTP and TTP) from the corresponding prodrug forms.

In conclusion, because of a successful cell membrane passage of the TriPPPro-compounds 3 and subsequent intracellular enzymatic hydrolysis, which led to the direct intracellular formation of phosphorylated d4T metabolites such as d4TTP 19 or at least d4TDP 6, marked anti-HIV activity in CEM/TK⁻ cell cultures was observed while the parent nucleoside d4T 1 lacked significant activity in this cell assay. Thus, although the TriPPPro-compounds are still charged at the phosphate groups, obviously the modification at the γ-phosphate group by lipophilic, bioreversible moieties gives the molecule sufficient lipophilicity to penetrate the cell membrane. To the best of our knowledge, we provided the first direct proof of the successful application of masked triphosphates that obviously are able to efficiently enter the cells and to directly deliver a higher phosphate derivative, most likely d4TTP 19. Because the concept should be generally applicable to natural nucleosides and a broad variety of nucleoside analogues, a novel way to deliver the corresponding bioactive triphosphate form of these nucleosides without any need for further enzymatically catalysed phosphorylation has been discovered. This concept seems to be very interesting for application with nucleoside analogues that show severe limitations in their activation to give the corresponding NTPs. Moreover, we are convinced that this approach is not limited to HIV treatment but can also be used for other viral targets and cancer and can also be used as a delivery for non-natural NTPs as biochemical tools in Chemical Biology approaches.

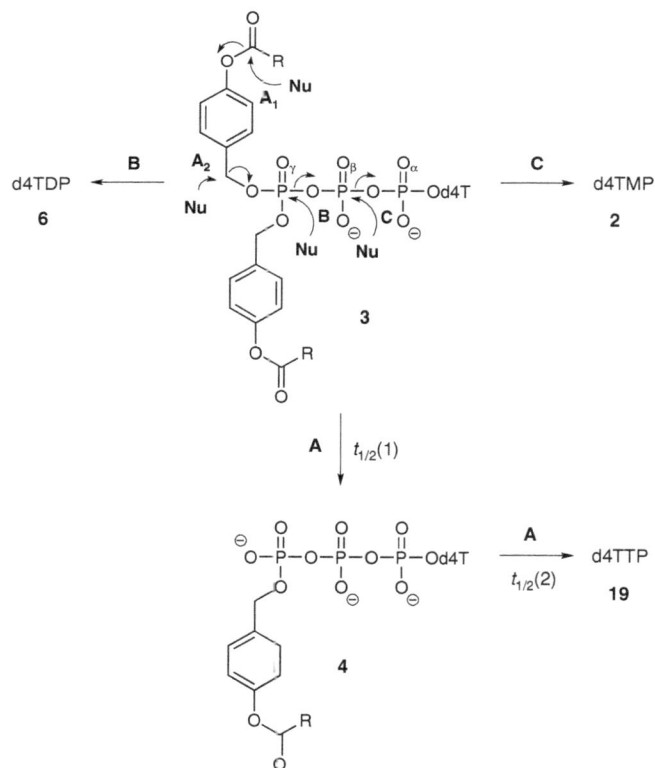

Figure 6 | Chemical hydrolysis pathways for TriPPPro-d4TTPs 3.
A_{1+2} delivery of d4TTP **19**; B release of d4TDP **6** by cleavage of the phosphoanhydride bond between β- and γ-phosphate; C release of d4TMP **2** by cleavage of phosphoanhydride bond between α- and β-phosphate.

Methods

General. All reactions were carried out under dry conditions and at room temperature. *Solvents and reagents*: Acetonitrile, THF and DMF were purchased from Acros Organics (Extra Dry over molecular sieves) and dried with activated molecular sieves. Triethylamine and N,N-diisopropylethylamine were refluxed over CaH_2 for 3 days and distilled under nitrogen. 5-Chlorosaligenylchlorophosphite **8** and 5-nitrosaligenylchlorophosphite **18** were synthesized according to the literature and **8** freshly distilled before use[48]. All further reagents commercially available were used as received. *Thin-layer chromatography*: For TLC Macherey–Nagel precoated TLC sheets Alugram Xtra SIL G/UV254 were used; sugar-containing compounds were visualized with sugar spray reagent (4-methoxybenzaldehyde/ EtOH/concentrated sulphuric acid/glacial acetic acid in ratio 5/90/5/0.1 v/v) and phosphate-containing compounds with ammonium molybdate solution (1 g $(NH_4)_6Mo_7O_{24}$ 4 H_2O in 7 ml semiconcentrated nitric acid and 13 ml water) followed by tin(II)chloride solution (0.1 g $SnCl_2$ 2 H_2O in 20 ml 0.5 mol l^{-1} hydrochloric acid). *Preparative chromatography*: The preparative TLCs were accomplished with a chromatotron (Harrison Research, Model 7,924T) using glass plates coated with 2 or 4 mm layers of Merck 60 PF$_{254}$ silica gel. *Column chromatography*: Normal phase column chromatography was performed with Macherey–Nagel silica gel 60 M (0.04–0.063 mm). *Automatic RP-18 chromatography*: For reverse-phase chromatography, an Intershim Puriflash 430 in combination with Chromabond Flash RS40 C_{18}ec was used. *High-performance liquid chromatography*: HPLC was required for analytical studies and monitoring reactions. It was performed using a VWR-Hitachi LaChromElite HPLC system (L-2130, L-2200, L-2455) and EzChromElite software, equipped with a Nucleodur 100–5 C_{18}ec or Nucleodur 100–5 C_8ec (Macherey–Nagel). Acetonitrile for HPLC was obtained from VWR (HPLC grade) and ultrapure water using Sartorius Aurium pro (Sartopore 0.2 μm, UV detector). Tetra-n-butylammonium acetate solution (2 mM; TBAA, pH 6.3) or 10 mM triethylammonium acetate (TEAA, pH 6.2) were used for buffering. *Method A*: Nucleodur 100–5 C_{18}ec; 0–20 min: TBAA buffer/acetonitrile gradient (5–80%); 20–30 min: buffer/acetonitrile (80%); 30– 33 min: buffer/acetonitrile (80–5%); 33–38 min: buffer/acetonitrile (5%); flow: 1 ml min^{-1}. *Method B*: Nucleodur 100–5 C_{18}ec; 0–20 min: TEAA buffer/ acetonitrile gradient (5–90%); 20–30 min: buffer/acetonitrile (90%); 30–33 min: buffer/acetonitrile (90–5%); 33–38 min: buffer/acetonitrile (5%); flow 1 ml min^{-1}. *Method C*: Nucleodur 100–5 C_8ec; 0–25 min: TBAA buffer/acetonitrile gradient (5–80%); 25–30 min: buffer/acetonitrile (80%); 30–33 min: buffer/acetonitrile (80–5%); 33–38 min: buffer/acetonitrile (5%); flow: 1 ml min^{-1}.

Nuclear Magnetic Resonance: NMR spectra were recorded at room temperature in an automation mode with a Varian Gemini 2000BB, Bruker Fourier 300, Bruker AMX 400, Bruker DRX 500 or Bruker AVIII 600. All ^{1}H- and ^{13}C-NMR chemical shifts ($δ$) are quoted in parts per million (p.p.m.) downfield from TMS and calibrated on solvent signal. The ^{31}P-NMR chemical shifts (proton decoupled) are also quoted in p.p.m. using phosphoric acid as the external standard. *Mass spectrometry*: high resolution mass spectrometry (HRMS and electrospray ionization (ESI) mass spectra were acquired with a VG Analytical Finnigan ThermoQuest MAT 95 XL spectrometer. MALDI measurements (matrix: 9-aminoacridine (9AA)) were performed with a Bruker UltraflexXtreme spectrometer. *Infrared spectroscopy*: IR spectra were recorded on a Bruker Alpha P FT-IR at room temperature in the range of 400–4,000 cm^{-1}.

General procedure A: preparation of 4-acyloxybenzyl alcohols 9.

4-Hydroxybenzyl alcohol **10** (1.1 eq.) and triethylamine (1.0 eq.) in THF were cooled down to 0 °C. The corresponding acyl chloride (1.0 eq.) in THF was added dropwise and the mixture stirred for 1–2 h. The precipitate was removed by filtration and the solvent evaporated in vacuum. The residue was diluted with CH_2Cl_2 and washed once with saturated sodium bicarbonate solution and once with water. The organic layer was dried with Na_2SO_4 and the solvent was removed in vaccum. The crude material was purified using column chromatography to give compound **9**.

The syntheses and characterization of 4-(hydroxymethyl)phenylalkanoates **9a-k** were described previously[33].

4-(Hydroxymethyl)phenylmethylcarbonate 9l.

General procedure A with 4.0 g 4-hydroxybenzyl alcohol **10** (33 mmol, 1.1 eq.), 4.1 ml triethylamine (3.0 g, 30 mmol, 1.0 eq.) dissolved in 35 ml THF and dropwise addition of 2.3 ml methyl chloroformate (2.8 g, 30 mmol, 1.0 eq.) in 20 ml THF at 0 °C. Reaction time was 1.5 h at room temperature (rt). Column chromatography (petroleum ether 50–70/ethyl acetate 4:3 v/v). Yield: 4.6 g (25 mmol, 85%) colourless oil. TLC (petroleum ether 50–70/ethyl acetate 3:2 v/v): $R_f = 0.35$; ^{1}H-NMR (400 MHz, dimethylsulphoxide (DMSO)-d_6): $δ$ 7.39–7.31 (m, 2H), 7.20–7.13 (m, 2H), 5.22 (t, $J = 5.7$ Hz, 1H), 4.50 (d, $J = 5.8$ Hz, 2H), 3.82 (s, 3H); ^{13}C-NMR (101 MHz, DMSO-d_6): $δ$ 153.7, 149.5, 140.5, 127.5, 121.4, 62.3, 55.4; infrared red (IR): 3,375, 2,959, 2,873, 1,758, 1,254, 1,210 cm^{-1}; HRMS (ESI$^+$, m/z): [M + Na]$^+$ calcd. for $C_9H_{10}O_4$, 205.0471; found, 205.0337.

4-(Hydroxymethyl)phenyloctylcarbonate 9m.

General procedure A with 3.1 g 4-hydroxybenzyl alcohol **10** (25 mmol, 1.1 eq.), 3.1 ml triethylamine (2.3 g, 23 mmol, 1.0 eq.) dissolved in 35 ml THF and dropwise addition of 4.4 ml octyl chloroformate (4.4 g, 23 mmol, 1.0 eq.) in 20 ml THF at 0 °C. Reaction time was 1.5 h at rt. Column chromatography (petroleum ether 50–70/ethyl acetate 4:3 v/v). Yield: 5.3 g (19 mmol, 84%) colourless oil. TLC (PE/EE 3:1 v/v): $R_f = 0.45$; ^{1}H-NMR (300 MHz, DMSO-d_6): $δ$ 7.39–7.31 (m, 2H), 7.21–7.12 (m, 2H), 5.22 (t, $J = 5.7$ Hz, 1H), 4.49 (d, $J = 5.7$ Hz, 2H), 4.18 (t, $^3J_{HH} = 6.6$ Hz, 2H), 1.72–1.58 (m, 2H),

1.41–1.18 (m, 10H), 0.87 (t, $J = 6.7$ Hz, 3H); ^{13}C-NMR (75 MHz, DMSO-d_6): $δ$ 153.2, 149.5, 140.4, 127.5, 120.8, 68.5, 62.3, 31.2, 28.6, 28.0, 25.2, 22.1, 28.6, 14.0; IR: 3,377, 2,955, 2,856, 1,758, 1,247, 1,210 cm^{-1}; HRMS (ESI$^+$, m/z): [M + Na]$^+$ calcd. for $C_{16}H_{24}O_4$, 303.1567; found, 303.1568.

4-(Hydroxymethyl)phenyldodecylcarbonate 9n.

General procedure A with 4.1 g 4-hydroxybenzyl alcohol **10** (33 mmol, 1.1 eq.), 4.0 ml triethylamine (2.9 g, 30 mmol, 1.0 eq.) dissolved in 40 ml THF and dropwise addition of 8.1 ml dodecyl chloroformate (7.5 g, 30 mmol, 1.0 eq.) in 20 ml THF at 0 °C. Reaction time was 1.5 h at rt. Column chromatography (petroleum ether (PE) 50–70/ethyl acetate (EE) 4:1 v/v). Yield: 7.7 g (23 mmol, 76%) colourless oil. TLC (PE/EE 3:1 v/v): $R_f = 0.48$; ^{1}H-NMR (300 MHz, CDCl$_3$): $δ$ 7.42–7.33 (m, 2H), 7.21–7.12 (m, 2H), 4.68 (s, 2H), 4.24 (t, $J = 6.7$ Hz, 2H), 1.81–1.69 (m, 2H), 1.47–1.19 (m, 18H), 0.88 (t, $J = 6.7$ Hz, 3H); ^{13}C-NMR (75 MHz, CDCl$_3$): $δ$ 153.9, 150.7, 138.8, 128.2, 121.1, 69.2, 64.8, 32.1, 29.8, 29.7, 29.6, 29.5, 29.3, 28.7, 25.8, 22.8, 28.6, 14.3; IR: 3,355, 2,917, 2,848, 1,747, 1,273 cm^{-1}; HRMS (ESI$^+$, m/z): [M + Na]$^+$ calcd. for $C_{20}H_{34}O_4$, 359.2193; found, 359.2195.

4-((($tert$-Butyldimethylsilyl)oxy)methyl)phenol 11.

4-Hydroxybenzyl alcohol **10** (5.1 g; 41 mmol, 1.0 eq.), dissolved in 40 ml DMF, was converted with 6.8 g $tert$-butyldimethylsilyl chloride (45 mmol, 1.1 eq.) and 6.1 g imidazole (89 mmol, 2.2 eq.). After 17 h the solvent was removed by evaporation. The crude product was dissolved in CH_2Cl_2 and washed with 0.1 M HCl. The organic phase was dried over Na_2SO_4, filtered and the solvent was removed by evaporation. Column chromatography (petroleum ether 50–70/ethyl acetate 6:1 v/v). Yield: 7.9 g (33 mmol, 81%) colourless oil. TLC (PE/EE 4:1 v/v): $R_f = 0.34$; ^{1}H-NMR (300 MHz, DMSO-d_6): $δ$ 9.28 (s, 1H), 7.12–7.06 (m, 2H), 6.74–6.68 (m, 2H), 4.56 (s, 2H), 0.87 (s, 9H), 0.04 (s, 6H); ^{13}C-NMR (75 MHz, DMSO-d_6): $δ$ 139.2, 131.6, 127.5, 114.6, 64.0, 25.6, 17.6, -5.4; IR: 3,355, 2,954, 2,857, 1,707, 1,515 cm^{-1}; HRMS (ESI$^+$, m/z): [M + Na]$^+$ calcd. for $C_{13}H_{22}O_2Si$, 261.1287; found, 261.1285.

4-((($tert$-Butyldimethylsilyl)oxy)methyl)phenyl-(4-nitrophenyl)-carbonate 12.

Compound **11** (7.6 g; 32 mmol, 1.0 eq.) was dissolved in 100 ml CH_2Cl_2. 4-Nitrophenyl chloroformate (12.8 g, 64 mmol, 2.0 eq.) was added slowly to the reaction flask and the mixture was kept for 1 h at rt. Then, for consumption of the excess of chloroformate and for facilitation of purification, 7.5 ml tri(ethylene glycol) monomethyl ether (7.9 g, 48 mmol, 1.5 eq.) was added. After 20 min the solution was diluted with CH_2Cl_2 and washed with 1 M HCl. The organic phase was dried over Na_2SO_4, filtered and the solvent was removed by evaporation. Column chromatography (petroleum ether 50–70/ethyl acetate 6:1 v/v). Yield: 6.8 g (17 mmol, 53%) colourless solid. TLC (PE/EE 6:1 v/v): $R_f = 0.73$; ^{1}H-NMR (400 MHz, DMSO-d_6): $δ$ 8.38–8.33 (m, 2H), 7.73–7.67 (m, 2H), 7.43–7.36 (m, 4H), 4.73 (s, 2H), 0.91 (s, 9H), 0.09 (s, 6H); ^{13}C-NMR (101 MHz, DMSO-d_6): $δ$ 155.2, 150.7, 149.3, 145.4, 139.6, 127.2, 125.4, 122.7, 120.9, 64.0, 25.8, 18.0, -5.3; IR: 2,954, 2,929, 2,857, 1,768, 1,265 cm^{-1}; HRMS (ESI$^+$, m/z): [M + Na]$^+$ calcd. for $C_{20}H_{25}NO_6Si$, 426.1349; found, 426.1340.

$tert$-Butylmethyl(2-(methylamino)ethyl)-carbamate 13.

A flask containing 4.6 ml N,N-dimethylethylendiamine (3.7 g, 42 mmol, 3.8 eq.) in 40 ml CH_2Cl_2 was cooled to 0 °C. A solution of 2.4 g di-$tert$-butyl dicarbonate (11 mmol, 1.0 eq.) in 20 ml CH_2Cl_2 was added dropwise and, following the reaction mixture, was allowed to warm to rt. After 16 h, the solvent was removed in vacuum. The product was extracted with ethyl acetate/water (2:1 v/v) and washed with saturated aqueous $NaHCO_3$. The organic phase was dried over Na_2SO_4, filtered and the solvent was removed by evaporation. Yield: 1.6 g (8.6 mmol, 78%) yellowish oil. ^{1}H-NMR (600 MHz, CDCl$_3$): $δ$ 3.35–3.25 (m, 2H, rotamers), 2.85 (s, 3H), 2.70 (t, $J = 6.7$ Hz, 2H), 2.42 (s, 3H), 1.43 (s, 9H); ^{13}C-NMR (151 MHz, CDCl$_3$): $δ$ 156.1, 79.5, 49.8, 48.8 + 48.3 (rotamers), 36.4, 34.9 + 34.8 (rotamers), 28.6; IR: 2,974, 2,931, 1,687, 1,154 cm^{-1}; HRMS (ESI$^+$, m/z): [M + Na]$^+$ calcd. for $C_9H_{20}N_2O_2$, 211.1417; found, 211.1411.

4-(Hydroxymethyl)phenyl-methyl(2-(methylamino)ethyl)-carbamate 14.

At 0 °C to a stirred solution of 1.6 g compound **13** (8.6 mmol, 1.2 eq.), 1.9 ml diisopropylethylamine (1.4 g, 11 mmol, 1.6 eq.) and catalytic amounts of 4-dimethylaminophenol in 30 ml toluene 2.8 g activated carbonate **12** (7.0 mmol, 1.0 eq.) was added. The reaction mixture was allowed to warm to rt and stirred for 16 h. The solution was diluted with ethyl acetate and washed with 1 M HCl, followed by saturated aqueous $NaHCO_3$. The organic phase was dried over Na_2SO_4, filtered and the solvent was removed by evaporation. For deprotection the residue was redissolved in a mixture of CH_2Cl_2/trifluoroacetic acid (1:1 v/v). After 1 h the volatile components were removed by evaporation and the residue was co-evaporated twice with toluene. The crude material was purified by automatic RP-18 chromatography (water/acetonitrile gradient). Yield: 1.6 g (6.9 mmol, 98%) yellowish oil. TLC (CH_2Cl_2/MeOH 4:1 v/v): $R_f = 0.67$; ^{1}H-NMR (400 MHz, DMSO-d_6): $δ$ 8.72, 8.62 (br.s, 2H, rotamers), 7.34–7.28 (m, 2H), 7.14–7.07 (m, 2H), 4.48 (s, 2H), 3.69, 3.57 (t, $J = 6.0$ Hz, 2H, rotamers), 3.24–3.10 (m, 2H, rotamers), 3.05, 2.93 (s, 3H, rotamers), 2.68–2.57 (m, 3H, rotamers); ^{13}C-NMR (101 MHz, DMSO-d_6): $δ$ 154.7 + 153.8 (rotamers), 149.9, 139.7, 127.2, 121.7 + 121.4 (rotamers), 62.4,

46.3 + 46.0 (rotamers), 45.2, 34.6 + 34.4 (rotamers), 32.9 + 32.8 (rotamers); IR: 3,401, 2,975, 2,871, 1,671, 1,172 cm^{-1}; HRMS (ESI$^+$, m/z): [M + Na]$^+$ calcd. for C$_{12}$H$_{18}$N$_2$O$_3$, 239.1390; found, 239.1391.

General procedure B: preparation of bis-methylcarbamates 15.

4-(Hydroxymethyl)phenylcarbamate 14 (1.0 eq.) was dissolved in THF and cooled down to 0 °C. After addition of imidazole (1.3 eq.) and TMSCl (1.2 eq.) the mixture was stirred for 2 h. Triethylamine (3.1 eq.) and the corresponding alkyl chloroformate (3.0 eq.) were added. The reaction was kept for 1.5 h at rt and then diluted with 30 ml of 1 vol% concentrated (12 M) HCl in EtOH for desilylation. The solution was stirred for 1 h and the solvent evaporated in vacuum. The residue was dissolved in CH$_2$Cl$_2$ and washed with saturated aqueous NaHCO$_3$. The organic phase was dried over Na$_2$SO$_4$, filtered and the solvent was removed in vacuum. The crude material was purified using column chromatography.

n-Butyl-(4-(hydroxymethyl)phenyl)ethane-1,2-diylbis(methylcarbamate) 15o.

General procedure B with 2.1 g 14 (8.8 mmol, 1.0 eq.), 0.78 g imidazole (11 mmol, 1.3 eq.), 1.3 ml TMSCl (1.1 g, 11 mmol, 1.2 eq.), 3.8 ml triethylamine (2.8 g, 27 mmol, 3.1 eq.), 3.4 ml butyl chloroformate (3.6 g, 26 mmol, 3.0 eq.) dissolved in 15 ml THF. Column chromatography (petroleum ether 50–70/ethyl acetate 1:1 v/v). Yield: 1.8 g (19 mmol, 59%) colourless oil. TLC (CH$_2$Cl$_2$/MeOH 9:1 v/v): R$_f$ = 0.56; ^{1}H-NMR (400 MHz, DMSO-d$_6$): δ 7.34–7.27 (m, 2H), 7.04–6.97 (m, 2H), 5.17 (t, J = 5.6 Hz, 1H), 4.48 (d, J = 4.3 Hz, 2H), 4.02–3.91 (m, 2H), 3.57–3.40 (m, 4H, rotamers), 3.02, 2.90 (s, 3H, rotamers), 2.90–2.82 (m, 3H, rotamers), 1.60–1.44 (m, 2H, rotamers), 1.39–1.22 (m, 2H, rotamers), 0.87, 0.80 (t, J = 7.3 Hz, 3H, rotamers); ^{13}C-NMR (101 MHz, DMSO-d$_6$): δ 155.8, 153.9, 150.0, 139.3, 127.2, 121.4 + 121.3 (rotamers), 64.5 + 64.4 (rotamers), 62.4, 46.5 + 46.2 (rotamers), 46.0 + 45.6 (rotamers), 35.2 + 35.0 (rotamers), 34.7 + 34.5 (rotamers), 30.6 + 30.6 (rotamers), 18.6, 13.6; IR: 3,445, 2,958, 2,933, 1,694, 1,202 cm^{-1}; HRMS (ESI$^+$, m/z): [M + H]$^+$ calcd. for C$_{17}$H$_{26}$N$_2$O$_5$, 339.1914; found, 339.1918.

n-Octyl-(4-(hydroxymethyl)phenyl)ethane-1,2-diylbis(methylcarbamate) 15p.

General procedure B with 0.86 g 14 (3.6 mmol, 1.0 eq.), 0.32 g imidazole (4.7 mmol, 1.3 eq.), 0.55 ml TMSCl (0.47 g, 4.3 mmol, 1.2 eq.), 1.6 ml triethylamine (1.1 g, 11 mmol, 3.1 eq.), 2.1 ml octyl chloroformate (2.1 g, 11 mmol, 3.0 eq.) dissolved in 5 ml THF. Column chromatography (petroleum ether 50–70/ethyl acetate 1:1 v/v). Yield: 0.72 g (1.8 mmol, 51%) colourless oil. TLC (CH$_2$Cl$_2$/MeOH 9:1 v/v): R$_f$ = 0.60; ^{1}H-NMR (400 MHz, DMSO-d$_6$): δ 7.34–7.27 (m, 2H), 7.02–6.98 (m, 2H), 5.17 (t, J = 5.7 Hz, 1H), 4.47 (d, J = 5.6 Hz, 2H), 4.01–3.90 (m, 2H), 3.57–3.39 (m, 4H, rotamers), 3.02, 2.90 (s, 3H, rotamers), 2.90–2.81 (m, 3H, rotamers), 1.62–1.44 (m, 2H, rotamers), 1.36–1.12 (m, 10H), 0.89–0.80 (m, 3H, rotamers); ^{13}C-NMR (101 MHz, DMSO-d$_6$): δ 155.7, 154.0, 150.0, 139.2, 127.2, 121.4 + 121.3 (rotamers), 64.8 + 64.7 (rotamers), 62.4, 46.5 + 46.2 (rotamers), 45.9 + 45.5 (rotamers), 34.6 + 34.5 (rotamers), 31.2, 28.7, 28.6 + 28.6 (rotamers), 25.4, 22.0, 13.9; IR: 3,447, 2,926, 2,856, 1,698, 1,203 cm^{-1}; HRMS (ESI$^+$, m/z): [M + H]$^+$ calcd. for C$_{21}$H$_{34}$N$_2$O$_5$, 395.2540; found, 395.2540.

n-Dodecyl-(4-(hydroxymethyl)phenyl)ethane-1,2-diylbis(methylcarbamate) 15q.

General procedure B with 0.95 g 14 (4.0 mmol, 1.0 eq.), 0.35 g imidazole (5.2 mmol, 1.3 eq.), 0.61 ml TMSCl (0.52 g, 4.8 mmol, 1.2 eq.), 1.7 ml triethylamin (1.3 g, 12 mmol, 3.1 eq.), 3.2 ml dodecyl chloroformate (3.0 g, 12 mmol, 3.0 eq.) dissolved in 15 ml THF. Column chromatography (petroleum ether 50–70/ethyl acetate 1:1 v/v). Yield: 0.75 g (1.7 mmol, 42%) colourless oil. TLC (CH$_2$Cl$_2$/MeOH 9:1 v/v): R$_f$ = 0.65; ^{1}H-NMR (400 MHz, CDCl$_3$): δ (p.p.m.) = 7.36–7.31 (m, 2H), 7.10–7.05 (m, 2H), 4.64 (s, 2H), 4.12–4.02 (m, 2H), 3.63–3.44 (m, 4H), 3.15–2.89 (s, 6H, rotamers), 1.68–1.54 (m, 2H, rotamers), 1.43–1.13 (m, 10H), 0.88 (t, J = 6.8 Hz, 3H); ^{13}C-NMR (101 MHz, CDCl$_3$): δ 157.1, 154.9, 151.0, 138.3, 128.0, 121.9 + 121.3 (rotamers), 65.9 + 65.8 (rotamers), 64.9, 47.4 + 47.3 (rotamers), 47.1 + 46.4 (rotamers), 35.4 + 35.3 (rotamers), 32.1, 29.8, 29.7, 29.7, 29.5 + 29.5 (rotamers), 29.4, 29.2, 29.2, 26.1, 22.8, 14.2; IR: 3,459, 2,923, 1,699, 1,203 cm^{-1}; HRMS (ESI$^+$, m/z): [M + H]$^+$ calcd. for C$_{25}$H$_{42}$N$_2$O$_5$, 451.3172; found, 451.3167.

General procedure C: preparation of bis-(4-acyloxybenzyl)-N,N-diisopropylphosphoramidites 5.

Dichloro-N,N-diisopropylphosphoramidite (1.0 eq.) was dissolved in THF and cooled to 0 °C. Triethylamine (2.3 eq.) and the corresponding 4-acyloxybenzylalcohol 9 (2.1–2.2 eq.) in THF were added dropwise. The reaction mixture was kept at 0 °C for 18–24 h. After filtration, the solvent was removed by evaporation. The crude products were purified either using column chromatography or using preparative TLC (chromatotron).

The syntheses and characterization of Bis-(4-acyloxybenzyl)-N,N-diisopropyl-phosphoramidite 5a–k were described previously[33].

Bis-(4-methyloxycarbonyloxybenzyl)-N,N-diisopropylaminophosphoramidite 5l.

General procedure C with 0.74 g dichloro-N,N-diisopropylphosphoramidite (3.7 mmol, 1.0 eq.) dissolved in 15 ml THF, 1.2 ml triethylamine (0.85 g, 8.4 mmol, 2.3 eq.) and 1.5 g 4-(hydroxymethyl)phenylmethylcarbonate (8.2 mmol, 2.2 eq.) in 15 ml THF. The crude product was purified by preparative TLC (petroleum ether 50–70/ethyl acetate 4:1 v/v + 5% Et$_3$N). Yield: 1.5 g (3.0 mmol, 82%) colourless oil. TLC (PE/EE 1:1 v/v + 5% Et$_3$N): R$_f$ = 0.77; ^{1}H-NMR (300 MHz, DMSO-d$_6$): δ 7.42–7.34 (m, 4H), 7.18–7.07 (m, 4H), 4.78–4.61 (m, 4H), 3.82 (s, 6H), 3.72–3.57 (m, 2H), 1.16 (d, J = 6.8 Hz, 12H); ^{13}C-NMR (75 MHz, DMSO-d$_6$): δ 153.7, 149.9, 137.2 (d, J = 7.4 Hz), 128.0, 121.1, 64.1 (d, J = 18.1 Hz), 55.4, 42.6 (d, J = 12.5 Hz), 24.4 (d, J = 6.7 Hz); ^{31}P-NMR (202 MHz, DMSO-d$_6$): δ 147.5; IR: 2,965, 2,916, 1,760, 1,200, 1,126 cm^{-1}; HRMS (ESI$^+$, m/z): [M + H]$^+$ calcd. for C$_{24}$H$_{32}$NO$_8$P, 494.1938; found, 494.2276.

Bis-(4-octyloxycarbonyloxybenzyl)-N,N-diisopropylaminophosphoramidite 5m.

General procedure C with 0.76 g dichloro-N,N-diisopropylphosphoramidite (3.8 mmol, 1.0 eq.) dissolved in 15 ml THF, 1.3 ml triethylamine (0.88 g, 8.7 mmol, 2.3 eq.) and 2.3 g 4-(hydroxymethyl)phenyloctylcarbonate (8.3 mmol, 2.2 eq.) in 15 ml THF. The crude product was purified by preparative TLC (petroleum ether 50–70/ethyl acetate 6:1 v/v + 5% Et$_3$N). Yield: 2.2 g (3.2 mmol, 83%) colourless oil. TLC (PE/EE 6:1 v/v + 5% Et$_3$N): R$_f$ = 0.43; ^{1}H-NMR (300 MHz, CDCl$_3$): δ 7.39–7.31 (m, 4H), 7.20–7.13 (m, 4H), 4.80–4.62 (m, 4H), 4.24 (t, J = 6.7 Hz, 4H), 3.69 (dquint, J = 10.0 Hz, J = 6.8 Hz, 2H), 1.82–1.66 (m, 4H), 1.48–1.23 (m, 16H), 1.20 (d, J = 6.8 Hz, 12H), 0.89 (t, J = 6.7 Hz, 6H); ^{13}C-NMR (75 MHz, CDCl$_3$): δ 153.9, 150.4, 137.4 (d, J = 7.5 Hz), 128.2, 121.0, 69.1, 64.9 (d, J = 18.7 Hz), 42.2 (d, J = 12.6 Hz), 31.9, 29.3, 29.3, 25.8, 22.8, 28.7, 24.8 (d, J = 7.6 Hz), 14.2; ^{31}P-NMR (202 MHz, CDCl$_3$): δ 148.0; IR: 2,961, 2,926, 1,759, 1,215 cm^{-1}; HRMS (ESI$^+$, m/z): [M + H]$^+$ calcd. for C$_{38}$H$_{60}$NO$_8$P, 690.4129; found, 690.4086.

Bis-(4-dodecyloxycarbonyloxybenzyl)-N,N-diisopropylaminophosphoramidite 5n.

General procedure C with 0.50 g dichloro-N,N-diisopropylphosphoramidite (2.5 mmol, 1.0 eq.) dissolved in 14 ml THF, 0.80 ml triethylamine (0.58 g, 5.8 mmol, 2.3 eq.) and 1.8 g 4-(hydroxymethyl)phenyldodecylcarbonate (5.2 mmol, 2.1 eq.) in 10 ml THF. The crude product was purified using preparative TLC (petroleum ether 50–70/ethyl acetate 10:1 v/v + 5% Et$_3$N). Yield: 1.8 g (2.2 mmol, 88%) colourless solid. TLC (PE/EE 6:1 v/v + 5% Et$_3$N): R$_f$ = 0.53; ^{1}H-NMR (300 MHz, CDCl$_3$): δ 7.39–7.32 (m, 4H), 7.17–7.09 (m, 4H), 4.80–4.62 (m, 4H), 4.24 (t, J = 6.7 Hz, 4H), 3.75–3.57 (m, 2H), 1.80–1.67 (m, 4H), 1.47–1.23 (m, 36H), 1.20 (d, J = 6.8 Hz, 12H), 0.88 (t, J = 6.7 Hz, 6H); ^{13}C-NMR (75 MHz, CDCl$_3$): δ 153.9, 150.4, 137.4 (d, J = 7.8 Hz), 128.2, 121.0, 69.1, 64.9 (d, J = 18.2 Hz), 43.2 (d, J = 12.5 Hz), 32.1, 29.8, 29.7, 29.6, 29.5, 29.4, 25.8, 22.8, 28.6, 24.8 (d, J = 7.4 Hz), 14.3; ^{31}P-NMR (162 MHz, CDCl$_3$): δ 148.0; IR: 2,961, 2,923, 2,853, 1,760, 1,216 cm^{-1}; HRMS (ESI$^+$, m/z): [M + H]$^+$ calcd. for C$_{46}$H$_{76}$NO$_8$P, 802.5381; found, 802.5352.

Bis-(4-(butyl-ethan-1,2-diylbis(methylcarbamate))-oxybenzyl)-N,N-diisopropylaminophosphoramidite 5o.

General procedure C with 0.20 g dichloro-N,N-diisopropylphosphoramidite (0.99 mmol, 1.0 eq.) dissolved in 4 ml THF, 0.32 ml triethylamine (0.23 g, 2.3 mmol, 2.3 eq.) and 0.75 g compound 15o (2.2 mmol, 2.2 eq.) in 5 ml THF. The crude product was purified using column chromatography (petroleum ether 50–70/ethyl acetate 1:1 v/v + 5% Et$_3$N). Yield: 0.49 g (0.61 mmol, 62%) colourless oil. TLC (PE/EE 1:1 v/v + 5% Et$_3$N): R$_f$ = 0.30; ^{1}H-NMR (400 MHz, CDCl$_3$): δ 7.39–7.30 (m, 4H), 7.10–7.01 (m, 4H), 4.78–4.60 (m, 4H), 4.14–4.02 (m, 4H), 3.76–3.61 (m, 2H), 3.62–3.42 (m, 8H, rotamers), 3.15–2.89 (m, 12H, rotamers), 1.65–1.56 (m, 4H, rotamers), 1.46–1.30 (m, 4H, rotamers), 1.19 (d, J = 6.9 Hz, 12H), 0.93, 0.88 (t, J = 7.4 Hz, 6H, rotamers); ^{13}C-NMR (101 MHz, CDCl$_3$): δ 156.9, 154.8, 150.5, 136.5, 128.0, 121.6 + 121.6 (rotamers), 65.7 + 65.6 (rotamers), 65.0 (d, J = 18.1 Hz), 47.8 + 47.4 (rotamers), 47.0 + 46.4 (rotamers), 43.3 (d, J = 12.2 Hz), 35.4 + 35.3 (rotamers), 35.2 + 34.8 (rotamers), 31.3 + 31.3 (rotamers), 24.8 (d, J = 7.5 Hz), 19.3, 13.9; ^{31}P-NMR (162 MHz, CDCl$_3$): δ 147.4; IR: 2,962, 2,932, 2,871, 1,719, 1,695, 1,199 cm^{-1}; HRMS (ESI$^+$, m/z): [M + H]$^+$ calcd. for C$_{40}$H$_{64}$N$_5$O$_{10}$P, 806.4464; found, 806.4440.

Bis-(4-(octyl-ethan-1,2-diylbis(methylcarbamate))-oxybenzyl)-N,N-diisopropylaminophosphoramidite 5p.

General procedure C with 0.14 g dichloro-N,N-diisopropylphosphoramidite (0.71 mmol, 1.0 eq.) dissolved in 10 ml THF, 0.23 ml triethylamine (0.17 g, 1.6 mmol, 2.3 eq.) and 0.59 g compound 15p (1.5 mmol, 2.1 eq.) in 5 ml THF. The crude product was purified using column chromatography (petroleum ether 50–70/ethyl acetate 1:1 v/v + 5% Et$_3$N). Yield: 0.59 g (0.64 mmol, 90%) colourless oil. TLC (PE/EE 1:1 v/v + 5% Et$_3$N): R$_f$ = 0.41; ^{1}H-NMR (400 MHz, CDCl$_3$): δ 7.37–7.29 (m, 4H), 7.10–7.02 (m, 4H), 4.78–4.61 (m, 4H), 4.12–4.02 (m, 4H), 3.74–3.63 (m, 2H), 3.62–3.43 (m, 8H, rotamers), 3.15–2.89 (m, 12H, rotamers), 1.69–1.55 (m, 4H, rotamers), 1.40–1.19 (m, 36H, rotamers), 1.19 (d, J = 6.8 Hz, 12H), 0.87 (t, J = 6.8 Hz, 6H, H-n, rotamers); ^{13}C-NMR (101 MHz, CDCl$_3$): δ 156.6, 154.8, 150.7, 136.6, 128.0, 121.6 + 121.5 (rotamers), 65.9 + 65.8 (rotamers), 65.0 (d, J = 18.0 Hz), 47.8 + 47.4 (rotamers), 47.0 + 46.4 (rotamers), 43.2 (d, J = 12.6 Hz), 35.4 + 35.3 (rotamers), 35.1 + 34.8 (rotamers), 31.9, 29.4, 29.3, 29.2 + 29.2 (rotamers), 26.1, 24.8 (d, J = 7.2 Hz), 22.8, 14.2; ^{31}P-NMR (162 MHz, CDCl$_3$): δ 147.7; IR: 2,958, 2,927, 2,856, 1,722, 1,699, 1,202 cm^{-1}; HRMS (ESI$^+$, m/z): [M + H]$^+$ calcd. for C$_{48}$H$_{80}$N$_5$O$_{10}$P, 918.5716; found, 918.6124.

Bis-(4-(dodecyl-ethan-1,2-diylbis(methylcarbamate))-oxybenzyl)-*N,N*-di*iso*-propylaminophosphoramidite 5q. General procedure C with 0.15 g dichloro-*N,N*-di*iso*propylphosphoramidite (0.75 mmol, 1.0 eq.) dissolved in 3 ml THF, 0.24 ml triethylamine (0.17 g, 1.7 mmol, 2.3 eq.) and 0.71 g compound **15q** (1.6 mmol, 2.1 eq.) in 5 ml THF. The crude product was purified using column chromatography (petroleum ether 50–70/ethyl acetate 1:1 v/v + 5% Et_3N). Yield: 0.37 g (0.36 mmol, 48%) colourless oil. TLC (PE/EE 1:1 v/v + 5% Et_3N): $R_f = 0.50$; ^{1}H-NMR (600 MHz, $CDCl_3$): δ 7.36–7.30 (*m*, 4H), 7.08–7.03 (*m*, 4H), 4.76–4.62 (*m*, 4H), 4.11–4.02 (*m*, 4H), 3.73–3.62 (*m*, 2H), 3.61–3.42 (*m*, 8H, rotamers), 3.14–2.90 (*m*, 12H, rotamers), 1.67–1.56 (*m*, 4H, rotamers), 1.37–1.21 (*m*, 36H), 1.19 (*d*, $J = 6.8$ Hz, 12H), 0.87 (*t*, $J = 6.9$ Hz, 6H, rotamers); ^{13}C-NMR (101 MHz, $CDCl_3$): δ 157.0, 154.7, 150.7 + 150.6 (rotamers), 136.6, 128.0 + 128.0 (*d*, $J = 2.6$ Hz), 121.6 + 121.5 (rotamers), 65.9 + 65.8 (rotamers), 65.0 (*d*, $J = 18.3$ Hz), 47.4 + 47.3 (rotamers), 46.9 + 46.4 (rotamers), 43.2 (*d*, $J = 12.3$ Hz), 35.4, 35.3 (rotamers), 35.0 + 34.6 (rotamers), 32.0, 29.8, 29.7, 29.7, 29.7, 29.5, 29.4, 29.2 + 29.2 (rotamers), 26.1, 24.8 (*d*, $J = 7.4$ Hz), 22.8, 14.2; ^{31}P-NMR (162 MHz, $CDCl_3$): δ 147.3; IR: 2,923, 2,853, 1,721, 1,699, 1,200 cm^{-1}; HRMS (ESI$^+$, *m/z*): $[M+H]^+$ calcd. for $C_{48}H_{80}N_5O_{10}P$, 1030.6982; found, 1030.6968.

5-Chloro-*cyclo*Sal-3′-deoxy-2′,3′-didehydrothymidine monophosphate 7. To a suspension of 0.50 g d4T **1** (2.2 mmol, 1.0 eq.) in 8 ml, acetonitrile was added 0.53 ml di*iso*propylethlyamine (0.54 g, 3.1 mmol, 1.4 eq.) followed by 0.60 g 5-chlorosaligenylchlorophosphite **8** (2.7 mmol, 1.2 eq.). The reaction mixture was stirred for 3 h and subsequently cooled to 0 °C. By addition of a 5.5-M solution of 0.57 ml *tert*-butylhydroperoxide in *n*-decane (3.1 mmol, 1.4 eq.) the phosphite was oxidized for 20 min. The solvent was removed in vacuum. The residue was redissolved in CH_2Cl_2 and washed with 1 M ammonium acetate solution. The organic phase was dried over Na_2SO_4, filtered and the solvent was removed by evaporation. The crude product was purified using column chromatography (CH_2Cl_2/MeOH 9:1 v/v). Yield: 0.91 g (2.1 mmol, 97%) colourless foam as a mixture of two diastereomers. TLC (CH_2Cl_2/MeOH 9:1 v/v): $R_f = 0.29$; ^{1}H-NMR (500 MHz, $CDCl_3$): δ 8.92, 8.92 (br.s, 1H, diasteromers), 7.33–7.26 (*m*, 1H, ds), 7.20, 7.18 (*s*, 1H, ds), 7.12–7.07 (*m*, 1H, ds), 7.04–6.95 (*m*, 2H, ds), 6.40–6.32 (*m*, 1H, ds), 5.94, 5.94 (*d*, $J = 5.8$ Hz, ds), 5.43–5.18 (*m*, 2H, ds), 5.06–4.99 (*m*, 1H, ds), 4.47–4.30 (*m*, 2H, ds), 1.82, 1.73 (*s*, 3H, ds); ^{13}C-NMR (126 MHz, $CDCl_3$): δ 163.9 + 163.8 (diastereomers), 150.9 + 150.8 (ds), 148.7 + 148.7 (ds), 135.8 + 135.6 (ds), 132.8 + 132.7 (ds), 130.3 + 130.3 (ds), 130.1 + 130.1 (ds), 128.1 + 128.0 (ds), 125.7 + 125.6 (ds), 122.3 + 122.3 (ds), 120.1 + 120.0 (*d*, $J = 5.3$ Hz, ds), 111.5 + 111.4 (ds), 90.0 + 89.9 (ds), 84.6 + 84.5 (ds), 68.7 + 68.6 (ds), 68.1 + 67.9 (*d*, $J = 6.7$ Hz, ds), 12.4 + 12.3 (ds); ^{31}P-NMR (162 MHz, $CDCl_3$): δ −9.80, −9.87 (*s*, diastereomers); IR: 3,168, 3,050, 2,886, 1,684 cm^{-1}; HRMS (ESI$^+$, *m/z*): $[M+H]^+$ calcd. for $C_{17}H_{16}ClN_2O_7P$, 449.0276; found, 449.0287.

3′-Deoxy-2′,3′-didehydrothymidinediphosphate 6 (d4TDP, tetra-*n*-butylammonium salt). *cyclo*Sal-triester **7** (1.1 g; 2.5 mmol, 1.0 eq.) was dissolved in 10 ml DMF and added dropwise to a solution of 2.1 g mono-(tetra-*n*-butylammonium)-phosphate (6.2 mmol, 2.5 eq.) in 12 ml DMF. After 16 h, the solvent was removed in vacuum. The residue was extracted with ethyl acetate/water followed by freeze-drying of the aqueous phase. The crude product was purified using automatic RP-18 chromatography (water/acetonitrile gradient: 5–100%, 0–90 min, flow 1 ml min^{-1}). The purification had to repeat for complete removement of the excess of the monophosphate salt. Yield: 0.78 g (0.90 mmol, 36%, 2 × Bu_4N^+) colourless solid. TLC (*iso*propanol/NH_3/water 4:1:2.5 v/v/v): $R_f = 0.16$; ^{1}H-NMR (300 MHz, D_2O): δ 7.60 (*d*, $J = 1.3$ Hz, 1H), 6.93 (dt, $J = 3.3$ Hz, $J = 1.7$ Hz, 1H), 6.48 (dt, $J = 6.2$ Hz, $J = 1.8$ Hz, 1H), 5.91 (ddd, $J = 6.1$ Hz, $J = 2.4$ Hz, $J = 1.4$ Hz, 1H), 5.10–5.04 (*m*, 1H), 4.11 (dt, $J = 6.2$ Hz, $J = 3.3$ Hz, 2H), 3.25–3.05 (*m*, 16H), 1.86 (*d*, $J = 1.3$ Hz, 3H), 1.73–1.49 (*m*, 16H), 1.22 (sext, $J = 7.4$ Hz, 16H), 0.91 (*t*, $J = 7.3$ Hz, 24H); ^{13}C-NMR (75 MHz, D_2O): δ 166.8, 152.2, 138.1, 134.2, 125.1, 111.2, 89.8, 85.8 (*d*, $J = 8.5$ Hz), 66.2 (*d*, $J = 5.6$ Hz), 58.0, 23.0, 19.0, 12.8, 11.4; ^{31}P-NMR (162 MHz, D_2O): δ −8.32 (*d*, $J = 21.7$ Hz), −11.23 (*d*, $J = 21.7$ Hz); IR: 3,220, 1,645, 1,486 cm^{-1}; MALDI-MS (ESI$^+$, *m/z*): $[M\text{-}H]^-$ calcd. for $C_{10}H_{14}N_2O_{10}P_2$, 383.005; found, 382.928.

General procedure D: preparation of γ-bis(4-alkanoyloxybenzyl)-d4TTPs 3. D4TDP **6** (1.0 eq.) were once co-evaporated with DMF and then dissolved in acetonitrile. Phosphoramidites **5** (1.7–2.0 eq.) were added and the solvent removed in vacuum quantitatively. The residue was redissolved in a minimum of acetonitrile or in a mixture of acetonitrile/THF (1:1), and the reaction was started by addition of a 0.25-M solution of DCI in acetonitrile (1.2–1.4 eq.). After stirring for 1 min the reaction was cooled to −10 °C, and a 5.5 M solution of *t*-BuOOH in *n*-decane (2.1–2.2 eq.) was added for oxidation. The mixture was stirred for 20 min and the volatile components were removed in vacuum. The reaction was monitored with HPLC. If the conversion of d4TDP was not complete, the procedure was repeated as described above. The crude products were purified by automatic RP-18 flash chromatography followed by an ion exchange to the ammonium form with Dowex 50WX8 cation exchange resin and a second RP-18 chromatography (**3a–g,l–q**). For elution water/acetonitrile (5–100%, 0–40 min, flow 1 ml min^{-1}) or water/THF gradients (5–80%, 0–40 min, flow 1 ml min^{-1} were used. Product-containing fractions were pooled and the organic solvent evaporated. The remaining aqueous solutions were freeze-dried and the desired product obtained as colourless solids.

γ-Bis-(4-acetyloxybenzyl)-d4TTP 3a (ammonium salt). General procedure D with 86 mg d4TDP **6** (99 μmol, 1.0 eq.), 92 mg **5a** (0.20 mmol, 2.0 eq.), 0.55 ml 0.25 M solution of DCI in acetonitrile (0.14 mmol, 1.4 eq.), 40 μl 5.5 M solution of *t*-BuOOH in *n*-decane (0.22 mmol, 2.2 eq.) in 0.7 ml acetonitrile. The crude product was purified using automatic RP-18 chromatography (water/acetonitrile gradient). Yield: 46 mg (58 μmol, 59%) colourless solid. UV (HPLC): $\lambda_{max} = 265$ nm; HPLC: $t_R = 11.00$ min (method A); 8.75 min (method B); ^{1}H-NMR (400 MHz, CD_3OD): δ 7.67 (*d*, $J = 1.3$ Hz, 1H), 7.46–7.40 (*m*, 4H), 7.13–7.06 (*m*, 4H), 6.94 (dt, $J = 3.4$ Hz, $J = 1.8$ Hz, 1H), 6.48 (dt, $J = 5.9$ Hz, $J = 1.9$ Hz, 1H), 5.82 (dt, $J = 5.9$ Hz, $J = 1.9$ Hz, 1H), 5.18 (*d*, $J = 8.1$ Hz, 4H), 4.99–4.93 (*m*, 1H), 4.32–4.17 (*m*, 2H), 2.30 (*s*, 6H), 1.92 (*d*, $J = 1.3$ Hz, 3H); ^{13}C-NMR (101 MHz, CD_3OD): δ 171.1, 166.5, 152.8, 152.3, 138.7, 134.9, 134.9 (d, $J = 6.8$ Hz), 130.4 (*d*, $J = 2.7$ Hz), 127.3, 122.9, 112.0, 90.8, 87.1 (*d*, $J = 8.8$ Hz), 70.3 (*d*, $J = 6.1$ Hz), 67.6, 20.9, 12.5; ^{31}P-NMR (162 MHz, CD_3OD): δ −11.69 (*d*, $J = 19.4$ Hz), −13.11 (*d*, $J = 17.1$ Hz), −23.51 (*t*, $J = 17.8$ Hz); IR: 3,191, 2,988, 1,756, 1,687, 1,193 cm^{-1}; MALDI-MS (*m/z*): $[M\text{-}H]^-$ calcd. for $C_{28}H_{31}N_2O_{17}P_3$, 759.076; found, 759.131.

γ-Bis-(4-propanoyloxybenzyl)-d4TTP 3b (ammonium salt). General procedure D with 87 mg d4TDP **6** (0.10 mmol, 1.0 eq.), 93 mg **5b** (0.20 mmol, 2.0 eq.), 0.48 ml 0.25 M solution of DCI in acetonitrile (0.12 mmol, 1.2 eq.), 38 μl 5.5 M solution of *t*-BuOOH in *n*-decane (0.21 mmol, 2.1 eq.) in 0.5 ml acetonitrile. The crude product was purified using automatic RP-18 chromatography (water/acetonitrile gradient). Yield: 35 mg (43 μmol, 43%) colourless solid. UV (HPLC): $\lambda_{max} = 265$ nm; HPLC: $t_R = 11.83$ min (method A); 10.09 min (method B); ^{1}H-NMR (200 MHz, CD_3OD): δ 7.63 (*d*, $J = 1.3$ Hz, 1H), 7.44–7.32 (*m*, 4H), 7.09–6.99 (*m*, 4H), 6.90 (dt, $J = 3.4$ Hz, $J = 1.6$ Hz, 1H), 6.43 (dt, $J = 5.9$ Hz, $J = 1.7$ Hz, 1H), 5.77 (ddd, $J = 5.9$ Hz, $J = 2.4$ Hz, $J = 1.4$ Hz, 1H), 5.12 (*d*, $J = 8.0$ Hz, 4H), 4.94–4.89 (*m*, 1H), 4.31–4.08 (*m*, 2H), 2.58 (*q*, $J = 7.5$ Hz, 4H), 1.86 (*d*, $J = 1.3$ Hz, 3H), 1.20 (*t*, $J = 7.5$ Hz, 6H); ^{13}C-NMR (75 MHz, CD_3OD): δ 174.5, 166.5, 152.8, 152.4, 138.7, 135.7, 134.9 (*d*, $J = 7.6$ Hz), 130.4 (*d*, $J = 2.4$ Hz), 127.2, 122.9, 112.0, 90.8, 87.2 (*d*, $J = 9.0$ Hz), 70.3 (*d*, $J = 5.6$ Hz), 67.6 (*d*, $J = 6.3$ Hz), 28.3, 12.5, 9.3; ^{31}P-NMR (81 MHz, CD_3OD): δ −11.76 (*d*, $J = 19.4$ Hz), −13.19 (*d*, $J = 17.1$ Hz), −23.51 (*t*, $J = 18.4$ Hz); IR: 3,195, 2,987, 1,758, 1,691, 1,254 cm^{-1}; MALDI-MS (*m/z*): $[M\text{-}H]^-$ calcd. for $C_{30}H_{35}N_2O_{17}P_3$, 787.108; found, 787.275.

γ-Bis-(4-pentanoyloxybenzyl)-d4TTP 3c (ammonium salt). General procedure D with 90 mg d4TDP **6** (0.10 mmol, 1.0 eq.), 0.11 g **5c** (0.21 mmol, 2.0 eq.), 0.50 ml 0.25 M solution of DCI in acetonitrile (0.13 mmol, 1.2 eq.), 40 μl 5.5 M solution of *t*-BuOOH in *n*-decane (0.21 mmol, 2.1 eq.) in 0.5 ml acetonitrile. The crude product was purified using automatic RP-18 chromatography (water/acetonitrile gradient). Yield: 43 mg (49 μmol, 47%) colourless solid. UV (HPLC): $\lambda_{max} = 265$ nm; HPLC: $t_R = 13.61$ min (method A); ^{1}H-NMR (400 MHz, CD_3OD): δ 7.59 (*d*, $J = 1.5$ Hz, 1H), 7.38–7.32 (*m*, 4H), 7.04–6.97 (*m*, 4H), 6.87 (dt, $J = 3.4$ Hz, $J = 1.7$ Hz, 1H), 6.39 (dt, $J = 5.9$ Hz, $J = 1.8$ Hz, 1H), 5.77 (ddd, $J = 5.9$ Hz, $J = 2.4$ Hz, $J = 1.4$ Hz, 1H), 5.12 (*d*, $J = 8.1$ Hz, 4H), 4.94–4.84 (*m*, 1H), 4.26–4.08 (*m*, 2H), 2.57–2.50 (*m*, 4H), 1.84 (*d*, $J = 1.5$ Hz, 3H), 1.71–1.61 (*m*, 4H), 1.47–1.26 (*m*, 4H), 0.93 (*t*, $J = 7.4$ Hz, 6H); ^{13}C-NMR (101 MHz, CD_3OD): δ 173.8, 166.5, 152.7, 152.3, 138.6, 135.6, 134.8 (*d*, $J = 7.3$ Hz), 130.5 (*d*, $J = 3.1$ Hz), 127.2, 122.9, 112.0, 90.8, 87.1 (*d*, $J = 8.8$ Hz), 70.4 (dd, $J = 6.0$ Hz, $J = 2.1$ Hz), 67.9 (*d*, $J = 5.4$ Hz), 34.7, 28.1, 23.2, 14.1, 12.5; ^{31}P-NMR (81 MHz, CD_3OD): δ −11.76 (*d*, $J = 19.3$ Hz), −13.19 (*d*, $J = 17.1$ Hz), −23.51 (*t*, $J = 18.2$ Hz); IR: 3,183, 2,959, 1,755, 1,687, 1,219 cm^{-1}; MALDI-MS (*m/z*): $[M\text{-}H]^-$ calcd. for $C_{34}H_{43}N_2O_{17}P_3$, 843.170; found, 843.267.

γ-Bis-(4-heptanoyloxybenzyl)-d4TTP 3d (ammonium salt). General procedure D with 99 mg d4TDP **6** (0.11 mmol, 1.0 eq.), 0.14 g **5d** (0.23 mmol, 2.0 eq.), 0.55 ml 0.25 M solution of DCI in acetonitrile (0.14 mmol, 1.2 eq.), 44 μl 5.5 M solution of *t*-BuOOH in *n*-decane (0.24 mmol, 2.1 eq.) in 0.5 ml acetonitrile. The crude product was purified using automatic RP-18 chromatography (water/acetonitrile gradient). Yield: 41 mg (44 μmol, 40%) colourless solid. UV (HPLC): $\lambda_{max} = 265$ nm; HPLC: $t_R = 15.40$ min (method A); ^{1}H-NMR (400 MHz, CD_3OD): δ 7.68 (*d*, $J = 1.2$ Hz, 1H), 7.46–7.39 (*m*, 4H), 7.11–7.05 (*m*, 4H), 6.95 (dt, $J = 3.4$ Hz, $J = 1.6$ Hz, 1H), 6.48 (dt, $J = 6.1$ Hz, $J = 1.7$ Hz, 1H), 5.86–5.80 (*m*, 1H), 5.18 (*d*, $J = 8.2$ Hz, 4H), 5.01–4.94 (*m*, 1H), 4.34–4.16 (*m*, 2H), 2.60 (*t*, $J = 7.4$ Hz, 4H), 1.92 (*d*, $J = 1.2$ Hz, 3H), 1.76 (quint, $J = 7.4$ Hz, 4H), 1.51–1.34 (*m*, 12H), 0.96 (*t*, $J = 6.8$ Hz, 6H); ^{13}C-NMR (101 MHz, CD_3OD): δ 173.8, 166.5, 152.8, 152.3, 138.4, 135.8, 134.9 (*d*, $J = 7.8$ Hz), 130.5 (*d*, $J = 2.9$ Hz), 127.2, 122.9, 112.1, 90.8, 87.2 (*d*, $J = 8.9$ Hz), 70.4 (*d*, $J = 6.8$ Hz), 67.9 (*d*, $J = 4.9$ Hz), 35.0, 32.7, 29.9, 23.6, 25.9, 14.4, 12.5; ^{31}P-NMR (162 MHz, CD_3OD): δ −11.64 (br.s), −13.08 (*d*, $J = 17.5$ Hz), −23.47 (br.s); IR: 3,190, 2,928, 1,756, 1,689, 1,250 cm^{-1}; MALDI-MS (*m/z*): $[M\text{-}H]^-$ calcd. for $C_{38}H_{51}N_2O_{17}P_3$, 899.233; found, 899.229.

γ-Bis-(4-nonanoyloxybenzyl)-d4TTP 3e (ammonium salt). General procedure D with 0.15 g d4TDP **6** (0.17 mmol, 1.0 eq.), 0.22 g **5e** (0.34 mmol, 2.0 eq.), 0.88 ml 0.25 M solution of DCI in acetonitrile (0.22 mmol, 1.3 eq.), 68 μl 5.5 M solution of *t*-BuOOH in *n*-decane (0.37 mmol, 2.2 eq.) in 3 ml acetonitrile. The crude product was purified using automatic RP-18 chromatography (water/acetonitrile gradient). Yield: 70 mg (71 µmol, 42%) beige solid. UV (HPLC): λ_{max} = 265 nm; HPLC: t_R = 17.31 min (method A); ^{1}H-NMR (300 MHz, CD_3OD): δ 7.65 (*d*, *J* = 1.3 Hz, 1H), 7.42–7.35 (*m*, 4H), 7.07–7.00 (*m*, 4H), 6.92 (dt, *J* = 3.5 Hz, *J* = 1.6 Hz, 1H), 6.45 (dt, *J* = 6.1 Hz, *J* = 1.7 Hz, 1H), 5.79 (ddd, *J* = 6.0 Hz, *J* = 2.4 Hz, *J* = 1.7 Hz, 1H), 5.14 (*d*, *J* = 8.1 Hz, 4H), 4.96–4.90 (*m*, 1H), 4.31–4.13 (*m*, 2H), 2.57 (*t*, *J* = 7.4 Hz, 4H), 1.88 (*d*, *J* = 1.3 Hz, 3H), 1.72 (quint, *J* = 7.3 Hz, 4H), 1.49–1.24 (*m*, 20H), 0.96–0.85 (*m*, 6H); ^{13}C-NMR (75 MHz, CD_3OD): δ 173.4, 166.5, 152.9, 152.3, 138.4, 135.8, 134.5, 130.2 (*d*, *J* = 2.4 Hz), 126.9, 122.6, 111.9, 90.5, 86.8 (*d*, *J* = 9.5 Hz), 70.1 (*d*, *J* = 5.2 Hz), 67.6 (*d*, *J* = 5.6 Hz), 34.7, 32.7, 30.1, 30.1, 29.9, 25.7, 23.5, 14.2, 12.2; ^{31}P-NMR (162 MHz, CD_3OD): δ − 11.83 (*d*, *J* = 20.1 Hz), − 3.28 (*d*, *J* = 17.5 Hz), − 23.82 (*t*, *J* = 18.8 Hz); IR: 3,192, 3,062, 2,926, 1,757, 1,694, 1,250 cm^{-1}; MALDI-MS (*m/z*): [M-H]$^-$ calcd. for $C_{42}H_{59}N_2O_{17}P_3$, 955.295; found, 955.296.

γ-Bis-(4-decanoyloxybenzyl)-d4TTP 3f. General procedure D with 71 mg d4TDP **6** (82 µmol, 1.0 eq.), 0.11 g **5f** (0.16 mmol, 2.0 eq.), 0.40 ml 0.25 M solution of DCI in acetonitrile (0.10 mmol, 1.2 eq.), 32 µl 5.5 M solution of *t*-BuOOH in *n*-decane (0.18 mmol, 2.2 eq.) in 1.2 ml acetonitrile. The crude product was purified using automatic RP-18 chromatography (water/acetonitrile gradient). Yield: 23 mg (21 µmol, 26%) colourless solid (counterions: 0.2 × Bu_4N^+, 1.8 × NH_4^+). UV (HPLC): λ_{max} = 265 nm; HPLC: t_R = 18.06 min (method A); ^{1}H-NMR (400 MHz, CD_3OD): δ 7.69 (*d*, *J* = 1.4 Hz, 1H), 7.46–7.39 (*m*, 4H), 7.12–7.05 (*m*, 4H), 6.96 (dt, *J* = 3.4 Hz, *J* = 1.6 Hz, 1H), 6.50 (dt, *J* = 6.0 Hz, *J* = 1.7 Hz, 1H), 5.86–5.81 (*m*, 1H), 5.19 (*d*, *J* = 8.1 Hz, 4H), 5.00–4.95 (*m*, 1H), 4.35–4.17 (*m*, 2H), 3.30–3.23 (*m*, 1.5H), 2.61 (*t*, *J* = 7.4 Hz, 4H), 1.93 (*d*, *J* = 1.4 Hz, 3H), 1.76 (quint, *J* = 7.3 Hz, 4H), 1.73–1.64 (*m*, 1.5H), 1.52–1.28 (*m*, 25.5H), 1.06 (*t*, *J* = 7.4 Hz, 2.3H), 0.97–0.90 (*m*, 6H); ^{13}C-NMR (101 MHz, CD_3OD): δ 173.7, 166.7, 152.6, 152.6, 138.7, 135.8, 135.0 (*d*, *J* = 7.8 Hz), 130.5 (*d*, *J* = 2.9 Hz), 127.1, 122.9, 112.1, 90.9, 87.2 (*d*, *J* = 9.7 Hz), 70.4 (dd, *J* = 5.6 Hz, *J* = 1.7 Hz), 67.9 (*d*, *J* = 4.8 Hz), 59.5, 35.0, 33.0, 30.6, 30.4, 30.4, 30.2, 26.0, 23.7, 24.8, 19.4, 14.4, 13.9, 12.5; ^{31}P-NMR (162 MHz, CD_3OD): δ − 11.80 (*d*, *J* = 19.9 Hz), − 13.07 (*d*, *J* = 17.5 Hz), − 23.82 (br.s); IR: 3,174, 2,925, 1,758, 1,690, 1,249 cm^{-1}; MALDI-MS (*m/z*): [M-H]$^-$ calcd. for $C_{44}H_{63}N_2O_{17}P_3$, 983.327; found, 983.512.

γ-Bis-(4-dodecanoyloxybenzyl)-d4TTP 3g. General procedure D with 74 mg d4TDP **6** (85 µmol, 1.0 eq.), 0.13 g **5g** (0.17 mmol, 2.0 eq.), 0.41 ml 0.25 M solution of DCI in acetonitrile (0.11 mmol, 1.2 eq.), 33 µl 5.5 M solution of *t*-BuOOH in *n*-decane (0.18 mmol, 2.1 eq.) in 1.2 ml acetonitrile and 1.0 ml THF. The crude product was purified by automatic RP-18 chromatography (water/acetonitrile gradient). Yield: 44 mg (37 µmol, 44%) colourless solid (counterions: 1.6 × Bu_4N^+, 0.4 × NH_4^+). UV (HPLC): λ_{max} = 265 nm; HPLC: t_R = 20.15 min (method A); ^{1}H-NMR (400 MHz, CD_3OD): δ 7.74 (*d*, *J* = 1.5 Hz, 1H), 7.47–7.39 (*m*, 4H), 7.10–7.03 (*m*, 4H), 6.96 (dt, *J* = 3.4 Hz, *J* = 1.6 Hz, 1H), 6.56 (dt, *J* = 6.0 Hz, *J* = 1.8 Hz, 1H), 5.83–5.78 (*m*, 1H), 5.22 (dd, *J* = 8.0 Hz, *J* = 2.0 Hz, 4H), 5.01–4.95 (*m*, 1H), 4.43–4.19 (*m*, 2H), 3.31–3.19 (*m*, 12.8H), 2.61 (*t*, *J* = 7.4 Hz, 4H), 1.93 (*d*, *J* = 1.5 Hz, 3H), 1.76 (quint, *J* = 6.7 Hz, 4H), 1.73–1.63 (*m*, 12.8H), 1.44 (sext, *J* = 7.4 Hz, 12.8H), 1.51–1.28 (*m*, 32H), 1.05 (*t*, *J* = 7.4 Hz, 19.2H), 0.98–0.89 (*m*, 6H); ^{13}C-NMR (101 MHz, CD_3OD): δ 173.7, 166.5, 152.8, 152.2, 138.8, 136.2, 135.2 (*d*, *J* = 7.8 Hz), 130.5 (*d*, *J* = 2.8 Hz), 126.9, 122.8, 112.1, 90.8, 87.4 (*d*, *J* = 6.3 Hz), 70.4 (*d*, *J* = 5.7 Hz), 67.8, 59.4, 35.0, 33.1, 30.7, 30.7, 30.6, 30.4, 30.4, 30.2, 26.0, 23.7, 24.8, 20.7, 14.5, 14.0, 12.5; ^{31}P-NMR (162 MHz, CD_3OD): δ − 11.91 (br.s), − 13.28 (*d*, *J* = 17.6 Hz), − 3.99 (br.s); IR: 3,203, 2,925, 1,757, 1,690, 1,262 cm^{-1}; MALDI-MS (*m/z*): [M-H]$^-$ calcd. for $C_{48}H_{69}N_2O_{17}P_3$, 1039.389; found, 1039.561.

γ-Bis-(4-tetradecanoyloxybenzyl)-d4TTP 3h. General procedure D with 48 mg d4TDP **6** (53 µmol, 1.0 eq.), 85 mg **5h** (0.11 mmol, 2.0 eq.), 0.28 ml 0.25 M solution of DCI in acetonitrile (69 µmol, 1.3 eq.), 21 µl 5.5 M solution of *t*-BuOOH in *n*-decane (0.12 mmol, 2.2 eq.) in 0.5 ml acetonitrile and 0.7 ml THF. The reaction was restarted once. The crude product was purified using automatic RP-18 chromatography (water/THF gradient). Yield: 72 mg (37 µmol, 70% (exclusive contamination)) colourless solid (counterions: 1.0 × Bu_4N^+, 1.0 × $DIPAH^+$), contaminated with Bu_4N^+ and diisopropylammonium salts. UV (HPLC): λ_{max} = 265 nm; HPLC: t_R = 22.22 min (method A); ^{1}H-NMR (300 MHz, THF-d_8): δ 10.10 (*s*, 1H), 7.88 (*d*, *J* = 1.2 Hz, 1H), 7.53–7.44 (*m*, 4H), 7.04–6.96 (*m*, 4H), 6.91 (dt, *J* = 3.3 Hz, *J* = 1.6 Hz, 1H), 6.62 (dt, *J* = 5.9 Hz, *J* = 1.7 Hz, 1H), 5.61–5.56 (*m*, 1H), 5.26–5.17 (*m*, 4H), 4.85–4.78 (*m*, 1H), 4.44–4.31 (*m*, 1H), 4.14–4.01 (*m*, 1H), 3.50–3.39 (*m*, 8H), 3.33–2.85 (*m*, 2H), 2.52 (*t*, *J* = 7.5 Hz, 4H), 1.91 (*d*, *J* = 1.2 Hz, 3H), 1.77–1.59 (*m*, 12H), 1.50–1.23 (*m*, 60H), 0.94 (*t*, *J* = 7.4 Hz, 12H), 0.89 (*t*, *J* = 6.8 Hz, 6H); ^{13}C-NMR (75 MHz, THF-d_8): δ 172.2, 164.9, 152.1, 151.8, 138.2, 136.9, 136.1 (*d*, *J* = 8.5 Hz), 130.1 (*d*, *J* = 1.6 Hz), 126.2, 122.3, 111.3, 90.1, 87.8 (*d*, *J* = 8.5 Hz), 69.2 (*d*, *J* = 5.4 Hz), 67.2, 59.3, 47.2, 34.9, 33.1, 30.8, 30.8, 30.8, 30.8, 30.7, 30.5, 30.5, 30.2, 26.0, 25.0, 23.8, 20.7, 19.9, 14.6, 14.4, 12.8; ^{31}P-NMR (162 MHz, THF-d_8): δ − 14.16 (*d*, *J* = 20.8 Hz), − 14.65 (*d*, *J* = 17.8 Hz), − 23.82 (*t*, *J* = 19.1 Hz); IR: 3,400, 2,924, 1,757, 1,689, 1,263 cm^{-1}; MALDI-MS (*m/z*): [M-H]$^-$ calcd. for $C_{52}H_{79}N_2O_{17}P_3$, 1095.452; found, 1095.503.

γ-Bis-(4-hexadecanoyloxybenzyl)-d4TTP 3i. General procedure D with 90 mg d4TDP **6** (0.10 mmol, 1.0 eq.), 0.18 g **5i** (0.21 mmol, 2.0 eq.), 0.50 ml 0.25 M solution of DCI in acetonitrile (0.13 mmol, 1.3 eq.), 42 µl 5.5 M solution of *t*-BuOOH in *n*-decane (0.23 mmol, 2.2 eq.) in 0.3 ml acetonitrile and 0.9 ml THF. The reaction was restarted once. The crude product was purified using automatic RP-18 chromatography (water/THF gradient). Yield: 96 mg (64 µmol, 62%) colourless solid (counterions: 1.0 × Bu_4N^+, 1.0 × $DIPAH^+$). UV (HPLC): λ_{max} = 265 nm; HPLC: t_R = 23.28 min (method A); ^{1}H-NMR (500 MHz, THF-d_8): δ 10.22 (*s*, 1H), 7.88 (*d*, *J* = 1.3 Hz, 1H), 7.48–7.42 (*m*, 4H), 7.05–6.99 (*m*, 4H), 6.92 (dt, *J* = 3.4 Hz, *J* = 1.6 Hz, 1H), 6.55 (dt, *J* = 5.8 Hz, *J* = 1.6 Hz, 1H), 5.67–5.61 (*m*, 1H), 5.22–5.13 (*m*, 4H), 4.87–4.82 (*m*, 1H), 4.38–4.29 (*m*, 1H), 4.15–4.07 (*m*, 1H), 3.43–3.27 (*m*, 8H), 3.31–3.15 (*m*, 2H), 2.53 (*t*, *J* = 7.5 Hz, 4H), 1.90 (*d*, *J* = 1.0 Hz, 3H), 1.74–1.62 (*m*, 12H), 1.48–1.20 (*m*, 68H), 0.95 (*t*, *J* = 7.2 Hz, 12H), 0.89 (*t*, *J* = 6.8 Hzm, 6H); ^{13}C-NMR (75 MHz, THF-d_8): δ 172.1, 164.9, 152.1, 152.0, 137.8, 136.3, 135.5 (*d*, *J* = 8.6 Hz), 130.1, 126.6, 122.5, 111.3, 90.2, 87.3 (*d*, *J* = 7.7 Hz), 69.4 (*d*, *J* = 7.2 Hz), 67.0, 59.3, 47.4, 34.9, 33.0, 30.8, 30.8, 30.8, 30.8, 30.7, 30.5, 30.5, 30.2, 26.1, 24.8, 23.6, 20.7, 19.8, 14.6, 14.4, 12.8; ^{31}P-NMR (202 MHz, THF-d_8): δ − 12.56 (*d*, *J* = 19.6 Hz), − 13.38 (*d*, *J* = 17.5 Hz), − 24.17 (*t*, *J* = 18.5 Hz); IR: 2,987, 2,916, 1,756, 1,691, 1,251 cm^{-1}; MALDI-MS (*m/z*): [M-H]$^-$ calcd. for $C_{56}H_{85}N_2O_{17}P_3$, 1151.515; found, 1151.663.

γ-Bis-(4-octadecanoyloxybenzyl)-d4TTP 3j. General procedure D with 87 mg d4TDP **6** (0.10 mmol, 1.0 eq.), 0.19 g **5j** (0.20 mmol, 2.0 eq.), 0.52 ml 0.25 M solution of DCI in acetonitrile (0.13 mmol, 1.3 eq.), 38 µl 5.5 M solution of *t*-BuOOH in *n*-decane (0.21 mmol, 2.1 eq.) in 0.3 ml acetonitrile and 0.9 ml THF. The reaction was restarted once. The crude product was purified using automatic RP-18 chromatography (water/THF gradient). Yield: 69 mg (44 µmol, 44%) colourless solid (counterions: 1.0 × Bu_4N^+, 1.0 × $DIPAH^+$).

UV (HPLC): λ_{max} = 265 nm; HPLC: t_R = 19.45 min (method C); ^{1}H-NMR (300 MHz, THF-d_8): δ 10.16 (*s*, 1H), 7.84 (*d*, *J* = 1.4 Hz, 1H), 7.50–7.41 (*m*, 4H), 7.05–6.96 (*m*, 4H), 6.91 (dt, *J* = 3.3 Hz, *J* = 1.5 Hz, 1H), 6.62–6.53 (*m*, 1H), 5.65–5.57 (*m*, 1H), 5.24–5.13 (*m*, 4H), 4.89–4.79 (*m*, 1H), 4.43–4.30 (*m*, 1H), 4.17–4.04 (*m*, 1H), 3.51–3.28 (*m*, 8H), 3.30–3.09 (*m*, 2H), 2.51 (*t*, *J* = 7.4 Hz, 4H), 1.91 (*d*, *J* = 0.7 Hz, 3H), 1.77–1.60 (*m*, 13H), 1.49–1.19 (*m*, 76H), 1.00–0.82 (*m*, 18H); ^{13}C-NMR (75 MHz, THF-d_8): δ 172.1, 164.8, 152.1, 151.9, 138.0, 136.6, 135.8 (*d*, *J* = 7.8 Hz), 130.1, 126.5, 122.4, 111.3, 90.2, 87.5 (*d*, *J* = 8.4 Hz), 69.2 (*d*, *J* = 5.3 Hz), 67.1, 59.3, 47.2, 34.9, 33.1, 30.8, 30.8, 30.7, 30.5, 30.5, 30.3, 26.0, 24.9, 23.8, 20.8, 19.8, 14.6, 14.4, 12.8; ^{31}P-NMR (162 MHz, THF-d_8): δ − 12.74 (*d*, *J* = 19.2 Hz), − 12.83 (*d*, *J* = 18.3 Hz), − 23.46 (*t*, *J* = 18.7 Hz); IR: 2,959, 2,916, 1,756, 1,688, 1,252 cm^{-1}; MALDI-MS (*m/z*): [M-H]$^-$ calcd. for $C_{60}H_{95}N_2O_{17}P_3$, 1207.577; found, 1207.670.

γ-Bis(4-(*Z*)-octadec-9-enoyloxybenzyl)-d4TTP 3k. General procedure D with 96 mg d4TDP **6** (0.11 mmol, 1.0 eq.), 0.20 g **5k** (0.22 mmol, 2.0 eq.), 0.53 ml 0.25 M solution of DCI in acetonitrile (0.13 mmol, 1.2 eq.), 42 µl 5.5 M solution of *t*-BuOOH in *n*-decane (0.23 mmol, 2.1 eq.) in 0.3 ml acetonitrile and 0.9 ml THF. The reaction was restarted once. The crude product was purified using automatic RP-18 chromatography (water/THF gradient). Yield: 99 mg (64 µmol, 58%) colourless solid (counterions: 1.0 × Bu_4N^+, 1.0 × $DIPAH^+$). UV (HPLC): λ_{max} = 265 nm; HPLC: t_R = 22.92 min (method A); ^{1}H-NMR (300 MHz, THF-d_8): δ 10.20 (*s*, 1H), 7.86 (*s*, 1H), 7.52–7.42 (*m*, 4H), 7.07–6.96 (*m*, 4H), 6.94–6.88 (*m*, 1H), 6.67–6.53 (*m*, 1H), 5.68–5.54 (*m*, 1H), 5.44–5.27 (*m*, 4H), 5.24–5.14 (*m*, 4H), 4.90–4.79 (*m*, 1H), 4.43–4.31 (*m*, 1H), 4.18–4.03 (*m*, 1H), 3.57–3.25 (*m*, 8H), 3.32–3.02 (*m*, 2H), 2.52 (*t*, *J* = 7.5 Hz, 4H), 2.14–1.95 (*m*, 8H), 1.91 (*s*, 3H), 1.80–1.58 (*m*, 12H), 1.54–1.16 (*m*, 60H), 1.05–0.75 (*m*, 18H); ^{13}C-NMR (75 MHz, THF-d_8): δ 172.1, 164.8, 152.1, 151.9, 138.0, 137.3, 135.9 (*d*, *J* = 7.9 Hz), 130.7, 130.7, 130.1 (*d*, *J* = 1.5 Hz), 126.3, 122.4, 111.2, 90.2, 87.6 (*d*, *J* = 8.8 Hz), 69.1, 67.1, 59.3, 47.2, 34.9, 33.0, 30.9, 30.7, 30.5, 30.4, 30.3, 30.2, 28.2, 28.2, 25.9, 25.0, 23.7, 20.8, 19.8, 14.7, 14.4, 12.8; ^{31}P-NMR (162 MHz, THF-d_8): δ − 14.44 (*d*, *J* = 19.0 Hz), − 14.94 (*d*, *J* = 18.0 Hz), − 25.55 (*t*, *J* = 18.5 Hz); IR: 3,358, 2,965, 2,924, 1,757, 1,689, 1,262 cm^{-1}; MALDI-MS (*m/z*): [M-H]$^-$ calcd. for $C_{60}H_{91}N_2O_{17}P_3$, 1203.557; found, 1203.546.

γ-Bis-(4-methyloxycarbonyloxybenzyl)-d4TTP 3l (ammonium salt). General procedure D with 99 mg d4TDP **6** (0.11 mmol, 1.0 eq.), 0.11 g **5l** (0.23 mmol, 2.0 eq.), 0.59 ml 0.25 M solution of DCI in acetonitrile (0.15 mmol, 1.3 eq.), 46 µl 5.5 M solution of *t*-BuOOH in *n*-decane (0.25 mmol, 2.2 eq.) in 0.7 ml acetonitrile. The crude product was purified using automatic RP-18 chromatography (water/acetonitrile gradient). Yield: 49 mg (59 µmol, 52%) colourless solid. UV (HPLC): λ_{max} = 265 nm; HPLC: t_R = 11.28 min (method A); 9.17 min (method B); ^{1}H-NMR (400 MHz, CD_3OD): δ 7.68 (*d*, *J* = 1.2 Hz, 1H), 7.43–7.38 (*m*, 4H), 7.16–7.11 (*m*, 4H), 6.92 (dt, *J* = 3.4 Hz, *J* = 1.8 Hz, 1H), 6.47 (dt, *J* = 6.0 Hz, *J* = 1.7 Hz, 1H), 5.82 (ddd, *J* = 6.1 Hz, *J* = 2.5 Hz, *J* = 1.4 Hz, 1H), 5.18 (*d*, *J* = 8.0 Hz, 4H), 4.96–4.90 (*m*, 1H), 4.31–4.15 (*m*, 2H), 3.86 (*s*, 6H), 1.88 (*d*, *J* = 1.2 Hz, 3H); ^{13}C-NMR (101 MHz, CD_3OD): δ 166.7, 155.7, 152.8, 152.7, 138.7, 135.8, 135.4 (*d*, *J* = 7.6 Hz), 130.5 (*d*, *J* = 3.5 Hz), 127.1, 122.3, 112.1, 90.8, 87.3 (*d*, *J* = 9.5 Hz), 70.3 (dd, *J* = 5.8 Hz, *J* = 2.1 Hz), 67.6 (*d*, *J* = 5.9 Hz), 56.0, 12.5; ^{31}P-NMR (162 MHz, CD_3OD): δ − 11.79 (*d*, *J* = 19.8 Hz), − 13.23 (*d*, *J* = 17.6 Hz), − 23.71

(*t*, $J = 18.5$ Hz); IR: 3,191, 3,050, 1,764, 1,692, 1,263 cm^{-1}; MALDI-MS (*m/z*): [M-H]$^-$ calcd. for $C_{28}H_{31}N_2O_{19}P_3$, 791.066; found, 791.003.

γ-Bis-(4-octyloxycarbonyloxybenzyl)-d4TTP 3m. General procedure D with 0.11 g d4TDP **6** (0.13 mmol, 1.0 eq.), 0.18 g **5m** (0.26 mmol, 2.0 eq.), 0.68 ml 0.25 M solution of DCI in acetonitrile (0.17 mmol, 1.3 eq.), 53 µl 5.5 M solution of *t*-BuOOH in *n*-decane (0.29 mmol, 2.2 eq.) in 0.7 ml acetonitrile. The crude product was purified using automatic RP-18 chromatography (water/acetonitrile gradient). Yield: 75 mg (69 µmol, 52%) colourless solid (counterions: 0.3 × Bu_4N^+, 1.7 × NH_4^+). UV (HPLC): $\lambda_{max} = 265$ nm; HPLC: $t_R = 16.72$ min (method A); ^{1}H-NMR (400 MHz, CD_3OD): δ 7.65 (d, $J = 1.1$ Hz, 1H), 7.43MALDI-MS (*m/z*): [M-H]$^-$ calcd7.36 (*m*, 4H), 7.17MALDI-MS (*m/z*): [M-H]$^-$ calcd7.09 (*m*, 4H), 6.91 (dt, $J = 3.5$ Hz, $J = 1.9$ Hz, 1H), 6.44 (dt, $J = 6.0$ Hz, $J = 1.8$ Hz, 1H), 5.82 (ddd, $J = 6.0$ Hz, $J = 2.4$ Hz, $J = 1.3$ Hz, 1H), 5.14 (d, $J = 8.2$ Hz, 4H), 4.96–4.90 (*m*, 1H), 4.29–4.13 (*m*, 2H), 4.22 (*t*, $J = 6.6$ Hz, 4H), 3.25–3.15 (*m*, 2.5H), 1.88 (d, $J = 1.1$ Hz, 3H), 1.77–1.64 (*m*, 4H), 1.67–1.57 (*m*, 2.5H), 1.47–1.22 (*m*, 22.5H), 1.00 (*t*, $J = 7.3$ Hz, 3.8H), 0.90 (*t*, $J = 6.7$ Hz, 6H); ^{13}C-NMR (101 MHz, CD_3OD): δ 166.5, 155.1, 152.7, 152.7, 138.6, 135.7, 135.2 (d, $J = 7.6$ Hz), 130.5 (d, $J = 2.3$ Hz), 127.2, 122.3, 112.0, 90.8, 87.3 (d, $J = 9.5$ Hz), 70.3 (dd, $J = 5.4$ Hz, $J = 1.4$ Hz), 70.0, 67.8 (d, $J = 5.6$ Hz), 59.4, 32.9, 30.3, 30.3, 29.7, 26.8, 24.7, 23.7, 20.7, 14.5, 14.0, 12.5; ^{31}P-NMR (162 MHz, CD_3OD): δ −11.68 (d, $J = 19.3$ Hz), −13.15 (d, $J = 16.1$ Hz), −23.53 (*t*, $J = 18.0$ Hz); IR: 3,198, 2,926, 1,760, 1,690, 1,250 cm^{-1}; MALDI-MS (*m/z*): [M-H]$^-$ calcd. for $C_{42}H_{59}N_2O_{19}P_3$, 987.285; found, 987.396.

γ-Bis-(4-dodecyloxycarbonyloxybenzyl)-d4TTP 3n. General procedure D with 80 mg d4TDP **6** (92 µmol, 1.0 eq.), 0.15 g **5n** (0.19 mmol, 2.0 eq.), 0.48 ml 0.25 M solution of DCI in acetonitrile (0.12 mmol, 1.3 eq.), 37 µl 5.5 M solution of t-BuOOH in *n*-decane (0.20 mmol, 2.1 eq.) in 0.5 ml acetonitrile and 0.5 ml THF. The crude product was purified using automatic RP-18 chromatography (water/acetonitrile gradient). Yield: 52 mg (38 µmol, 41%) colourless solid (counterions: 1.1 × Bu_4N^+, 0.9 × NH_4^+). UV (HPLC): $\lambda_{max} = 265$ nm; HPLC: $t_R = 20.53$ min (method A); ^{1}H-NMR (300 MHz, CD_3OD): δ 7.70 (*d*, $J = 1.3$ Hz, 1H), 7.43–7.36 (*m*, 4H), 7.19–7.11 (*m*, 4H), 6.94 (dt, $J = 3.4$ Hz, $J = 1.7$ Hz, 1H), 6.52 (dt, $J = 6.0$ Hz, $J = 1.8$ Hz, 1H), 5.80 (ddd, $J = 6.0$ Hz, $J = 2.4$ Hz, $J = 1.4$ Hz, 1H), 5.19 (*d*, $J = 8.0$ Hz, 4H), 5.00–4.93 (*m*, 1H), 4.37–4.15 (*m*, 2H), 4.25 (*t*, $J = 6.6$ Hz, 4H), 3.29–3.14 (*m*, 9H), 1.92 (*d*, $J = 1.3$ Hz, 3H), 1.80–1.66 (*m*, 4H), 1.71–1.58 (*m*, 9H), 1.50–1.25 (*m*, 45H), 1.03 (*t*, $J = 7.4$ Hz, 13.5H), 0.92 (*t*, $J = 6.6$ Hz, 6H); ^{13}C-NMR (75 MHz, CD_3OD): δ 166.5, 155.1, 152.7, 152.6, 138.7, 136.0, 135.4 (*d*, $J = 7.8$ Hz), 130.5 (*d*, $J = 2.4$ Hz), 127.0, 122.3, 112.1, 90.8, 87.3 (*d*, $J = 9.2$ Hz), 70.2 (*d*, $J = 5.6$ Hz), 70.0, 67.8 (*d*, $J = 6.0$ Hz), 59.5, 33.1, 30.8, 30.7, 30.6, 30.5, 30.3, 29.7, 26.8, 24.8, 23.7, 20.7, 19.4, 14.5, 13.9, 12.5; ^{31}P-NMR (162 MHz, CD_3OD): δ −12.07 (*d*, $J = 21.7$ Hz), −13.38 (*d*, $J = 18.1$ Hz), −24.20 (dd, $J = 21.7$ Hz, $J = 18.1$ Hz); IR: 2,923, 1,760, 1,689, 1,248 cm^{-1}; MALDI-MS (*m/z*): [M-H]$^-$ calcd. for $C_{50}H_{75}N_2O_{19}P_3$, 1099.410; found, 1099.083.

γ-Bis-(4-(butyl-ethane-1,2-diylbis(methylcarbamate))-oxybenzyl)-d4TTP 3o (ammonium salt). General procedure D with 75 mg d4TDP **6** (87 µmol, 1.0 eq.), 0.12 g **5o** (0.15 mmol, 1.7 eq.), 0.45 ml 0.25 M solution of DCI in acetonitrile (0.11 mmol, 1.3 eq.), 32 µl 5.5 M solution of *t*-BuOOH in *n*-decane (0.18 mmol, 2.1 eq.) in 1.5 ml acetonitrile. The crude product was purified using automatic RP-18 chromatography (water/acetonitrile gradient). Yield: 68 mg (60 µmol, 69%) colourless solid. UV (HPLC): $\lambda_{max} = 265$ nm; HPLC: $t_R = 12.88$ min (method A); ^{1}H-NMR (400 MHz, CD_3OD): δ 7.68 (*d*, $J = 1.0$ Hz, 1H), 7.48–7.42 (*m*, 4H), 7.15–7.09 (*m*, 4H, rotamers), 6.96 (dt, $J = 3.5$ Hz, $J = 1.7$ Hz, 1H), 6.49 (dt, $J = 6.1$ Hz, $J = 1.7$ Hz, 1H), 5.86–5.82 (*m*, 1H), 5.22–5.16 (*m*, 4H), 5.00–4.96 (*m*, 1H), 4.34–4.19 (*m*, 2H), 4.17–4.05 (*m*, 4H), 3.71–3.53 (*m*, 8H, rotamers), 3.15–2.96 (*m*, 12H), 1.93 (*d*, $J = 1.0$ Hz, 3H), 1.72–1.56 (*m*, 4H, rotamers), 1.50–1.34 (*m*, 4H, rotamers), 0.96, 0.90 (*t*, $J = 7.4$ Hz, 6H, rotamers); ^{13}C-NMR (101 MHz, CD_3OD): δ 166.5, 158.3, 156.4, 152.8, 152.7, 138.6, 135.7, 134.6, 130.4 (*d*, $J = 2.7$ Hz), 127.2, 123.1 + 122.9 (rotamers), 112.0 (C-5), 90.8 (C-1′), 87.2 (*d*, $J = 9.1$ Hz), 70.4 (dd, $J = 5.4$ Hz, $J = 2.5$ Hz), 67.9 (*d*, $J = 5.8$ Hz), 66.8 + 66.6 (rotamers), 48.1 + 47.8 (rotamers), 47.6 + 47.3 (rotamers), 35.5 + 35.0 (rotamers), 32.2 + 32.2 (rotamers), 20.2, 14.1 + 14.1 (rotamers), 12.5; ^{31}P-NMR (162 MHz, CD_3OD): δ −11.72 (d, $J = 19.5$ Hz), −13.16 (*d*, $J = 17.8$ Hz), −23.55 (*t*, $J = 18.1$ Hz); IR: 3,191, 1,959, 1,687, 1,204 cm^{-1}; MALDI-MS (*m/z*): [M-H]$^-$ calcd. for $C_{44}H_{63}N_6O_{21}P_3$, 1103.319; found, 1103.383.

γ-Bis-(4-(octyl-ethane-1,2-diylbis(methylcarbamate))-oxybenzyl)-d4TTP 3p (ammonium salt). General procedure D with 80 mg d4TDP **6** (92 µmol, 1.0 eq.), 0.15 g **5p** (0.16 mmol, 1.7 eq.), 0.48 ml 0.25 M solution of DCI in acetonitrile (0.12 mmol, 1.3 eq.), 37 µl 5.5 M solution of *t*-BuOOH in *n*-decane (0.20 mmol, 2.2 eq.) in 0.8 ml acetonitrile. The crude product was purified using automatic RP-18 chromatography (water/acetonitrile gradient). Yield: 73 mg (58 µmol, 63%) colourless solid. UV (HPLC): $\lambda_{max} = 265$ nm; HPLC: $t_R = 15.98$ min (method A); ^{1}H-NMR (400 MHz, CD_3OD): δ 7.69 (br.s, 1H), 7.47–7.42 (*m*, 4H), 7.15–7.08 (*m*, 4H, rotamers), 6.96 (dt, $J = 3.5$ Hz, $J = 1.6$ Hz, 1H), 6.49 (dt, $J = 6.0$ Hz, $J = 1.7$ Hz, 1H), 5.83 (dt, $J = 6.0$ Hz, $J = 1.7$ Hz, 1H), 5.22–5.16 (*m*, 4H), 5.00–4.96 (*m*, 1H), 4.34–4.19 (*m*, 2H), 4.15–4.05 (*m*, 4H), 3.72–3.53 (*m*, 8H, rotamers), 3.18–2.96 (*m*, 12H), 1.93 (*s*, 3H, H-7), 1.74–1.59 (*m*, 4H, rotamers), 1.47–1.22 (*m*, 20H), 0.92 (*t*, $J = 6.2$ Hz, 6H); ^{13}C-NMR (101 MHz, CD_3OD): δ 166.3, 158.4, 156.5, 152.8, 152.8, 138.6, 135.7, 134.6, 130.4 (*d*, $J = 2.7$ Hz), 127.2, 123.2 + 123.0 (rotamers), 112.0, 90.8, 87.2 (*d*, $J = 9.2$ Hz), 70.5–70.3 (*m*), 67.9 (*d*, $J = 5.9$ Hz), 67.1 + 66.9 (rotamers), 48.2 + 47.9 (rotamers), 47.6 + 47.3 (rotamers), 35.5 + 35.4 (rotamers), 35.2 + 35.0 (rotamers), 32.9, 30.3, 30.3, 30.2 + 30.1 (rotamers), 27.0, 23.7, 14.5, 12.5; ^{31}P-NMR (162 MHz, CD_3OD): δ −11.71 (*d*, $J = 19.2$ Hz), −13.16 (*d*, $J = 16.7$ Hz), −3.54 (br.s, $J = 17.2$ Hz); IR: 3,190, 2,925, 0,693, 1,205 cm^{-1}; MALDI-MS (*m/z*): [M-H]$^-$ calcd. for $C_{52}H_{79}N_6O_{21}P_3$, 1215.444; found, 1215.630.

γ-Bis-(4-(dodecyl-ethane-1,2-diylbis(methylcarbamate))-oxybenzyl)-d4TTP 3q (ammonium salt). General procedure D with 78 mg d4TDP **6** (90 µmol, 1.0 eq.), 0.22 g **5q** (0.15 mmol, 1.7 eq.), 0.47 ml 0.25 M solution of DCI in acetonitrile (0.12 mmol, 1.3 eq.), 36 µl 5.5 M solution of *t*-BuOOH in *n*-decane (0.20 mmol, 2.2 eq.) in 3.0 ml acetonitrile. The crude product was purified using automatic RP-18 chromatography (water/acetonitrile gradient). Yield: 36 mg (26 µmol, 29%) colourless solid. UV (HPLC): $\lambda_{max} = 265$ nm; HPLC: $t_R = 19.04$ min (method A); ^{1}H-NMR (400 MHz, CD_3OD): δ 7.66 (br.s, 1H), 7.46–7.39 (*m*, 4H), 7.13–7.06 (*m*, 4H, rotamers), 6.95–6.92 (*m*, 1H), 6.47 (dt, $J = 6.1$ Hz, $J = 1.7$ Hz, 1H), 5.83–5.79 (*m*, 1H), 5.20–5.13 (*m*, 4H), 4.98–4.93 (*m*, 1H), 4.33–4.16 (*m*, 2H), 4.14–4.01 (*m*, 4H), 3.71–3.53 (*m*, 8H, rotamers), 3.17–2.93 (*m*, 12H), 1.91 (*s*, 3H), 1.72–1.55 (*m*, 4H, rotamers), 1.45–1.21 (*m*, 36H), 0.91 (*t*, $J = 6.6$ Hz, 6H); ^{13}C-NMR (101 MHz, CD_3OD): δ 166.4, 158.3, 156.4, 152.8, 152.7, 138.6, 135.7, 134.7–134.4 (*m*), 130.4 (*d*, $J = 2.5$ Hz), 127.2, 123.2 + 123.0 (rotamers), 112.5, 90.8, 87.2 (*d*, $J = 9.2$ Hz), 70.4 (dd, $J = 5.3$ Hz, $J = 2.2$ Hz), 67.9 (*d*, $J = 5.0$ Hz), 67.1 + 66.9 (rotamers), 48.2 + 47.9 (rotamers), 47.6 + 47.3 (rotamers), 35.5 + 35.4 (rotamers), 35.2 + 34.9 (rotamers), 33.1, 30.7, 30.7, 30.6, 30.5, 30.4, 30.3, 30.2 + 30.1 (rotamers), 27.0, 23.7, 14.5, 12.5; ^{31}P-NMR (162 MHz, CD_3OD): δ −11.74 (br.s), −13.10 (*d*, $J = 16.1$ Hz), −23.51 (br.s); IR: 3,191, 2,922, 1,697, 1,205 cm^{-1}; MALDI-MS (*m/z*): [M-H]$^-$ calcd. for $C_{60}H_{95}N_6O_{21}P_3$, 1327.569; found, 1327.607.

General procedure E: preparation of 5-Nitro-*cyclo*Sal-(4-alkanoyloxybenzyl)-monophosphates 17. Corresponding 4-alkanoyloxybenzyl alcohol **9** (1.0 eq.) and 2.2 eq. di*iso*propylethylamine were dissolved in acetonitrile or THF and cooled to −20 °C. After dropwise addition of 2.0 eq., 5-nitrosaligenylchlorophosphite **18**, dissolved in acetonitrile or THF, the reaction mixture was allowed to warm to rt. The solution was kept at this temperature for 2 h. For oxidation, oxone (4.0 eq.) dissolved in water was added. The mixture was stirred for 15 min and immediately extracted with ethyl acetate. The organic phase was dried over Na_2SO_4, filtered and the solvent was removed by evaporation. The crude products were purified using preparative TLC (chromatotron).

5-Nitro-*cyclo*Sal-(4-acetyloxybenzyl)-monophosphate 17a. General procedure E with a solution of 0.11 g 4-(hydroxymethyl)phenylacetate **9a** (0.67 mmol, 1.0 eq.) and 0.25 ml di*iso*propylethylamine (0.19 g, 1.5 mmol, 2.2 eq.) dissolved in 12 ml acetonitrile, 0.31 g 5-nitrosaligenylchlorophosphite **18** (1.3 mmol, 2.0 eq.) dissolved in 15 ml acetonitrile. For oxidation 1.7 g oxone (2.7 mmol, 4.0 eq.) were used. The crude product was purified using preparative TLC (CH_2Cl_2/MeOH 19:1 v/v + 0.1% HOAc). Yield: 0.12 g (0.31 mmol, 46%) yellowish oil. TLC (PE/EE 1:1 v/v + 0.1% HOAc): $R_f = 0.45$; ^{1}H-NMR (300 MHz, $CDCl_3$): δ 8.15–8.05 (*m*, 1H), 7.99–7.94 (*m*, 1H), 7.38–7.29 (*m*, 2H), 7.08–6.95 (*m*, 3H), 5.42–5.27 (*m*, 2H), 5.18 (*d*, $J = 10.1$ Hz, 2H), 2.25 (*s*, 3H); ^{13}C-NMR (75 MHz, $CDCl_3$): δ 172.2, 154.3 (*d*, $J = 6.8$ Hz), 151.2, 143.8, 132.2 (*d*, $J = 5.6$ Hz), 129.6, 125.4, 122.0, 121.4, 121.4, 119.7 (*d*, $J = 9.2$ Hz), 70.2 (*d*, $J = 6.0$ Hz), 67.9 (*d*, $J = 7.1$ Hz), 21.0; ^{31}P-NMR (162 MHz, $CDCl_3$): δ −10.30; IR: 3,075, 1,753, 1,193 cm^{-1}; HRMS (ESI$^+$, *m/z*): [M + Na]$^+$ calcd. for $C_{16}H_{14}NO_8P$, 402.0349; found, 402.0306.

5-Nitro-*cyclo*Sal-(4-nonanoyloxybenzyl)-monophosphate 17e. General procedure E with a solution of 0.39 g 4-(hydroxymethyl)phenylnonanoate **9e** (1.5 mmol, 1.0 eq.) and 0.55 ml di*iso*propylethylamine (0.42 g, 3.3 mmol, 2.2 eq.) dissolved in 10 ml acetonitrile, 0.69 g 5-nitrosaligenylchlorophosphite **18** (3.0 mmol, 2.0 eq.) dissolved in 20 ml acetonitrile. For oxidation, 3.6 g oxone (5.9 mmol, 4.0 eq.) was used. The crude product was purified using preparative TLC (CH_2Cl_2/MeOH 19:1 v/v + 0.1% HOAc). Yield: 0.57 g (1.2 mmol, 80%) beige solid. TLC (PE/EE 1:1 v/v + 0.1% HOAc): $R_f = 0.66$; ^{1}H-NMR (300 MHz, $CDCl_3$): δ 8.19–8.11 (*m*, 1H), 8.02–7.95 (*m*, 1H), 7.42–7.32 (*m*, 2H), 7.12–6.98 (*m*, 3H), 5.45–5.29 (*m*, 2H), 5.22 (*d*, $J = 10.3$ Hz, 2H), 2.54 (*t*, $J = 7.5$ Hz, 2H), 1.74 (quint, $J = 7.5$ Hz, 2H), 1.46–1.17 (*m*, 10H), 0.87 (*t*, $J = 6.8$ Hz, 3H); ^{13}C-NMR (75 MHz, $CDCl_3$): δ 172.2, 154.6 (*d*, $J = 6.9$ Hz), 151.5, 143.9, 132.2 (*d*, $J = 5.7$ Hz), 129.8, 125.6 (*d*, $J = 1.4$ Hz), 122.3, 121.6, 121.4, 119.9 (*d*, $J = 9.1$ Hz), 70.4 (*d*, $J = 5.6$ Hz), 67.9 (*d*, $J = 6.8$ Hz), 34.4, 31.9, 29.3, 29.2, 29.2, 24.9, 22.7, 14.2; ^{31}P-NMR (81 MHz, $CDCl_3$): δ −10.73; IR: 2,921, 2,852, 1,749 cm^{-1}; HRMS (ESI$^+$, *m/z*): [M + Na]$^+$ calcd. for $C_{23}H_{28}NO_8P$, 500.1445; found, 500.1469.

5-Nitro-*cyclo*Sal-(4-octadecanoyloxybenzyl)-monophosphate 17j. General procedure E with a solution of 0.43 g 4-(hydroxymethyl)phenyloctadecanoate **9j** (1.1 mmol, 1.0 eq.) and 0.38 ml di*iso*propylethylamine (0.29 g, 2.2 mmol, 2.0 eq.) dissolved in 20 ml THF, 0.69 g 5-nitrosaligenylchlorophosphite **18** (1.7 mmol,

1.5 eq.) dissolved in 15 ml THF. For oxidation, 2.0 g oxone (3.3 mmol, 3.0 eq.) was used. The crude product was purified using preparative TLC (CH$_2$Cl$_2$/MeOH 30:1 v/v + 0.1% HOAc). Yield: 0.58 g (0.96 mmol, 87%) yellowish solid. TLC (PE/EE 1:1 v/v + 0.1% HOAc): R_f = 0.72; ^{1}H-NMR (400 MHz, CDCl$_3$): δ 8.19–8.14 (m, 1H), 8.00 (d, J = 2.7 Hz, 1H), 7.41–7.35 (m, 2H), 7.10–7.02 (m, 3H), 5.43–5.29 (m, 2H), 5.23 (d, J = 10.4 Hz, 2H), 2.55 (t, J = 7.5 Hz, 2H), 1.74 (quint, J = 7.5 Hz, 2H), 1.46–1.19 (m, 28H), 0.87 (t, J = 6.8 Hz, 3H); ^{13}C-NMR (75 MHz, CDCl$_3$): δ 172.2, 154.6, 151.6, 144.0, 132.2 (d, J = 5.5 Hz), 129.9, 125.7, 122.2, 121.6, 121.3, 120.0 (d, J = 9.4 Hz), 70.5 (d, J = 5.8 Hz), 68.1 (d, J = 7.1 Hz), 34.5, 32.0, 29.8, 29.8, 29.7, 29.6, 29.5, 29.4, 29.2, 25.0, 22.8, 14.2; ^{31}P-NMR (162 MHz, CDCl$_3$): δ − 10.30; IR: 2,955, 2,849, 1,746 cm^{-1}; HRMS (ESI$^+$, m/z): [M + Na]$^+$ calcd. for C$_{32}$H$_{46}$NO$_8$P, 626.2853; found, 626.2821.

General procedure F: preparation of γ-mono(4-alkanoyloxybenzyl)-d4TTP 4.

d4TDP 6 (1.0 eq.) was co-evaporated with DMF and dried in vacuum for 2 h. Then, 2.0–2.5 eq. of the corresponding 5-nitro-cycloSal-(4-alkanoyloxybenzyl)-mono-phosphate 17 was dissolved in a minimum of DMF followed by a dropwise addition to the nucleotide 8 dissolved in DMF. The reaction was stirred at rt for 20 h, and the solvent was removed under reduced pressure. The residue was dissolved in CH$_2$Cl$_2$/ammonium acetate (1 M). The layers were separated and the aqueous layer was freeze-dried. The crude product thus obtained was purified using automatic RP-18 chromatography (water/acetonitrile gradient). Subsequently, the cations were exchanged to ammonium ions using Dowex 50WX8 (ammonium form) cation exchange resin followed by a second RP-18 chromatography.

γ-Mono-(4-acetyloxybenzyl)-d4TTP 4a (ammonium salt).

General procedure F with 70 mg d4TDP 6 (81 μmol, 1.0 eq.) in 1.0 ml DMF and 77 mg 5-nitro-cycloSal-(4-acetyloxybenzyl)-monophosphate 17a (0.20 mmol, 2.5 eq.) in 0.5 ml DMF. Yield: 16 mg (24 μmol, 30%) colourless solid. UV (HPLC): λ_{max} = 265 nm; HPLC: t_R = 10.88 min (method A), 5.23 min (method B); ^{1}H-NMR (400 MHz, CD$_3$OD): δ 7.69 (d, J = 1.2 Hz, 1H), 7.52–7.48 (m, 2H), 7.10–7.04 (m, 2H), 6.95 (dt, J = 3.5 Hz, J = 1.6 Hz, 1H), 6.53 (dt, J = 6.0 Hz, J = 1.7 Hz, 1H), 5.85 (ddd, J = 6.1 Hz, J = 2.4 Hz, J = 1.7 Hz, 1H), 5.07 (d, J = 6.2 Hz, 2H), 5.02–4.97 (m, 1H), 4.32–4.17 (m, 2H), 2.29 (s, 3H), 1.93 (d, J = 1.2 Hz, 3H); ^{13}C-NMR (101 MHz, CD$_3$OD): δ 171.3, 166.7, 153.0, 151.7, 138.7, 137.4 (d, J = 8.7 Hz), 135.9, 129.7, 127.0, 122.5, 112.0, 90.9, 87.3 (d, J = 9.1 Hz), 68.2 (d, J = 5.3 Hz), 67.8 (d, J = 6.1 Hz), 20.9, 12.5; ^{31}P-NMR (162 MHz, CD$_3$OD): δ − 10.95 (d, J = 19.0 Hz), − 11.27 (d, J = 18.8 Hz), − 22.04 (t, J = 18.8 Hz); IR: 3,190, 2,988, 1,687, 1,663, 1,217 cm^{-1}; MALDI-MS (m/z): [M-H]$^-$ calcd. for C$_{19}$H$_{23}$N$_2$O$_{15}$P$_3$, 611.024; found, 611.044.

γ-Mono-(4-nonanoyloxybenzyl)-d4TTP 4e (ammonium salt).

General procedure F with 57 mg d4TDP 6 (66 μmol, 1.0 eq.) in 1.0 ml DMF and 63 mg 5-nitro-cycloSal-(4-nonanoyloxybenzyl)-monophosphate 17e (0.13 mmol, 2.0 eq.) in 0.5 ml DMF. Yield: 15 mg (20 μmol, 30%) colourless solid. UV (HPLC): λ_{max} = 265 nm; HPLC: t_R = 13.03 min (method A); ^{1}H-NMR (400 MHz, CD$_3$OD): δ 7.70 (d, J = 1.4 Hz, 1H), 7.53–7.47 (m, 2H), 7.08–7.03 (m, 2H), 6.96 (dt, J = 3.4 Hz, J = 1.6 Hz, 1H), 6.53 (dt, J = 5.9 Hz, J = 1.7 Hz, 1H), 5.88–5.82 (m, 1H), 5.08 (d, J = 6.1 Hz, 2H), 5.02–4.97 (m, 1H), 4.34–4.17 (m, 2H), 2.60 (t, J = 7.4 Hz, 2H), 1.94 (s, 3H), 1.76 (quint, J = 7.3 Hz, 2H), 1.50–1.29 (m, 10H), 0.94 (t, J = 6.7 Hz, 3H); ^{13}C-NMR (101 MHz, CD$_3$OD): δ 173.9, 166.5, 152.8, 151.7, 138.7, 137.4, 135.9, 129.7, 127.0, 122.5, 112.0, 90.9, 87.3 (d, J = 5.2 Hz), 68.2 (d, J = 5.3 Hz), 67.8 (d, J = 5.4 Hz), 35.0, 33.0, 30.4, 30.2, 26.0, 23.7, 14.4, 12.5; ^{31}P-NMR (162 MHz, CD$_3$OD): δ − 10.99 (d, J = 19.5 Hz), − 11.31 (d, J = 18.8 Hz), − 22.12 (t, J = 18.7 Hz); IR: 3,258, 2,973, 1,691, 1,066 cm^{-1}; MALDI-MS (m/z): [M-H]$^-$ calcd. for C$_{26}$H$_{37}$N$_2$O$_{15}$P$_3$, 709.133; found, 709.238.

γ-Mono-(4-octadecanoyloxybenzyl)-d4TTP 4j (ammonium salt).

General procedure F with 56 mg d4TDP 6 (65 μmol, 1.0 eq.) in 1.0 ml DMF and 98 mg 5-nitro-cycloSal-(4-octa-decanoyloxybenzyl)-monophosphate 17j (0.16 mmol, 2.5 eq.) in 0.5 ml DMF. Yield: 15 mg (17 μmol, 26%) colourless solid. UV (HPLC): λ_{max} = 265 nm; HPLC: t_R = 14.79 min (method A); ^{1}H-NMR (400 MHz, CD$_3$OD): δ 7.70 (d, J = 1.3 Hz, 1H), 7.55–7.47 (m, 2H), 7.10–7.02 (m, 2H), 6.96 (dt, J = 3.4 Hz, J = 1.6 Hz, 1H), 6.53 (dt, J = 6.0 Hz, J = 1.7 Hz, 1H), 5.87–5.83 (m, 1H), 5.09 (d, J = 5.8 Hz, 2H), 5.02–4.97 (m, 1H), 4.36–4.16 (m, 2H), 2.60 (t, J = 7.4 Hz, 2H), 1.94 (d, J = 1.3 Hz, 3H), 1.76 (quint, J = 7.3 Hz, 2H), 1.52–1.27 (m, 28H), 0.93 (t, J = 6.6 Hz, 3H); ^{13}C-NMR (101 MHz, CD$_3$OD): δ 174.0, 166.6, 152.8, 151.7, 138.7, 137.2 (d, J = 7.6 Hz), 135.9, 129.8, 127.1, 122.5, 112.0, 90.9, 87.2 (d, J = 8.1 Hz), 68.3, 67.8, 35.0, 33.0, 30.8, 30.7, 30.6, 30.5, 30.4, 30.2, 26.0, 23.7, 14.4, 12.5; ^{31}P-NMR (162 MHz, CD$_3$OD): δ − 11.14 (d, J = 18.2 Hz), − 11.44 (d, J = 19.9 Hz), − 23.82 (t, J = 18.6 Hz); IR: 3,209, 3,066, 2,925, 1,757, 1,704, 1,251 cm^{-1}; MALDI-MS (m/z): [M-H]$^-$ calcd. for C$_{35}$H$_{55}$N$_2$O$_{15}$P$_3$, 835.274; found, 835.398.

3′-O-Acetylthymidine 20.

The synthesis was carried out as described previously[53].
TLC (CH$_2$Cl$_2$/MeOH 9:1): R_f = 0.59; ^{1}H-NMR (400 MHz, DMSO-d_6): δ 11.32 (br.s, 1H), 7.73 (d, J = 1.4 Hz, 1H), 6.17 (dd, J = 8.7 Hz, J = 5.9 Hz, 1H), 5.24–5.19 (m, 1H), 5.20 (t, J = 5.1 Hz, 1H), 3.99–3.95 (m, 1H), 3.62 (dd, J = 5.3 Hz, J = 3.5 Hz, 2H), 2.33–2.15 (m, 2H), 2.06 (s, 3H), 1.78 (d, J = 1.4 Hz, 3H); ^{13}C-NMR (101 MHz,

DMSO-d_6): δ 170.0, 163.7, 150.5, 135.8, 109.7, 84.6, 83.7, 74.7, 61.3, 36.5, 20.8, 12.3. IR: 3,468, 3,181, 1,706, 1,659 cm^{-1}; HRMS (m/z): [M + Na]$^+$ calcd. for C$_{12}$H$_{16}$N$_2$O$_5$, 307.0901; found, 307.0882.

Thymidine diphosphate 22 (TDP, tetra-n-butylammonium salt).

To a suspension of 1.4 g 3′-O-acetylthymidine 20 (1.8 mmol, 1.0 eq.) in 30 ml acetonitrile, 1.3 ml diisopropylethylamine (0.98 g, 7.6 mmol, 1.5 eq.) was added, followed by 1.4 g 5-chlorosaligenylchlorophosphite 8 (6.1 mmol, 1.2 eq.). The reaction mixture was stirred at 0 °C. By addition of 1.4 ml of a 5.5-M solution of tert-butylhydroperoxide in n-decane (7.6 mmol, 1.5 eq.) the phosphite was oxidized for 20 min. The solvent was removed in vacuum. The residue was redissolved in CH$_2$Cl$_2$ and washed with 1 M ammonium acetate solution. The organic phase was dried over Na$_2$SO$_4$, filtered and the solvent was removed under reduced pressure. The product 21 (quantitative conversion) was used for further steps without purification.

5-chloro-cycloSal-3′-O-acetyl-thymidinemonophosphate 21 (0.51 g; 1.0 mmol, 1.0 eq.) was reacted with 0.89 g mono-(tetra-n-butylammonium)-monophosphate (2.6 mmol, 2.5 eq.) in 10 ml DMF. After being stirred for 20 h, the solvent was removed in vacuum and the residue was redissolved in a mixture of methanol/water/tetra-n-butylammoniumhydroxide solution (40%) in water (7:3:1 v/v/v). The reaction mixture was stirred for 17 h for deacetylation, followed by removal of the solvent in vacuum. After extraction with water/ethyl acetate, the separated aqueous layer was freeze-dried. The crude product was purified using RP-18 chromatography (water/acetonitrile gradient: 8:1 to 4:1 v/v). Yield: 0.46 g (0.52 mmol, 59%, 2 × Bu$_4$N$^+$) colourless solid. TLC (isopropanol/NH$_3$/water 4:1:2.5 v/v/v): R_f = 0.19; ^{1}H-NMR (300 MHz, D$_2$O): δ 7.76 (d, J = 1.4 Hz, 1H), 6.32 (dd, J = 7.6 Hz, J = 6.4 Hz, 1H), 4.67–4.58 (m, 1H), 4.22–4.08 (m, 3H), 3.30–2.25 (m, 16H), 2.43–2.24 (m, 2H), 1.91 (d, J = 1.4 Hz, 3H), 1.74–1.51 (m, 16H), 1.35 (sext, J = 7.4 Hz, 16H), 0.93 (t, J = 7.3 Hz, 24H); ^{13}C-NMR (75 MHz, D$_2$O): δ 166.3, 151.6, 137.3, 111.7, 85.5, 84.9, 71.0, 65.3, 58.1, 38.6, 23.1, 19.1, 12.8, 11.6; ^{31}P-NMR (162 MHz, D$_2$O): δ − 10.89 (d, J = 20.0 Hz), − 11.53 (d, J = 20.0 Hz); IR: 3,165, 2,960, 2,875, 1,683 cm^{-1}; HRMS (ESI$^+$, m/z): [M + H]$^+$ calcd. for C$_{10}$H$_{16}$N$_2$O$_{11}$P$_2$, 401.016; found, 400.789.

γ-Bis-(4-nonanoyloxybenzyl)-TTP 3r (ammonium salt).

General procedure D with 0.11 g TDP 22 (0.13 mmol, 1.0 eq.), 0.17 g 5e (0.25 mmol, 2.0 eq.), 0.66 ml 0.25 M DCI solution (0.17 mmol, 1.3 eq.), 46 μl 5.5 M solution of t-BuOOH in n-decane (0.25 mmol, 2.0 eq.) in 0.7 ml acetonitrile. The crude product was purified using automatic RP-18 chromatography (water/acetonitrile gradient). Yield: 95 mg (94 μmol, 74%) colourless solid. UV (HPLC): λ_{max} = 266 nm; HPLC: t_R = 16.56 min (method A); ^{1}H-NMR (300 MHz, CD$_3$OD): δ 7.83 (d, J = 1.3 Hz, 1H), 7.42–7.33 (m, 4H), 7.03–6.96 (m, 4H), 6.28 (dd, J = 7.6 Hz, J = 6.0 Hz, 1H), 5.17 (d, J = 8.0 Hz, 4H), 4.65–4.58 (m, 1H), 4.30 (ddd, J = 11.4 Hz, J = 5.9 Hz, J = 2.8 Hz, 1H), 4.24–4.14 (m, 1H), 4.01–3.90 (m, 1H), 2.54 (t, J = 7.4 Hz, 4H), 2.31–2.18 (m, 1H), 2.12 (ddd, J = 13.5 Hz, J = 6.1 Hz, J = 3.3 Hz, 1H), 1.89 (d, J = 1.3 Hz, 3H), 1.75–1.51 (m, 4H), 1.47–1.21 (m, 20H), 0.93 (t, J = 6.7 Hz, 6H); ^{13}C-NMR (75 MHz, CD$_3$OD): δ 173.7, 166.7, 152.4, 152.2, 138.3, 135.2 (d, J = 7.1 Hz), 130.5, 122.8, 112.0, 87.6, 85.8, 72.2, 70.2 (d, J = 5.4 Hz), 67.0, 40.5, 35.0, 33.0, 30.4, 30.3, 30.2, 26.0, 23.7, 14.5, 12.7; ^{31}P-NMR (162 MHz, CD$_3$OD): δ − 13.62 (d, J = 22.0 Hz), − 15.17 (d, J = 17.8 Hz), − 23.67 (d, J = 20.0 Hz); IR: 3,182, 2,924, 1,755, 1,688 cm^{-1}; MALDI-MS (m/z): [M-H]$^-$ calcd. for C$_{42}$H$_{61}$N$_2$O$_{18}$P$_3$, 973.306; found, 973.491.

Chemical hydrolysis of TriPPPro-d4TTP compounds 3a–q and intermediates 4a,e,j.

Stock solutions (50 mM in DMSO-d_6) of the appropriate compounds were prepared. After dilution of 11 μl with 100 μl Millipore water and 189 μl DMSO-d_6 to 1.9 mM hydrolysis solutions the reaction was started by the addition of 300 μl PBS (50 mM, pH 7.3). The solution was incubated at 37 °C in a thermomixer. An initial aliquot (25 μl) was taken directly and analysed by analytical HPLC at 265–266 nm. Further aliquots were taken for monitoring the kinetic hydrolysis. The exponential decay curves (pseudo-first order) based on absolute integral values were calculated with commercially available software (OriginPro 9.0G) and yielded the half-lives $t_{1/2}$(1) and $t_{1/2}$(2) of the prodrugs via one determination.

Enzymatic hydrolysis of TriPPPro-d4TTP compounds 3a–n and intermediates 4a,e,j with PLE.

Overall, 20 μl of the appropriate 50 mM DMSO-d_6 stock solution were diluted to 6.0 mM by addition of 83.3 μl DMSO-d_6 as well as 83.3 μl Millipore water. Furthermore, 140 μl of the 6.0 mM solution was diluted with 105 μl DMSO-d_6 and 700 μl 50 mM PBS buffer. The reaction was started by addition of 52.5 μl of PLE in PBS buffer (3 mg ml^{-1}) and the mixture was incubated at 37 °C in a thermomixer. At different times, aliquots (125 μl) were taken and treated as follows: (a) for 3a–g,l,m and 4a,e the reaction was stopped by addition to 132.5 μl MeOH. The mixture was kept for 5 min on ice followed by centrifugation for 5 min (13,000 r.p.m.). The supernatant was filtered (Chromafil RC-20/15 MS, 0.2 μm) and stored in liquid nitrogen. (b) For 3h,i,k,n and 4j, the sample was directly frozen in liquid nitrogen. The solution was defrosted followed by ultrasonication for 10 min. After centrifugation for 5 min, the supernatant was filtered (Chromafil AO-20/3, 0.2 μm) and stored at − 196 °C. (c) For 3j, the mixture was diluted with 70 μl THF

(HPLC grade) and frozen in liquid nitrogen followed by defrosting, ultrasonication, centrifugation, filtration and stored as described for (b).

Samples were defrosted and 50–80 µl were subjected to HPLC analysis. The calculation of $t_{1/2}$ was performed analogously to that for the chemical hydrolysis studies.

Enzyme-catalysed hydrolysis of Tri*PPP*ro-d4TTP compounds 3a–n and intermediates 4a,e,j in CEM cell extracts. A volume of 10 µl of the appropriate 50 mM DMSO-d_6 stock solution was diluted to 6.0 mM hydrolysis solution by addition of 73.3 µl DMSO-d_6. Seven different samples including 10 µl water and 10 µl hydrolysis solution were prepared. The reaction was started by addition of 50 µl human CEM cell extract and the mixture was incubated at 37 °C for different time periods of hydrolysis. The work-up depended on the particular compound: (a) for 3a–f,l,m,p and 4a,e the reactions were stopped by addition of 150 µl MeOH. The solution was kept on ice for 5 min followed by centrifugation for 5 min (13,000 r.p.m.). The supernatants were filtered (Chromafil RC-20/15 MS, 0.2 µm) and stored in liquid nitrogen. (b) For 3g–i,k,n and 4j, the samples were directly frozen in liquid nitrogen. The solution was defrosted followed by ultrasonication for 10 min. After centrifugation for 5 min the supernatants were filtered (Chromafil AO-20/3, 0.2 µm) and stored at −196 °C. (c) For 3j the mixture was diluted with 70 µl THF (HPLC grade) and frozen in liquid nitrogen followed by defrosting, ultrasonication, centrifugation, filtration and stored as described for (b). Samples were defrosted and 50–80 µl were subjected to HPLC analysis. The calculation of $t_{1/2}$ was performed analogously to that for the chemical hydrolysis studies.

Preparation of cell extracts. Human CD_4^+ T-lymphocyte CEM cells were grown in RPMI-1640-based cell culture medium to a final density of ∼3·10⁶ cells ml⁻¹. Then, cells were centrifuged for 10 min at 1,250 r.p.m. at 4 °C, washed twice with cold PBS and the pellet was resuspended at 10⁸ cells ml⁻¹ and sonicated (Hielscher Ultrasound Techn., 100% amplitude, three·times for 10 s) to destroy cell integrity. The resulting cell suspension was then centrifuged at 10,000 r.p.m. to remove cell debris, and the supernatant divided into aliquots before being frozen at −80 °C and used.

Anti-HIV activity assay. Inhibition of HIV-1(III$_B$)- and HIV-2(ROD)-induced cytopathicity in wild-type CEM/0 and TK-deficient CEM/TK⁻ cell cultures was measured in microtitre 96-well plates containing ∼3 × 10⁵ CEM cells ml⁻¹ infected with 100 CCID$_{50}$ of HIV per millilitre and containing appropriate dilutions of the test compounds. After 4−5 days of incubation at 37 °C in a CO$_2$-controlled humidified atmosphere, CEM giant (syncytium) cell formation was examined microscopically. The EC$_{50}$ (50% effective concentration) was defined as the compound concentration required to inhibit HIV-induced giant cell formation by 50%.

Primer extension reactions. The used polymerase HIV RT was obtained from Roboklon. The primer and template were purchased from Life Technologies.

Primer sequence:
5′-TTGGATAGGAGGAAGTCCTGGTTGC-3′
Template sequence:
5′-AGACAAACCTATCCTCCTTCAGGACCAACG-3′
The primer extension assays were performed under the following conditions: The primer was labelled using [γ³²P]-ATP according to standard techniques. After 5-min incubation at 95 °C in 20 mM Tris-HCl (pH 7.6) and 50 mM NaCl, the hybridization/annealing of the primer to the template strand was achieved by a cooling phase from 95 to 20 °C over 3 h. The final assay solution (20 µl) consists of 2.5 µM dNTPs or hydrolysate, 1 × reaction buffer (50 mM Tris-HCl (pH 8.6), 10 mM MgCl$_2$ and 40 mM KCl), 0.02 µM of hybridization and 0.2 units of the enzyme, which was incubated at 37 °C for 10 min. The reaction was stopped by heating up to 80 °C for 3 min. The assays were separated using a denaturing PAGE (15%). The results were visualized by phosphorimaging.

References

1. Jordheim, L. P., Durantel, D., Zoulim, F. & Dumontet, C. Advances in the development of nucleoside and nucleotide analogues for cancer and viral diseases. *Nat. Rev. Drug Discov.* **12**, 447–464 (2013).
2. Deval, J. Antimicrobial strategies: inhibition of viral polymerases by 3′-hydroxyl nucleosides. *Drugs* **69**, 151–166 (2009).
3. Chilar, T. & Ray, A. S. Nucleoside and nucleotide HIV reverse transcriptase inhibitors: 25 years after zidovudine. *Antiviral Res.* **85**, 39–58 (2010).
4. El Safadi, Y., Vivet-Boudou, V. & Marquet, R. HIV-1 reverse transcriptase inhibitors. *Microbiol. Biotechnol.* **75**, 723–737 (2007).
5. Burton, J. R. & Everson, G. T. HCV NS5B polymerase inhibitors. *Clin. Liver Dis.* **13**, 453–465 (2009).
6. De Clercq, E. Antiviral drugs in current clinical use. *J. Clin. Virol.* **30**, 115–133 (2004).
7. Schader, S. M. & Wainberg, M. A. Insights into HIV-1 pathogenesis through drug discovery: 30 years of basic research and concerns for the future. *HIV AIDS Rev.* **10**, 91–98 (2011).
8. Balzarini, J., Herdewijn, P. & De Clercq, E. Differential patterns of intracellular metabolism of 2′,3′-didehydro-2′,3′-dideoxythymidine and 3′-azido-2′,3′-dideoxythymidine, two potent anti-human immunodeficiency virus compounds. *J. Biol. Chem.* **264**, 6127–6133 (1989).
9. Ho, H.-T. & Hitchcock, M. J. M. Cellular pharmacology of 2′,3′-Dideoxy-2′, 3′-didehydrothymidine, a nucleoside analog active against human immunodeficiency virus. *Antimicrob. Agents Chemother.* **33**, 344–349 (1987).
10. Balzarini, J. et al. The in vitro and in vivo anti-retrovirus activity, and intracellular metabolism of 3′-azido-2′,3′-dideoxythymidine are highly dependent on the cell species. *Biochem. Pharmacol.* **37**, 2065–2068 (1988).
11. McKenna, C. E., Kashemirov, B. A., Peterson, L. W. & Goodman, M. F. Modifications to the dNTP triphosphate moiety: from mechanistic probes for DNA polymerases to antiviral and anti-cancer drug design. *Biochim. Biophys. Acta* **1804**, 1223–1230 (2010).
12. Freeman, S. & Ross, K. C. Prodrug design for phosphates and phosphonates. *Prog. Med. Chem.* **34**, 112–142 (1997).
13. Van Rompay, A. R., Johansson, M. & Karlsson, A. Phosphorylation of nucleosides and nucleoside analogs by mammalian nucleoside monophosphate kinases. *Pharmacol. Ther.* **87**, 189–198 (2000).
14. Meier, C., Knispel, T., De Clercq, E. & Balzarini, J. *CycloSal*-Pro-nucleotides (*cyclo*Sal-NMP) of 2′,3′-dideoxyadenosine (ddA) and 2′,3′-dideoxy-2′, 3′-didehydroadenosine (d4A): synthesis and antiviral evaluation of a highly efficient delivery system. *J. Med. Chem.* **42**, 1604–1614 (1999).
15. Meier, C., Lomp, A., Meerbach, A. & Wutzler, P. *CycloSal*-BVDUMP pronucleotides: how to convert an antiviral-inactive nucleoside analogue into a bioactive compound against EBV. *J. Med. Chem.* **45**, 5157–5172 (2002).
16. Wagner, C. R., Iyer, V. V. & McIntee, E. J. Pronucleotides: toward the in vivo delivery of antiviral and anticancer nucleotides. *Med. Res. Rev.* **20**, 417–451 (2000).
17. Mutahir, Z. et al. Thymidine kinase 1 regulatory fine-tuning through tetramer formation. *FEBS J.* **280**, 1531–1541 (2013).
18. Hecker, S. J. & Erion, M. D. Prodrugs of phosphates and phosphonates. *J. Med. Chem.* **51**, 2328–2345 (2008).
19. Pradere, U., Garnier-Amblard, E. C., Coats, S. J., Amblard, F. & Schinazi, R. F. Synthesis of nucleoside phosphate and phosphonate prodrugs. *Chem. Rev.* **114**, 9154–9218 (2014).
20. Ho, H.-T. & Hitchcock, J. M. Cellular pharmacology of 2′,3′-dideoxy-2′, 3′-didehydrothymidine, a nucleoside analog active against human immunodeficiency virus. *Antimicrob. Agents Chemother.* **33**, 844–849 (1989).
21. Zhang, Y., Gao, Y., Wen, X. & Ma, H. Current strategies for improving oral absorption of nucleoside analogues. *Asian J. Pharm. Sci.* **9**, 65–74 (2014).
22. Cahard, D., McGuigan, C. & J. Balzarini, J. Aryloxyphosphoramidate triesters as pro-tides. *Mini Rev. Med. Chem.* **4**, 371–381 (2004).
23. Meier, C. & Balzarini, J. Application of the cycloSal-prodrug approach for improving the biological potential of phosphorylated biomolecules. *Antiviral Res.* **71**, 282–292 (2006).
24. Meier, C. CycloSal phosphates as chemical trojan horses for intracellular nucleotide and glycosylmonophosphate delivery-chemistry meets biology. *Eur. J. Org. Chem.* **5**, 1081–1102 (2006).
25. Meier, C., Lorey, M., De Clercq, E. & Balzarini, J. *Cyclo*Sal-2′,3′-dideoxy-2′, 3′-didehydrothymidine monophosphate (*cyclo*Sal-d4TMP): synthesis and antiviral evaluation of a new d4TMP delivery system. *J. Med. Chem.* **41**, 1417–1427 (1998).
26. Jessen, H. J., Balzarini, J. & Meier, C. Intracellular trapping of *cyclo*Sal-pronucleotides: modification of prodrugs with amino acid esters. *J. Med. Chem.* **51**, 6592–6598 (2008).
27. Gisch, N., Balzarini, J. & Meier, C. Doubly loaded *cyclo*Saligenyl-pronucleotides. 5,5′-Bis(*cyclo*Saligenyl-2′,3′-dideoxy-2′,3′-didehydrothymidine monophosphates). *J. Med. Chem.* **52**, 3464–3473 (2009).
28. Krylov, I. S., Kashemirov, B. A., Hilfinger, J. M. & McKenna, C. E. Evolution of an amino acid based prodrug approach: stay tuned. *Mol. Pharm.* **10**, 445–458 (2013).
29. Furman, P. A. et al. Phosphorylation of 3′-azido-3′-deoxythymidine and selective interaction of the 5′-triphosphate with human immunodeficiency virus reverse transcriptase. *Proc. Natl Acad. Sci. USA* **83**, 8333–8337 (1986).
30. Törnevik, Y., Ullman, B., Balzarini, J., Wahren, B. & Eriksson, S. Cytotoxicity of 3′-azido-3′-deoxythymidine correlates with 3′-azidothymidine-5′-monophosphate (AZTMP) levels, whereas antihuman immunodeficiency virus (HIV) activity correlates with 3′-azidothymidine-5′-triphosphate (AZTTP) levels in cultured CEM T-lymphoblastoid cells. *Biochem. Pharmacol.* **49**, 829–837 (1995).
31. Mackman, R. L. et al. Synthesis and anti-HIV activity of cyclic pyrimidine phosphonomethoxy nucleosides and their prodrugs: a comparison of phosphonates and corresponding nucleosides. *Nucleosides Nucleotides Nucleic Acids* **26**, 573–577 (2007).
32. Jessen, H. J., Schulz, T., Balzarini, J. & Meier, C. Bioreversible protection of nucleoside diphosphates. *Angew. Chem. Int. Ed. Engl.* **47**, 8719–8722 (2008).
33. Schulz, T., Balzarini, J. & Meier, C. The DiPPro approach: synthesis, hydrolysis, and antiviral activity of lipophilic d4T diphosphate prodrugs. *ChemMedChem.* **9**, 762–775 (2014).

34. Pertenbreiter, F., Balzarini, J. & Meier, C. Nucleoside mono- and diphosphate prodrugs of 2′,3′-dideoxyuridine and 2′,3′-dideoxy-2′,3′-didehydrouridine. *ChemMedChem.* **10**, 94–106 (2015).

35. Weinschenk, L., Schols, D., Balzarini, J. & Meier, C. Nucleoside diphosphate prodrugs: non-symmetric DiPPro-nucleotides. *J. Med. Chem.* **58**, 6114–6130 (2015).

36. Sienaert, R. et al. Specific recognition of the bicyclic pyrimidine nucleoside analogs, a new class of highly potent and selective inhibitors of varicella-zoster virus (VZV), by the VZV-encoded thymidine kinase. *Mol. Pharmacol.* **61**, 249–254 (2002).

37. Tan, X., Chu, C. K. & Boudinot, F. D. Development and optimization of anti-HIV nucleoside analogs and prodrugs: a review of their cellular pharmacology, structure-activity relationships and pharmacokinetics. *Adv. Drug Deliv. Rev.* **39**, 117–151 (1999).

38. Bonnaffé, D., Dupraz, B., Ughetto-Monfrin, J., Namane, A. & Dinh, T. H. Synthesis of acyl pyrophosphates - application to the synthesis of nucleotide lipophilic prodrugs. *Tetrahedron Lett.* **36**, 531–534 (1995).

39. Kreimeyer, A., Andrè, F., Gouyette, C. & Dinh, T. H. Transmembrane transport of adenosine 5′-triphosphate using a lipophilic cholesteryl derivative. *Angew. Chem. Int. Ed. Engl.* **37**, 2853–2855 (1998).

40. Kumar, S. et al. Terminal phosphate labeled nucleotides: synthesis, applications, and linker effect on incorporation by DNA polymerases. *Nucleosides Nucleotides Nucleic Acids* **24**, 401–408 (2005).

41. Sood, A. et al. Terminal phosphate-labeled nucleotides with improved substrate properties for homogeneous nucleic acid assays. *J. Am. Chem. Soc.* **127**, 2394–2395 (2005).

42. Vinogradov, S. V., Kohli, E. & Zeman, A. D. Comparison of nanogel drug carriers and their formulations with nucleoside 5′-triphosphates. *Pharm. Res.* **23**, 920–930 (2006).

43. Galmarini, C. M. et al. Polymeric nanogels containing the triphosphate form of cytotoxic nucleoside analogues show antitumor activity against breast and colorectal cancer cell lines. *Mol. Cancer Ther.* **7**, 3373–3380 (2008).

44. Peters, G. J., Adema, A. D., Bijnsdorp, I. V. & Sandvold, M. L. Lipophilic prodrugs and formulations of conventional (deoxy)nucleoside and fluoropyrimidine analogs in cancer. *Nucleosides Nucleotides Nucleic Acids* **30**, 1168–1180 (2011).

45. Menger, F. M., Guo, Y. & Lee, A. S. Synthesis of a lipid peptide drug conjugateN-4-(acylpeptidyl)-ara-C. *Bioconjugate Chem.* **5**, 162–166 (1994).

46. Ibrahim, S. S., Boudinot, F. D., Schinazi, R. F. & Chu, C. K. Physicochemical properties, bioconversion and disposition of lipophilic prodrugs of 2′,3′-dideoxycytidine. *Antiviral Chem. Chemother.* **7**, 167–172 (1996).

47. Horwitz, J. P., Chua, J., Da Rooge, M. A., Noel, M. & Klundt, I. L. Nucleosides. IX. The formation of 2′,2′-unsaturated pyrimidine nucleosides via a novel beta-elimination reaction. *J. Org. Chem.* **31**, 205–211 (1966).

48. Warnecke, S. & Meier, C. Synthesis of nucleoside di- and triphosphates and dinucleoside polyphosphates with cycloSal-nucleotides. *J. Org. Chem.* **74**, 3024–3030 (2009).

49. DeWit, M. W. & Gillies, E. R. A cascade biodegradable polymer based on alternating cyclization and elimination reactions. *J. Am. Chem. Soc.* **131**, 18327–18334 (2009).

50. Bonnaffé, D., Dupraz, B., Ughetto-Monfrin, J., Namane, A. & Dinh, T. H. Potential lipophilic nucleotide prodrugs- synthesis, hydrolysis and antiviral activity of AZT and d4T acyl nucleotides. *J. Org. Chem.* **61**, 895–902 (1996).

51. Sarac, I. & Meier, C. Efficient automated solid-phase synthesis of DNA and RNA 5′-triphosphates. *Chem. Eur. J.* **21**, 1–7 (2015).

52. Tonn, V. C. & Meier, C. Solid-phase synthesis of (Poly)phosphorylated Nucleosides and conjugates. *Chem. Eur. J.* **17**, 9832–9842 (2011).

53. Wolf, S., Zismann, T., Lunau, N. & Meier, C. Reliable synthesis of various nucleoside diphosphate glycopyranoses. *Chem. Eur. J* **15**, 7656–7664 (2009).

Acknowledgements

We are grateful to Lizette van Berckelaer, Ria Van Berwaer, Kristien Minner, Sandra Claes and Evelyne Van Kerckhove for excellent technical assistance. The work conducted by C.M. has been supported by the Deutsche Forschungsgemeinschaft (DFG; Me1161/13-1) and that of D.S. and J.B. has been supported by the KU Leuven (GOA 15/19 TBA).

Author contributions

C.M. headed the project; T.G. performed the chemical synthesis; T.D.d.O. contributed with the biochemical assays and D.S. and J.B. carried out the antiviral testing of the synthesized compounds. All authors were involved in the preparation of the manuscript.

Additional information

Permissions

List of Contributors

Rommie E. Amaro, Robert V. Swift and Lane Votapka
Department of Pharmaceutical Sciences, Computer Science and Chemistry, University of California, Irvine, California 92697, USA

Wilfred W. Li
National Biomedical Computation Resource, University of California, San Diego, La Jolla, California 92093, USA

Ross C. Walker
Department of Chemistry and Biocwhemistry, San Diego Supercomputer Center, University of California, San Diego, La Jolla , California 92093, USA

Robin M. Bush
Department of Ecology and Evolutionary Biology, University of California, Irvine, California 92697, USA

Milan Bergeron-Brlek, Michael Meanwell and Robert Britton
Department of Chemistry, Simon Fraser University, Burnaby, British Columbia, Canada

Steen U. Hansen, Gavin J. Miller and John M. Gardiner
Faculty of EPS, School of Chemistry, Manchester Institute of Biotechnology, The University of Manchester, 131 Princess Street, Manchester M1 7DN, UK

Claire Cole, Graham Rushton, Egle Avizienyte and Gordon C. Jayson
School of Cancer and Enabling Sciences, The University of Manchester, Wilmslow Road, Manchester M20 4BX, UK

J.M. Dubach, C. Vinegoni, R. Mazitschek, P. Fumene Feruglio and R. Weissleder
Center for System Biology, Massachusetts General Hospital and Harvard Medical School, Richard B. Simches Research Center, 185 Cambridge Street, Boston, Massachusetts 02114, USA

L.A. Cameron
Dana-Farber Cancer Institute, Department of Pediatric Oncology, 450 Brookline Ave., Boston, Massachusetts 02215, USA

Mi Liu and Jean- Christophe Leroux
Institute of Pharmaceutical Sciences, Department of Chemistry and Applied Biosciences, Swiss Federal Institute of Technology Zurich (ETH Zurich), Zurich 8093, Switzerland.

Pål Johansen and Franziska Zabel
Department of Dermatology, University Hospital Zurich, Zurich 8091, Switzerland

Marc A. Gauthier
Institute of Pharmaceutical Sciences, Department of Chemistry and Applied Biosciences, Swiss Federal Institute of Technology Zurich (ETH Zurich), Zurich 8093, Switzerland
Institut National de la Recherche Scientifique (INRS), EMT Research Center, Varennes, Quebec J3X 1S2, Canada

Madhavan Nair, Rakesh Guduru, Jeongmin Hong and Vidya Sagar
Department of Immunology, Center for Personalized Nanomedicine, Herbert Wertheim College of Medicine, Florida International University, Miami, Florida 33174, USA

Ping Liang
Department of Electrical Engineering, University of California, Riverside, California 92521, USA

Sakhrat Khizroev
Department of Immunology, Center for Personalized Nanomedicine, Herbert Wertheim College of Medicine, Florida International University, Miami, Florida 33174, USA
Department of Electrical Engineering, University of California, Riverside, California 92521, USA

James Allen Frank, Martin Sumser and Dirk Trauner
Department of Chemistry and Center for Integrated Protein Science, Ludwig Maximilians University Munich, Butenandtstrasse 5–13, Munich 81377, Germany

Mirko Moroni and Gary R. Lewin
Molecular Physiology of Somatic Sensation, Max Delbrück Center for Molecular Medicine, Berlin 13125, Germany

Rabih Moshourab
Department of Anesthesiology, Campus Charité Mitte und Virchow Klinikum, Charité Universita"tsmedizin Berlin, Augustburgerplatz 1, Berlin 13353, Germany

Akhil B. Vaidya, Joanne M. Morrisey, Sudipta Das, Thomas M. Daly, Lawrence W. Bergman and
Sandhya Kortagere
Department of Microbiology and Immunology, Center for Molecular Parasitology, Drexel University College of Medicine, 2900 Queen Lane, Philadelphia, Pennsylvania 190129, USA

Zhongsheng Zhang, Marcin Stasiak and Erkang Fan
Department of Biochemistry, University ofWashington, Box 357350, Seattle,Washington 98195, USA

Thomas D. Otto and Matthew Berriman
Wellcome Trust Sanger Institute, Hinxton, Cambridge CB101SA, UK

Natalie J. Spillman and Kiaran Kirk
Research School of Biology, The Australian National University, Canberra, Australian Capital Territory 0200, Australia

Matthew Wyvratt, Peter Siegl and Jeremy Burrows
Medicines for Malaria Venture, PO Box 1826, 20Rt de Pr-Bois, Geneva 15 1215, Switzerland

Jutta Marfurt and Grennady Wirjanata
Division of Global and Tropical Health, Menzies School of Health Research and Charles Darwin University, PO Box 41096, Casuarina, Northern Territory 0811, Australia

Boni F. Sebayang
Eijkman Institute for Molecular Biology, Jl. Diponegoro 69, Jakarta 10430, Indonesia

Ric N. Price
Division of Global and Tropical Health, Menzies School of Health Research and Charles Darwin University, PO Box 41096, Casuarina, Northern Territory 0811, Australia
Nuffield Department of Clinical Medicine, Centre for Tropical Medicine, University of Oxford, Oxford OX3 7LJ, UK

Arnab Chatterjee and Advait Nagle
Genomics Institute of the Novartis Research Foundation, 10675 John Jay Hopkins Drive, San Diego, California 92121, USA

Susan A. Charman
Center for Drug Candidate Optimisation, Monash University, 381 Royal Parade, Parkville, Victoria 3052, Australia

In˜igo Angulo-Barturen, Santiago 100Ferrer, María Belén Jiménez-Díaz, María Santos Martínez and Francisco Javier Gamo
GlaxoSmithKline, Malaria Support Group, Calle Severo Ochoa 2, Tres Cantos 28760, Spain

Vicky M. Avery
Eskitis Institute, Griffith University, Don Young Road, Nathan, Queensland 4111, Australia

Andrea Ruecker and Michael Delves
Department of Life Sciences, South Kensington Campus, Imperial College, London SW7 2AZ, UK

Lorena Mendive-Tapia
Institute for Research in Biomedicine, Barcelona Science Park, Baldiri Reixac 10-12, 08028 Barcelona, Spain
Department of Organic Chemistry, University of Barcelona, Martí i Franqués 1-11, 08028 Barcelona, Spain.
CIBER-BBN, Networking Centre on Bioengineering, Biomaterials and Nanomedicine.

Sara Preciado
Department of Organic Chemistry, University of Barcelona, Martí i Franqués 1-11, 08028 Barcelona, Spain

Jesús García
Institute for Research in Biomedicine, Barcelona Science Park, Baldiri Reixac 10-12, 08028 Barcelona, Spain

Rosario Ramón and Nicola Kielland
Barcelona Science Park, Baldiri Reixac 10-12, 08028 Barcelona, Spain

Fernando Albericio
Institute for Research in Biomedicine, Barcelona Science Park, Baldiri Reixac 10-12, 08028 Barcelona, Spain
Department of Organic Chemistry, University of Barcelona, Martí i Franqués 1-11, 08028 Barcelona, Spain
CIBER-BBN, Networking Centre on Bioengineering, Biomaterials and Nanomedicine School of Chemistry, Yachay Tech, Yachay City of Knowledge, 100119 Urcuqui, Ecuador

Rodolfo Lavilla
Barcelona Science Park, Baldiri Reixac 10-12, 08028 Barcelona, Spain
Laboratory of Organic Chemistry, Faculty of Pharmacy, University of Barcelona, Avda. Joan XXII s.n., 08028 Barcelona, Spain

Soosung Kang
Department of Chemistry, Chemistry of Life Processes Institute, and Center for Molecular Innovation and Drug Discovery, Northwestern University, Evanston, Illinois 60208, USA

D. James Surmeier
Department of Physiology, Feinberg School of Medicine, Northwestern University, Chicago, Illinois 60611, USA

Garry Cooper
Department of Chemistry, Chemistry of Life Processes Institute, and Center for Molecular Innovation and Drug Discovery, Northwestern University, Evanston, Illinois 60208, USA
Department of Physiology, Feinberg School of Medicine, Northwestern University, Chicago, Illinois 60611, USA

Sara F. Dunne and Brendon Dusel
High-Throughput Analysis Laboratory, Chemistry of Life Processes Institute, Northwestern University, Evanston, Illinois 60208, USA

Chi-Hao Luan
High-Throughput Analysis Laboratory, Chemistry of Life Processes Institute, Northwestern University, Evanston, Illinois 60208, USA

Richard B. Silverman
Department of Chemistry, Chemistry of Life Processes Institute, and Center for Molecular Innovation and Drug Discovery, Northwestern University, Evanston, Illinois 60208, USA
Department of Molecular Biosciences, Chemistry of Life Processes Institute, and Center for Molecular Innovation and Drug Discovery, Northwestern University, Evanston, Illinois 60208, USA

Aline Dantas de Araujo, Irina Vetter, Zoltan Dekan, Markus Muttenthaler, JingJing Wan, Richard J. Lewis, Glenn F. King and Paul F. Alewood
Institute for Molecular Bioscience, The University of Queensland, St Lucia, Queensland 4072, Australia

Mehdi Mobli
Institute for Molecular Bioscience, The University of Queensland, St Lucia, Queensland 4072, Australia
Centre for Advanced Imaging, The University of Queensland, St Lucia, Queensland 4072, Australia

Joel Castro and Andrea M. Harrington
Nerve-Gut Research Laboratory, Discipline of Medicine, The University of Adelaide, Adelaide, South Australia 5000, Australia

Department of Gastroenterology & Hepatology, Hanson Institute, Royal Adelaide Hospital, Adelaide, South Australia 5000, Australia

Stuart M. Brierley
Nerve-Gut Research Laboratory, Discipline of Medicine, The University of Adelaide, Adelaide, South Australia 5000, Australia
Department of Gastroenterology & Hepatology, Hanson Institute, Royal Adelaide Hospital, Adelaide, South Australia 5000, Australia
Discipline of Physiology, Faculty of Health Sciences, The University of Adelaide, Adelaide, South Australia 5000, Australia

Mariano Stornaiuolo, Prakash Rucktooa, Alexander Fish and Titia K. Sixma
Division of Biochemistry and Center for Biomedical Genetics, Netherlands Cancer Institute, Plesmanlaan 121, 1066 CX Amsterdam, The Netherlands

Gerdien E. De Kloe, Ewald S. Edink and Iwan J. P. de Esch
Division of Medicinal Chemistry, Faculty of Sciences, Amsterdam Institute for Molecules, Medicines and Systems, VU University Amsterdam, De Boelelaan 1083, 1081 HV Amsterdam, The Netherlands

René van Elk and August B. Smit
Department of Molecular and Cellular Neurobiology, Center for Neurogenomics and Cognitive Research, VU University, 1081 HVAmsterdam, The Netherlands

Daniel Bertrand
HiQScreenSa`rl, 6, rue de Compois, 1222 Vésenaz, Geneva, Switzerland

JiříSchimer and Jan Konvalinka
Institute of Organic Chemistry and Biochemistry, Academy of Sciences of the Czech Republic, Gilead Sciences and IOCB Research Center, Flemingovo n.2, 166 10, Prague 6, Czech Republic
Department of Biochemistry, Faculty of Science, Charles University in Prague, Hlavova 8, 128 43, Prague 2, Czech Republic

Marcela Pávová and Maria Anders
Institute of Organic Chemistry and Biochemistry, Academy of Sciences of the Czech Republic, Gilead Sciences and IOCB Research Center, Flemingovo n.2, 166 10, Prague 6, Czech Republic
Department of Infectious Diseases, Virology, University Hospital Heidelberg, Im Neuenheimer Feld 324, 69120 Heidelberg, Germany

Petr Pachl, PavelŠ ácha, Petr Cígler, JanWeber, Pavel

Majer and Pavlína Řeza´čová
Institute of Organic Chemistry and Biochemistry, Academy of Sciences of the Czech Republic, Gilead Sciences and IOCB Research Center, Flemingovo n.2, 166 10, Prague 6, Czech Republic
Department of Biochemistry, Faculty of Science, Charles University in Prague, Hlavova 8, 128 43, Prague 2, Czech Republic

Hans-Georg Kräusslich and Barbara Müller
Department of Infectious Diseases, Virology, University Hospital Heidelberg, Im Neuenheimer Feld 324, 69120 Heidelberg, Germany Molecular Medicine Partnership Unit, Heidelberg, Germany

Jingbo Xiao, Catherine Z. Chen, Noel Southall, Xin Hu, Raisa E. Jones, Marc Ferrer, Wei Zheng, and Juan J. Marugan
NIH Chemical Genomics Center, Discovery Innovation, National Center for Advancing Translational Sciences, National Institutes of Health, 9800 Medical Center Drive, Rockville, Maryland 20850, USA

Zaohua Huang and Alexander I. Agoulnik
Department of Human and Molecular Genetics, HerbertWertheim College of Medicine, Florida International University, 11200 SW 8th Street, Miami, Florida 33199, USA

Irina U. Agoulnik
Department of Cellular Biology and Pharmacology, Herbert Wertheim College of Medicine, Florida International University, 11200 SW 8th Street, Miami, Florida 33199, USA

Donald A. Winkelmann
Department of Pathology and Laboratory Medicine, Robert Wood Johnson Medical School, Rutgers University, Piscataway, New Jersey 08854, USA

Eva Forgacs
Department of Physiological Sciences, Eastern Virginia Medical School, Norfolk, Virginia 23507, USA

Matthew T. Miller
Center for Advanced Biotechnology and Medicine, RobertWood Johnson Medical School, Rutgers University, Piscataway, New Jersey 08854, USA

Ann M. Stock
Center for Advanced Biotechnology and Medicine, RobertWood Johnson Medical School, Rutgers University, Piscataway, New Jersey 08854, USA
Department of Biochemistry and Molecular Biology, Robert Wood Johnson Medical School, Rutgers

University, Piscataway, New Jersey 08854, USA

Tsuyoshi Sekitani
Department of Electrical and Electronic Engineering, The University of Tokyo, 7-3-1 Hongo Bunkyo-ku, Tokyo 113-8656, Japan
The Institute of Scientific and Industrial Research, Osaka University, 8-1, Mihogaoka, Ibaraki, Osaka 567-0047, Japan

Tomoyuki Yokota and Yusuke Inoue, Masaki Sekino
Department of Electrical and Electronic Engineering, The University of Tokyo, 7-3-1 Hongo Bunkyo-ku, Tokyo 113-8656, Japan

Kazunori Kuribara
Department of Applied Physics, The University of Tokyo, 7-3-1 Hongo, Bunkyo-ku, Tokyo 113-8656, Japan

Martin Kaltenbrunner
Department of Electrical and Electronic Engineering, The University of Tokyo, 7-3-1 Hongo Bunkyo-ku, Tokyo 113-8656, Japan
4 Soft Matter Physics, Linz Institute of Technology LIT, Johannes Kepler University Linz, Altenbergerstrasse 69, Linz 4040, Austria

Takanori Fukushima
Chemical Resource Laboratory, Tokyo Institute of Technology, 4259R1-1, Nagatsuda, Midoriku, Yokohama, Kanagawa 226-8503, Japan

Takashi Isoyama and Yusuke Abe
Department of Biomedical Engineering, Graduate School of Medicine, The University of Tokyo, 7-3-1 Hongo, Bunkyo-ku, Tokyo 113-8656, Japan

Hiroshi Onodera
Department of Electrical and Electronic Engineering, The University of Tokyo, 7-3-1 Hongo Bunkyo-ku, Tokyo 113-8656, Japan

Takao Someya
Department of Electrical and Electronic Engineering, The University of Tokyo, 7-3-1 Hongo Bunkyo-ku, Tokyo 113-8656, Japan
Department of Applied Physics, The University of Tokyo, 7-3-1 Hongo, Bunkyo-ku, Tokyo 113-8656, Japan
Photon Science Center, The University of Tokyo, 7-3-1 Hongo, Bunkyo-ku, Tokyo 113-8656, Japan

Yoshiyuki Soeda, Misato Yoshikawa, Akio Sumioka, Akihiko Takashima and Tetsuya Kimura

Department of Aging Neurobiology, National Center for Geriatrics and Gerontology, Obu, Aichi 474-8511, Japan

Osborne F.X. Almeida
Department of Stress Neurology and Neurogenesis, Max Planck Institute of Psychiatry, Kraepelinstrasse, 2-10, Munich 80804, Germany

Sumihiro Maeda
Gladstone Institute of Neurological Disease, University of California, San Francisco, California 94158-2261, USA

Hiroyuki Osada and Yasumitsu Kondoh
Chemical Biology Research Group, RIKEN Center for Sustainable Resource Science (CSRS), RIKEN, Wako, Saitama 351-0198, Japan
Antibiotics Laboratory, Advanced Science Institute, RIKEN, Wako, Saitama 351-0198, Japan

Akiko Saito
Graduate School of Engineering, Osaka Electro-communication University (OECU), 18-8 Hatsu-cho, Osaka 572-8530, Japan

Tomohiro Miyasaka
Department of Neuropathology, Faculty of Life and Medical Sciences, Doshisha University, Kyotanabe, Kyoto 610-0394, Japan

Masaaki Suzuki
Department of Clinical and Experimental Neuroimaging, Center for Development of Advanced Medicine for Dementia, National Center for Geriatrics and Gerontology, Obu, Aichi 474-8511, Japan

Hiroko Koyama
Division of Regeneration and Advanced Medical Science, Gifu University Graduate School of Medicine, Gifu 501-1194, Japan

Yuji Yoshiike
Alzheimer's Disease Project Team, National Center for Geriatrics and Gerontology, Obu, Aichi 474-8511, Japan

Hachiro Sugimoto
Laboratory of Structural Neuropathology, Graduate School of Brain Science, Doshisha University, Kizugawa, Kyoto 619-0225, Japan

Yasuo Ihara
Department of Neuropathology, Faculty of Life and Medical Sciences, Doshisha University, Kyotanabe, Kyoto 610-0394, Japan

Laboratory of Cognition and Aging, Doshisha University, Kizugawa 619-0225, Japan

Chul-Jin Lee, Qinglin Wu, Javaria Najeeb and Jinshi Zhao
Department of Biochemistry, Duke University Medical Center, Durham, North Carolina 27710, USA

Xiaofei Liang
Department of Chemistry, Duke University, Durham, North Carolina 27708, USA

Marie Titecat, Florent Sebbane and Nadine Lemaitre
Inserm, Univ. Lille, CHU Lille, Institut Pasteur de Lille, CNRS, U1019-UMR 8204-CIIL-Center for Infection and Immunity of Lille, F-59000 Lille, France

Ramesh Gopalaswamy
Department of Chemistry, Duke University, Durham, North Carolina 27708, USA.

Eric J. Toone and Pei Zhou
Department of Biochemistry, Duke University Medical Center, Durham, North Carolina 27710, USA
Department of Chemistry, Duke University, Durham, North Carolina 27708, USA

Marco Grossi and Marina Morgunova
Department of Pharmaceutical and Medicinal Chemistry, Royal College of Surgeons in Ireland, 123 St Stephen's Green, Dublin 2, Ireland

Shane Cheung
Department of Pharmaceutical and Medicinal Chemistry, Royal College of Surgeons in Ireland, 123 St Stephen's Green, Dublin 2, Ireland
School of Chemistry and Chemical Biology, Conway Institute, University College Dublin, Belfield, Dublin

Dimitri Scholz, Emer Conroy and Marta Terrile
School of Biomolecular and Biomedical Science, Conway Institute of Biomolecular and Biomedical Research, University College Dublin, Belfield, Dublin 4, Ireland

Angela Panarella and Jeremy C. Simpson
School of Biology and Environmental Science, Conway Institute of Biomolecular and Biomedical Research, University College Dublin, Belfield, Dublin 4, Ireland

William M. Gallagher and Donal F. O'Shea
Department of Pharmaceutical and Medicinal Chemistry, Royal College of Surgeons in Ireland, 123 St Stephen's Green, Dublin 2, Ireland
School of Chemistry and Chemical Biology, Conway Institute, University College Dublin, Belfield, Dublin 4, Ireland

Tristan Gollnest, Thiago Dinis de Oliveira and Chris Meier
Institute of Organic Chemistry, Department of Chemistry, Faculty of Sciences, University of Hamburg, Martin-Luther-King-Platz 6, D-20146 Hamburg, Germany

Dominique Schols and Jan Balzarini
Department of Microbiology and Immunology, Laboratory of Virology and Chemotherapy, Rega Institute for Medical Research, KU Leuven,Minderbroedersstraat 10, B-3000 Leuven, Belgium

Index

www.ingramcontent.com/pod-product-compliance
Lightning Source LLC
Chambersburg PA
CBHW080630200326
41458CB00013B/4576

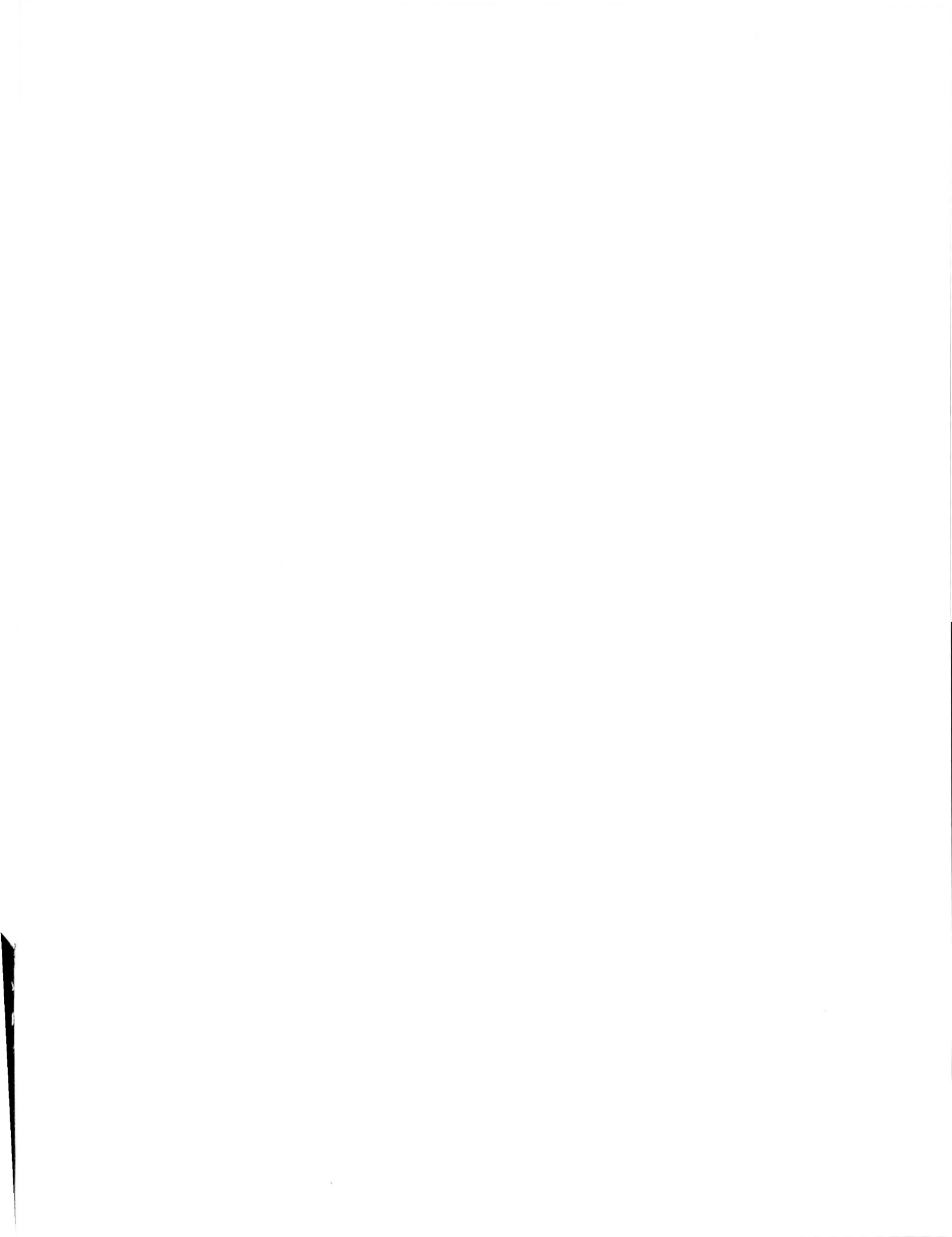